Bioelectronics

Bioelectronics is emerging as a new area of research where electronics can selectively detect, record, and monitor physiological signals. This is a rapidly expanding area of medical research that relies heavily on multidisciplinary technology development and cutting-edge research in chemical, biological, engineering, and physical science. This book provides extensive information on the (i) fundamental concepts of bioelectronics; (ii) materials for the developments of bioelectronics such as implantable electronics, self-powered devices, bioelectronic sensors, flexible bioelectronics, etc.; and (iii) an overview of the trends and gathering of the latest bioelectronic progress. This book will broaden our knowledge about newer technologies and processes used in bioelectronics.

Series in Materials Science and Engineering

The series publishes cutting-edge monographs and foundational textbooks for inter-disciplinary materials science and engineering. It is aimed at undergraduate- and graduate-level students, as well as practicing scientists and engineers. Its purpose is to address the connections between properties, structure, synthesis, processing, characterization, and performance of materials.

Conductive Polymers: Electrical Interactions in Cell Biology and Medicine
Ze Zhang, Mahmoud Rouabhia, Simon E. Moulton, Eds.

Silicon Nanomaterials Sourcebook, Two-Volume Set
Klaus D. Sattler, Ed.

Advanced Thermoelectrics: Materials, Contacts, Devices, and Systems
Zhifeng Ren, Yucheng Lan, Qinyong Zhang

Fundamentals of Ceramics, Second Edition
Michel Barsoum

Flame Retardant Polymeric Materials, A Handbook
Xin Wang and Yuan Hu

2D Materials for Infrared and Terahertz Detectors
Antoni Rogalski

Fundamentals of Fibre Reinforced Composite Materials
A. R Bunsell. S. Joannes, A. Thionnet

Fundamentals of Low Dimensional Magnets
Ram K Gupta, Sanjay R Mishra, Tuan Anh Nguyen

Emerging Applications of Low Dimensional Magnets
Ram K Gupta, Sanjay R Mishra, Tuan Anh Nguyen

Handbook of Silicon Carbide Materials and Devices
Zhe Chuan Feng

Bioelectronics: Materials, Technologies, and Emerging Applications
Ram K. Gupta and Anuj Kumar, Eds.

Series Preface

The series publishes cutting-edge monographs and foundational textbooks for inter-disciplinary materials science and engineering.

Its purpose is to address the connections between properties, structure, synthesis, pro-cessing, characterization, and performance of materials. The subject matter of individual volumes spans fundamental theory, computational modeling, and experimental methods used for design, modeling, and practical applications. The series encompasses thin films, surfaces, and interfaces, and the full spectrum of material types, including biomaterials, energy materials, metals, semiconductors, optoelectronic materials, ceramics, magnetic materials, superconductors, nanomaterials, composites, and polymers.

It is aimed at undergraduate- and graduate-level students, as well as practicing scientists and engineers.

Proposals for new volumes in the series may be directed to Carolina Antunes, Commissioning Editor at CRC Press, Taylor & Francis Group (Carolina.Antunes@tandf.co.uk).

Bioelectronics
Materials, Technologies, and Emerging Applications

Edited by
Anuj Kumar and Ram K. Gupta

CRC Press
Taylor & Francis Group
Boca Raton London New York

CRC Press is an imprint of the
Taylor & Francis Group, an **informa** business

Cover image: Ryzhi/Shutterstock

First edition published 2023
by CRC Press
6000 Broken Sound Parkway NW, Suite 300, Boca Raton, FL 33487-2742

and by CRC Press
4 Park Square, Milton Park, Abingdon, Oxon, OX14 4RN

CRC Press is an imprint of Taylor & Francis Group, LLC

© 2023 Taylor & Francis Group, LLC

Reasonable efforts have been made to publish reliable data and information, but the author and publisher cannot assume responsibility for the validity of all materials or the consequences of their use. The authors and publishers have attempted to trace the copyright holders of all material reproduced in this publication and apologize to copyright holders if permission to publish in this form has not been obtained. If any copyright material has not been acknowledged please write and let us know so we may rectify in any future reprint.

Except as permitted under U.S. Copyright Law, no part of this book may be reprinted, reproduced, transmitted, or utilized in any form by any electronic, mechanical, or other means, now known or hereafter invented, including photocopying, microfilming, and recording, or in any information storage or retrieval system, without written permission from the publishers.

For permission to photocopy or use material electronically from this work, access www.copyright.com or contact the Copyright Clearance Center, Inc. (CCC), 222 Rosewood Drive, Danvers, MA 01923, 978-750-8400. For works that are not available on CCC please contact mpkbookspermissions@tandf.co.uk

Trademark notice: Product or corporate names may be trademarks or registered trademarks and are used only for identification and explanation without intent to infringe.

Library of Congress Cataloguing-in-Publication Data
Names: Gupta, Ram K., editor. | Kumar, Anuj, Dr. editor.
Title: Bioelectronics : materials, technologies, and emerging applications / edited by Ram K. Gupta and Anuj Kumar.
Other titles: Bioelectronics (Gupta)
Description: First edition. | Boca Raton : CRC Press, 2023. | Includes bibliographical references and index.
Identifiers: LCCN 2022025753 | ISBN 9781032203133 (hardback) | ISBN 9781032203423 (paperback) | ISBN 9781003263265 (ebook)
Subjects: MESH: Electronics, Medical | Biosensing Techniques--instrumentation | Biomedical Engineering | Nanotechnology
Classification: LCC R857.B54 | NLM QT 36.2 | DDC 610.28--dc23/eng/20220912
LC record available at https://lccn.loc.gov/2022025753

ISBN: 978-1-032-20313-3 (hbk)
ISBN: 978-1-032-20342-3 (pbk)
ISBN: 978-1-003-26326-5 (ebk)

DOI: 10.1201/9781003263265

Typeset in Palatino
by MPS Limited, Dehradun

Contents

About the Editors

Dr. Anuj Kumar is an assistant professor at GLA University, Mathura, India. His research focus is on molecular as well M-N-C electrocatalysts for H_2, O_2, and CO_2 involving electrocatalysis, nanomaterials, nanocomposites, fuel cells, water electrolyzers, nano-sensors, bio-inorganic chemistry, and macrocyclic chemistry. He has published more than 80 articles in reputed peer-reviewed international journals. He has also contributed more than 12 book chapters to Elsevier, Springer, CRC Press, and Bentham Science book series. For outstanding contribution in his research field, he has been the recipient of "Best Young Scientist Award 2021" from the Tamil Nadu Association of Intellectuals and Faculty (TAIF) and GRBS Educational Charitable Trust, India, and the "Young Researcher Award 2020" by Central Education Growth and Research (CEGR), India. He is serving as a section editor, guest editor, and editorial board member for various journals.

Dr. Ram Gupta is an associate professor at Pittsburg State University. Dr. Gupta's research focuses on nanomagnetism, nanomaterials, green energy production and storage using conducting polymers and composites, electrocatalysts for fuel cells, optoelectronics and photovoltaics devices, organic-inorganic hetero-junctions for sensors, bio-based polymers, bio-compatible nanofibers for tissue regeneration, scaffold and antibacterial applications, and biodegradable metallic implants. Dr. Gupta published over 250 peer-reviewed articles, made over 300 national/international/regional presentations, chaired many sessions at national/international meetings, and edited/written several books/chapters for leading publishers. He has received over $2.5 million for research and educational activities from external agencies. He is serving as an associate editor, guest editor, and editorial board member for various journals.

Contributors

Prashanth S. Adarakatti
Department of Chemistry
SVM Arts, Science and Commerce College
  (affiliated to Rani Channamma
  University)
Karnataka, India

Darko Kwabena Adu
Department of Pharmaceutical Chemistry
College of Health Sciences
University of KwaZulu-Natal,
  Westville Campus
Durban, South Africa

John Alake
Department of Pharmaceutical
  Chemistry
College of Health Sciences
University of KwaZulu-Natal,
  Westville Campus
Durban, South Africa

Nazlı Albayrak
School of Medicine
Acibadem M. A. Aydınlar University
Istanbul, Turkey

A. Alhadhrami
Department of Chemistry,
  Faculty of Science
Taif University
Al Hawiyah, Saudi Arabia

Fahad Ali
Division of Analytical Chemistry
Bahauddin Zakariya University
Multan, Punjab, Pakistan

Abdulraheem S.A. Almalki
Department of Chemistry,
  Faculty of Science
Taif University
Al Hawiyah, Saudi Arabia

Khairunnisa Amreen
Micro-electromechanical systems (MEMS)
Microfluidics and Nanoelectronics Lab
Department of Electrical and Electronics
  Engineering
Birla Institute of Technology and
  Science Pilani
Jharkhand, India

Ajith Mohan Arjun
School of Materials Science and
  Engineering
National Institute of Technology Calicut
Kerala, India

Mamoni Banerjee
Rajendra Mishra school of Engineering and
  Entrepreneurship
Indian Institute of Technology Kharagpur
West Bengal, India

Alejandro Barragán-Ocaña
Center for Economic, Administrative and
  Social Research (CIECAS)
National Polytechnic Institute (IPN)
Mexico City, Mexico

Anna Batueva
Natural Sciences Department
Udmurt State University
Izhevsk, Udmurt Republic, Russia

Mario Birkholz
IHP – Leibniz Institut für innovative
  Mikroelektronik
Frankfurt (Oder), Germany

Leila Bousmaha-Marroki
Department of Biology, Faculty of Natural
  and Life Sciences
University Djillali Liabes
Sidi Bel Abbès, Algeria;
Laboratory of Research in Environment
  and Health, Faculty of Medicine
University Djillali Liabes
Sidi Bel Abbès, Algeria

Emilio Bucio
Departamento de Química de Radiaciones
  y Radioquímica, Instituto de Ciencias
  Nucleares
Universidad Nacional Autónoma de México
Circuito Exterior, Ciudad Universitaria
Mexico City, México

Jeong-Woo Choi
Department of Chemical & Biomolecular
  Engineering
Sogang University, Mapo-Gu
Seoul, Republic of Korea

Marc Dandin
Department of Electrical and Computer
  Engineering
Carnegie Mellon University
Pittsburgh, USA

Sobhi Daniel
Postgraduate and Research Department of
  Chemistry
T.M. Jacob Memorial Govt. College
Manimalakunnu, Ernakulam, India

Apurba Das
Department of Physics
D. K. College
Mirza, Assam, India;
Department of Physics
Indian Institute of Technology Guwahati
Guwahati, Assam, India

María de los Ángeles Olvera-Treviño
Faculty of Chemistry
National Autonomous University of
  Mexico (UNAM)
Metrology Unit
Mexico City, Mexico

Fahimeh Dehghandehnavi
Department of Electrical and Computer
  Engineering
Carnegie Mellon University
Pittsburgh, USA

Santanu Dhara
School of Medical Science and Technology
Indian Institute of Technology Kharagpur
West Bengal, India

P.K. Diwan
Department of Applied Science
UIET, Kurukshetra University
Kurukshetra, India

Pamu Dobbidi
Department of Physics
D. K. College Mirza
Assam, India

Lorena Duarte-Peña
Departamento de Química de Radiaciones
  y Radioquímica
Instituto de Ciencias Nucleares
Universidad Nacional Autónoma de
  México
Circuito Exterior, Ciudad Universitaria
Mexico City, México

Sinem Özlem Enginler
Department of Obstetrics and Gynecology,
  Faculty of Veterinary Medicine
Istanbul University-Cerrahpasa
Avcılar, Istanbul, Turkey

Batool Fatima
Department of Biochemistry
Bahauddin Zakariya University
Multan, Pakistan

Muhammad Umer Farooq
Division of Analytical Chemistry
Bahauddin Zakariya University
Multan, Punjab, Pakistan

Kiran Kumar Garlapati
Center for Interdisciplinary Programs
Indian Institute of Technology Hyderabad
Hyderabad, India

Yann Gilpin
Department of Electrical and Computer
  Engineering
Carnegie Mellon University
Pittsburgh, USA

Sanket Goel
Micro-electromechanical systems (MEMS)
Microfluidics and Nanoelectronics Lab
Department of Electrical and Electronics
  Engineering
Birla Institute of Technology and Science
  Pilani
Jharkhand, India

Praveena Malliyil Gopi
Postgraduate and Research Department of
  Physics
Maharaja's College
Ernakulam, India

Ram K. Gupta
Department of Chemistry
National Institute for Materials Advancement
Pittsburg State University
Pittsburg, USA

Manjeet Harijan
Department of Chemistry
Mahila Mahavidyalaya
Banaras Hindu University
Varanasi, India

Dilshad Hussain
International Centre for Chemical and
  Biological Sciences
HEJ Research Institute of Chemistry
University of Karachi
Karachi, Pakistan

Shumaila Ibraheem
Institute for Advanced Study
Shenzhen University
Shenzhen, Guangdong, China

Blessing Wisdom Ike
Department of Pharmaceutical Chemistry
College of Health Sciences
University of KwaZulu-Natal,
  Westville Campus
Durban, South Africa

Shagun Kainth
Virginia Tech Center for Excellence in
  Emerging Materials
Thapar Institute of Engineering &
  Technology
Patiala, India

Selcan Karakuş
Department of Chemistry,
  Faculty of Engineering
Istanbul University-Cerrahpasa
Avcılar, Istanbul, Turkey

Rajshekhar Karpoormath
Department of Pharmaceutical Chemistry
College of Health Sciences
University of KwaZulu-Natal,
  Westville Campus
Durban, South Africa

Naeem Akhtar Khan
IRCBM
COMSAT University Islamabad
Lahore, Punjab, Pakistan

Jayshree Khedkar
Department of Chemistry
Shri Anand College
Pathardi, Ahmednagar, India

Jinmyeong Kim
Department of Chemical Engineering
Kwangwoon University, Kwangwoon-Ro,
  Nowon-Gu
Seoul, Republic of Korea

Gaurav Kulkarni
School of Medical Science and
  Technology
Indian Institute of Technology
  Kharagpur
West Bengal, India

Anuj Kumar
Nano-Technology Research Laboratory
Department of Chemistry
GLA University
Mathura, Uttar Pradesh, India

Guglielmo Lanzani
Department of Physics
Politecnico di Milano, Piazza Leonardo da Vinci
Milano, Italy;
Center for Nanoscience and Technology
Istituto Italiano di Tecnologia Via Giovanni Pascoli
Milano, Italy

Taek Lee
Department of Chemical Engineering
Kwangwoon University, 20 Kwangwoon-Ro, Nowon-Gu
Seoul, Republic of Korea

Joungpyo Lim
Department of Chemical & Biomolecular Engineering
Sogang University
Seoul, Republic of Korea

Ching-Yi Lin
Department of Electrical and Computer Engineering
Carnegie Mellon University
Pittsburgh, USA

Kai-Chun Lin
Department of Electrical and Computer Engineering
Carnegie Mellon University
Pittsburgh, USA

Felipe López-Saucedo
Departamento de Química de Radiaciones y Radioquímica
Instituto de Ciencias Nucleares
Universidad Nacional Autónoma de México
Circuito Exterior, Ciudad Universitaria
Mexico City, México

Saadat Majeed
Division of Analytical Chemistry
Bahauddin Zakariya University
Multan, Punjab, Pakistan

S. G. Manjushree
Department of Chemistry
Siddaganga Institute of Technology
Karnataka, India

Ahmed Marroki
Department of Biology, Faculty of Natural and Life Sciences
University Djillali Liabes
Sidi Bel Abbès, Algeria;
Laboratory of Molecular Biology and Microbial Genetic, Faculty of Natural and Life Sciences
University Oran1
Oran, Algeria

Nicole McFarlane
Min H. Kao Department of Electrical Engineering and Computer Science
University of Tennessee
Knoxville, USA

Alessandra S. Menandro
Laboratory of Hybrid Materials, Institute of Environmental, Chemical, and Pharmaceutical Sciences
Federal University of São Paulo
São Paulo, Brazil

Mohammed Essac Mohamed
Postgraduate and Research Department of Physics, Maharaja's College
Ernakulam, India

Noorhashimah Mohamad Nor
School of Materials and Mineral Resources Engineering
Universiti Sains Malaysia, Nibong Tebal
Penang, Malaysia

Muhammad Najam-ul-Haq
Institute of Chemical Sciences
Bahauddin Zakariya University
Multan, Pakistan

Sayed Tayyab Raza Naqvi
Division of Analytical Chemistry
Bahauddin Zakariya University
Multan, Punjab, Pakistan

Zondi Nate
Department of Pharmaceutical Chemistry
College of Health Sciences
University of KwaZulu-Natal
South Africa;
Department of biotechnology & Chemistry
Vaal University of Technology
Vanderbijlpark, South Africa

Atul Kumar Ojha
School of Medical Science and Technology
Indian Institute of Technology Kharagpur
West Bengal, India

Anil M. Palve
Department of Chemistry, Mahatma Phule
    ASC College
Panvel, Navi-Mumbai, India

Giuseppe M. Paternò
Department of Physics
Politecnico di Milano, Piazza Leonardo da
    Vinci
Milano, Italy;
Center for Nanoscience and Technology
Istituto Italiano di Tecnologia, Via
    Giovanni Pascoli
Milano, Italy

Jhansi L. Parimi
Rajiv Gandhi School of Intellectual Property
Indian Institute of Technology Kharagpur
West Bengal, India

Giovana A. Parolin
Laboratory of Hybrid Materials
Institute of Environmental, Chemical, and
    Pharmaceutical Sciences
Federal University of São Paulo
São Paulo, Brazil

Laura O. Péres
Laboratory of Hybrid Materials
Institute of Environmental, Chemical, and
    Pharmaceutical Sciences
Federal University of São Paulo
São Paulo, Brazil

Ragavi Rajasekaran
School of Medical Science and Technology
Indian Institute of Technology Kharagpur
India;
Rajendra Mishra school of Engineering and
    Entrepreneurship
Indian Institute of Technology Kharagpur
West Bengal, India

Nurul Hidayah Ramli
School of Materials and Mineral Resources
    Engineering
Universiti Sains Malaysia, Nibong Tebal
Penang, Malaysia

Pathath Abdul Rasheed
Department of Biological Sciences and
    Engineering
Indian Institute of Technology Palakkad
Kerala, India

Khairunisak Abdul Razak
School of Materials and Mineral Resources
    Engineering
Universiti Sains Malaysia, Nibong Tebal
Penang, Malaysia

Rebeca R. Rodrigues
Laboratory of Hybrid Materials, Institute
    of Environmental, Chemical, and
    Pharmaceutical Sciences
Federal University of São Paulo
São Paulo, Brazil

Ummama Saeed
Department of Biochemistry
Bahauddin Zakariya University
Multan, Pakistan

Baisakhee Saha
School of Medical Science and Technology
Indian Institute of Technology Kharagpur
West Bengal, India

Md. Sakibur Sajal
Department of Electrical and Computer
    Engineering
Carnegie Mellon University
Pittsburgh, USA

Julián E. Sánchez-Velandia
Grupo Fitoquímica Universidad Javeriana
Pontificia Universidad Javeriana, Bogotá
Colombia;
Grupo de Investigación Catálisis Ambiental
Facultad de Ingeniería
Universidad de Antioquia
Medellín, Colombia

Piyush Sharma
Virginia Tech Center for Excellence in
  Emerging Materials
Thapar Institute of Engineering & Technology
Patiala, India

Minkyu Shin
Department of Chemical & Biomolecular
  Engineering
Sogang University, Mapo-Gu,
Seoul, Republic of Korea

Paz Silva-Borjas
Center for Economic
Administrative and Social Research (CIECAS)
National Polytechnic Institute (IPN)
Mexico City, Mexico

Meenakshi Singh
Department of Chemistry
Mahila Mahavidyalaya
Banaras Hindu University
Varanasi, India

Ritu Singh
Department of Chemistry
Mahila Mahavidyalaya
Banaras Hindu University
Varanasi, India

Akriti Srivastava
Department of Chemistry
Mahila Mahavidyalaya
Banaras Hindu University
Varanasi, India

Ghulam Yasin
Institute for Advanced Study
Shenzhen University
Shenzhen, Guangdong, China

Jinho Yoon
Department of Chemical and Biomolecular
  Engineering
Sogang University, Mapo-Gu,
Seoul, Republic of Korea

Nor Dyana Zakaria
NanoBiotechnology Research and
  Innovation (NanoBRI)
INFORMM Universiti Sains Malaysia
Penang, Malaysia

1

Introduction to Bioelectronics

Anuj Kumar

Nano-Technology Research Laboratory, Department of Chemistry, GLA University, Mathura, Uttar Pradesh, India

Shumaila Ibraheem and Ghulam Yasin

Institute for Advanced Study, Shenzhen University, Shenzhen, Guangdong, China

Ram K. Gupta

Department of Chemistry, National Institute for Materials Advancement, Pittsburg State University, Pittsburg, USA

CONTENTS

1.1 Introduction

Many diseases existed in ancient times that people could not identify or could only detect at a mature phase, and as a result, a large number of people died either unattended or lately attended when the chances of recovery were low. Even though many detection devices have been developed that can greatly assist in recovering even from fatal diseases due to early detection, there is still a great deal of scope to be discovered to address this issue for today's generation and generations to come due to the drastic improvement in quality research over the years. Biological phenomena and electrical principles are

DOI: 10.1201/9781003263265-1

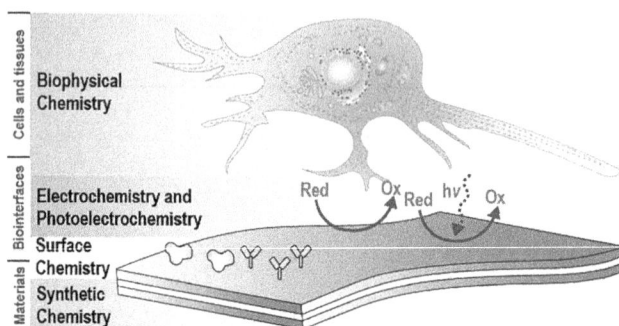

FIGURE 1.1
The chemical aspects of bioelectronics. Reproduced with permission [1]. Copyrights (2020), Royal Society of Chemistry.

brought together in the topic of bioelectronics, which can be used to establish a bridge between electronic devices and biological science, potentially opening up new technology for medical advancement. Bioelectronics, a rapidly expanding area of medical research, relies heavily on multidisciplinary technology development and cutting-edge research in chemical, biological, engineering, and physical science as shown in Figure 1.1. For example, features of bioelectronics components such as potential, impedance, and charge transport may be monitored to determine the source of a bioreaction by analyzing its surface resistance or resonance frequency, among other things. When a biological event happens, the electronic materials may be used to test how well they work in the presence of the event. With electrical components, it is possible to develop a second sort of bioelectronic system, which aids biomaterials in performing their activities. Likewise, biosensors capable to transform biological processes into electrical signals create a new domain in bioelectronics. Because of these advancements, bioelectronic scientists are inventing numerous gadgets for replacing ill-fated body parts to offer humans a new life to live. Using artificial body parts, these technologies can recognize complex brain impulses and translate them into normal physical actions. In addition, these newly created bioelectronics devices are potentially able to sense various abnormalities to alert the immune system to prepare for designing a defense protocol. At the molecular, cellular, tissue, and system levels, our understanding of biology and the basis of illness is rapidly improving.

In the coming years, as semiconductor devices shrink and become more useful, scientists expect to develop implantable prostheses that improve quality of life, lab-on-a-chip tools that enable sensitive and selective detection of infections, biomarkers for diseases, portable and cheaper imaging tools. However, the aging population in affluent nations, rising healthcare costs, and limited access to medical treatment in less developed and rural areas are driving demand for new developments in this sector. On the other hand, it has become increasingly important in recent years to investigate and build bioelectronic circuits. Incorporating similarities between biological processes and electronic circuits or combining biomaterials with electrical components can be used to develop these circuits. A bioelectronic system is designed such that electronic components may be utilized to steer biomaterials toward their intended uses. Biomaterials may be created by genetic engineering or bioengineering, allowing for the generation of novel enzymes and protein receptors, as well as the manufacturing of monoclonal antibodies or aptamers for non-biological substrates such as metals and metalloids. These materials and electrical components can be mixed in a variety of functional units to get the desired effect.

This chapter presents an overview of bioelectronics' underlying theory and practical applications, focusing on fundamental concepts, materials, fabrication, and testing of bioelectronic tools.

1.2 Fundamental Concepts of Bioelectronics

Multidisciplinary research fields including electrical engineering, biology, chemical, and physical science, and material science are required to fully realize the promise of bioelectronics. Even though the field of bioelectronic medicine is still in its infancy, the opportunities and hopes it inspires are vast. A revolution in medical practice, not an innovation, is what bioelectronic medicine is all about. New bioelectronics disciplines have the potential to have an enormous influence on a wide range of national priorities, including healthcare and medicine, homeland security, forensics, and environmental and food supply protection. The synergy between electronics and biology might be greatly enhanced with the evolution of electronic technology to the atomic scale, as well as major advances in system, cell, and molecular biology. A lab-on-a-chip for a clinic for medical diagnosis, and real-time detection of biological agents would eliminate the need for a laboratory in the next decades. This section will introduce the reader to the principles of working with bio-interfaces, which are junctions between different materials and biological structures. The discussion of the size and time of interactions, material selection, and the basic biophysical ideas is highlighted to explain how biological events happen and how their signals can be interpreted in terms of bioelectronics.

1.2.1 Bioelectronics with a Size Scale

When designing the bio-interfaces, it is important to consider the length scale of the interface to effectively address the relevant biological events. These can range from the large area with non-specific modulation to micro-sensing and everything in between (Figure 1.2a). Electrodes with a large surface area were the first such device developed and still in use. There are many more frequently used advanced techniques available like electroencephalography (EEG) to record brain activity through the scalp, electrocardiography (ECG) to monitor cardiac activity, and electromyography (EMG) to record skeletal muscle activity [2].

The advances in materials research have opened the door to the possibility of constructing probes with higher resolution that can be placed closer to the active cells, enabling the creation of smaller and less invasive devices to be built. The first phase was the development of direct bio-interfaces with a single organ, which was completed in two stages. The second step was the establishment of indirect bio-interfaces with a single organ. Because of these efforts, artificial pacemakers, cochlear implants, and deep-brain stimulation probes have all been produced, and they have helped millions of people live longer, better lives. Probes have shortened in size and grown more adaptable, which has resulted in an improvement in the biocompatibility of electrical devices [3–5]. They opened up an entirely new viewpoint on the study of cell physiology since micron-sized devices were able to detect local electric potential deep within tissues while also interacting with small groups of cells, making them an invaluable tool in the field. To operate at this scale, it is required to consider major chemical interactions between the materials

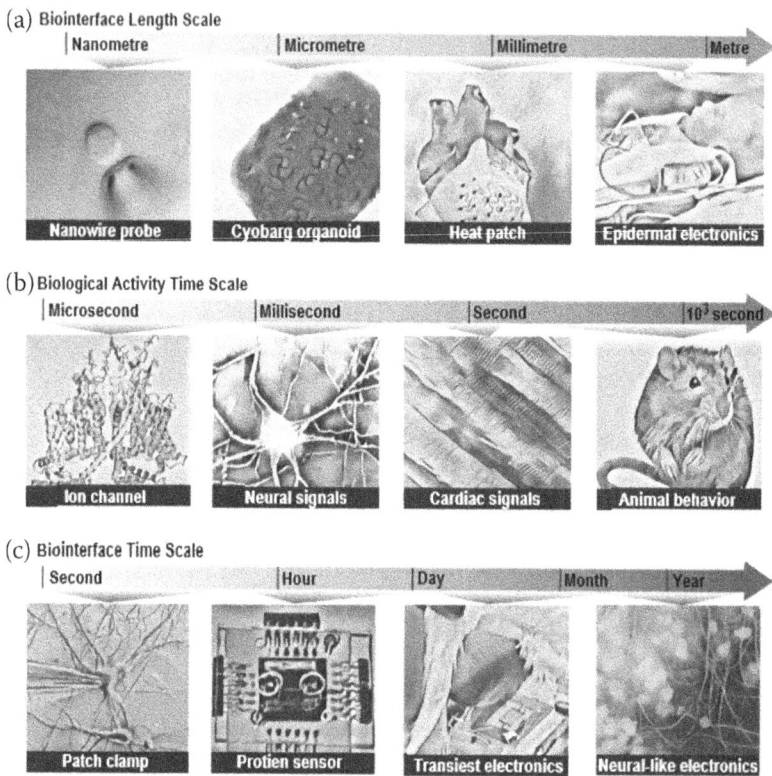

FIGURE 1.2
(a–c) The illustration of length and time scales in bioelectronics as well as bioelectrical studies. Reproduced with permission [1]. Copyrights (2020), Royal Society of Chemistry.

and the tissues, such as adhesion forces. Extracellular and intracellular interfaces between single cells may now be generated with high accuracy using devices that are now accessible at the cutting edge of technology [6–9]. The possibility exists that future studies in this area will offer methods for manipulating certain organelles, or even studies on specific cell components such as microfilaments or ion channels, among other things.

1.2.2 Timing in Bioelectronics

Both sequential and sequential with regard to time are valid approaches to analyzing the essential time scales in bioelectronics research. It is necessary to examine the length of time that the device and biological system are in contact with one another to have a better understanding of how biological signals are created (Figure 1.2b, c). The ability of the device to respond at a high frequency is required when engaging with highly active cells such as neurons or cardiac muscles, which can generate an action potential in milliseconds or less. The time at which the desired process occurs determines the kinetics of the recording or stimulation that is used. When it comes to slower physiological processes like bone regeneration, a different set of considerations must be taken into account when building devices to sense or activate such processes. Interfacial chemistry is important because it can influence both the stability of an interface and the resulting immune response. Devices with the capacity to impact chemical transduction must also consider the significant delay in signal transmission and processing that happens during these processes, which can last anywhere from minutes to hours [1,10].

The duration of time that expects the bio-interface to remain operational is another independent time scale. The time used for interfacing might range from relatively brief studies to long-term implantation for clinical purposes, depending on the application. Bio-interfaces utilized in the study of individual physiological processes may only remain operational for a brief time [11]. They are employed to investigate single physiological interactions and then discarded after a short period. As a result, these sorts of trials do not need significant investigations into the stability and biocompatibility of the materials. Working with the tissues or cell cultures, maintaining stable bio-interfaces becomes a major consideration. In this situation, it becomes necessary for the devices to preserve their integrity to analyze new interactions in the bio-interface that are not related to the device's intended function. The consequences of uncontrolled cell growth or enhanced cytotoxicity, for example, resulting from the disintegration of the device, must be overlooked. Similarly, it is consequently crucial to consider the chemical composition of such devices, as well as the reactivity of the materials that make up their construction. The immune system's response to the presence of a foreign body must also be taken into account when dealing with applications that need the implantation of a device into an organism [12,13].

On the other hand, for the long-term integration of bioelectronics with a host body, excellent stability and biocompatibility are critical considerations. The construction of chronic brain interfaces is an important example of an application that necessitates long-term integration and integration of several technologies. Because of the fragile nature of brain tissue, it is not only more sensitive to intrusive probes but also has a limited ability to regenerate, making the replacement of worn bioelectronic devices with new ones an impractical option. When probes are removed and reinserted, they induce permanent trauma that can result in the buildup of deadly damage over time [14,15].

1.2.3 Transductions of Signals

The signal production and transmission techniques utilized by biological systems are significantly different from those used by conventional electronics. Electrons immediately transmit electronic charges in classical conductors such as metals, which is why they carry the majority of electric charge [16]. The bulk of the electric current carried by biological systems, which are rich in water, ions, and organic matter, is caused by ionic fluxes. Because these two forms of conduction are fundamentally different, the construction of a specialized interface over which signals may be delivered and received is required (Figure 1.3a, b) [1]. An increase in ion fluxes caused by a rapid release of ions, also known as an action potential, permits electrically active cells to interact with one another. It is sustained by active transport and an imbalance in the concentration of ions, often K^+ and Na^+, between the insides of cells and their external environment (which is usually negative). Electrochemical [17], optoelectronic [11] or photo-electronic [18], photo-thermal [19], transistor-based sensing processes [20], as well as the stimulation with molecular [21] and optical signals [22], or the transduction of mechanical signals [23], can be used to understand the transduction of bio-signals.

1.2.4 Mechanism of Bioelectronics

Because practically all body organs and functions are regulated by brain circuits that communicate by electrical impulses, they should potentially be able to comprehend the

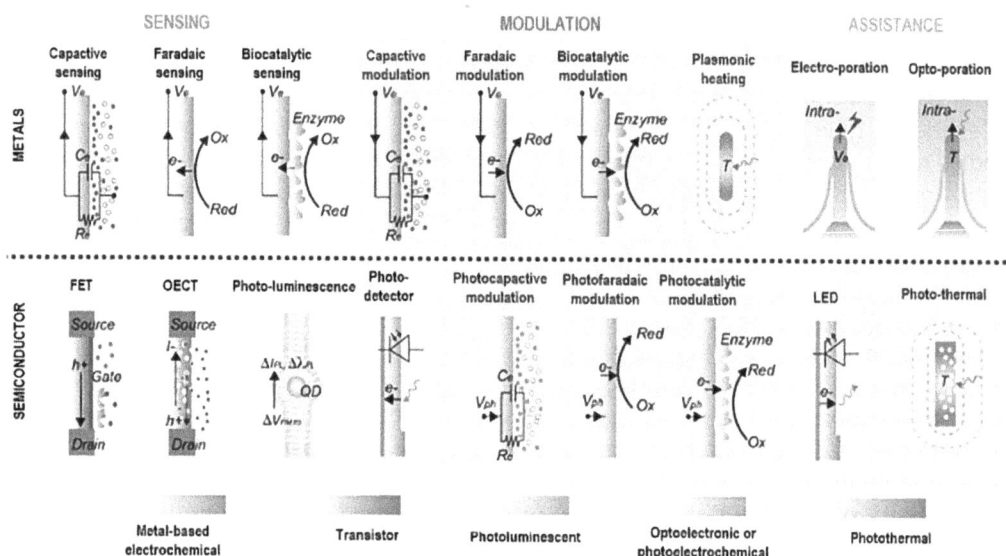

FIGURE 1.3

A systematic representation of (a) metal-based electrodes for the capturing as well as installation of capacitive, faradaic, and biocatalytic currents, and (b) field-effect and organic electrochemical transistors (FET and OECT, respectively) for sensing bioelectric signals. Reproduced with permission [1]. Copyright (2020), Royal Society of Chemistry.

electrical language used by disorders. Theoretically, it may be possible to correct the problem by using tiny electrodes to activate or block the faulty circuits. Researchers could potentially manipulate a wide variety of bodily functions using this method of micro-manipulation of the nervous system, which involves sending impulses (action potentials) to specific cells within neural circuits. These applications include controlling appetite or blood pressure, as well as stimulating the release of insulin in response to rising blood sugar levels. An invasive procedure will likely be necessary to identify and block the nerve bundles carrying different signals from the peripheral nervous system to the brain that are implicated in certain disorders. Preventing the different signals from being discharged in the brain will have a greater effect than previously assumed [24]. The following are a few noteworthy areas for bioelectronics: (i) gaining an understanding of the interactions between molecules, cells, and electronics; (ii) recognizing and understanding cellular responses to stimulus, as well as their variations (electrical, mechanical, chemical, thermal, and the like); (iii) the ability to collect and analyze critical data on the state of biomolecules and cells (chemical, physical, structural, and functional data); (iv) the ability to monitor, in real time, the biochemistry of a single cell or a population of cells, which necessitates an understanding of the interactions between molecules; (v) the ability to give treatment materials and stimuli in real time that are suitable; and (vi) capability of concurrently detecting, identifying, and quantifying hundreds of distinct biomarkers [25].

1.2.5 Materials' Reactivity

Environmental conditions that are volatile and difficult to plan and manage for the formation of bio-interfaces are common in nature. There is a wide variety of pH values present in the cells and tissues present on the materials, as well as variable ion concentrations and a spectrum of chemicals and biomolecules – the majority of which are chemically active. To ensure that devices remain chemically stable and electrically functional over an extended period, it is necessary to consider the chemical processes that occur throughout the device's operation while designing the device, which can either be undesirable or desirable, depending on the use. A thorough analysis of the material's chemical characteristics enables it to be properly tuned in terms of its stability [1].

1.3 Innovative Technologies in Bioelectronics

There are mainly two innovative technologies actively engaged in bioelectronics. The first one is bioelectronics corporation as a leader in non-invasive electroceuticals and the manufacturer of an industry-leading family of disposable, drug-free pain therapy devices, including ActiPatch® Therapy (an over-the-counter treatment for back pain and other musculoskeletal complaints), RecoveryRx® Devices (for chronic and post-operative wound care), Allay® Menstrual Pain Therapy, and HealFast® Therapy (for dogs and cats). The second one is electroCore medical technology. This is a non-implanted device called GammaCore that stimulates the vagal nerve as a way of treating cluster headaches and migraines in Canada, Germany, the United Kingdom, and other areas of Europe. The non-invasive gadget is also being developed for use in other conditions such as epilepsy, asthma, irritable bowel syndrome, and potentially Alzheimer's disease [24].

The design of electronic medical devices using wireless power transfer has been accomplished by Stanford engineers, who have devised a method of wirelessly transferring electricity deep into the body, and using this power to operate minute electronic medical devices. Furthermore, it raised the prospect that this technology might pave the way for a new style of medicine that would allow physicians to treat diseases using electrical devices rather than pharmaceuticals in the future. Electronic pulses, rather than medications, are used to treat migraine headaches by ElexroCore. ElexroCore has created a portable device that relieves migraine headaches instead of using pharmaceuticals. A device called the GammaCore, which looks like an electric razor and is put against the neck, where it stimulates the vagus nerve, is referred to as electroceuticals or bioelectronics in the scientific literature. The electrical pulses aid in the management of a chemical known as glutamate, which has been related to migraines in certain studies [26].

1.4 Materials and Their Classifications in Bioelectronics

1.4.1 Bioelectronics with Inorganic Semiconductors

Inorganic semiconductors are frequently employed in the study of electronic and photonic bio-interfaces, as well as in a variety of other applications. A few examples of high-performance electronic applications include electronic sensing, signal amplification, transduction, etc. Scientists have taken a special interest in Si-based semiconductors, in particular, because of their biocompatibility and the fact that they have undergone extensive microfabrication development. Si has high charge carrier mobilities, which results in short response times and great sensitivity of the devices [27]. This property, when used in bioelectronic devices, allows for the precise probing of complex biological dynamics. Si is straightforwardly used to manufacture a variety of designs at various sizes, ranging from the nanoscale to the macroscale. This sort of multiscale material management is well suited to the multiscale application of varied biological components and enables integration with a wide range of biological systems, as demonstrated in the case study. A more specific example is the administration of Si-based 1D nanostructures into neuronal cultures or tissues in a drug-like manner while maintaining high spatial resolution. Si-based 1D nanostructures have improved mechanical flexibility, in addition to carrier transport capacity [6].

Furthermore, photonic energy may be turned into electrical energy once it has been absorbed by silicon semiconductors. Si-based materials are frequently surrounded by biological fluids when used in cell cultures or as implants, leading to the production of interfaces between the two materials, which are known as semiconductor/saline interfaces. It is possible that in the presence of light, this will result in transient photocapacitive modulation of cells or tissues or longer-lasting photofaradic reactions in which cells or tissues are harmed. The participation of electrons and holes in cathodic and anodic processes, respectively, makes these processes more efficient [28].

Palanker et al. developed a series of photovoltaic retinal implants, in which the high-pixel-density devices provide local control of rat retinal neurons, with the hope of recovering vision one day. When developing nano-bioelectronic devices, it is vital to boost the photovoltaic or photoelectrochemical impact of these devices to improve photostimulation by these devices [29,30]. Parameswaran et al. [31] observed that dopant alteration and surface chemistry of the Si-based nanostructures might increase their efficacy as neuromodulators by a factor of two, compared to the control group (Figure 1.4a). They used coaxial p-type/intrinsic/n-type (p–i–n) Si-based nanowires (Si-NWs) to regulate primary rat dorsal root ganglion neurons by photo-electrochemical processes. Each Si-NWs was made of a core nanowire doped with p, an interlayer of intrinsic Si, and an n-doped shell. Further experiments demonstrated that the inclusion of distributed atomic Au on the sidewalls of Si-NWs might significantly boost the generation of photo-electrochemical currents and, as a result, the efficacy of neuro-modulation (Figure 1.4b).

Another study, conducted by Jiang et al. [27], looked at 2D p–i–n Si membranes that were adorned with noble metal nanoparticles (such as Au, Ag, and Pt) to get deposited on their surfaces via electroless deposition. They came to a similar conclusion. A considerable increase in the generation of photo-electrochemical currents was seen when metal-decorated p–i–n membranes were used, with the increase being at least an order of magnitude. Consequently, visual stimulation of the cerebral cortex, as well as behavior control, were both significantly improved (Figure 1.4c). In addition, the researchers believe that Si photovoltaic devices can play a significant role in the ultrasensitive detection of biometric signals. Yokota et al. [33] have reported an imager constructed of low-temperature polycrystalline silicon (LTPS) thin-film transistors (TFTs), which can read out modest photocurrents of less than 10 μA while producing very little background noise. Polycrystalline silicon (polySi) was transformed into an amorphous silicon film (a-Si) by the use of excimer laser annealing, which was then utilized to fabricate the TFT readout circuits. For the design of the TFT readout circuits, the silicon oxide (SiO) film, silicon nitride film (SiN), and amorphous silicon film (a-Si) films were all employed. When used in conjunction with sensitive biological detectors, the imager is capable of electrically detecting and calibrating the movement of the device based on fingerprint or vein feature points, which is particularly useful in medical applications.

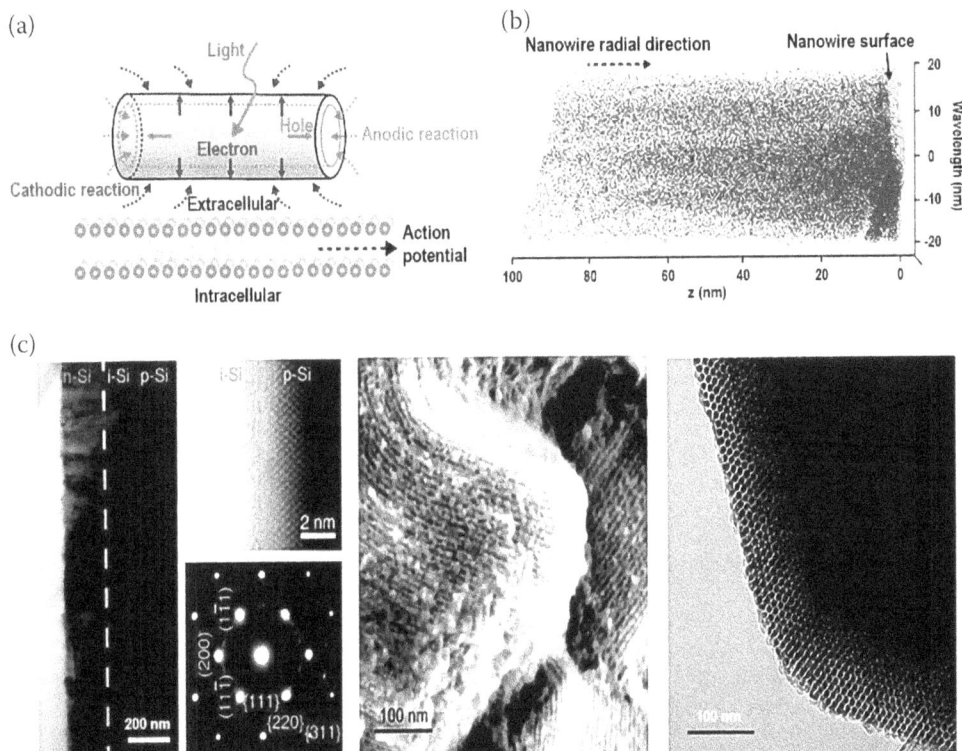

(a)

(b)

(c)

FIGURE 1.4
(a) The illustration of coaxial p-type/intrinsic/n-type (p–i–n) Si-NWs architecture for photo-electrochemical extracellular modulation of neuron membrane potential. Reproduced with permission [27]. Copyright (2018), Springer Nature. (b) The tomographic representation of atomic probe of diffused gold on Si-NWs architecture's sidewalls. Reproduced with permission [31]. Copyright (2018), Springer Nature. (c) TEM/SEM images showing the cross-section along with diffraction pattern of Si-NWs architecture. Reproduced with permission [32]. Copyright (2018), Springer Nature.

1.4.2 Bioelectronics with Organic Semiconductor

Organic semiconductors have proven to be an excellent candidate for flexible and stretchable bioelectronic applications, particularly in biosensors and biomedical devices, due to a combination of their low-temperature solution-phase processability, good mechanical deformability, and applicable charge transport properties. Organic bioelectronics that is mechanically compliant, whether in contact with the skin or implanted into tissues, can aid to lessen discomfort and other negative outcomes that can arise as a result of the mechanical mismatch between the device and the body [34]. Furthermore, because many organic semiconductors are self-healing and biodegradable, they are particularly well suited for use in wearable and injectable bioelectronics applications, such as cardiac monitoring. It will be necessary to consider many variables when developing the next generation of organic bioelectronics, including the balance between mechanical deformability and device mobility, long-term stability under physiological conditions, stretching and bending durability, among other things [35,36].

On the other hand, surface functionalization may also be utilized to produce bio-recognition (Figure 1.5a, b) [37]. Mulla et al. [38] employed monomeric porcine odorant-binding proteins (pOBPs) as ligands in a capacitive coupled p-type organic FET

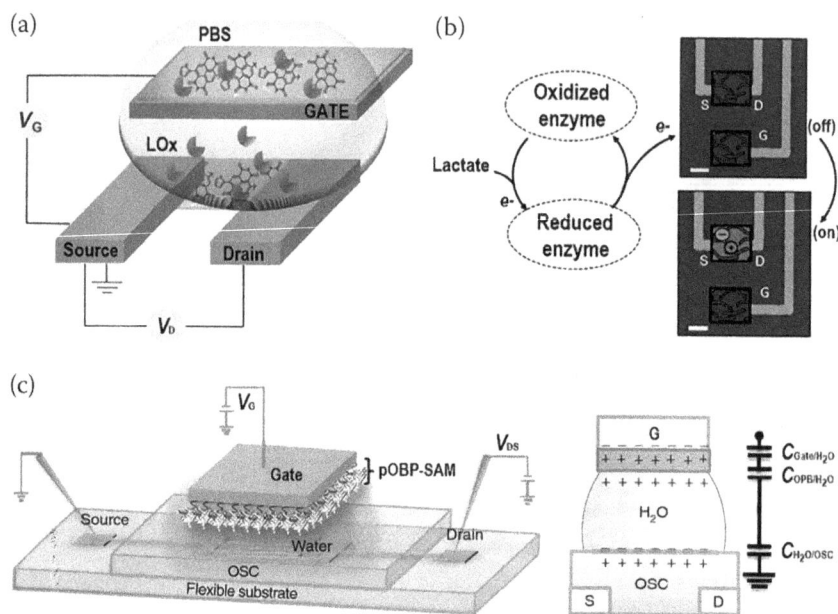

FIGURE 1.5
(a) A schematic representation for the bio-functionalization of OECTs with enzyme, (b) the immobilization of LOx enzyme on the gate electrode of transistors for sensing selectivity enhancement. Reproduced with permission [37]. Copyright (2018), American Association for the Advancement of Science Publishing Group. (c) A schematic representation and (d) working mechanism of a capacitively coupled p-type organic FET with pOBPs as ligands. Reproduced with permission [38]. Copyright (2015), Springer Nature.

(polymer, PBTTT-C14) device and organized them on the metal gate of the device. With this method, it is possible to detect pico-molar concentrations of OBPs, which may then be used to determine chiral differential interactions in OBPs with high selectivity and specificity (Figure 1.5c, d). Through the use of small capacitance changes associated with ligand-protein complex formation, it is possible to calculate free-energy balances from conformational events, such as the interaction of chiral (S)-(+)-carvone enantiomers with OBPs, with high accuracy. While pOBPs are negatively charged in pure water, the chiral molecules have a dipole moment and physically connect to the pOBPs. In contrast, pOBPs are positively charged in pure water, and the chiral molecules have a dipole moment and physically bind to the pOBPs.

1.4.3 Bioelectronics with Inorganic Conductors

Metals-based materials are the most frequently used conductive inorganic materials in bioelectronic devices, as well as for the development of a wide range of bioelectronic devices. New advances in chemistry are necessary to improve the conductivity, biocompatibility, chemical stability, and workability of these materials, and their manufacturing and patterning capabilities, to improve the performance of next-generation bioelectronics. For instance, platinum nanoparticles (Pt NPs) are often used as a decorative coating on other materials to give reactive sites while also increasing the overall properties of the substance. When Pt NPs are exposed to liquid metals, they exhibit a significant attraction to them, resulting in a homogenous dispersion of the liquid metal across Pt NPs-coated carbon nanotubes [39]. This composite metal exhibits mechanical and electrical characteristics that are superior to those of pure Pt NPs. This composite may be used to print high-resolution 3D structures. Thus, the fabrication of future 3D wearable bioelectronics with improved mechanical and electrical characteristics will be possible in the future. Because of their enormous surface area, Pt NPs-decorated Si composites have the potential to provide cathodal charge storage capacities of B50 mCcm^2, which are comparable to those of strongly doped organic electrode coatings. Aside from providing superior catalytic performance over hydrogen peroxide, Pt NPs significantly improve the current density and detection sensitivity of graphene-based glutamate and glucose sensors [40].

In another study, to monitor the intracellular action potentials in excitable cells such as neurons and cardiomyocytes, Au-based nano-pillar with a mushroom-shaped have also been demonstrated to be capable of recording subthreshold synaptic activity and action potentials in vitro with minimal invasiveness for days at a time, which is 50 times longer than the typical patch-clamp techniques [41]. Researchers discovered that mushroom-shaped Au micro-electrodes significantly improved membrane engulfment, which is advantageous for their application because it results in the formation of high resistance seals between the interfaced cell and the electrodes [42].

1.4.4 Bioelectronics with Nanocarbons

Nanocarbons like graphene and carbon nanotubes (CNTs) are valued in bioelectronics due to their exceptional chemical stability, biocompatibility, recyclability, great mechanical flexibility, a huge surface area, and a broad electro-mechanical range. Nanocarbons are used in the fabrication of fiber-like probes for biomedical applications. Energy storage and electrochemical sensing are examples of electrochemical technologies using these carbon materials. In addition, carbon microelectrodes with a conductive coating have been used for high-resolution measurements. With an increase in synaptic activity as well as in vesicles, oxidation of carbon fiber in a cell or near a cell can also take place [28,43].

1.4.5 Bioelectronics with Organic Conductors

Making conducting materials that are both very flexible and mechanically robust is one of the most challenging difficulties faced by researchers working on bioelectronics in the past few decades. In comparison to the majority of inorganic conducting materials currently on the market, organic conducting materials, such as conjugated polymers and hydrogels, have the potential to be more biocompatible and easier to manufacture [44,45]. The conductive polymers have been discovered for use in flexible electronics, and only a few have been used for bioelectronics applications. Current research is mostly focused on three materials, namely poly(3,4-ethylenedioxythiophene)poly(styrene sulfonate) (PEDOT-PSS), polypyrrole (PPy), and polyaniline (PANI) in particular [46].

The development of synthetic approaches to increase the purity of PEDOT-PSS is important due to the risk that additives may impair the material homogeneity and introduce the possibility of cytotoxicity. Because of the collapse of the fibrillary structure, which decreases the conductivity of pure PEDOT-PSS hydrogels when synthesized under normal conditions, it is difficult to obtain a consistent result in the laboratory (Figure 1.6a) [46]. Purified PEDOT-PSS may be produced using a process developed by Luet al. [46] that maintains the desired features like the material's stability, flexibility, and conductivity. Adding DMSO to aqueous PEDOT-PSS, they were able to form interconnected and pure PEDOT-PSS nano-fibrils (Figure 1.6b). At the end of the process, a dry phase-separated

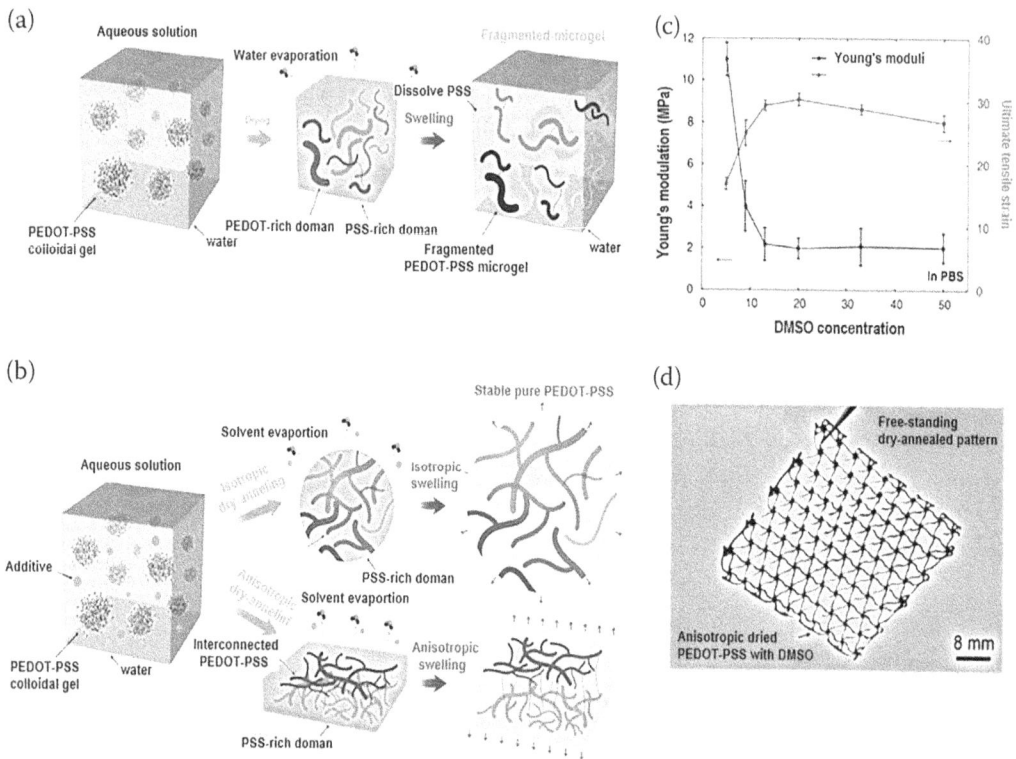

FIGURE 1.6
Schematic representation of (a) PEDOT: PSS domain aggregation via water evaporation, (b) morphology for fibril domain in PEDOT: PSS hydrogel with DMSO as a de-hydrating agent, (c) the curves for Young's moduli and ultimate tensile strains in PEDOT: PSS, and (d) the representation of PEDOT: PSS with a free-standing pattern. Reproduced with permission [46]. Copyright (2019), Springer Nature.

system was generated, which, when maintained in a well-spaced network, maintained its connectivity even after the hydrophilic PSS domains have been rehydrated. The amount of DMSO used in these gels, as well as the duration of the dry annealing process, may be varied to get the mechanical properties that are needed (Figure 1.6c). It is important to note that this technology is compatible with inkjet printing and allows for the fabrication of patterns in a short amount of time (Figure 1.6d).

A combination of PEDOT-PSS and polyethylenimine (PEI) was developed by Cea et al. [47] to produce a biocompatible material. The active channel of this novel material is composed mostly of PEDOT-PSS, PEI, and D-sorbitol. In this study, D-sorbitol was utilized as a biocompatible stabilizer to boost the hydration and mobility of ions. However, the interaction between PEDOT-PSS and PEI resulted in the development of unique electrical characteristics (Figure 1.7a). PEI was responsible for electron transfer and reduction of PEDOT through the creation of PEI-PSS complexes. It also causes de-doping in PEDOT, which results in a decrease in its conductivity. When a gate bias is applied, PEI becomes protonated and releases PSS, which, when bound to PEDOT, restores conductivity in the device under consideration. "Channel" is a term that refers to the passage of information through a channel. The resultant material is extremely stable, and the redox reaction is nearly perfect in terms of reversibility. The materials discovered may be easily produced using a typical lithographic technique to generate thin and flexible

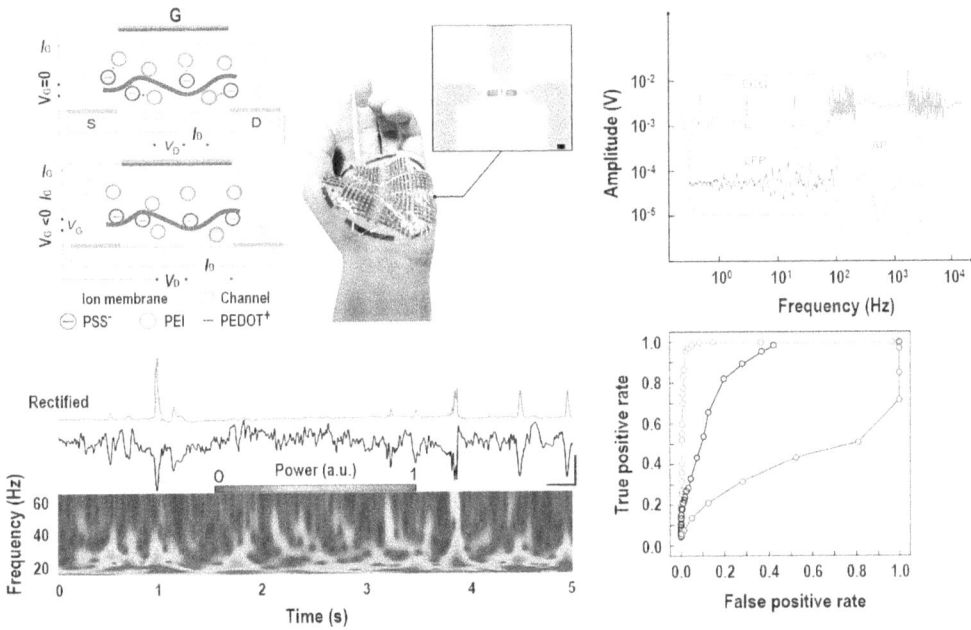

FIGURE 1.7
A systematic representation of (a) e-IGT device function, (b) e-IGT device installed in a human hand, (c) signal response displayed by e-IGT-based electronic devices, (d) its output, and (e) corresponding operating curves. Reproduced with permission [47]. Copyright (2020), Springer Nature.

membranes, which is a straightforward process (Figure 1.7b). It was determined that the application of the prepared material could be demonstrated by recording a variety of distinct bioelectronic signals (Figure 1.7c). In this study, IGTs were employed for non-linear signal amplification of high-fidelity detection of epileptic discharges to establish long-term in-vivo biocompatibility (Figure 1.7d) [47]. When compared to traditional approaches, such local nonlinear amplifiers demonstrated both a high response rate as well as better detection quality (Figure 1.7e). The devices were stable for more than two weeks after being implanted and delivered high-quality recordings from animals that were free to move around. This work demonstrated how chemical principles may be used for the realization of additional functions while simultaneously protecting the stability and biocompatibility of the device in a biomedical environment.

1.5 Conclusions

To sum up, in recent years, there has been an increased interest in the use of electronics technology in biology and medicine. Pacemakers, as well as almost the whole medical imaging sector, are examples of this. The research that enabled these applications arose from a variety of scientific and technical fields. Nevertheless, the word "bioelectronics" has lately gained popularity as a more general phrase to characterize this diverse field of study. In bioelectronics, there is significant potential for breakthroughs that are based on perspectives from a wide range of diverse domains. Partnerships in bioelectronics within the natural sciences are no different than collaborations between scientists and researchers in other disciplines of study. Through the use of a certain approach, materials with similar chemistries but different functionality may be used in combination to develop bioelectronic devices that have capabilities to exceed the capabilities of either material alone. In the vast majority of cases, such strategies will provide extremely valuable insights into the situation.

The utilization of hard-soft composites to lessen the impact of mechanical mismatch between a device and a tissue, while simultaneously enabling unique sensing and stimulation avenues, serves as a mechanical example of this concept. Furthermore, discoveries in disciplines that are adjacent to bioelectronics have the added benefit of opening up a wide range of new possibilities for bioelectronics applications. One of the most often discussed topics in the realm of energy input techniques with a good spatiotemporal resolution, such as acoustic, optical, and magnetic impulses, is the application of these techniques to dramatically enhance the localization of different therapies. New technologies are required to successfully construct structures at the nanoscale, and new metrology and using biological assemblages for nanoscale manufacturing are hot topics right now. Fabrication of complex physical features onto substrates with essential dimensions of less than 1 nm, development of metrology instruments for testing and measuring nanoscale features, and surfaces for controlling antibody and antigen-binding are being developed.

Despite the significant advancements in bioelectronics, to move bioelectronics ahead further, innovation is required in many broad areas, including measurements and analysis, fabrication, biocompatibility, and power sources. In general, these cross-cutting issues are caused by a lack of technological advancement, a lack of biological knowledge, or a combination of the two factors. To achieve the essential advances, it will be important to coordinate and bring together the expertise that exists across government agencies, university research institutes, and industry. Among the manufacturing issues are the development of improved sensors and the development of innovative fabrication processes. It is also difficult to merge numerous sensing technologies with integrated circuit technologies. Biosensors will play a critical part in addressing future bioelectronics needs, and increases in bandwidth and detection limits will be required to satisfy these expectations.

Developing a detailed bioelectronics roadmap with input from the government, academic institutions, and the private sector would be an excellent next step. Such a road map would allow for more effective planning and resource management, as well as an increase in the productivity and commercialization of bioelectronics research and development. Such an activity would establish and explain expected application-specific research metrics and metrology gaps and needs, as well as timescales for research, development, and prototyping, as well as upcoming market and commercialization opportunities and challenges in bioelectronics. To build synergistic combinations of some of the recent results presented in this chapter, we predict that chemical considerations will be used successfully soon, with considerable success being achieved in bioelectronics. Moreover, the following shortcomings are also necessary for the development of this field: (i) understanding molecule/cell-electronic interactions; (ii) understanding cellular reactions to a stimulus; and (iii) researchers must understand how molecules interact with each other to deliver appropriate therapeutic materials and stimuli in real time and can detect, identify, and quantify thousands of biomarkers simultaneously. Collaboration between the electronics and biomedical device industries, as well as university and government research groups, will hasten the transition of this interdisciplinary research to commercial devices. Leadership from diverse fields must be prepared to commit to collaborative activities when multidisciplinary input is required for success.

References

1. Y. Fang, L. Meng, A. Prominski, E.N. Schaumann, M. Seebald, B. Tian, Recent advances in bioelectronics chemistry. *Chemical Society Reviews* 2020, *49* (22), 7978–8035.
2. A.H. Moffa, D. Martin, A. Alonzo, D. Bennabi, D.M. Blumberger, I.M. Benseñor, Z. Daskalakis, F. Fregni, E. Haffen, S.H. Lisanby, Efficacy and acceptability of transcranial direct current stimulation (tDCS) for major depressive disorder: An individual patient data meta-analysis. *Progress in Neuro-Psychopharmacology Biological Psychiatry* 2020, *99*, 109836.
3. A. Chortos, J. Liu, Z. Bao, Pursuing prosthetic electronic skin. *Nature Materials* 2016, *15* (9), 937–950.
4. G. Hong, T.-M. Fu, M. Qiao, R.D. Viveros, X. Yang, T. Zhou, J.M. Lee, H.-G. Park, J.R. Sanes, C.M. Lieber, A method for single-neuron chronic recording from the retina in awake mice. *Science* 2018, *360* (6396), 1447–1451.
5. G. Hong, C.M. Lieber, Novel electrode technologies for neural recordings. *Nature Reviews Neuroscience* 2019, *20* (6), 330–345.
6. R. Chen, A. Canales, P. Anikeeva, Neural recording and modulation technologies. *Nature Reviews Materials* 2017, *2* (2), 1–16.
7. N. Obidin, F. Tasnim, C. Dagdeviren, The future of neuroimplantable devices: A materials science and regulatory perspective. *Advanced Materials* 2020, *32* (15), 1901482.
8. T.R. Ray, J. Choi, A.J. Bandodkar, S. Krishnan, P. Gutruf, L. Tian, R. Ghaffari, J.A. Rogers, Bio-integrated wearable systems: A comprehensive review. *Chemical Reviews* 2019, *119* (8), 5461–5533.
9. J. Shi, C. Clayton, B. Tian, Nano-enabled cellular engineering for bioelectric studies. *Nano Research* 2020, *13* (5), 1214–1227.
10. R. Chen, G. Romero, M.G. Christiansen, A. Mohr, P. Anikeeva, Wireless magnetothermal deep brain stimulation. *Science* 2015, *347* (6229), 1477–1480.
11. Y. Jiang, R. Parameswaran, X. Li, J.L. Carvalho-de-Souza, X. Gao, L. Meng, F. Bezanilla, G.M. Shepherd, B. Tian, Nongenetic optical neuromodulation with silicon-based materials. *Nature Protocols* 2019, *14* (5), 1339–1376.
12. R. Parameswaran, K. Koehler, M.Y. Rotenberg, M.J. Burke, J. Kim, K.-Y. Jeong, B. Hissa, M.D. Paul, K. Moreno, N. Sarma, Optical stimulation of cardiac cells with a polymer-supported silicon nanowire matrix. *Proceedings of the National Academy of Sciences* 2019, *116* (2), 413–421.
13. S. Yoo, S. Hong, Y. Choi, J.-H. Park, Y. Nam, Photothermal inhibition of neural activity with near-infrared-sensitive nanotransducers. *ACS Nano* 2014, *8* (8), 8040–8049.
14. J.L. Carvalho-de-Souza, B.I. Pinto, D.R. Pepperberg, F. Bezanilla, Optocapacitive generation of action potentials by microsecond laser pulses of nanojoule energy. *Biophysical Journal* 2018, *114* (2), 283–288.
15. J.L. Carvalho-de-Souza, J.S. Treger, B. Dang, S.B.H. Kent, D.R. Pepperberg, F. Bezanilla, Photosensitivity of neurons enabled by cell-targeted gold nanoparticles. *Neuron* 2015, *86* (1), 207–217.
16. R. Plonsey, R. Barr, Bioelectricity: A quantitative approach. Springer Science & Business Media. 2007. ISBN-13 : 978-0387488646
17. H. Yuk, B. Lu, X. Zhao, Hydrogel bioelectronics. *Chemical Society Reviews* 2019, *48* (6), 1642–1667.
18. N. Zhang, F. Huang, S. Zhao, X. Lv, Y. Zhou, S. Xiang, S. Xu, Y. Li, G. Chen, C. Tao, Photo-rechargeable fabrics as sustainable and robust power sources for wearable bioelectronics. *Matter* 2020, *2* (5), 1260–1269.
19. E. Miyako, C. Hosokawa, M. Kojima; M. Yudasaka, R. Funahashi, I. Oishi, Y. Hagihara, M. Shichiri, M. Takashima, K. Nishio, A. Photo-thermal-electrical converter based on carbon nanotubes for bioelectronic applications. *Angewandte Chemie International Edition* 2011, *50* (51), 12266–12270.

20. M.Y. Lee, H.R. Lee, C.H. Park, S.G. Han, J.H. Oh, Organic transistor-based chemical sensors for wearable bioelectronics. *Accounts of Chemical Research* 2018, *51* (11), 2829–2838.
21. F. Fu, J. Wang, H. Zeng, J. Yu, Functional conductive hydrogels for bioelectronics. *ACS Materials Letters* 2020, *2* (10), 1287–1301.
22. Y. Zhang, Z. Zhou, Z. Fan; S. Zhang, F. Zheng, K. Liu, Y. Zhang, Z. Shi, L. Chen, X. Li, Self-powered multifunctional transient bioelectronics. *Small* 2018, *14* (35), 1802050.
23. A.J. Bandodkar, D. Molinnus, O. Mirza, T. Guinovart, J.R. Windmiller, G. Valdés-Ramírez, F.J. Andrade, M.J. Schöning, J. Wang, Epidermal tattoo potentiometric sodium sensors with wireless signal transduction for continuous non-invasive sweat monitoring. *Biosensors Bioelectronics* 2014, *54*, 603–609.
24. S. Thonte, O.G. Bhusnure, V. Makanikar, O. Pravin, D. Sagar, Smart bioelectronics: The future of medicine is electric. *International Journal of Engineering Technology Science and Research* 2016, *3*, 43–53.
25. H. Lee, Y. Lee, C. Song, H.R. Cho, R. Ghaffari, T.K. Choi, K.H. Kim, Y.B. Lee, D. Ling, H. Lee, An endoscope with integrated transparent bioelectronics and theranostic nanoparticles for colon cancer treatment. *Nature Communications* 2015, *6* (1), 1–10.
26. J. Kim, S. Imani, W.R. de Araujo, J. Warchall, G. Valdés-Ramírez, T.R. Paixão, P.P. Mercier, J. Wang, Wearable salivary uric acid mouthguard biosensor with integrated wireless electronics. *Biosensors Bioelectronics* 2015, *74*, 1061–1068.
27. Y. Jiang, X. Li, B. Liu, J. Yi, Y. Fang, F. Shi, X. Gao, E. Sudzilovsky, R. Parameswaran, K. Koehler, Rational design of silicon structures for optically controlled multiscale biointerfaces. *Nature Biomedical Engineering* 2018, *2* (7), 508–521.
28. J.G. Roberts, E.C. Mitchell, L.E. Dunaway, G.S. McCarty, L.A. Sombers, Carbon-fiber nanoelectrodes for real-time discrimination of vesicle cargo in the native cellular environment. *ACS Nano* 2020, *14* (3), 2917–2926.
29. H. Lorach, G. Goetz, R. Smith, X. Lei, Y. Mandel, T. Kamins, K. Mathieson, P. Huie, J. Harris, A. Sher, Photovoltaic restoration of sight with high visual acuity. *Nature Medicine* 2015, *21* (5), 476–482.
30. L. Wang, K. Mathieson, T.I. Kamins, J.D. Loudin, L. Galambos, G. Goetz, A. Sher, Y. Mandel, P. Huie, D. Lavinsky, Photovoltaic retinal prosthesis: Implant fabrication and performance. *Journal of Neural Engineering* 2012, *9* (4), 046014.
31. R. Parameswaran, J.L. Carvalho-de-Souza, Y. Jiang, M.J. Burke, J.F. Zimmerman, K. Koehler, A.W. Phillips, J. Yi, E.J. Adams, F. Bezanilla, Photoelectrochemical modulation of neuronal activity with free-standing coaxial silicon nanowires. *Nature Nanotechnology* 2018, *13* (3), 260–266.
32. Y. Jiang, J.L. Carvalho-de-Souza, R.C. Wong, Z. Luo, D. Isheim, X. Zuo, A.W. Nicholls, I.W. Jung, J. Yue, D.-J. Liu, Heterogeneous silicon mesostructures for lipid-supported bioelectric interfaces. *Nature Materials* 2016, *15* (9), 1023–1030.
33. T. Yokota, T. Nakamura, H. Kato, M. Mochizuki, M. Tada, M. Uchida, S. Lee, M. Koizumi, W. Yukita, A. Takimoto, A conformable imager for biometric authentication and vital sign measurement. *Nature Electronics* 2020, *3* (2), 113–121.
34. J. Park, J. Kim, S.-Y. Kim, W.H. Cheong, J. Jang, Y.-G. Park, K. Na, Y.-T. Kim, J.H. Heo, C.Y. Lee, Soft, smart contact lenses with integrations of wireless circuits, glucose sensors, and displays. *Science Advances* 2018, *4* (1), 9841–9852.
35. Z. Ma, D. Kong, L. Pan, Z. Bao, Skin-inspired electronics: Emerging semiconductor devices and systems. *Journal of Semiconductors* 2020, *41* (4), 041601.
36. S. Wang, J. Xu, W. Wang, G.-J. N. Wang, R. Rastak, F. Molina-Lopez, J.W. Chung, S. Niu, V.R. Feig, J. Lopez, Skin electronics from scalable fabrication of an intrinsically stretchable transistor array. *Nature* 2018, *555* (7694), 83–88.
37. A.M. Pappa, D. Ohayon, A. Giovannitti, I.P. Maria, A. Savva, I. Uguz, J. Rivnay, I. McCulloch, R.M. Owens, S. Inal, Direct metabolite detection with an n-type accumulation mode organic electrochemical transistor. *Science Advances* 2018, *4* (6), eaat0911.

38. M.Y. Mulla, E. Tuccori, M. Magliulo, G. Lattanzi, G. Palazzo, K. Persaud, L. Torsi, Capacitance-modulated transistor detects odorant binding protein chiral interactions. *Nature Communications* 2015, 6 (1), 1–9.
39. Y.-G. Park, H. Min, H. Kim, A. Zhexembekova, C.Y. Lee, J.-U. Park, Three-dimensional, high-resolution printing of carbon nanotube/liquid metal composites with mechanical and electrical reinforcement. *Nano Letters* 2019, 19 (8), 4866–4872.
40. C. Tortiglione, M.R. Antognazza, A. Tino, C. Bossio, V. Marchesano, A. Bauduin, M. Zangoli, S.V. Morata, G. Lanzani, Semiconducting polymers are light nanotransducers in eyeless animals. *Science Advances* 2017, 3 (1), e1601699.
41. O.S. Abdullaeva, F. Balzer, M. Schulz, J. Parisi, A. Lützen, K. Dedek, M. Schiek, Organic photovoltaic sensors for photocapacitive stimulation of voltage-gated ion channels in neuroblastoma cells. *Advanced Functional Materials* 2019, 29 (21), 1805177.
42. A. Fendyur, N. Mazurski, J. Shappir, M.E. Spira, Formation of essential ultrastructural interface between cultured hippocampal cells and gold mushroom-shaped MEA-toward "IN-CELL" recordings from vertebrate neurons. *Frontiers in Neuroengineering* 2011, 4, 14.
43. N.T. Phan, X. Li, A.G. Ewing, Measuring synaptic vesicles using cellular electrochemistry and nanoscale molecular imaging. *Nature Reviews Chemistry* 2017, 1 (6), 1–18.
44. K. Feron, R. Lim, C. Sherwood, A. Keynes, A. Brichta, P.C. Dastoor, Organic bioelectronics: Materials and biocompatibility. *International Journal of Molecular Sciences* 2018, 19 (8), 2382.
45. C. Yang, Z. Suo, Hydrogel ionotronics. *Nature Reviews Materials* 2018, 3 (6), 125–142.
46. B. Lu, H. Yuk, S. Lin, N. Jian, K. Qu, J. Xu, X. Zhao, Pure PEDOT: PSS hydrogels. *Nature Communications* 2019, 10 (1), 1–10.
47. C. Cea, G. Spyropoulos, P. Jastrzebska-Perfect, J.J. Ferrero, J.N. Gelinas, D. Khodagholy, Enhancement-mode ion-based transistor as a comprehensive interface and real-time processing unit for in vivo electrophysiology. *Nature Materials* 2020, 19, 679–678.

2

Materials and Their Classifications in Bioelectronics

Lorena Duarte-Peña

Departamento de Química de Radiaciones y Radioquímica, Instituto de Ciencias Nucleares, Universidad Nacional Autónoma de México, Circuito Exterior, Ciudad Universitaria, Mexico City, México

Julián E. Sánchez-Velandia

Grupo Fitoquímica Universidad Javeriana, Pontificia Universidad Javeriana, Bogotá, Colombia

Grupo de Investigación Catálisis Ambiental, Facultad de Ingeniería, Universidad de Antioquia, Medellín, Colombia

Felipe López-Saucedo and Emilio Bucio

Departamento de Química de Radiaciones y Radioquímica, Instituto de Ciencias Nucleares, Universidad Nacional Autónoma de México, Circuito Exterior, Ciudad Universitaria, Mexico City, México

CONTENTS

2.1 Introduction

Humanity since its inception has used the materials around it to create tools to supply its needs, promoting the development and creation of increasingly specialized and durable

DOI: 10.1201/9781003263265-2

devices, which makes materials science an area essential for the development of society. The interest to understand how biological systems work has grown with the advancement of medicine and biology, seeking to monitor them, model them, and create tools that allow the sustainability and reparation of live tissues. The first functional equipment that successfully measured electrical signals produced by the body was the electrocardiogram in 1912 [1]; later appeared pacemaker, the first invasive device of this type, and transistors. Currently, the use of electronic devices to solve medical problems is extensive and continues to advance, such as systems for neural stimulation, vestibular implants, biosensors, and retinal prostheses.

In search of a reduction in the existing gap between synthetic systems (abiotic) and biological systems (biotic), bioelectronics was born, a multidisciplinary area that bonds electronics and biology, two highly developed sciences, and also requires the participation of different branches such as physics, chemistry, and materials science. Bioelectronics seeks to understand and know the biotic/abiotic interface to obtain information and achieve selective control of biological processes. The biotic/abiotic interface includes all the interactions between electronics and biological systems, whether to translate information, stimulate or control [2]. Within the study areas of bioelectronics, the development of translators that allow communication between living systems and electronic processing systems is of great interest since this type of device would allow the specific and controlled monitoring and regulation of the physiology and the functional processes in tissues, organs, and cells. A bioelectronics material must have electrical characteristics and also be non-toxic, biocompatible, and have comfortable mechanical properties for the application, for example, devices used on the skin should be flexible and breathable, implantable devices should adapt to the implant area and be bioabsorbable, and the wound treatment devices should inhibit bacterial growth [3].

Bioelectronics materials may be classified according to their composition or the application for which they were designed (Figure 2.1). In the first case, bioelectronics materials might be mainly inorganic and organic. Inorganic bioelectronics materials have been the most researched because inorganic materials are the main component of many electrical devices. The most common inorganic material for electronic and bioelectronics is silicon, a biocompatible semiconductor that shows high charge mobility and versatility in macro- and microfabrication methods [4]. Currently, inorganic bioelectronics focuses on the development of flexible inorganic materials, which allow the manufacturing of more comfortable and biocompatible devices, regarding this, transfer printing has been studied

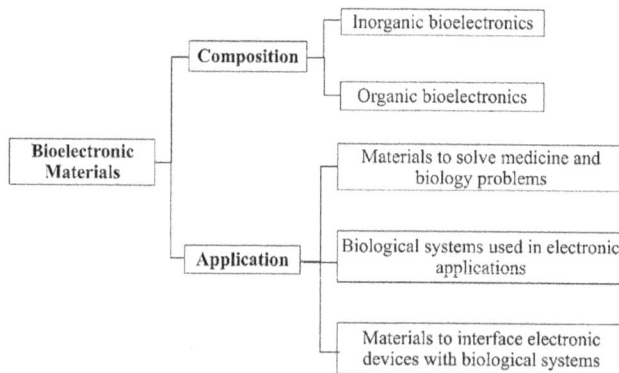

FIGURE 2.1
Classification scheme of bioelectronics materials according to their composition and their application.

to convert brittle inorganic materials into flexible systems, maintaining their electronic mobility and stability. In inorganic systems, flexibility may achieve by reducing the thickness and elasticity through the design of undulating structures; moreover, flexible inorganic systems are usually supported or encapsulated in polymeric materials [5]. On the other hand, organic bioelectronics materials are those based on carbon, generally conductive polymers or allotropes of carbon such as graphene or carbon nanotubes, these materials tend to have higher biocompatibility due to their mechanical properties are compatible with biological tissues; besides, they have greater versatility of manufacturing than inorganic materials.

In the classification according to the application, bioelectronics materials may be grouped into three areas; the electronic materials to solve medicine and biology problems, which include the detection and characterization of biological materials at the cellular and sub-cellular level, some examples are materials for electroactive scaffolds, photostimulation, or drug delivery; biological systems used in electronics application, i.e., new electronic components from biological systems; and materials to interface electronic devices with living systems, such as neural interface electrodes, optical implants, and biosensors for monitoring physiological functions, through the measurement of electrophysiological signals, biophysical signals (temperature, pressure) and signals biochemical (through body fluids) [6].

2.2 Classification of Bioelectronics Materials According to Their Composition

According to their composition, bioelectronics materials can be classified into organic or inorganic. Organic bioelectronics materials for technological applications are common because of their high biocompatibility. For example, semiconductors and conductors in electronics and microelectronics interact with biological tissues and usually require some flexibility and moldability, as well as strength and long cycle life. Therefore, a polymer matrix is the best option in delicate biological systems. On the other hand, inorganic semiconductors and conductors provide unique mechanical and conduction properties as supercapacitors used in bioelectronics tissues. Both inorganic and organic materials must have biocompatibility as well as functionality for their implementation in bioelectronics applications and subsequently in living tissue. This section shows the characteristics and the progress in the bioelectronics application of each material.

2.2.1 Inorganic Bioelectronics Materials

Among the existing materials, such based on inorganics represent an emerging and relevant area of research for application in bioelectronics. They can be configured to harmlessly dissolve, resorb or just degrade at nanometric/molecular scale, as temporary biomedical implants or environmental sensors. These kinds of materials have been proposed to manufacture deformable and flexible devices, with conductivity, semi-conductivity, or at least with transduction and energy storage [5]. Inorganic bioelectronics materials preparation is based on micro-fabrication (film deposition, lithography), and their successful application depends basically on the type of transfer of the inorganic function from the substrate to the desired target and a stable communication pathway between the nervous system and electronic devices [7].

Inorganic materials based on silicon, germanium, zinc oxide, and dielectrics present features as bioresorbable electronics, semiconductivity, and also can be dissolved in water. These parameters are considered as an important advantage in the context of the applications of biocompatibility and electronic because many biological processes involve ionic fluxes in an aqueous environment and the transduction or transformation of ionic signals into electronic ones [8]. An inorganic biomaterial can present different temporal linkers as an electronic device, and their dependence and response in the tissue will define their biocompatibility. In the same way, there are other important inorganic bio-materials related with the coordination polymers together with nanostructured materials, which have emerged as a solution for the current challenges in the preparation and ap-plication of structures that show fine crystals without impurities, high specific surface area, hierarchical pores, and thermic stability.

On the other hand, several metal oxides have been reported in the literature as pro-missory materials for bioelectronics applications. Among a lot of these oxides, zinc oxide (ZnO) has attracted considerable attention due to its exceptional properties such as low cost, high abundance, and wide bandgap [9]. The typical structure of ZnO consists of two forms: wurtzite and zincblende; however, wurtzite seems to be the most stable under ambient conditions. Besides, its polar ions (Zn^{2+} and O^{2}) make this solid interesting for photocatalytic applications and besides as excellent material in piezo electronics. In the same way, ZnO nanoparticles have been recently used for bioelectronics applications because they can be used as the active sites in several biological events defining the sensitivity and stability of the device where they will be applied. Different shapes of this oxide (from nanorods, nanotubes, nanosheets, nanodiscs, nanowalls, nanoflakes) present advantages with respect to the number of active sites providing fast electronic transfer and also creating an extra surface area with enhancing in its mechanical and electronic properties [10]. Similarly, indium-gallium-zinc oxide (IGZO) has been fabricated as Schottky diodes on a thiol-ene/acrylate shape memory polymer (SMP) that can endure mechanical strain with minimal to no loss in electrical performance [11]. In particular, IGZO has gained much attention due to its high mobility, low-temperature process compatibility, and insensitivity to visible light. In general, inorganic materials containing inert and semiconductors amorphous oxides have been a point of especial interest for bioelectronics. Among the properties of this kind of material are synthetic routes of low-cost, low-temperature, bias-stress stability, and processability.

Among the existing technologies, nanomaterials have been converted into an important topic for researchers of different areas. Fundamental differences are related to the size of nanometer-scale objects and their functions. In general, there are two ways to synthesize materials in the nano-scale: Bottom-up and top-down; the selection of one method over the other depends on the final requirements of the material and will define the synthetic strategy. Many nanomaterials have been reported to be active for implants, electronic devices, and sensors with exceptional mechanical, thermal, and optical properties. Several nanomaterials can fill the required properties to be used as bioelectronics, among them, inorganic nanoparticles that present large surface area, are inert, and have high me-chanical resistance.

2.2.2 Organic Bioelectronics Materials

Bioelectronics materials based on organic components represent the next step in the development of a high-efficiency biotic/biotic interface since they allow overcoming limitations associated with flexibility, softness, and malleability, features required to adjust electronic devices to biological systems, increasing their compatibility and effectiveness [12]. Besides, organic materials can be chemically modified and their manufacturing processes adapted to obtain the physical characteristics according to the application, therefore the organic bioelectronics material can have different displays as coatings, films, hydrogels, nanoparticles, etc. Another of their main advantages is that organic bioelectronics materials can be in direct contact with biological environments without suffering degradation or oxidation, which keeps the interface free of contaminants and extends the useful life of the devices [2]. Furthermore, unlike other systems in these, the transfer of charges not only occurs on the surface but also involves a three-dimensional character, which is given by the interaction of the charges with the polymeric network that can also swell facilitating the electronic transport. These characteristics make them tempting materials for the fabrication of biosensors and bioactuators.

Organic bioelectronics materials need the ability to transport charges, whereby molecules or polymers with high conjugation are generally used, which allow the mobility of charges through their electronic cloud formed by delocalized π electrons. Furthermore, these structures may increase their conductivity by mixing with agents that oxidized or reduced the conjugate bonds or doping them with p- or n-type conductors. Based on the density of transported charge and the material morphology, electronic organic materials can classify as semiconductors or conductors [13]. Polymers are particularly outstanding since allowing migration not only of electronics but also of ions due to their porosity and high flexibility, in addition, polymers might have charged groups in their structure, the so-called polyelectrolytes, which allows them to act as a transport channel of ions and compensate counterions that migrate under the action of an electric field. Polyelectrolytes can be polyanions or polycations being selective in terms of the charge of the transported ion; these characteristics make them useful in the manufacture of electrochemical membrane devices, electrochemical cells, organic electronic ion pumps, and ion bipolar transistors [14].

The mixed conducting polymers stand out within the organic bioelectronics materials because of can transport both electrons and ions. The former are transported by displacements in the delocalized electrons cloud, and the latter by diffusion between the polymer chains, which is improved by the swelling of the material. To exploit the full potential of this type of material, a strong ionic-electronic coupling so that the currents mutually induce each other is necessary; this behavior might be achieved by a redox process of electrochemical doping, where the mobile electronic charges are stabilized by the ions; organic bioelectronics materials are regularly used for the manufacture of organic electrochemical transistors that can translate amplified neuronal signals [15]. One of the common forms of polymers in bioelectronics devices is the hydrogels, which are three-dimensional networks of hydrophilic polymers that can swell in water and hold a large amount of water while maintaining the structure due to chemical or physical cross-linking of polymeric chains. This affinity with the aqueous systems and their excellent mechanical properties (such as rigidity, torsional vibration, and hardness) together with their conductivity properties make conductive hydrogels an excellent alternative for implantable bioelectronics and tissue engineering [16].

In contrast to inorganic bioelectronics materials, organic bioelectronics polymers have a lower overshoot that allows safe electrical stimulation of tissues. In addition, when these polymers are used together with electrical responsive materials can work as drug carriers or influence cell functions [17]. Nowadays, the most researched polymers in bioelectronics are poly(3,4-ethylene dioxythiophene): poly(styrene sulfonate) (PEDOT: PSS), polypyrroles (PPy), and polyanilines (PANI). Figure 2.2 show the molecular structures of these polymers. PEDOT: PSS is a mixed conducting copolymer where PEDOT is responsible for electronic

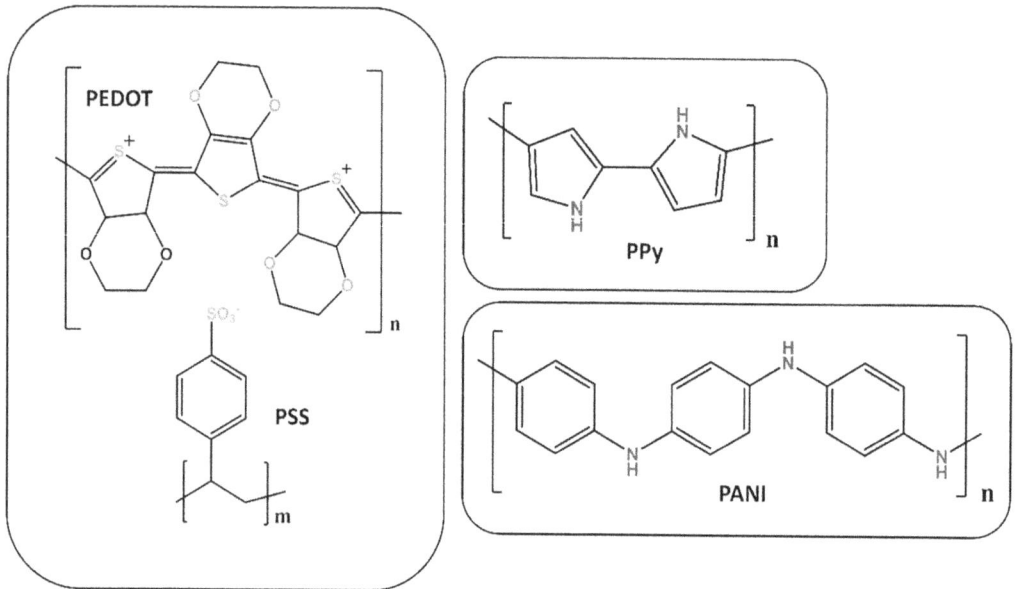

FIGURE 2.2
Molecular structures of the most used conductive polymers, PEDOT: PSS, PPy, and PANI.

conductivity and PSS for cation conductivity. This material has limitations due to its low mechanical stability, so it is used together with additives such as acrylamide and poly(vinyl alcohol), or in combination with higher mechanical resistant polymers, for example, Cuttaz et al. synthesized a composite material of PEDOT: PSS and polyurethane (PU), for the manufacture of flexible electrodes using laser micromachining, finding that dispersions of 10% to 15 % of PEDOT: PSS in PU achieve a balance between electrical and mechanical properties, helping to increase the neuronal cells survival compared to pristine PU [18]. PPys become conductors when oxidized due to the delocalized electrons cloud throughout the polymeric network; these materials also present biocompatibility, thermal stability, and ease of synthesis, characteristics that allowed the manufacture of actuators based on PPy films doped with BF_4^-, which have potential application in the manufacture of artificial muscles [19]. Finally, PANI is a low-cost conductive polymer due to its accessible synthesis, which retains the characteristics of biocompatibility and chemical stability. The PANI properties may be enhanced by combining it with secondary materials; for example, Cui et al. developed a chitosan-PANI patch that tries to modulate the electrophysiology of cardiac tissue and shows little inflammatory response in *in-vivo* assays [20].

Recent research works have sought the formulation of structures with multiple functions, which shows other characteristics in addition to charge transport, such as optically active, catalytic properties, or are self-repairing. So, Uzuncar et al. presented a PANI: PSS copolymer that was used for the fabrication of NH_4^+ sensors and urea biosensors by coupling with the enzyme urease, which showed high sensitivity and selectivity in modeled urine samples [21].

2.2.2.1 Allotropes of Carbon

In addition to conductive polymers, allotropes of carbon, such as graphene and carbon nanotubes (CNTs), are a good alternative for the development of bioelectronics detection

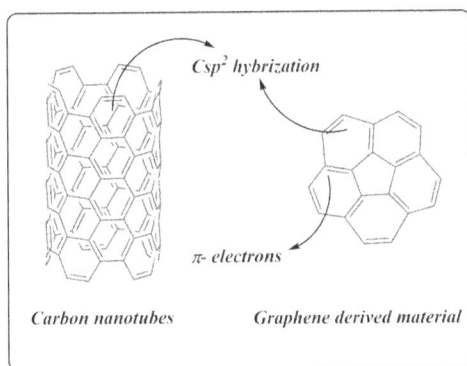

FIGURE 2.3
Carbon nanotubes and graphene-derived materials.

devices due to they are chemically stable, flexible, biocompatible, and have a high surface area and electrochemical versatility. Graphene (Figure 2.3) has become one of the most used 2D-nanomaterials in medicine, electronic engineering, and other fields. There are several graphene-derived materials such as graphitic carbon nitride (g-C_3N_4), boron nitride (BN), transition metal dichalcogenides (TMDs), transition metal oxides (TMOs), which are promissory to be applied as a new family of engineered nanomaterials for electronic devices [22]. Graphene presents a single or double layer of carbon, which is linked by different sp^2 hybridization and van der Waals interactions, its electric properties are given by the delocalized electrons, and its surface properties can be modified by the use of condensation or addition reactions, nucleophilic substitution among others. Graphene films may be used in combination with metallic microelectrodes, generating a synergistic effect that improves the electrochemical performance of the components; for example, Lee et al. developed patches for diabetes control based on a therapeutic feedback system that monitors glucose in sweat and uses a bilayer made up of a gold mesh and a gold-doped graphene film to transfer the electrical signal to stimulate the drug release, which showed the formation of a more efficient charge transfer interface than the individual layers [23].

CNTs are peculiar materials that are well ordered with a high aspect ratio and may be visualized as rolled-up structures of single or multiples sheets of graphene (Figure 2.3). Since their discovery, CNTs have been applied for applications in both biological and biomedical fields. In general, CNTs are one-dimensional (1D) tubular forms of sp^2 carbon networks, which also contain concentric graphitic shells and are typically 1–50 nm in diameter and micrometers in length [24]. Because of their π-delocalized electrons, electrical properties have been recognized in comparison with other reported materials. Although their low solubility in fluids has been a barrier for biomedical applications, the modification of CNTs' surface with hydrophilic organic/inorganic groups has made them facile to manipulate in physiological environments. Modification of CNTs' surface can be achieved by different pathways that include the typical impregnation (incipient/wetness physio-adsorption) and covalent attachment. CNTs also increase cell growth and adhesion, and they have been studied in transistors, self-repairing skins, and implantable microfibers due to their flexibility. Vitale et al. used CNT fiber electrodes for neuronal monitoring and stimulation, both in *in-vitro* and *in-vivo* tests; CNT electrodes showed a significant decrease in contact impedance with neurons in comparison with metallic electrodes; besides tests with Parkinsonian rodents, CNT electrodes showed the same stimulation efficiency as metal electrodes but with a lower inflammatory response [25].

The impregnation of active phases over the surface of carbon nanotubes or even over others such as graphene, polymers, and semiconductors is a well-known methodology that involves the use of organic/inorganic precursors containing the desired target (metals, amino acids, proteins, etc.). The dissolved precursors in water (or another solvent) are then added dropwise or in an excess of the solvent over the material. After constant stirring, the modified material is dried and then calcined to ensure the maximum anchoring or adsorption of the active phase or precursor on the surface. When an excess of solvent is used to further the active phase impregnation, coverage is usually deficient and dispersion is not good. When the volume is similar to the pore size (incipient impregnation), a monolayer of the active phase is dispersed over the surface, and final properties seem to change drastically. In both impregnation methodologies, incipient wetness and wetness, the interaction of the active phase with the surface is only by physical adsorption rather than chemical or covalent interaction. Thereby, other methodologies such as grafting or covalent anchoring are used to achieve a strong interaction between the desired target/active phase and the surface (generally given by the external groups as hydroxyls). On the other hand, grafting is crucial when a covalent interaction is required or desired. For the typical materials that require this strategy, a chemical bond is formed, and the energy to break them is larger than physisorption [26].

2.3 Classification of Bioelectronics Materials According to Their Application

Bioelectronics materials can also be classified according to their application. This classification is possibly one of the most logical for the end-user since associating groups or sets by application is natural for human beings. Classification of bioelectronics materials according to their application or interaction with a biological system is a specialized method to identify those materials with suitable thermal, electrical, and mechanical properties. Said materials for part of high-performance bioelectronics devices and disposables. For example, it has been found that conductive polymer coatings and silicon-based semiconductors conform to high-tech materials that can be accessed relatively easily for sophisticated electrical stimulation. In this section, the bioelectronics materials were classified according to their application as electronic materials to solve medicine and biology problems, materials for the use of biological systems in electronics, and materials to interface electronic devices with living systems.

2.3.1 Electronic Materials to Solve Medicine and Biology Problems

This section focuses on those materials that have been developed and approved by the FDA as inactive ingredients, such as poloxamer, polyvinylpyrrolidone, povidone, polylactide, polyethylene glycol, or polyvinyl alcohol, which have been proposed as alternatives to solve problems in medicine and biology and that are commonly found in medical devices, electroactive scaffolds, photosensitive materials, and in drug delivery systems.

Several physical factors such as toughness, mechanical properties, thermal resistance, or electrical stimuli-responsiveness are involved in the modulation of biometrics, so the next generation of bioelectronics devices is conceived from the versatility of manufactured materials. These devices include from electrocardiographs, cardiac pace-makers, defibrillators, blood pressure, and flow monitors to medical imaging systems. Some examples of new materials used in medicine are a polydimethylsiloxane microchip attached to a flexible printed board [27]; a 3D polydimethylsiloxane flexible matrix with a Ti layer deposited using radio-frequency-biased plasma [28]; a glass-based 96-well microelectrode array with microtiter plates supported on polymethylmethacrylate [29]; and a bioinorganic nanocomposite used for monitoring of cell redox-state formulated with DNA-MoS_2 and natural peptides [30]; all these devices seek the advance of the medicine and biology to understand, monitor, and control living systems.

2.3.1.1 Materials for Electroactive Scaffolding

Approaching the science of integral bioelectronics systems from a biomaterial scaffolds point of view is fundamental to reaching suitable tissue-electrode assemblages. A challenge of bioelectronics consists in the development of scaffolds able to mimic the native cell functions. Particularly for those types of cells that form part of sensible tissues, because in the case of damage they would be tuned or modulated by electrical stimulus; for example, in neural or muscular systems. Neurons, in this case, are sensitive to electrical stimulus, causing contraction and relaxation that, in case of damage, scaffolds are ideal to help in the restoration of tissue activity.

Tissue engineering is under continuous exploration in the matter of scaffolds; the foundation is to achieve a controlled electrical input for an action or response. The study of 3D scaffolds in cells is a more realistic point of view because the additional dimension provides results close to those observed in human organs. 3D scaffolds have the objective of being seeded with cell cultures to promote the growth of new cells and subsequently new healthy tissue. But as in anything related to bioelectronics, issues always arise, mainly those respecting differentiation, modulation of cell growth, and acceptance (hypoallergenic). Currently, most projects aim to develop 3D scaffolds in an attempt to emulate biological systems accurately. It is affordable to think that if the goal to achieve precise and well-structured scaffolds is complete, then another door of biotechnology would be unlocked [31]. For that reason, it is important to mention those promissory bioelectronics materials that comply with the basic requirements for 2D and 3D scaffolds such as a copolymer formed only by synthetic polymers, poly(ethylene glycol), and diacrylate-poly(acrylic acid) [32]; a copolymer using the absorbable poly-l-lactide modified with synthetic nanoparticles of polypyrrole [33]; a copolymer of biodegradable polycaprolactone modified with polyaniline [34]; a thermo responsiveness composite of the copolymer [poly(polyethylene glycol citrate-N-isopropylacrylamide)] modified with graphene oxide [35]; and a composite of exfoliated graphene and polyacrylamide [36].

2.3.1.2 Materials for Photostimulation

Organic and inorganic materials can induce photostimulation. This phenomenon may be exploited as an alternative for bioelectronics applications. New semiconductor and conductor materials are studied for their implementation in bioelectronics as components of pacemakers and other optoelectronic and mechanical therapies through optical stimulation. This promising method seizes the lights to the research about photons able to excite ion and molecular receptors to modulate, for example, cardiac cell disorders. Even if photostimulation is effective and noninvasive, the photostimulation yet faces some difficulties doing its clinic implementation is not completely viable, and it requires perfection to adapt the optical input to produce thermal or electrical responsiveness able to stimulate target cells selective and systematically.

Significant examples of materials that use electromagnetic radiation of UV and infrared to bioelectronics application are a light-responsive glass (regio-regular poly(3-hexylthiophene)) supported on indium tin oxide, abbreviated as ITO, which is a mixture of indium oxide (In_2O_3) and tin oxide (SnO_2), to manufacture of the mesoporous electrodes that work in aqueous solution [37]; a bio-syncretic phototransistor conformed of living HEK293 cells endowed with photosensitive ion channels supported on graphene to complete the phototransistor [38]; a composite with two types of semiconductors, polymer silicon nanowire (n-type) on the support of SU-8 (p-type), to optical stimulation of cardiac cells [39]; and a metal-organic "optrode" with a Pt black layer on a base of organic copolymer PEDOT/PSS to improve the neural monitoring [40]. Works presented are a sample of the future of bioelectronics materials.

2.3.1.3 Materials for Drug Administration

In drug administration, the vehicle takes a relevant role in oral medication such as pills, tablets, powders, as well as via epidermises such as gels and unguents. Even if the dosage is the most important factor, bioavailability depends on the success of treatments and a great percentage of bioavailability depends, subsequently, on vehicle or excipient. In fact, among different routes of administration, topical and oral medication bring the most diversity among new materials for excipients, such as microcapsules, hydrogels, temperature- and pH-responsive polymers, and even nanoporous surfaces. Materials for drug administration must reduce dosing frequency, improve therapeutic effects, and minimize side effects. For this reason, both traditional and new materials have been adopted by bioelectronics to create sophisticated devices worth mentioning are multipart systems, in the sense of a large number of components. Some representative examples of biocompatible materials for drug delivery are anti-inflammatory oral administration of antisense oligonucleotide using a microfluidics system Konjac glucomannan and gelatin methacryloyl [41]; a composite of microbeads with chitosan and magnetic nanoparticles loaded with antibiotic Vancomycin [42]; a glucose monitoring device for transdermal metformin (or chlorpropamide) delivery, the multi-component device comprises polydimethylsiloxane, and sensor contains poly(3,4-ethylene dioxythiophene), among other materials [43]; and programmable microspheres as a dexamethasone delivery system [44].

2.3.2 Biological Systems Used in Electronics Applications

Living systems have acquired the ability to synthesize materials with unique properties to selectively and efficiently carry out biological functions. This is the case of some derived from polyconjugates natural pigments and dyes, which show remarkable electronic properties and are essential for processes such as photosynthesis, charge transport, and control of free radicals. These materials are difficult to synthesize, so on some occasions, they are extracted from their natural environment to take advantage of them in the components manufacture of electronic devices. Furthermore, their structures may be employed as a model for the design of synthetic materials with mimetic properties to make electronic devices that can adapt to biological environments. Most of the essential electronic components, such as semiconductors and insulators, can be found in materials of natural origin [45].

Pigments, such as eumelanins, carotenoids, and indigo, are the better well-known natural semiconductors. Eumelanins are an ununiform group of conjugated macromolecules that

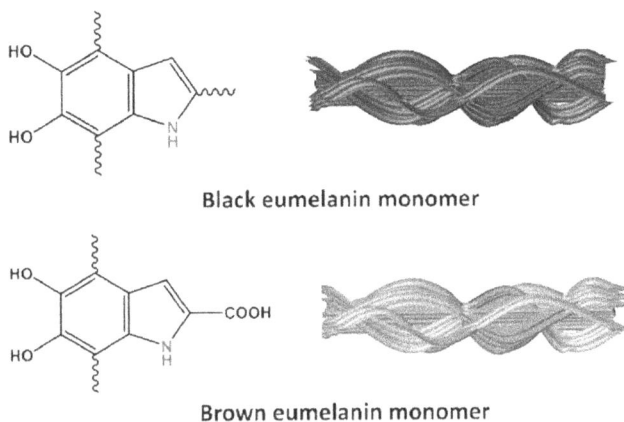

FIGURE 2.4
Structures of eumelanin monomers.

are obtained by the oxidative polymerization of 5,6-dihydroxyindoles and behave as amorphous semiconductors. Figure 2.4 shows the structure of eumelanins monomers. According to their structure at a biological level, these molecules have functionality as protective agents against UV radiation. Although their exact charge transport mechanism is unknown, some studies have shown that it occurs by cations mobility and depends on the system hydration. Thin films of eumelanins may be used for the fabrication of electronic devices such as photovoltaic devices, light-emitting diodes, organic electrochemical transistors, and sensing devices [46]. Wu and Hong developed a humidity sensor that uses dopamine-melanin thin films; the sensor showed response times around 0.45 s and a recovery time of 0.46 s, outperforming devices made of inorganic materials. Natural melanin is insoluble in practically all solvents, so they proposed a preparation method of dopamine-melanin oligomers by dopamine autoxidation induced polymerization, which at basic pH (>11) allowed the formation of water-soluble aggregates [47].

On the other hand, carotenoids are molecules of natural origin, low molecular weight, and high conjugation, which perform functions of antioxidant, pigmentation, and light capture in photosynthetic processes. Some carotenoids, such as β carotenes and bixin, have shown remarkable semiconductor properties. Although the use of carotenoids in bioelectronics is limited by their size, these may be employed as a template for the manufacture of efficient semiconductors [48]. Finally, indigo is a natural pigment found in some plants such as *Indigofera tinctoria* and snails of the *Hexaplex trunculus* family, but that is currently synthetically obtained. The electrical properties of indigo are given by its high aromaticity and have allowed its use in the design of bioelectronics devices [45,49].

In addition to semiconductors, there are also insulators of natural origin; for example, polypeptides and proteins that could be used for the formation of the dielectric film due to their monodisperse nature. Chang et al. used chicken egg albumin to make insulating films and networks, for thin-film transistors whose active phase was pentacene layers; these devices showed comparable electrical properties to the synthetic materials [50]. Deoxyribonucleic acid (DNA) can also be used for the fabrication of dielectric thin films, as the work of Yumusak et al. showed, who synthesized highly resistant thin films of DNA, from the cross-link of poly(phenyl isocyanate-co-formaldehyde) and DNA mix with a cationic surfactant [51].

2.3.3 Materials to Interface Electronic Devices with Living Systems

One of the main goals of bioelectronics is to achieve efficient communication between living systems and electronic devices. The biggest challenge of this objective is the development of interfaces that allow the union between different conduction modes since the most conventional electronic devices transport electric charge by electron mobility; while in living systems, charge transport takes place by ionic fluxes and it is strongly influenced by the water-rich biological medium. At a cellular level, communication occurs through the combination of mechanical, thermal, biological, chemical, and electrical signals; the electrical signals are given by peaks of flows of ions, mainly cations, which are released in response to differences in potential inside and outside the cell. When the ions are released, they alter the potential of the tissue, which induces communication. The integration between electrical devices and biological systems through capturing these signals allows the control of adhesion, proliferation, and apoptosis cellular. While at the tissue level, integration provides information on the biological functioning and allows the formation of regeneration structures, stimulation, drug release, and disease modeling. Specific applications of this technology include support for people with chronic brain diseases such as paralysis, artificial retinas, and new technologies to model, monitor, and influence cellular behavior [52].

In order to facilitate communication between the living and artificial systems, biotic/abiotic interfaces have been developed that serve as ionic/electronic couplers, which are usually composed of a hybrid circuit that facilitates interaction. In addition, current researches are searching for the development of artificial devices based on ion transport that allows greater affinity with nature. In both cases, the most common ion transport mechanisms in synthetic materials are the formation of an electrical double layer and electrochemical reactions. The former involves the redistribution of ions on the charged surface by electrostatic forces, which generates a local dipole field that allows the transport of ions and the detection and interpretation of biological signals (Figure 2.5); and the latter involves oxidation-reduction processes that allow the transfer of electrons. The organic electrical ion pumps (OEIPs) are an example of these ionic interfaces, which allow controlling the flow of ions in physiological processes. The OEIPs generally contain a film of a mixed conductive copolymer of PEDOT: PSS. In 2007, the first OEIP was published, which successfully allowed the transport of small cations. From this, the

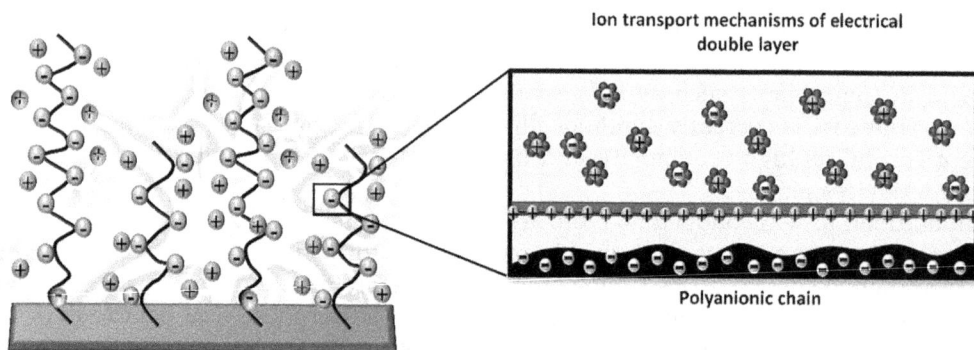

FIGURE 2.5
The schematization of the ion transport mechanism of the electrical double layer.

efficient transport of larger ions such as Na^+, K^+, Ca^{2+}, and charged neurotransmitters such as acetylcholine or with electrical dipoles such as aspartate and glutamate has been achieved. The efficiency of OIEPs has been tested both *in vitro* and *in vivo* [53].

Nervous system/electronic devices interfaces are of greatest interest in the electronic stimulation and translation systems since they would help in the diagnosis and treatment of many chronic conditions. Sensory input and processing of all body information, both external and internal, occur in the brain. Neurons are the basic processing units that communicate with electrical signals and the flow of ions and neurotransmitters. For example, Cea et al. developed an organic electrochemical transistor based on a reversible redox process in conjunction with an ion-conducting polymer, which allows the fabrication of long-term implants with high biocompatibility for the detection of epileptic discharges [54].

2.4 Conclusion

Bioelectronics is a developing science that has imposed challenges at the level of materials science, electronics, and biology, given the need to create tools that allow rapid, prolonged, and high-resolution interactions between biotic and abiotic systems, leading to the development of materials with mixed characteristics between electrical systems and living systems, such as ion transistors, biosensors, ion pumps, and neural implants. In this chapter, a detailed description of the different materials that may be used for the manufacture of bioelectronics devices and their classification according to composition and application, highlighting the new advances, the remains, and the perspectives of each one, was provided.

Acknowledgments

Lorena Duarte Peña (887494) acknowledges CONACyT for the doctoral scholarship. This work was supported by Dirección General de Asuntos del Personal Académico, Universidad nacional Autónoma de México (DGAPA-UNAM) [Grant IN202320] (Mexico).

References

1. C. Cajavilca, J. Varon, Willem Einthoven: The development of the human electrocardiogram, *Resuscitation*. 76 (2008) 325–328. 10.1016/j.resuscitation.2007.10.014.
2. J. Rivnay, R.M. Owens, G.G. Malliaras, The Rise of organic bioelectronics, *Chem. Mater.* 26 (2014) 679–685. 10.1021/cm4022003.
3. D.T. Simon, E.O. Gabrielsson, K. Tybrandt, M. Berggren, Organic bioelectronics: Bridging the signaling gap between biology and technology, *Chem. Rev.* 116 (2016) 13009–13041. 10.1021/acs.chemrev.6b00146.

4. Y. Fang, L. Meng, A. Prominski, E.N. Schaumann, M. Seebald, B. Tian, Recent advances in bioelectronics chemistry, *Chem. Soc. Rev.* 49 (2020) 7978–8035. 10.1039/d0cs00333f.
5. Y. Chen, Y. Zhang, Z. Liang, Y. Cao, Z. Han, X. Feng, Flexible inorganic bioelectronics, *Npj Flex. Electron.* 4 (2020) 1–20. 10.1038/s41528-020-0065-1.
6. K. Feron, R. Lim, C. Sherwood, A. Keynes, A. Brichta, P.C. Dastoor, Organic bioelectronics: Materials and biocompatibility, *Int. J. Mol. Sci.* 19 (2018) 1–21. 10.3390/ijms19082382.
7. A. Carlson, A.M. Bowen, Y. Huang, R.G. Nuzzo, J.A. Rogers, Transfer printing techniques for materials assembly and micro/nanodevice fabrication, *Adv. Mater.* 24 (2012) 5284–5318. 10.1002/adma.201201386.
8. S. Inal, J. Rivnay, A.O. Suiu, G.G. Malliaras, I. McCulloch, Conjugated polymers in bioelectronics, *Acc. Chem. Res.* 51 (2018) 1368–1376. 10.1021/acs.accounts.7b00624.
9. N.P. Shetti, S.D. Bukkitgar, K.R. Reddy, C.V. Reddy, T.M. Aminabhavi, ZnO-based nanostructured electrodes for electrochemical sensors and biosensors in biomedical applications, *Biosens. Bioelectron.* 141 (2019) 1–12. 10.1016/j.bios.2019.111417.
10. M.L.M. Napi, S.M. Sultan, R. Ismail, K.W. How, M.K. Ahmad, Electrochemical-based biosensors on different zinc oxide nanostructures: A review, *Materials (Basel).* 12 (2019) 1–34. 10.3390/ma12182985.
11. E. Guerrero, A. Polednik, M. Ecker, A. Joshi-Imre, W. Choi, G. Gutierrez-Heredia, W.E. Voit, J. Maeng, Indium–gallium–zinc oxide schottky diodes operating across the glass transition of stimuli-responsive polymers, *Adv. Electron. Mater.* 6 (2020) 1–8. 10.1002/aelm.201901210.
12. G. Malliaras, M.R. Abidian, Organic bioelectronic materials and devices, *Adv. Mater.* 27 (2015) 7492. 10.1002/adma.201504783.
13. J. Tropp, J. Rivnay, Design of biodegradable and biocompatible conjugated polymers for bioelectronics, *J. Mater. Chem. C.* 9 (2021) 13543–13556. 10.1039/d1tc03600a.
14. K. Svennersten, K.C. Larsson, M. Berggren, A. Richter-Dahlfors, Organic bioelectronics in nanomedicine, *Biochim. Biophys. Acta – Gen. Subj.* 1810 (2011) 276–285. 10.1016/j.bbagen.2010.10.001.
15. E. Macchia, L. Torsi, Organic biosensors and bioelectronics, in: P. Cosseddu, M. Caironi (Eds.), *Org. Flex. Electron.*, Woodhead Publishing, 2021: pp. 501–530. 10.1016/B978-0-12-818890-3.00017-5.
16. F. Fu, J. Wang, H. Zeng, J. Yu, Functional conductive hydrogels for bioelectronics, *ACS Mater. Lett.* 2 (2020) 1287–1301. 10.1021/acsmaterialslett.0c00309.
17. D. Ohayon, S. Inal, Organic bioelectronics: From functional materials to next-generation devices and power sources, *Adv. Mater.* 32 (2020) 2001439. 10.1002/adma.202001439.
18. E. Cuttaz, J. Goding, C. Vallejo-Giraldo, U. Aregueta-Robles, N. Lovell, D. Ghezzi, R.A. Green, Conductive elastomer composites for fully polymeric flexible bioelectronics, *Biomater. Sci.* 7 (2019) 1372–1385. 10.1039/C8BM01235K.
19. S. Hara, T. Zama, W. Takashima, K. Kaneto, Artificial muscles based on polypyrrole actuators with large strain and stress induced electrically, *Polym. J.* 36 (2004) 151–161. 10.1295/polymj.36.151.
20. C. Cui, N. Faraji, A. Lauto, L. Travaglini, J. Tonkin, D. Mahns, E. Humphrey, C. Terracciano, J.J. Gooding, J. Seidel, D. Mawad, A flexible polyaniline-based bioelectronic patch, *Biomater. Sci.* 6 (2018) 493–500. 10.1039/C7BM00880E.
21. S. Uzunçar, L. Meng, A.P.F. Turner, W.C. Mak, Processable and nanofibrous polyaniline:polystyrene-sulphonate (nano-PANI: PSS) for the fabrication of catalyst-free ammonium sensors and enzyme-coupled urea biosensors, *Biosens. Bioelectron.* 171 (2021) 112725. 10.1016/j.bios.2020.112725.
22. R. Antiochia, C. Tortolini, F. Tasca, L. Gorton, P. Bollella, Graphene and 2D-Like nanomaterials: Different biofunctionalization pathways for electrochemical biosensor development, in: A. Tiwari (Ed.), *Graphene Bioelectron.*, Elsevier Inc., 2018: pp. 1–35. 10.1016/B978-0-12-813349-1.00001-9.

23. H. Lee, T.K. Choi, Y.B. Lee, H.R. Cho, R. Ghaffari, L. Wang, H.J. Choi, T.D. Chung, N. Lu, T. Hyeon, S.H. Choi, D.-H. Kim, A graphene-based electrochemical device with thermo-responsive microneedles for diabetes monitoring and therapy, *Nat. Nanotechnol.* 11 (2016) 566–572. 10.1038/nnano.2016.38.

24. C.F. Sun, B. Meany, Y.H. WangCharacteristics and applications of carbon nanotubes with different numbers of walls, in: K., Tanaka, S., Iijima (Eds.), *Carbon Nanotub. Graphene, Second Edi*, Elsevier Ltd., 2014: pp. 313–339. 10.1016/B978-0-08-098232-8.00013-9.

25. F. Vitale, S.R. Summerson, B. Aazhang, C. Kemere, M. Pasquali, Neural stimulation and recording with bidirectional, soft carbon nanotube fiber microelectrodes, *ACS Nano.* 9 (2015) 4465–4474. 10.1021/acsnano.5b01060.

26. S.A. Khan, C.A. Vandervelden, S.L. Scott, B. Peters, Grafting metal complexes onto amorphous supports: From elementary steps to catalyst site populations: Via kernel regression, *React. Chem. Eng.* 5 (2020) 66–76. 10.1039/c9re00357f.

27. Y. Mermoud, M. Felder, J.D. Stucki, A.O. Stucki, O.T. Guenat, Microimpedance tomography system to monitor cell activity and membrane movements in a breathing lung-on-chip, *Sensors Actuators B Chem.* 255 (2018) 3647–3653. 10.1016/j.snb.2017.09.192.

28. H. Moon, B. Park, D. Hong, K.-S. Park, S. Lee, S. Kim, 3D-structured soft bioelectronic devices with crack-free metal patterns, *Sensors Actuators B Chem.* 343 (2021) 130123. 10.1016/j.snb.2021.130123.

29. S. Schmidt, R. Frank, D. Krinke, H.-G. Jahnke, A.A. Robitzki, Novel PMMA based 96-well microelectrode arrays for bioelectronic high throughput monitoring of cells in a live mode, *Biosens. Bioelectron.* 202 (2022) 114012. 10.1016/j.bios.2022.114012.

30. J. Yoon, M. Shin, D. Kim, J. Lim, H.-W. Kim, T. Kang, J.-W. Choi, Bionanohybrid composed of metalloprotein/DNA/MoS2/peptides to control the intracellular redox states of living cells and its applicability as a cell-based biomemory device, *Biosens. Bioelectron.* 196 (2022) 113725. 10.1016/j.bios.2021.113725.

31. Y. Guo, J. Huang, Y. Fang, H. Huang, J. Wu, 1D, 2D, and 3D scaffolds promoting angiogenesis for enhanced wound healing, *Chem. Eng. J.* (2022) 134690. 10.1016/j.cej.2022.134690.

32. K. Gupta, R. Patel, M. Dias, H. Ishaque, K. White, R. Olabisi, Development of an electroactive hydrogel as a scaffold for excitable tissues, *Int. J. Biomater.* 2021 (2021) 1–9. 10.1155/2021/6669504.

33. C. Ma, L. Jiang, Y. Wang, F. Gang, N. Xu, T. Li, Z. Liu, Y. Chi, X. Wang, L. Zhao, Q. Feng, X. Sun, 3D Printing of conductive tissue engineering scaffolds containing polypyrrole nanoparticles with different morphologies and concentrations, *Materials (Basel).* 12 (2019) 2491. 10.3390/ma12152491.

34. A. Wibowo, C. Vyas, G. Cooper, F. Qulub, R. Suratman, A.I. Mahyuddin, T. Dirgantara, P. Bartolo, 3D printing of polycaprolactone–polyaniline electroactive scaffolds for bone tissue engineering, *Materials (Basel).* 13 (2020) 512. 10.3390/ma13030512.

35. C. Zhao, Z. Zeng, N.T. Qazvini, X. Yu, R. Zhang, S. Yan, Y. Shu, Y. Zhu, C. Duan, E. Bishop, J. Lei, W. Zhang, C. Yang, K. Wu, Y. Wu, L. An, S. Huang, X. Ji, C. Gong, C. Yuan, L. Zhang, W. Liu, B. Huang, Y. Feng, B. Zhang, Z. Dai, Y. Shen, X. Wang, W. Luo, L. Oliveira, A. Athiviraham, M.J. Lee, J.M. Wolf, G.A. Ameer, R.R. Reid, T.-C. He, W. Huang, Thermoresponsive citrate-based graphene oxide scaffold enhances bone regeneration from BMP9-stimulated adipose-derived mesenchymal stem cells, *Biomater. Sci. Eng.* 4 (2018) 2943–2955. 10.1021/acsbiomaterials.8b00179.

36. C. Arndt, M. Hauck, I. Wacker, B. Zeller-Plumhoff, F. Rasch, M. Taale, A.S. Nia, X. Feng, R. Adelung, R.R. Schröder, F. Schütt, C. Selhuber-Unkel, Microengineered hollow graphene tube systems generate conductive hydrogels with extremely low filler concentration, *Nano Lett.* 21 (2021) 3690–3697. 10.1021/acs.nanolett.0c04375.

37. G. Tullii, A. Desii, C. Bossio, S. Bellani, M. Colombo, N. Martino, M.R. Antognazza, G. Lanzani, Bimodal functioning of a mesoporous, light sensitive polymer/electrolyte interface, *Org. Electron.* 46 (2017) 88–98. 10.1016/j.orgel.2017.04.007.

38. J. Yang, G. Li, W. Wang, J. Shi, M. Li, N. Xi, M. Zhang, L. Liu, A bio-syncretic phototransistor based on optogenetically engineered living cells, *Biosens. Bioelectron.* 178 (2021) 113050. 10.1016/j.bios.2021.113050.

39. R. Parameswaran, K. Koehler, M.Y. Rotenberg, M.J. Burke, J. Kim, K.-Y. Jeong, B. Hissa, M.D. Paul, K. Moreno, N. Sarma, T. Hayes, E. Sudzilovsky, H.-G. Park, B. Tian, Optical stimulation of cardiac cells with a polymer-supported silicon nanowire matrix, *Proc. Natl. Acad. Sci.* 116 (2019) 413–421. 10.1073/pnas.1816428115.

40. L.-C. Wang, M.-H. Wang, C.-F. Ge, B.-W. Ji, Z.-J. Guo, X.-L. Wang, B. Yang, C.-Y. Li, J.-Q. Liu, The use of a double-layer platinum black-conducting polymer coating for improvement of neural recording and mitigation of photoelectric artifact, *Biosens. Bioelectron.* 145 (2019) 111661. 10.1016/j.bios.2019.111661.

41. J. Gan, Y. Liu, L. Sun, W. Ma, G. Chen, C. Zhao, L. Wen, Y. Zhao, L. Sun, Orally administrated nucleotide-delivery particles from microfluidics for inflammatory bowel disease treatment, *Appl. Mater. Today.* 25 (2021) 101231. 10.1016/j.apmt.2021.101231.

42. A. Mohapatra, C. Wells, A. Jennings, M. Ghimire, S.R. Mishra, B.I. Morshed, Electric stimulus-responsive chitosan/MNP composite microbeads for a drug delivery system, *IEEE Trans. Biomed. Eng.* 67 (2020) 226–233. 10.1109/TBME.2019.2911579.

43. H. Lee, C. Song, Y.S. Hong, M.S. Kim, H.R. Cho, T. Kang, K. Shin, S.H. Choi, T. Hyeon, D.-H. Kim, Wearable/disposable sweat-based glucose monitoring device with multistage transdermal drug delivery module, *Sci. Adv.* 3 (2017) e1601314. 10.1126/sciadv.1601314.

44. M. Antensteiner, M. Khorrami, F. Fallahianbijan, A. Borhan, M.R. Abidian, Conducting polymer microcups for organic bioelectronics and drug delivery applications, *Adv. Mater.* 29 (2017) 1702576. 10.1002/adma.201702576.

45. M. Muskovich, C.J. Bettinger, Biomaterials-based electronics: Polymers and interfaces for biology and medicine, *Adv. Healthc. Mater.* 1 (2012) 248–266. 10.1002/adhm.201200071.

46. E. Vahidzadeh, A.P. Kalra, K. Shankar, Melanin-based electronics: From proton conductors to photovoltaics and beyond, *Biosens. Bioelectron.* 122 (2018) 127–139. 10.1016/j.bios.2018.09.026.

47. T.-F. Wu, J.-D. Hong, Synthesis of water-soluble dopamine–melanin for ultrasensitive and ultrafast humidity sensor, *Sensors Actuators B Chem.* 224 (2016) 178–184. 10.1016/j.snb.2015.10.015.

48. R.R. Burch, Y.-H. Dong, C. Fincher, M. Goldfinger, P.E. Rouviere, Electrical properties of polyunsaturated natural products: Field effect mobility of carotenoid polyenes, *Synth. Met.* 146 (2004) 43–46. 10.1016/j.synthmet.2004.06.014.

49. M. Irimia-Vladu, E.D. Głowacki, P.A. Troshin, G. Schwabegger, L. Leonat, D.K. Susarova, O. Krystal, M. Ullah, Y. Kanbur, M.A. Bodea, V.F. Razumov, H. Sitter, S. Bauer, N.S. Sariciftci, Indigo–A natural pigment for high performance ambipolar organic field effect transistors and circuits, *Adv. Mater.* 24 (2012) 375–380. 10.1002/adma.201102619.

50. J.-W. Chang, C.-G. Wang, C.-Y. Huang, T.-D. Tsai, T.-F. Guo, T.-C. Wen, Chicken albumen dielectrics in organic field-effect transistors, *Adv. Mater.* 23 (2011) 4077–4081. 10.1002/adma.201102124.

51. C. Yumusak, T.B. Singh, N.S. Sariciftci, J.G. Grote, Bio-organic field effect transistors based on crosslinked deoxyribonucleic acid (DNA) gate dielectric, *Appl. Phys. Lett.* 95 (2009) 1–3. 10.1063/1.3278592.

52. N. Yi, H. Cui, L.G. Zhang, H. Cheng, Integration of biological systems with electronic-mechanical assemblies, *Acta Biomater.* 95 (2019) 91–111. 10.1016/j.actbio.2019.04.032.

53. T. Yang, C. Xu, C. Liu, Y. Ye, Z. Sun, B. Wang, Z. Luo, Conductive polymer hydrogels crosslinked by electrostatic interaction with PEDOT:PSS dopant for bioelectronics application, *Chem. Eng. J.* 429 (2022) 1–10. 10.1016/j.cej.2021.132430.

54. C. Cea, G.D. Spyropoulos, P. Jastrzebska-Perfect, J.J. Ferrero, J.N. Gelinas, D. Khodagholy, Enhancement-mode ion-based transistor as a comprehensive interface and real-time processing unit for in vivo electrophysiology, *Nat. Mater.* 19 (2020) 679–686. 10.1038/s41563-020-0638-3.

3

2D Materials for Bioelectronics

Piyush Sharma and Shagun Kainth

Virginia Tech Center for Excellence in Emerging Materials, Thapar Institute of Engineering & Technology, Patiala, India

P.K. Diwan

Department of Applied Science, UIET, Kurukshetra University, Kurukshetra, India

CONTENTS

3.1 Introduction

The bioelectronic is a bridge between electronic and biological devices. Bioelectronics connects biological components such as proteins, antibodies, DNA, and cells with electronic

DOI: 10.1201/9781003263265-3

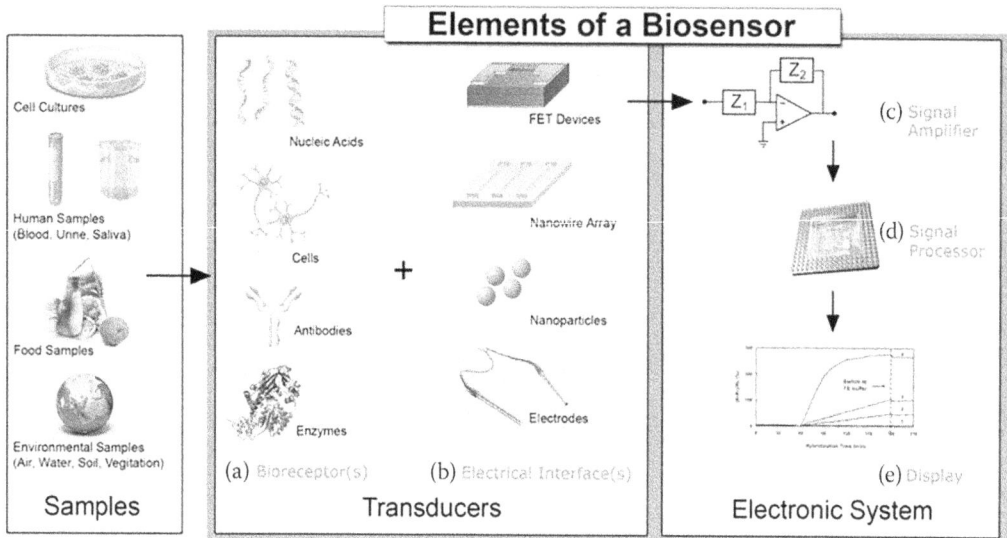

FIGURE 3.1

Various elements of bioelectronic devices. Adapted with permission from Ref. [5]. Copyright (2021) Copyright the Authors, some rights reserved; exclusive licensee [MDPI]. Distributed under a Creative Commons Attribution License 3.0 (CC BY) https://creativecommons.org/licenses/by/3.0/).

components including field-effect transistors (FETs), electrodes, electrode arrays, and optical resonators to create efficient biosensing devices [1]. These devices control and monitor biological processes and physiological responses through electrical/optical signals. Figure 3.1 shows the various elements of a bioelectronic device. Bioelectronics was first recognized by Galvani in the 1780s [2]. This experiment sparked a wave of new research into the role of electricity in biological processes. Later in 1843, the discovery of the action potential has open gateways for electrical stimulation into therapy through devices such as the cardiac pacemakers and implants [3]. In clinical practice, neuronal and cardiac stimulators relieved the pains of millions of patients suffering from cerebrovascular disease, epilepsy, Alzheimer's disease, Parkinson's disease, depression, and a variety of other neurological disorders [4].

Bioelectronic devices represent significant breakthroughs, yet there is still potential for development in terms of long-term stability. Current technology suffers from major incompatibilities at the interface between tissues and electronics in terms of chemical structure, Young's moduli, and electrical conductivity [6]. The stability of bioelectronic devices can be improved by minimizing mechanical mismatches between soft tissues and hard electronic devices. Moreover, the majority of electricity in the biological system is carried through ions rather than electrons. In water-rich conditions, the ions are highly conductive in comparison to electrons and holes. These dissimilarities restrict information flow between biology and electronics, limiting the extent and longevity of bioelectronic devices. Therefore, the scientific community has thought of hunting soft and ion-conducting materials to meet mechanical properties and boost electron-to-ion conversion at the biological contact [7].

In the current scenario, two-dimensional (2D) materials have pushed materials research to new heights. 2D materials have brought immense possibilities in composition, microstructures, and properties that make them a potential candidate for a wide range of applications [8]. Since the discovery of 2D graphene, the development of novel 2D materials has arisen as a fiercely contested topic in materials research. Material scientists

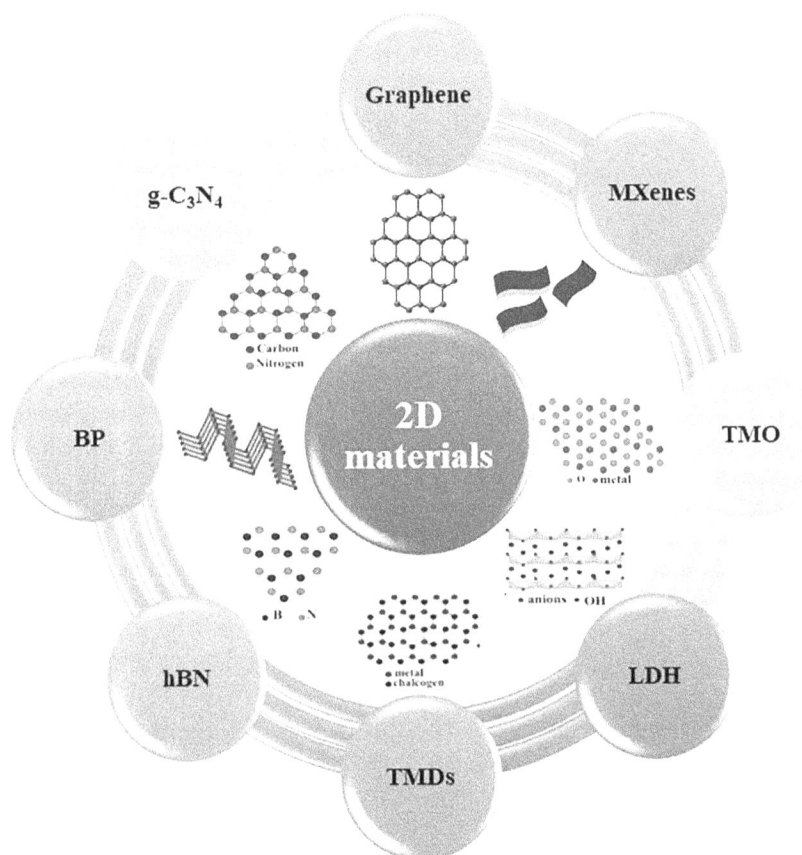

FIGURE 3.2
Types of two-dimensional (2D) materials.

made significant efforts that culminated in the discovery of various two-dimensional materials (Figure 3.2) including transition metal oxides (TMOs), layered double hydroxide (LDH), transition metal dichalcogenides (TMDs), hexagonal boron nitride (h-BN), black phosphorus (BP), g-C$_3$N$_4$, graphene, and MXenes [9]. Recently discovered 2D materials also demonstrated unique electronic and other physicochemical features, including high surface area, flexibility, excellent biocompatibility, durable interfacial connection with cells, proteins, biomolecules, and other bio-organisms. These materials have been employed for numerous applications, including biomedical science. Hence, unique features of 2D materials have immense potential for the development of bioelectronic devices. Herein, a detailed description related to key material's properties essential for bioelectronics, fabrication of 2D materials, and sensing mechanism are addressed. The chapter ended with emerging challenges and prospects of 2D materials for bioelectronics.

3.2 Key Properties of Materials for Bioelectronics

To design an efficient device, it is crucial to identify material properties required for targeted application. Current innovations in materials and design resulted in the development of biodegradable implantable medical devices. Materials for bioelectronic devices must be strong enough to withstand massive deformations while being flexible enough to be compatible with soft tissues. Such devices have made their way not just into biomedical research, but also into stretchy, flexible, and wearable electronics. To design an efficient bioelectronic device, the material's properties such as biocompatibility, shape conformance, electrical, optical, and mechanical properties must be considered.

3.2.1 Biocompatibility

Biocompatibility and safety are the fundamental concern to utilizing 2D materials–based bioelectronic devices for in-vivo biomedical applications. Even for in-vitro applications, the biocompatibility of the materials is also reviewed to find the extent of tolerance of various cell lines such as HeLa, 4T1, A549, 293T, MCF7, PC3. Typical examinations used to estimate the cell viability are the methyl thiazolyl tetrazolium, water-soluble tetrazolium, Alamar Blue, calcein acetoxymethyl/propidium iodide, and dihydroethidine. The toxic effect of materials on hemo-, histo-, and neuro systems must be examined before using them in biomedicine. In certain instances, in-vivo toxicity experiments were performed on rats or mice to understand material's toxicity in hemo-, histo-, and neuro systems. The compositional biocompatibility of bare transition metal dichalcogenides (TMDs) nanosheets (MoS_2, WS_2, and WSe_2) was evaluated by employing MTT and WST-8 tests on the A549 cell line [10]. The results demonstrated that WSe_2 was highly toxic (0.2 mg/mL) as compared to the other two even at a higher concentration (0.4 mg/mL). This designated that the biocompatibility of a 2D material also depends on its chemical composition.

The tunning chemical composition provides a possible gateway to modify the surface of 2D materials and improves their biocompatibility. Better biocompatibility was observed when the surface of molybdenum disulfide was modified through exfoliation in bovine serum albumin (BSA) (Figure 3.3) [11]. A schematic binding (Figure 3.3a) of BSA on the molybdenum disulfide layer was observed with benzene rings and disulfides. BSA and other polymeric compounds affect the biocompatibility, adsorption, and capacitance of MoS_2. BSA-modified MoS_2 showed higher biocompatibility (Figure 3.3b) in comparison to bulk and polymers adsorbed MoS_2. In addition, 2,4-D bounding with BSA-modified MoS_2 (Figure 3.3c) was better than bulk and other polymers modified MoS_2. The MoS_2 BSA nanosheets (Figure 3.3d) demonstrated higher specific capacitance. A similar approach has been extensively employed using smaller molecules and polymers including polyethylene glycol (PEG), BSA, poly(vinyl pyrrolidone) (PVP), glutathione, soybean phospholipid, and polyacrylic acid [11,12]. Surface treatment through these chemicals increases material stability under physiological conditions and improves biocompatibility at the expense of toxicity. Furthermore, coatings are used to improve the biocompatibility of TMDs. A mesoporous Si coating on PEG-modified $WS_2@Fe_3O_4$ demonstrated superior biocompatibility through 4T1, HeLa, and 293T cells up to 0.2 mg/mL dosage [13]. In addition, coated TMDs showed no noticeable damage or abnormalities in the organ. Recently discovered 2D Ti_3C_2 MXene nanosheets have also shown higher biocompatibility when encapsulated with soybean phospholipid [14]. The encapsulated MXene nanosheets have no noticeable toxic impact on 4T1 cells even at a higher dosage of 0.4 mg/mL.

The biocompatibility of black phosphorus (BP) quantum dots can be improved by modifying the synthesis protocol. Better biocompatibility and stability were observed when BP was synthesized through the liquid-phase exfoliation method and encapsulated with poly(lactic-co-glycolic acid) (PLGA) nanospheres [15]. BP encapsulated agarose hydrogel was tested for breast cancer therapy [16]. The results revealed that encapsulated

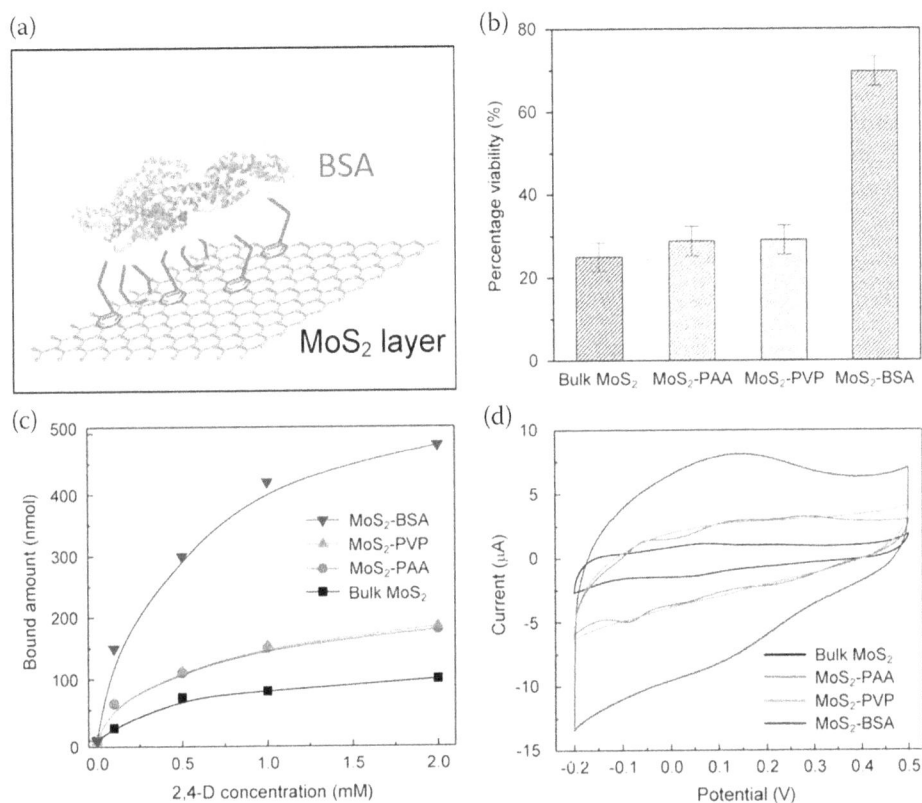

FIGURE 3.3
(a) Schematic representation of BSA-MoS$_2$ layer. (b) Comparison of biocompatibility in terms of the viability of bulk as well as modified MoS$_2$. (c) Bound amount of 2,4-D with bulk as well as modified MoS$_2$. (d) Cyclic voltammetry curves of bulk MoS$_2$ and various polymer-adsorbed MoS$_2$ nanosheets. Adapted with permission [11]. Copyright (2015) American Chemical Society.

BP possesses minute cytotoxicity in-vitro and no toxicity in-vivo. These hydrogels could be degraded and eliminated with urine. Additionally, the complexity of in-vivo applications affects the performance of bioelectronics based on 2D materials. The chemical stability of biofluids under in-vivo configuration is different as compared to ambient conditions. Apart from chemical stability, biofouling is a critical parameter that influences device performance. Since the complex biological components deposited on the sensor surface blocks the passage of target molecules. However, very few reports are available related to the biofouling of bioelectronic devices. It is believed that the coating approach might avoid problems associated with biofouling. Except for graphene, the exact interaction processes of 2D materials have seldom been documented, making full evaluations of the relevant biological impacts challenging.

3.2.2 Shape Conformation

To achieve stable interfaces between biological and electronic components, conformal electronic systems must be considered. The use of flexible and elastic substrates for 2D materials permits successful interfacing at the cell or tissue level. Though it is thought-provoking to conformably wrap complete organs (particularly the heart) to achieve a reliable interface for spatiotemporal mapping and stimulating cardiac physiology without interrupting the actions of cardiac muscle. In 2014, devices based on 3D integumental membranes were developed for high-density multipurpose recording, precise measurements, and activation of organs like brain and heart [17]. 3D printing was used to create a 3D heart structure with multipurpose electronics (pH, temperature, and strain sensors) and optoelectronic components. These accomplishments in implantable devices have considerable promise for biological and clinical research.

3.2.3 Electrical and Optical Properties

To design a bioelectronic device, the electrical properties of material play a vital role. Among a variety of materials, graphene has demonstrated excellent electrical properties. Even at room temperature, the graphene carrier mobility was found to be ~10,000 cm^2/Vs [18]. Some 2D materials emerged as intrinsic semi-conductors with carrier mobilities ~200 cm^2/Vs and bandgap ~1.8 eV for monolayer MoS_2 [19]. These materials are highly suitable for the development of the digital transistor. The chemical diversity of 2D materials offers ease to tune properties for the desired application. This opened new research avenues to design bioelectronic devices based on tunable 2D materials. Conley and co-workers [20] released an indirect bandgap in multi-layered and direct bandgap in monolayer 2D MoS_2. The bandgap of 2D materials is strongly influenced by the number of layers (Figure 3.4) [21]. Black phosphorous (BP) is also a 2D semiconductor and its bandgap varies (0.2–2.1 eV) with the thickness [22]. Single-layer BP along the zig-zag direction demonstrated higher carrier mobility (10,000–26,000 cm^2/Vs) [23].

Additionally, some of the 2D materials act as semiconductors and insulators such as MoS_2. The flakes of MoS_2 with odd layers possess piezoelectricity while MoS_2 flakes with even layers demonstrated no piezoelectric response [24]. Such materials with tunable electrical properties are promising to develop next-generation smart bioelectronic devices. To develop wearable bioelectronic devices, the optical properties of materials must be considered. A material should exhibit high visible light absorption, zero bandgap, and high carrier mobility. 2D semiconducting and insulating materials have shown a higher absorption coefficient. The absorption coefficient of 2D materials varies with the number of layers (Figure 3.5) [25].

3.2.4 Mechanical Properties

Mechanical properties are one of the significant and basic aspects of novel material investigation, development, and design. Regarding bioelectronics, the mechanical properties of material play a vital role. The material required for bioelectronic devices not only sustain substantial deformation but is also flexible enough to be compatible with tissues. In this scenario, 2D materials emerged as suitable candidates for bioelectronic devices. These materials possess higher strength due to strong in-plane covalent/ionic connections and good flexibility owing to their atomic thickness. Among 2D materials, graphene possesses the highest value of Young's modulus and fracture strength [26]. Other 2D materials have poor mechanical properties but are strong enough to be used for the fabrication of bioelectronic devices [27]. The 2D materials exhibit higher Young's modulus and fracture strength in comparison to 3D materials. The fracture strength of mono-layered 2D MoS_2 (~23 GPa) is found to be higher than steel [28]. This enables MoS_2 to withstand ~10 times larger strain in comparison to steel. The single crystalline structure of 2D materials at micro or nanoscale is responsible for

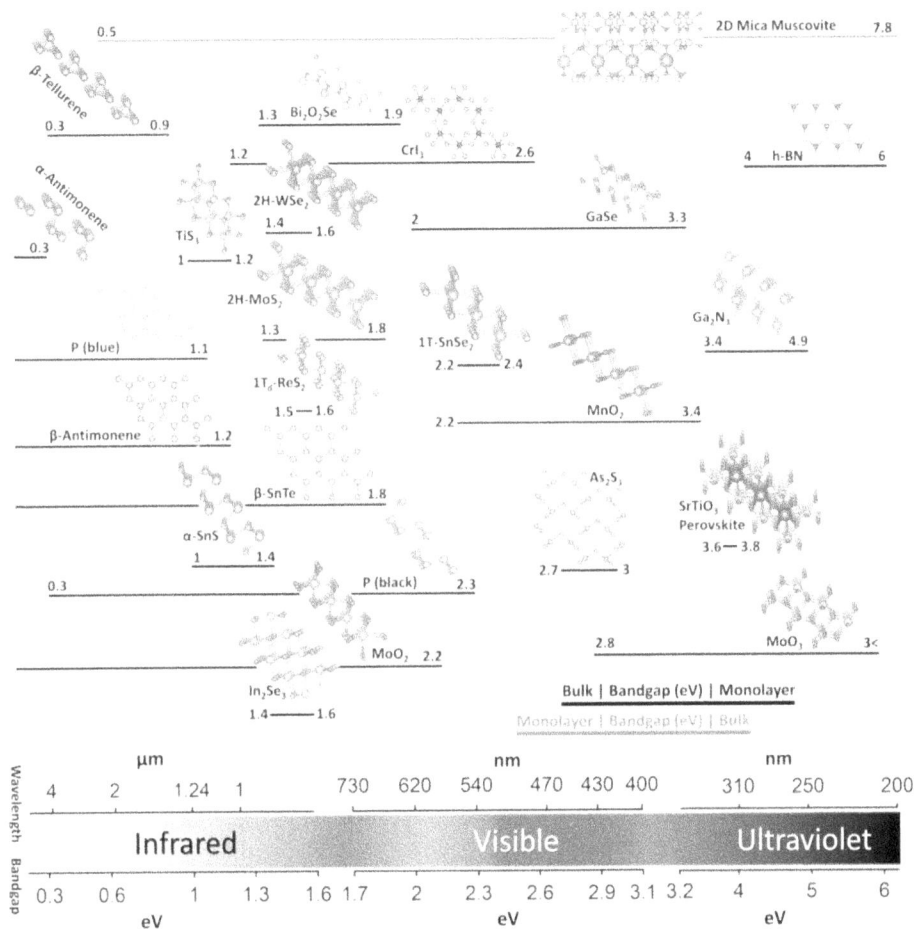

0.5 2D Mica Muscovite 7.8

β-Tellurene

0.3 0.9

1.3 Bi₂O₂Se 1.9

1.2 CrI₃ 2.6 4 h-BN 6

α-Antimonene

2H-WSe₂ GaSe 3.3

TiS₂ 1.4 ——— 1.6 2

0.3 1 ——— 1.2

2H-MoS₂

P (blue) 1.1 1.3 1.8 1T-SnSe₂ Ga₂N₃

1T₄-ReS₂ 2.2 ——— 2.4 3.4 4.9

β-Antimonene 1.2 1.5 — 1.6 MnO₂ 3.4

2.2 ———

β-SnTe 1.8 As₂S₃

α-SnS SrTiO₃ Perovskite

1 1.4 3.6 — 3.8

0.3 P (black) 2.3 2.7 ——— 3

MoO₃ 2.2 2.8 MoO₃ 3<

In₂Se₃ Bulk | Bandgap (eV) | Monolayer

1.4 ——— 1.6 Monolayer | Bandgap (eV) | Bulk

Wavelength

μm nm nm

4 2 1.24 1 730 620 540 470 430 400 310 250 200

Infrared **Visible** **Ultraviolet**

Bandgap

0.3 0.6 1 1.3 1.6 1.7 2 2.3 2.6 2.9 3.1 3.2 4 5 6

eV eV eV

FIGURE 3.4
Bandgap of 2D materials. Adapted with permission [21]. Copyright (2014) the Authors, some rights reserved; exclusive licensee [Nature]. Distributed under a Creative Commons Attribution License 4.0 (CC BY) https:// creativecommons.org/licenses/by/4.0/).

their excellent mechanical properties. In spite of their higher Young's modulus, the energy required to expand, bend, and shear them is very low due to their thickness of one or fewer atoms [29]. Consequently, 2D materials possess higher strength as well as good flexibility at the same time. Such materials are highly compatible with the development of bioelectronics that could connect and follow movements of body tissues.

3.3 Synthesis of 2D Materials for Bioelectronics

The performance of 2D material for bioelectronics significantly depends on its synthesis protocol. Numerous synthesis protocols have been proposed to prepare a variety of 2D materials. In contrast, 2D materials are prepared by two most common synthesis protocols, i.e., top-down and bottom-up approaches. Herein, recent advances and drawbacks of synthesis approaches are addressed.

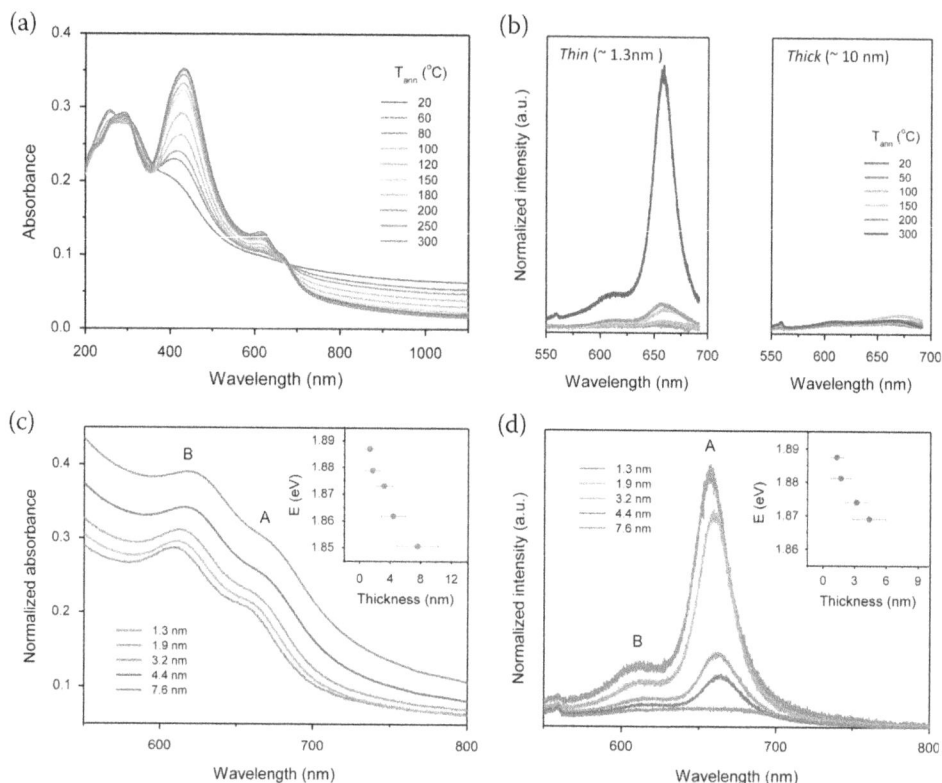

FIGURE 3.5

Absorption spectra of MoS$_2$ thin films having thicknesses varying from 1.3–7.6 nm. Inset shows the energy of excitation peak with respect to film thickness. Adapted with permission [25]. Copyright (2011) American Chemical Society.

3.3.1 Top-Down Synthesis Protocols

A mono or few-layered 2D material can be synthesized through top-down synthesis protocols. These protocols eliminate the van der Waals interactions in between the stacked layers of 2D materials. Several top-down synthesis protocols have been reported such as Scotch-tape, mechanical force-assisted liquid exfoliation, liquid exfoliation through ion intercalation and ion exchange, liquid exfoliation through oxidation/reduction, and liquid exfoliation through etching [30].

3.3.1.1 Scotch-Tape Protocol

Scotch-tape protocol is a conventional route to synthesize nanosheets of 2D materials. This method is also named as mechanical cleavage method. In this protocol, nanosheets are peeled off from the stacked layers of 2D materials by eliminating/weakening the van der Waals forces. The nanosheets are obtained in such a way that the in-plane covalent bonds remained unaffected. Scotch-tape protocol was coined by Geim and Novoselov [31] in 2004. They were the first to cleave a mono-layered graphene sheet from graphite. After this remarkable contribution, the scotch-tape protocol is used to prepare a wide range of 2D materials including h-BN, TMDs, antimonene, CuInP$_2$S$_6$, and BP from their bulk counterparts [32,33]. A schematic representation of graphene nanosheets synthesis

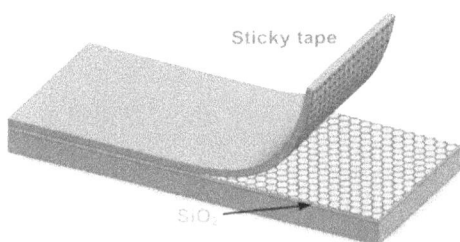

FIGURE 3.6
A schematic representation of nanosheets synthesis through Scotch-tape protocol. Adapted with permission [34]. Copyright (2012) Elsevier.

through the scotch-tape approach is shown in Figure 3.6 [34]. This protocol is chemical-free and nanosheets with clear surfaces and high crystal quality can be obtained. The drawback of this protocol is the low production rate and limited access to the production parameters due to manual processes.

3.3.1.2 Mechanical Force–Assisted Liquid Exfoliation

To obtain 2D nanomaterials, mechanical force–assisted liquid exfoliation methods emerge as an appropriate strategy to exfoliate stacked layers of material. In general, the mechanical force-assisted liquid exfoliation method is broadly classified on the behalf of sonication and shear force. The former method involves the sonication of a material dispersed in a solvent for exfoliation. The suspension obtained after sonication was further centrifuged to obtain 2D material. The sonication process induces mechanical forces in the liquid that eventually eliminate or weaken the van der Waals forces between the layers. This resulted in the formation of 2D materials without interrupting the covalent bonding of the layers. Furthermore, the exfoliation efficiency can be improved through the matching surface of layered material and solvent. Hernandez and coworkers [35] were the first to employ liquid exfoliation via sonication method without utilizing costly instruments and chemicals. Afterward, this method was modified and surfactant-assisted liquid exfoliation through sonication was introduced [36]. A graphical representation of sonication-assisted liquid exfoliation of graphite is presented in Figure 3.7. However, mechanical force–assisted liquid exfoliation suffers from certain drawbacks such as low production of mono-layered 2D materials, presence of defects on the sheets, and smaller lateral size of the exfoliated 2D material sheets.

To overcome these drawbacks, shear force–assisted liquid exfoliation has been introduced [37]. This approach allows the development of high shear rates in the liquid phase of bulk material. A simple shear force setup includes a mixing head and a rotor to produce 300 to 800 nm lateral size graphene and few-layered sheets of BPs. The choice of solvent, shear rate, and polymer additive further improve the exfoliation process. If the value of the shear rate is below 10^4 S^{-1} then the efficiency of exfoliation is low. As the shear rate increased above 10^4 S^{-1}, the efficiency of exfoliation improves significantly. Consequently, shear rate plays a vital role to obtain exfoliated 2D material nanosheets. The shear force–assisted exfoliation technique emerged as a promising protocol to produce 2D graphene at a large scale by utilizing rotating blade reactors.

3.3.1.3 Liquid Exfoliation Through Ion Intercalation and Ion Exchange

The ion intercalation protocol of liquid exfoliation is based on the idea of cation ion intercalation in the interlayer of bulk material. This enables weakening or eliminating van

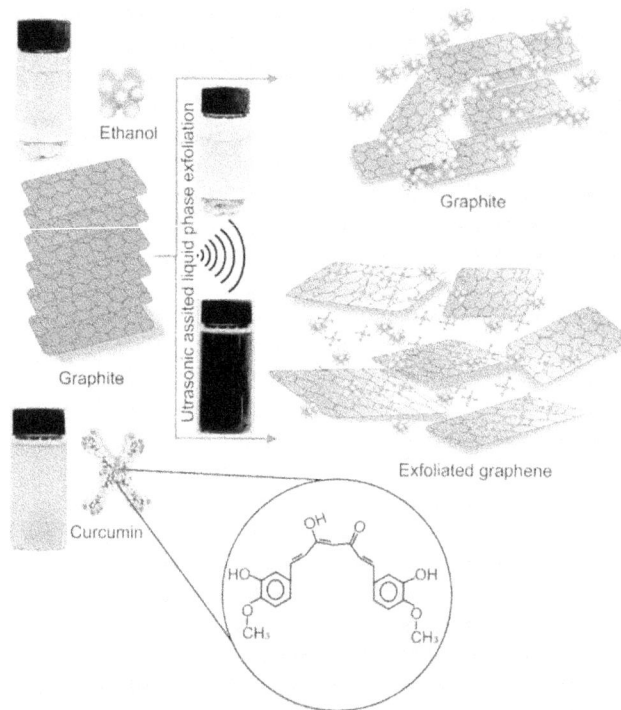

FIGURE 3.7
Liquid exfoliation of graphite via sonication to obtain graphene. Adapted with permission [36]. Copyright (2018) Elsevier.

der Waals force present in between stacked layers of bulk material. These intercalated compounds can be exfoliated by a modest sonication technique to mono- or few-layer sheets. In the majority of cases, hydrogen gas is produced due to a reaction between intercalated ions and water, which further promotes exfoliation. Through these methods, a high yield of 2D materials can be achieved [38]. Therefore, liquid exfoliation via ion intercalation is suitable to synthesize 2D materials for bioelectronics. Furthermore, the electrochemical ion intercalation method has been effectively employed to prepare a variety of 2D materials [38]. Figure 3.8 shows the schematic representation of 2D graphene synthesis through electrochemical assisted liquid exfoliation of graphite. In this method, electrochemical force and ions for intercalation act as the driving force [39]. The metallic foils coated with bulk material act as a cathode, while Li foils (intercalating ion) act as anodes. Under the applied voltage, the layered bulk material is intercalated with Li, and intercalated material is obtained on the electrodes. Afterward, the electrodes with intercalated material are washed and the obtained suspension was sonicated for exfoliation. Later, exfoliated material is centrifuged to obtain mono- or few-layered 2D material. This approach has many benefits such as high yield, flexibility in various conditions, and ecofriendly in nature. However, complexity and irreversibility are the two major drawbacks that restrict the widespread use of electrochemical intercalation.

Moreover, liquid exfoliation by cation or anion exchange is also utilized to synthesize 2D materials. Layered metal oxides and metal phosphorus trichalcogenides are frequently exfoliated through cation exchange [40]. In the process, the layered metal oxide is immersed in an acidic medium. This resulted in H^+ cation exchange and the formation of

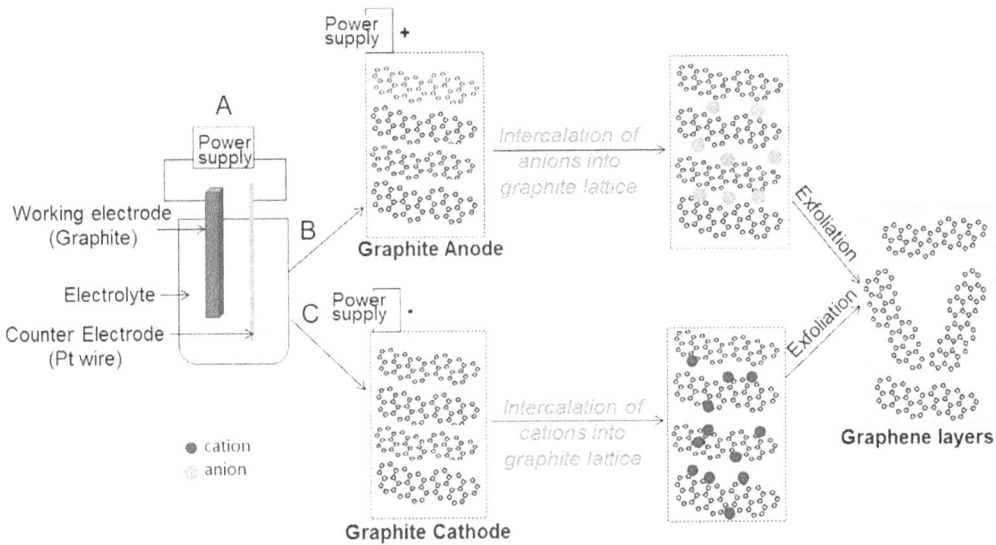

FIGURE 3.8
Electrochemical-assisted liquid exfoliation of graphite to obtain graphene. Adapted with permission [39]. Copyright (2020) Elsevier.

hydrated protonic compounds occur. These compounds are later substituted with orga-noammonium ions that led to the expansion of interlayer spacing between layers of bulk material. The expansion causes the exfoliation of the layered metal oxides with a positive surface charge. In the case of layered metal phosphorus trichalcogenides, the exfoliation process is slightly different. Firstly, metal phosphorus trichalcogenides are immersed in an alkali-based solution to replace the metal ions with K^+ ions to form intermediate compounds. Secondly, interlayer spacing is increased by exchanging K^+ ions with Li-ions. Finally, the exfoliation of metal phosphorus trichalcogenides is achieved. Furthermore, the anion exchange method is used to exfoliate layered double hydroxide [41]. The in-terlayers of one anion are exchanged with the other anion, resulting in the expansion of interlayer distance. Later, 2D materials are obtained from exchanged layered double hydroxides by sonicating or heating in organic solvents. Through this method, a high yield of 2D material can be achieved. Consequently, liquid exfoliation through the ion exchange method is suitable for the large-scale production of 2D materials.

3.3.1.4 Liquid Exfoliation Through Oxidation and Reduction

The preparation of 2D materials through liquid exfoliation by oxidation is extensively studied. The oxidation is performed by employing modified Hummer's method [42]. In the process, strong oxidizing agents are used to oxidized bulk material to obtain 2D materials. For instance, graphite is oxidized by using the mixture of $KMnO_4$ and H_2SO_4 to obtain graphene. The oxidation process led to the production of various oxygen-based functional groups including hydroxyl, carboxyl, and epoxy groups attached to the surface of graphene layers. These functional groups promote the expansion of the in-terlayer and weaken the van der Waals forces between graphite layers. Later, sonication is used to convert the expanded graphite oxide into mono- or few-layered graphene oxide sheets

3.3.1.5 Liquid Exfoliation Via Etching

This approach is successfully used to prepare 2D MXene via selective etching of their 3D counterparts, i.e., MAX phases [43]. The general formula for MAX phases in $M_{n+1}AX_n$, here M is transition metal, A is group IIIA or IVA metal, X is C or N and n is the integer. In this process, the bulk MAX phase is immersed in an etching agent to remove the A layer. The etching agents frequently used are hydrofluoric acid, hydrochloric acid, and lithium fluoride. Firstly, the MAX phases are etched to form MXenes attached with different functional groups (O, OH, F, H) depending upon the etching agent used. Later, the MXenes are intercalated by using different salts and organic compounds to increase the interlayer spacing. Finally, mono- or few-layered MXenes are obtained via sonication and centrifugation.

3.3.2 Bottom-Up Synthesis Protocols

2D materials can be frequently synthesized by two bottom-up approaches such as chemical vapor deposition (CVD) and wet-chemical synthesis methods.

3.3.2.1 Chemical Vapor Deposition

Thin films of 2D materials are widely prepared through the CVD technique [44]. In this method, a precursor in gas or vapor form reacts or decompose on a substrate at elevated temperature under vacuum condition. 2D sheets could be grown on the substrate without the aid of a catalyst. There are a variety of 2D materials are developed through the CVD technique including graphene, h-BN, TMDs, metal carbides, borophenes, antimonene, and silicene [44]. Somani and coworkers [45] were the first to propose a CVD technique for the synthesis of graphene. CVD method also offers ease to control the synthesis parameters to obtain 2D materials as compared to other techniques. In addition, a high yield of a 2D material with high purity and the least defect can be accomplished through the CVD technique. The major drawback of this technique is the higher production cost.

3.3.2.2 Wet-Chemical Synthesis

In this method, 2D materials are obtained via chemical reactions in a solution medium using a precursor at a particular condition. The wet-chemical route is highly preferable to develop 2D materials that one cannot develop through a top-down approach. A higher degree of control and excellent repeatability are the two key features of the wet-chemical synthesis route. There is a variety of wet-chemical synthesis methods such as solvothermal, hydrothermal, template synthesis, self-assembly, oriented attachment, hot-injection, and interface-mediated synthesis to prepare 2D materials [46].

3.4 Mechanism of Bioelectronic System

The transduction and sensing mechanisms of various 2D materials–based bioelectronic devices are addressed in this section. These devices include field-effect transistors (FETs), electrodes and electrode arrays, optical resonators, and multifunctional sensors [1]. In general, the biological elements provide signals related to the alternation of interfacial properties through biological activities. These signals are transduced to the readouts via electrical current, potential, conductance, impedance, and resonant frequency. For instance, a bioelectronic system can be functionalized when linker molecules are covalently connected to 2D materials–based sensors. The linker molecules are responsible for the identification of specificity, improving the transduction of signals, and amplifying the signals received from sensing elements. Though the covalent bonds between linker molecules and graphene alter the electrophysical properties of graphene from sp^2 to sp^3 bond and reduce carrier mobility [47]. In addition, non-covalent routes employ electrostatic, van der Waals, hydrophobic interactions between linker molecules and graphene. This route not only permits shallow functionalization via adsorption of different molecules but also results in a yield of non-specific adsorption. The problem of non-specific adsorption can be resolved through passivation that restricts non-functional sites through surfactants and stabilizing biomolecules [9].

3.4.1 Mechanism for Field-Effect Transistors

2D materials–based FETs possess configuration analogous to a solution-gated FET biosensor. In these devices, efficient gating could be achieved through an electrolyte. The conductance in such devices is controlled via the potential difference between a grounded electrode (drain) and a reference electrode. The measurement of source-drain current is determined in terms of gate voltage that shows the least value of source-drain current at a finite gate voltage, which is also known as the Dirac point. Conceptually, the sensing mechanism is governed by the combination of the electrostatic gating effect and the Schottky barrier [48,49]. The electrostatic gating effect could change transistor conductance due to an electrostatic disturbance caused by biomolecule adsorption. This also results in doping in graphene and alters the Dirac point [47]. In the case of the Schottky barrier mechanism, the adsorbed biomolecules at metal contact alter the variation between the work functions and conductive channel. This changes an asymmetric conductance in p- and n-branches of a source-drain current (I_{SD}) – gate voltage (V_G) plot. When the passivation on the conductive channel-metal contact occurs then the electrostatic gating effect dominates the Schottky barrier effect. The other mechanism involves variation in carrier mobility and decreased gate performance [50]. At the sensing site, adsorbed molecules adversely affect the mobility of the charge carrier. Moreover, less permittivity of adsorbed biomolecules in comparison to electrolytes led to a decrease in gate conductance and reduces the efficacy of gate. Compared to the electrostatic gating effects, these changes in carrier mobility and gate coupling are minimal. To develop 2D material-based FET devices for biomedical applications, the Debye length must be considered [51]. The Debye length is defined as a distance where surplus ions in an electrolyte screen the target and probe biomolecules. This length depends on the ionic composition of buffer solution, temperature, and dielectric constant. The larger distance from the surface of the FET device as compared to the Debye length, seldom affect the mobile charges. Consequently, the target and probe interaction must occur within the Debye length and the probe size should be lower than the Debye length. The limit of detection in FET devices depends on the buffer solution ionic strength and size of interacting biomolecules. This mechanism enables electrochemical and electrical sensing of DNA, biomolecules, and cells.

3.4.2 Mechanism for Nanopore-Based Bioelectronics

A nano-sized aperture on a thin film is used for sensing in nanopore-based bioelectronics. This mechanism is broadly used to sense DNA. In this mechanism, the electric potential is applied on the membrane sandwiched between two sections filled with electrolytes. This acts as the driving force to pass charged biomolecules via a nanopore, and provides controls of ionic current across nanopores. This way, information about the structure and motion of biomolecules could be determined. The nanopore-based bioelectronics is highly suitable for DNA sequencing due to its label-free and high efficiency for the analysis of single molecules. In other words, the variation in ion current depends on the nucleotide or base type passing through the nanopore. Accordingly, measuring variation in ionic current enables the estimation of the base sequence in a DNA molecule. The nanopore-based bioelectronics can be modified through the attachment of optical or electrical readout techniques. For DNA sequencing, graphene emerged as a promising candidate due to its thickness lies in between the spacing (0.32–0.52 nm) of nucleotide. However, cracks and defects in the graphene membrane could result in poor insulation and higher disturbance in ionic current. Beyond graphene, MoS_2, BN, and other heterogeneous-layered 2D materials are also studied for nanopore sensing.

3.4.3 Mechanism for Multi-Electrode Array-Based Bioelectronics

The multi-electrode arrays (MEAs) technology is extensively used in neuroscience to simultaneously record intra- or extracellular of a variety of neurons [52]. The action potential of a cell that controls the electrical behavior of neuro or cardio cells is recorded through electrodes. This action potential travels via a neuron's axon from a membrane region to a neighboring active area and the inactive membrane potential towards a barrier for activation. To estimate neural signals effectively, the velocity of conduction plays a vital role. The conduction velocity is directly proportional to the axoplasm resistivity and the membrane capacitance. The extracellular signals produced by cells are detected when MEAs electrodes are placed over the cell. The MEAs enable to map of the neuronal network as the function of physiological and pathological. To date, ~10,000 electrodes are placed in an MEA chip for in-vitro recordings, while only ~100 electrodes for in-vivo recordings [53]. In addition, the extracellular signals are several times smaller than intracellular signals, making it challenging to record them with less noise.

3.4.4 Mechanism for Optical Resonator-Integrated Bioelectronics

To sense the interactions of biomolecules, graphene integrated with surface plasmon resonance (SPR) based biosensor is employed. In this sensor, the detection of biomolecular interactions is accomplished via a subsequent change in the refractive index near the detection surface [54]. This variation alters the resonance wavelength. A shift in resonance is optically determined through the attenuated total reflection (ATR) method. Graphene enhances the efficiency of the SPR sensor by increasing biomolecule adsorption on the graphene surface. When the micro/nanoribbons or patterned graphenes are integrated with a SPR sensor, then unusual electrical and optical properties are observed. The features of resonant absorption and tunability of properties via electrostatic gating of patterned graphenes have brought new research avenues to develop bioelectronic devices with high sensitivity and label-free detection.

3.4.5 Mechanism for Multifunctional Sensor Array-Based Bioelectronics

A multipurpose sensing/stimulating system is newly examined as an alternative to a single functional component system [55]. In the area of cardiology and neuroscience, simultaneous measuring and stimulating several physiological parameters is crucial for powerful mapping capacity. Such bioelectronic devices comprise temperature, pH, and mechanical strain sensors, optical stimulators, and thermal/electrical actuators. Multifunctional sensor array-based bioelectronic devices have a great deal of promise to realize non-invasive biomedical implants. In addition, these devices could be used for epidermal electronics and provide data to evaluate disease and clinical monitoring.

3.5 Emerging Challenges and Future Prospective

Bioelectronics applications of 2D materials face several obstacles, despite the considerable progress achieved in the synthesis and processing of these materials for electrical applications. To be compatible with soft tissues, bioelectronic devices need materials that are both robust and flexible. The material's biocompatibility, shape conformity, mechanical, electrical, optical, and thermal properties must be taken into account while developing a bioelectronic device. The performance of 2D materials–based bioelectronic devices also depends on the synthesis protocol of 2D materials. It is emergent to hunt easy and green synthesis protocols to develop 2D materials having suitable interfaces compatible with biomolecules and tissues. To attain this aim, researchers should focus their efforts on easy surface modification of 2D materials using targeted molecules. It is also critical to note that certain 2D materials (MoS_2, BPs, and MXenes) have unacceptable interfacial stabilities. Therefore, the antioxidant properties of these materials must be improved via interface protection strategies. Such improvements result in the utilization of these materials for long-term in-vitro and i- vivo exposure to physiological fluids.

Another challenge is the scaling-up of present single prototype devices to array-level or batch-level devices. This significantly demands the synthesis of wafer-scale, highly uniform, and defect-controlled 2D materials except for graphene (which has been unsuccessful until now). In addition, it is still difficult to prevent the deterioration of these devices due to contamination during processing. The mechanical and chemical stability of these materials may need future development of specific patterning, modification, or packaging processes. Furthermore, a variety of bioelectronic devices may be integrated to create multifaceted bioelectric systems capable of performing a wide range of tasks. Consequently, greater efforts are required to make 2D materials compete with conventional bioelectronic materials. Additionally, the identification of individual biomolecules amid a vast number of interferents is still difficult for 2D materials–based bioelectronics. It is also important to pay attention to 2D materials–based bioelectronics that possesses specific bio-interactions on targeted cells, and even pathogens. Hence, the practical application potential in therapeutic domains may be pushed ahead.

References

1. B. Wang, Y. Sun, H. Ding, X. Zhao, L. Zhang, J. Bai, K. Liu, Bioelectronics-related 2D materials beyond graphene: Fundamentals, properties, and applications, *Adv. Funct. Mater.* 30 (2020). https://doi.org/10.1002/adfm.202003732

2. L. Galvani, D.H.D. Roller, Commentary on the effect of electricity on muscular motion, *Am. J. Phys.* 22 (2005) 40.
3. I. Tasaki, Physiology and electrochemistry of nerve fibers, *Physiol. Electrochem. Nerve Fibers.* (1982). ISBN 978-0-12-683780-3.
4. M. Jia, M. Rolandi, Soft and ion-conducting materials in bioelectronics: From conducting polymers to hydrogels, *Adv. Healthc. Mater.* 9 (2020) 1901372.
5. D. Grieshaber, R. MacKenzie, J. Vörös, E. Reimhult, Electrochemical biosensors – Sensor principles and architectures, *Sensors.* 8 (2008) 1400–1458.
6. H. Yuk, B. Lu, X. Zhao, Hydrogel bioelectronics, *Chem. Soc. Rev.* 48 (2019) 1642–1667.
7. T. Nezakati, A. Seifalian, A. Tan, A.M. Seifalian, Conductive polymers: Opportunities and challenges in biomedical applications, *Chem. Rev.* 118 (2018) 6766–6843.
8. H.W. Guo, Z. Hu, Z.B. Liu, J.G. Tian, Stacking of 2D materials, *Adv. Funct. Mater.* 31 (2021). https://doi.org/10.1002/adfm.202007810
9. P. Kang, M.C. Wang, S. Nam, Bioelectronics with two-dimensional materials, *Microelectron. Eng.* 161 (2016) 18–35.
10. W.Z. Teo, E.L.K. Chng, Z. Sofer, M. Pumera, Cytotoxicity of exfoliated transition-metal dichalcogenides (MoS_2, WS_2, and WSe_2) is lower than that of graphene and its analogues, *Chem. – A Eur. J.* 20 (2014) 9627–9632.
11. G. Guan et al., Protein induces layer-by-layer exfoliation of transition metal dichalcogenides, *J. Am. Chem. Soc.* 137 (2015) 6152–6155.
12. X. Li, Y. Gong, X. Zhou, H. Jin, H. Yan, S. Wang, J. Liu, Facile synthesis of soybean phospholipid-encapsulated MoS_2 nanosheets for efficient in vitro and in vivo photothermal regression of breast tumor, *Int. J. Nanomedicine.* 11 (2016) 1819–1833.
13. G. Yang, H. Gong, T. Liu, X. Sun, L. Cheng, Z. Liu, Two-dimensional magnetic $WS_2@Fe_3O_4$ nanocomposite with mesoporous silica coating for drug delivery and imaging-guided therapy of cancer, *Biomaterials.* 60 (2015) 62–71.
14. H. Lin, X. Wang, L. Yu, Y. Chen, J. Shi, Two-dimensional ultrathin MXene ceramic nanosheets for photothermal conversion, *Nano Lett.* 17 (2017) 384–391.
15. J. Shao et al., Biodegradable black phosphorus-based nanospheres for in vivo photothermal cancer therapy, *Nat. Commun.* 7 (2016). Article number: 12967.
16. M. Qiu et al., Novel concept of the smart NIR-light-controlled drug release of black phosphorus nanostructure for cancer therapy, *Proc. Natl. Acad. Sci. U. S. A.* 115 (2018) 501–506.
17. L. Xu et al., 3D multifunctional integumentary membranes for spatiotemporal cardiac measurements and stimulation across the entire epicardium, *Nat. Commun.* 5 (2014) 3329.
18. K.S. Novoselov et al., Electric field in atomically thin carbon films, *Science.* 306(80) (2004) 666–669.
19. T. Liu et al., Crested two-dimensional transistors, *Nat. Nanotechnol.* 14 (2019) 223–226.
20. H.J. Conley, B. Wang, J.I. Ziegler, R.F. Haglund, S.T. Pantelides, K.I. Bolotin, Bandgap engineering of strained monolayer and bilayer MoS2, *Nano Lett.* 13 (2013) 3626–3630.
21. A. Chaves et al., Bandgap engineering of two-dimensional semiconductor materials, *Npj 2D Mater. Appl.* 4 (2020) 29.
22. L. Li et al., Black phosphorus field-effect transistors, *Nat. Nanotechnol.* 9(5) (2014) 372–377.
23. J. Qiao, X. Kong, Z.X. Hu, F. Yang, W. Ji, High-mobility transport anisotropy and linear dichroism in few-layer black phosphorus, *Nat. Commun.* 51(5) (2014) 1–7.
24. W. Wu et al., Piezoelectricity of single-atomic-layer MoS2 for energy conversion and piezotronics, *Nature.* 514 (2014) 470–474.
25. G. Eda, H. Yamaguchi, D. Voiry, T. Fujita, M. Chen, M. Chhowalla, Photoluminescence from chemically exfoliated MoS 2, *Nano Lett.* 11 (2011) 5111–5116.
26. C. Lee, X. Wei, J.W. Kysar, J. Hone, Measurement of the elastic properties and intrinsic strength of monolayer graphene, *Science.* 321(80) (2008) 385–388.

27. A. Falin et al., Mechanical properties of atomically thin boron nitride and the role of inter-layer interactions, *Nat. Commun.* 8(81) (2017) 1–9.
28. S. Bertolazzi, J. Brivio, A. Kis, Stretching and breaking of ultrathin MoS 2, *ACS Nano.* 5 (2011) 9703–9709.
29. Y. Wei, B. Wang, J. Wu, R. Yang, M.L. Dunn, Bending rigidity and gaussian bending stiffness of single-layered graphene, *Nano Lett.* 13 (2012) 26–30.
30. A.J. Mannix, B. Kiraly, M.C. Hersam, N.P. Guisinger, Synthesis and chemistry of elemental 2D materials, *Nat. Rev. Chem.* 1(12) (2017) 1–14.
31. A.K. Geim, K.S. Novoselov, The rise of graphene, *Nat. Mater.* 6 (2007) 183–191.
32. F. Liu et al., Optoelectronic properties of atomically thin ReSSe with weak interlayer cou-pling, *Nanoscale.* 8 (2016) 5826–5834.
33. P. Ares, J.J. Palacios, G. Abellán, J. Gómez-Herrero, F. Zamora, Recent progress on anti-monene: A new bidimensional material, *Adv. Mater.* 30 (2018) 1703771.
34. F. Bonaccorso, A. Lombardo, T. Hasan, Z. Sun, L. Colombo, A.C. Ferrari, Production and processing of graphene and 2d crystals, *Mater. Today.* 15 (2012) 564–589.
35. Y. Hernandez et al., High-yield production of graphene by liquid-phase exfoliation of gra-phite, *Nat. Nanotechnol.* 3(39) (2008) 563–568.
36. R. Navik, Y. Gai, W. Wang, Y. Zhao, Curcumin-assisted ultrasound exfoliation of graphite to graphene in ethanol, *Ultrason. Sonochem.* 48 (2018) 96–102.
37. K.R. Paton et al., Scalable production of large quantities of defect-free few-layer graphene by shear exfoliation in liquids, *Nat. Mater.* 13(136) (2014) 624–630.
38. V. Nicolosi, M. Chhowalla, M.G. Kanatzidis, M.S. Strano, J.N. Coleman, liquid exfoliation of layered materials, *Science.* 340 (2013). DOI: 10.1126/science.1226419.
39. A. Agrawal, G.C. Yi, Sample pretreatment with graphene materials, *Compr. Anal. Chem.* 91 (2020) 21–47.
40. M. Osada, T. Sasaki, Nanosheet architectonics: A hierarchically structured assembly for tailored fusion materials, *Polym. J.* 47(2015) 89–98.
41. Q. Wang, D. Ohare, Recent advances in the synthesis and application of layered double hydroxide (LDH) nanosheets, *Chem. Rev.* 112 (2012) 4124–4155.
42. W.S. Hummers, R.E. Offeman, Preparation of graphitic oxide, *J. Am. Chem. Soc.* 80 (2002) 1339.
43. M. Naguib, V.N. Mochalin, M.W. Barsoum, Y. Gogotsi, 25th anniversary article: MXenes: A new family of two-dimensional materials, *Adv. Mater.* 26 (2014) 992–1005.
44. J. Jiang et al., Synergistic additive-mediated CVD growth and chemical modification of 2D materials, *Chem. Soc. Rev.* 48 (2019) 4639–4654.
45. P.R. Somani, S.P. Somani, M. Umeno, Planer nano-graphenes from camphor by CVD, *Chem. Phys. Lett.* 430 (2006) 56–59.
46. C. Tan, H. Zhang, Wet-chemical synthesis and applications of non-layer structured two-dimensional nanomaterials, *Nat. Commun.* 6(61) (2015) 1–13.
47. Y. Liu, X. Dong, P. Chen, Biological and chemical sensors based on graphene materials, *Chem. Soc. Rev.* 41 (2012) 2283–2307.
48. A.B. Artyukhin, M. Stadermann, R.W. Friddle, P. Stroeve, O. Bakajin, A. Noy, Controlled electrostatic gating of carbon nanotube FET devices, *Nano Lett.* 6 (2006) 2080–2085.
49. L.G. Ee et al., DNA sensing by field-effect transistors based on networks of carbon nano-tubes, *J. Am. Chem. Soc.* 129 (2007) 14427–14432.
50. D.S. Hecht, R.J.A. Ramirez, M. Briman, E. Artukovic, K.S. Chichak, J.F. Stoddart, G. Grüner, Bioinspired detection of light using a porphyrin-sensitized single-wall nanotube field effect transistor, *Nano Lett.* 6 (2006) 2031–2036.
51. Y. Ohno, K. Maehashi, K. Matsumoto, Label-free biosensors based on aptamer-modified graphene field-effect transistors, *J. Am. Chem. Soc.* 132 (2010) 18012–18013.
52. P. Connolly, P. Clark, A.S.G. Curtis, J.A.T. Dow, C.D.W. Wilkinson, An Extracellular mi-croelectrode Array for monitoring electrogenic cells in culture, *Biosens. Bioelectron.* 5 (1990) 223–234.

53. L. Berdondini, K. Imfeld, A. MacCione, M. Tedesco, S. Neukom, M. Koudelka-Hep, S. Martinoia, Active pixel sensor array for high spatio-temporal resolution electrophysiological recordings from single cell to large scale neuronal networks, *Lab Chip.* 9 (2009) 2644–2651.
54. E. Petryayeva, U.J. Krull, Localized surface plasmon resonance: Nanostructures, bioassays and biosensing—A review, *Anal. Chim. Acta.* 706 (2011) 8–24.
55. Y. Hattori et al., Multifunctional skin-like electronics for quantitative, clinical monitoring of cutaneous wound healing, *Adv. Healthc. Mater.* 3 (2014) 1597–1607.

4

Materials for Organic Bioelectronics

Giuseppe M. Paternò and Guglielmo Lanzani

Department of Physics, Politecnico di Milano, Piazza Leonardo da Vinci, Milano, Italy

Center for Nanoscience and Technology, Istituto Italiano di Tecnologia, Via Giovanni Pascoli, Milano, Italy

CONTENTS

4.1 Introduction

Bioelectronic materials for abiotic/biotic interfaces are extensively used for triggering and probing biological processes, ultimately owing to their ability to modulate the polarization state of cells. This can occur through various physical and chemical phenomena, usually involving the injection/generation of charges and/or heat, the displacement of ions, and the occurrence of red-ox reactions. Since Galvani's early experiments with frog legs date back to the end of the 17th century, the electrical excitability of biological tissues has a rich scientific history. In particular, in the last three decades, a wide community including chemists, physicists, biologists, and engineers steered their attention to the development of new abiotic/biotic interfaces to realize efficient communication between biological and electrical signals, with the final aim to build up devices that are fully biocompatible and conformable. Some recent and important developments in the field of

DOI: 10.1201/9781003263265-4

bioelectronic materials include advanced materials synthesis, bacterial, neural, and cardiac interfaces, function recovery and gain (*i.e.* vision and auditory system), and photo-
tactic guidance of animaloid soft robots or cyborgs [1–3].

For decades, inorganic materials have been routinely used in clinical settings and basic
research to stimulate and record signals from cells and tissues. These include both metals
and semiconducting systems. For the former case, most applications usually rely on metal
electrodes (*i.e.* made of Au, Pt, and Pd) that enable direct electrical stimulation of cells and
tissues and, more recently, on nanostructures, *i.e.* gold nanorods and nanoparticles [4],
which allows photoelectrical/thermal stimulation. Silicon represents another popular
semiconducting bioelectronic material, given its large availability and relatively low
toxicity. Recently, the use of silicon nanowires has been proposed to achieve optically
induced neuronal firing [5]. However, inorganic bioelectronic materials are relatively far
from living matter, for instance in regards to conformability, stiffness, and, in many cases,
biocompatibility. Furthermore, while conventional electronics is based on electron conduction, bioelectricity usually consists of ionic currents and stems from differences in
ionic concentration that are regulated by the activity of ion channels. Those discrepancies
in mechanical, compositional, and electrical properties between inorganic materials and
biological matter demand an alternative approach in bioelectronic materials.

On the other hand, the increasing number of studies reporting striking results using
organic semiconductors make these materials a competitive alternative in this field [3].
From the biocompatibility side, these systems are kin to proteins, carbohydrates, and
nucleic acids, as well as being biodegradable, soft, and conformable. On the functional
side, they can sustain both electronic and ionic transport and can be easily functionalized
to enable specific excitation and probing capabilities. Organic bioelectronics has strongly
benefitted from the advances in the field of organic semiconductors, driven mainly by the
development of organic light-emitting diodes [6], solar cells [7,8], and transistors [9].
Briefly, these materials exhibit semiconducting behavior owing to their delocalized
π-electron system. Chemical doping of organic semiconductors to highly conductive
states, either p-type or less frequently n-type, can be achieved via the addition of an
oxidizing or reducing agent. Doping can also occur when ions from an electrolyte enter
an organic film or vice versa. In this case, the compensating charge is supplied by
an electrode and the process is called "electrochemical doping." Apart from largely
π-delocalized polymers, also small molecules with different degrees of conjugation and
photochemical properties have been employed for the modification of the abiotic/biotic
interface. These include the use of conjugated oligomers, organic pigments, and
membrane-targeting photochromic materials for direct neuronal stimulation. Last but not
least, carbon-based nanomaterials such as graphene and carbon-nanotubes have also
attracted increasing attention recently. Their use has gained momentum owing to the
spectacular developments in the field of graphene derivatives and general 2D materials.

Therefore, given their ability to interface effectively with biological matter, organic materials have entered quietly but steadily the realm of bioelectronics. From the seminal review
by Magnus Berggren and Agneta Richter-Dahlfors in which the term "organic bioelectronics" was coined [10], the field has recorded many advances in material synthesis/design,
with several dozen groups in Europe, the Americas, Asia, and Australia that are active in the
field. The scope of this chapter is to give an overview of the most employed organic materials
as abiotic bioelectronic interfaces. Our motivation stems from the fact that bioelectronics is a
field that is limited by the materials that transduce signals across the biotic/abiotic interface.
For this reason, several breakthrough results in the field of organic bioelectronics have been
fueled by progress in materials chemistry and physics.

4.2 Why Organic Materials are Suitable for Bioelectronics

Before starting our discussion on the most used organic materials for bioelectronics, a useful exercise is to identify their peculiarities and rationalize whether they match with the requirements for bioelectronic applications. In this case, we reckon that an instructive comparison is between organic and inorganic materials. To highlight the most prominent differences, we select conjugated polymers and silicon as archetypical examples for organic and inorganic materials, respectively (Figure 4.1). The first difference lies in the connectivity, with silicon exhibiting a strong network of covalent bonds, in which each silicon atom shares valence electrons with the other four neighboring atoms. On the other hand, conjugated polymers and, in general, organic solids are made of different molecular blocks that however interact with each other via relatively weak non-covalent van der Waals forces. This implies that organic materials are "softer" and more disordered than their inorganic counterparts, in terms of the crystalline arrangement, excitation landscape, and charge transport. However, such a disordered and soft nature can be seen as an advantage, since intermolecular interactions and non-covalent bonding are the tools that nature uses to make life possible (DNA double helix, proteins folding/unfolding, and so on). This is the first feature that makes organic semiconductors more similar to biological matter than inorganic systems and, alongside their analogous chemical composition with cells and tissues, renders them inherently biocompatible. It is worth saying that biocompatibility cannot be universally defined, as the same material can elicit different toxicological responses depending on the type of cells and tissues under investigation.

Other bioelectronically relevant properties of organic semiconductors arise directly and indirectly from their softness. First, organic semiconductors usually offer a facile chemical modification, due to the power and versatility of chemical synthesis. Electronic, optical, and mechanical properties of organic semiconductors can be usually tailored via direct alteration of the π-conjugated backbone, and/or via modification of their side groups. In this regard, this latter aspect is extremely useful with the view to tune organic semiconductors'

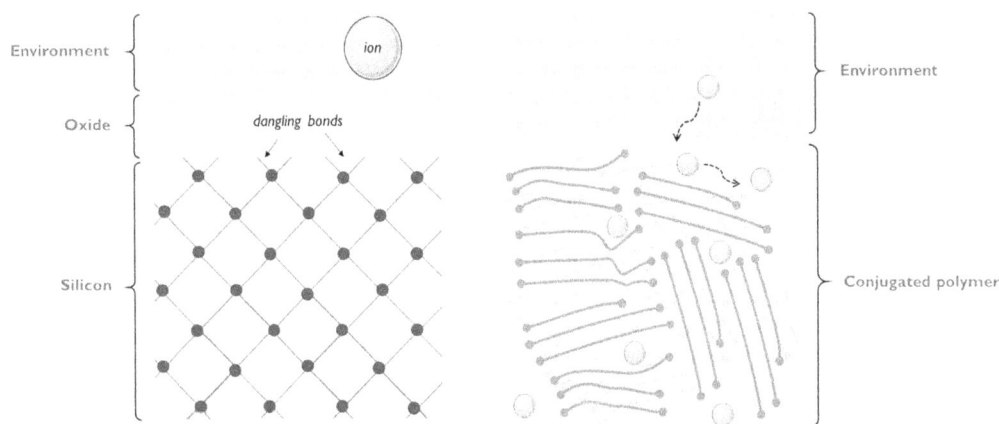

FIGURE 4.1
Simplified schematic of inorganic and organic semiconductors. We selected silicon and conjugated polymers as archetypical examples of the two classes of materials. Note that the size of hydrated ions is meant to be equal in both cartoons (for silicon and conjugated polymers), while they appear to be smaller in the organic schematic due to the different length scales.

biodegradability, which can be modified via the insertion of specific chemical groups in the conjugated polymer backbone [11]. Furthermore, one can exploit weak intermolecular forces to control their arrangement at the molecular level. This enables the formation of a wealth of morphologies and structures from the same material (i.e. from single crystals to semicrystalline films and nanoparticles) that can show different bioelectronic performances. Finally, their softness in terms of intermolecular forces enables their processability from solution and at a low temperature. This property not only permits to fabrication of bioelectronic devices in a large variety of substrates with high conformability and low stiffness but also maintains the functionality of cells and tissues during device fabrication. In this context, it is worth reporting the work of Torsi and collaborators, showing that the organic active material can be deposited on top of biological materials without damaging them [12].

Second, the large free volume provided by the non-covalent forces allows for ion penetration and transport in the organic material. In addition, hydrophilic organic films can swell upon the incorporation of water molecules, an effect that enhances ion permeation. The possibility to transport both electrons and ions is indeed one of the most important properties of organic semiconductors since it implies that the entire bulk of the material, and not just its surface, can participate in the interaction with the biological environment. To be more specific, the fact that organic materials usually exhibit oxide-free interfaces represents an important asset since this effect increases further the contact between the material and the biological environment and, consequently, ion exchanges. Again, this property stems from the fact that organic semiconductors do not expose dangling covalent bonds at the interface that can react with oxygen, while inorganics do. This appealing feature can be exploited to develop effective biosensors and bioactuators, such as organic electronic ion pumps (OEIP) [13] and organic electrochemical transistors (OECT) [14]. In particular, this latter device was introduced by Mark Wrighton and collaborators in 1984 [15] and relies on the use of an organic semiconductor as an oxide-free channel layer. In OECT, ions from the electrolyte penetrate the volume of the polymer film and change its conductance. In 2013, Malliaras and coworkers have exploited this device configuration to record brain activity in a rat model for epilepsy [16].

Finally, in organic semiconductors excitations are strongly coupled to their lattice. For instance, inorganic semiconductors the addition/removal of charges does not affect the lattice appreciably, while in organics this leads to lattice distortion, with the corresponding quasi-particles, which deform and polarize the surrounding lattice, called polarons. This also means that ionic doping from electrolyte solution can cause large dimensional changes in the organic material, implying that doping has a strong influence across the abiotic/biotic interface. As an example, Malliaras and coworkers have shown that the red-ox state of a conjugated polymer can influence the fibronectin conformation, which is an important cell adhesion protein [17], as a result, that can enable the preparation of substrates for cells culturing exhibiting a different degree of stickiness that can be tuned by the external bias.

However, organic materials come with some disadvantages, which have been or are being tackled currently by the concerted action of chemists, physicists, and materials scientists. We believe that one of the most important issues is material stability in biological environments since organic semiconductors show usually degradation upon exposure to water and oxygen. In addition, some conjugated polymers are water-soluble, and therefore they must be stabilized to avoid deformation or delamination upon immersion in physiological electrolytes. This is a crucial aspect since the materials must ensure their electrical stability for many cycles of operation to secure accurate electrical

TABLE 4.1

Summary of Advantages and Disadvantages of the Material Groups Used in Bioelectronics

	Advantages	Disadvantages
Metals	• Good stability • Established processing and functionalization methods • Easy fabrication of nanostructures (*i.e.* colloidal nanoparticles) • High crystallinity • Low toxicity in many cases • High electrical stability	• Mechanical mismatch at the biotic interface • Electronic mismatch at the biotic interface • High stiffness • Low conformability
Inorganic semiconductors	• Good stability • Established processing • High crystallinity in most cases • Easy fabrication of nanostructures (*i.e.* colloidal nanoparticles) • Tunable optoelectronic properties (doping) • Easy surface functionalization	• Mechanical mismatch at the biotic interface • Electronic mismatch at the biotic interface • Presence of the oxide layer at the surface • High stiffness • Low conformability • Cytotoxicity in many cases
Organic semiconductors	• High affinity with biological matter and biocompatibility • Low temperature solution process • Large variety of structures and morphologies • Tunable optoelectronic and mechanical properties • Conformable and stretchable materials • Ionic and electronic conduction • Oxide-free materials	• Low stability in air and in biological settings • Low crystallinity • Low charge carrier mobility

stimulation or probing of biological events. The most successful example of stable and efficient bioelectronic material is poly(3,4-ethylenedioxythiophene) polystyrene sulfonate (PEDOT:PSS), which is widely used in bioelectronics due to its stability under biological conditions, as well as its commercial availability, and excellent mixed ionic and electronic conduction properties [2]. The most important advantages and disadvantages of organic and inorganic materials are summarized in Table 4.1.

4.3 Conjugated Polymers

Conjugated polymers (CPs) are the workhorse materials for organic bioelectronics. For this reason, there are a wealth of studies in which these systems are employed as bioelectronic transducers. Thus, we do not aim at giving a detailed list of reports on CPs for

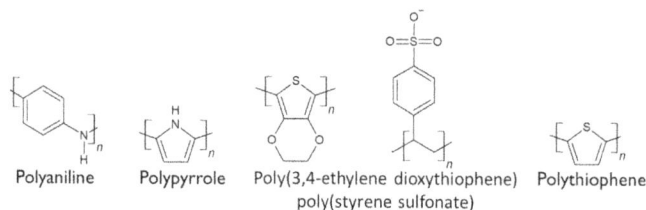

FIGURE 4.2
Chemical structure of the most commonly used conjugated polymers for bioelectronics applications.

bioelectronics, rather we want to provide an overview of the main class of CPs that are representative of the entire literature on the field. The most used CPs in bioelectronics are displayed in Figure 4.2. The first two CPs employed as organic semiconductors were polyanilines (PANIs) and polypyrroles (PPys), while poly(3,4-ethylene dioxythiophene): poly(styrene sulfonate) (PEDOT:PSS) and polythiophenes (PThs) were introduced more recently. Note that PANIs, PPys, and PEDOT:PSS are conductive polymers, while PThs display a semiconducting behavior.

4.3.1 Polyaniline

PANI is an important conductive polymer that has been used extensively in bioelectronics. Despite its relatively good bioelectronic properties, PANI exhibits some disadvantages, such as its limited solubility in many solvents and its poor conductivity at high pH values. This latter issue has been solved by adding crystalline nanocellulose to PANI (CNC-PANI): the high density of hydroxyl groups of the nanocellulose stabilizes the polymer structure via hydrogen bonding [18]. A very recent and interesting example of the use of PANI as an abiotic interface has been reported by Deisseroth, Bao, and coworkers [19]. Here, the authors show that modification of neurons with conductive PANI, which is synthesized by genetically instructing cells, increased their membrane capacitance and decreased spike number. In addition, this method was also applied *in vivo*, to modify the motor functions of *Caenorhabditis elegans*. Although this approach can pose some cytotoxicity issues due to the monomer or radical side products, it can pave the way towards the development of biocompatible hybrids that are directly synthesized by cells.

4.3.2 Polypyrrole

PPy represents another important class of conductive polymers, owing to the easiness of its synthesis, high biocompatibility, and environmental stability [20]. This material is usually produced as conductive monolithic sheets that display appreciable mechanical strain upon application of an external bias. This property has rendered PPys a perfect choice for the fabrication of artificial muscles or mechano-modulators [21]. Despite these sheets being intrinsically stretchable, they do not adhere effectively to cells and tissues due to their hydrophobicity. This is a serious disadvantage since to efficiently sense or stimulate a desired target molecule or cell, the device must be able to integrate with the bio-target. To overcome this issue, PPys have been often coupled to other stretchable materials, such as hyaluronic acid and poly(dimethylsiloxane) (PDMS) [20]. In regards to PPys applications, Golabi et al. studied the effect of PPy ion dopants on bacterial differentiation. In particular, the authors found that the adhesion of specific bacterial strains

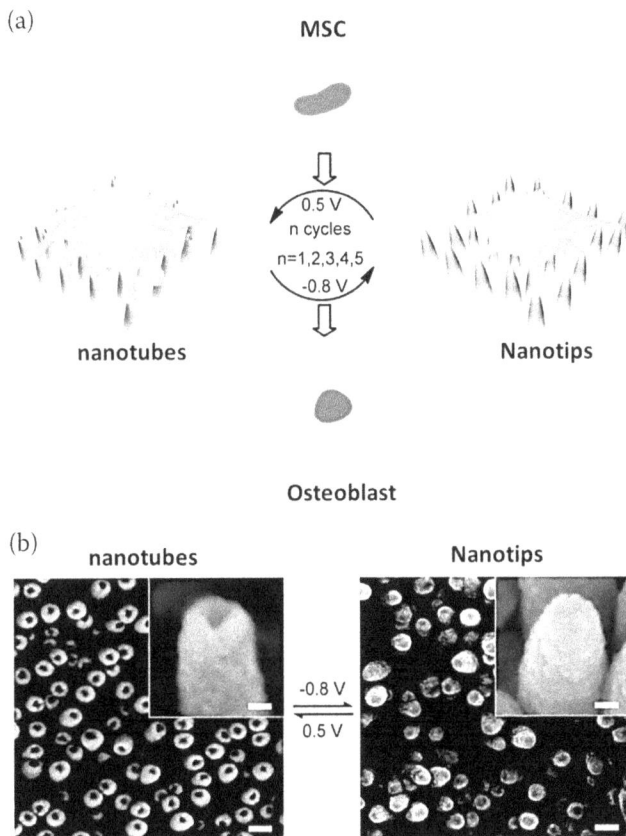

FIGURE 4.3
(a) Illustration of switching between the nanotube/nanotip on a PPy array upon redox switching. (b) Scanning electron microscopy images of the nano-morphology switching scale bars, 100 nm. The insets show magnified nanostructures. Scale bars, 20 nm. Adapted with permission [23]. Copyright (2017) American Chemical Society.

is strongly dependent on the dopant type [22]. This study can be exploited to build up new platforms for label-free bacterial differentiation, as well as for monitoring the bacterial population. The electroactivity of PPys has been exploited to achieve mechano-transduction in mesenchymal stem cells. In particular, Jiang and collaborators showed that the nano-morphology of a Ppy array can be switched between highly adhesive hydrophobic nanotubes and poorly adhesive hydrophilic nanotips via electrochemical oxidation/reduction (Figure 4.3) [23].

4.3.3 Poly(3,4-Ethylene Dioxythiophene): Polystyrene Sulfonate

PEDOT:PSS is perhaps the most employed conductive polymer in bioelectronics, owing to its conductivity, stability, biocompatibility, and excellent mixed electronic and ionic conduction. Specifically, PEDOT is conductive but virtually insoluble in water, while the addition of the negatively charged sulfonate groups of PSS increases PEDOT solubility and dispersibility via Coulomb interactions. In this ionomer mixture form, PEDOT:PSS is thus highly processable and biocompatible, allowing the formation of biocompatible and stable hydrogels, whose conductivity can be largely tuned by using a variety of dopants [24]. Note that PSS is an insulator, hence most research efforts have been devoted to minimizing PSS interference in the PEDOT interchain π-π interaction, whose accounts for the overall PEDOT:PSS conductivity via holes polarons/bipolarons hopping. For this reason, most PEDOT: PSS-based materials are prepared as composites with additives, which permit to maximization of the formation of hydrophobic fibers and, consequently, PEDOT:PSS conductivity. For instance, sodium dodecyl sulfate has been used to remove the insulating PSS, an effect that enhances interconnectivity between PEDOT chains [25]. The versatility of PEDOT:PSS to be mixed with a variety of materials has been exploited for a range of applications. For instance, Bonfiglio and collaborators have built up conductive textile based on PEDOT:PSS electrodes that can be employed as a wearable electro-cardiogram system [26]. Furthermore, PEDOT:PSS can be fabricated as a thin film, which can be transferred onto elastic substrates, such as PDMS. This can preserve the high conductivity of pristine PEDOT:PSS, while ensuring the mechanical stability offered by the presence of the substrate. Moreover, to enhance the adhesive properties of PEDOT:PSS, Gan et al. have synthesized nanosheets by blending them with polydopamine-reduced sulfonated graphene oxide [27], which are redox-active due to the abundant catechol groups and can be implanted for biosignals detection *in vivo*. Besides its good ion and electron mobility for organic electrochemical transistors and all the above-mentioned properties, PEDOT:PSS can be used effectively as a coating layer for metal electrodes, an effect that reduces interface capacitance, enhances tissue integration, and increases surface area. In this regard, it is useful reporting the review article by Green et al. on the use of conductive polymers to modify metal electrodes for developing effective long-term implants for neurostimulation [28].

4.3.4 Polythiophene

Polythiophene derivatives have been the work-horse organic semiconducting materials in solar cells for at least two decades. The photophysical/chemical properties that have determined PThs success as photovoltaic materials have also driven its broad application in bioelectronics as a photo transducer for cells stimulation. For these peculiar reasons, in this section, we mostly focus on these aspects. The coexistence of different stimulation mechanisms in PThs and, in general, π-conjugated materials stems from the deactivation pathways occurring upon photoexcitation to the excited states, namely: i) radiative and non-radiative recombination of excitons, with the latter effect contributing to the release of thermal energy; ii) exciton dissociation into free charges leading to the generation of polarons. These long-lived species (μs up to ms) can contribute to either the build-up of an electrical polarization at the abiotic/biotic interface, thus leading to a photocapacitive effect, or electrochemical faradaic phenomena. For instance, nanoparticles consisting of the prototypical organic photovoltaics polymer poly(3-hexylthiophene) (P3HT) have been used as light transducers in eyeless animals, namely, *Hydra vulgaris* [29]. Provided that at the light intensities used in this study the authors could rule out the involvement of any thermal effect, the formation of a stable population of polarons with consequent electrical effect appears to be the most probable scenario. In particular, polymer chains are closely packed in nanoparticles, allowing interchain interactions that, in turn, can favor delocalization and stabilization of charged species. Conversely, in P3HT thin films that offer a much larger coupling surface, the stimulation mechanism has been also ascribed to a convolution of thermal and electrical phenomena [30]. For instance, our group has recently exploited such an effect to optically enhance the contraction rate of a human and patient-specific cardiac *in vitro* cell model [31].

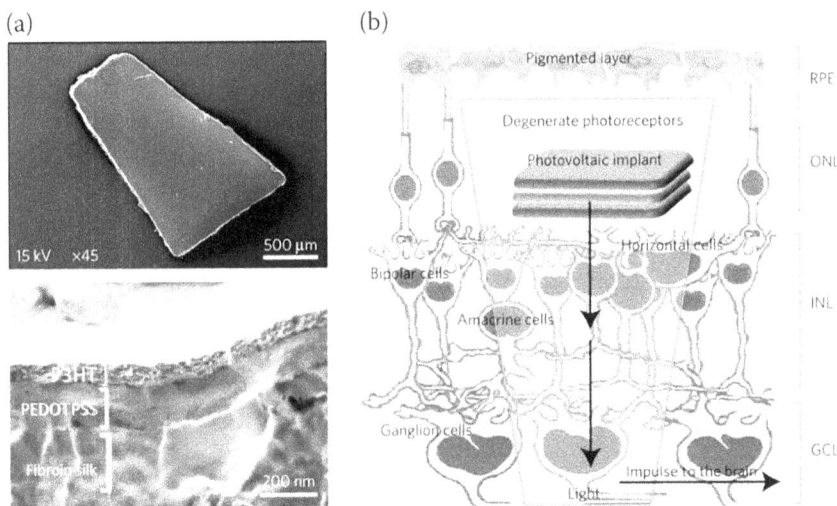

FIGURE 4.4
(a) Scanning electron microscopy images of the prosthetic device (top) and of its cross-section. (b) Scheme of the implant approach. Adapted with permission [34]. Copyright (2017) Springer Nature.

The use of PThs as phototransducers for neurostimulation has opened new and exciting avenues for rescuing biological functions and treating diseases [32,33], including their use as retinal prostheses. In this case, PThs offers important advantages as compared with other materials, namely photovoltaic functioning, high biocompatibility, mechanical resilience, and a relatively high light sensitivity. In this regard, Maya-Vetencourt et al. have developed a P3HT-based device composed of a flexible and highly conformable silk substrate covered with photoactive layers (Figure 4.4), which was able to rescue vision in dystrophic rats [34]. The further evolution of such an approach was the development of injectable P3HT sub-micro particles in suspension. This approach simplifies the surgery and provides a much better and diffuse retina coverage [35]. These results have inspired other works, such as the work of Ghezzi et al., in which the prostheses are composed of a P3HT/PCBM layer over a PDMS substrate [36]. Other works employ either organic pigments or semiconducting carbon nanotubes and will be described in the relevant sections below.

4.4 Small Molecules

Traditionally, small molecules have been employed widely in bioelectronics to modify chemically the surface of electrodes, *i.e.* to enhance cell-to-electrode attachment and electron transfer [37]. Some relevant examples relate to microbial fuel cells, whose efficiency greatly depends on bacteria-electrode attachment. For instance, Cheng et al. reported the ammonia treatment of neutral carbon cloth at elevated temperature, which leads to the improvement of the start-up time and power production in mixed culture microbial fuel cells [38]. Apart from these applications in which small molecules are employed as passive components, in the last couple of decades, they have been increasingly used as active bioelectronic systems, *i.e.* for triggering bioelectric signaling.

This is the case of π-conjugated molecules and oligomers, which are being utilized to trigger electron injection or for photostimulation. In this section, we will focus on three main classes of photosensitive bioelectronic molecules: conjugated oligomers, organic dyes/pigments, and photoswitches.

4.4.1 Conjugated Oligomers

Conjugated oligoelectrolytes (COEs) consist of a π-delocalized backbone and ionic pendant groups, have been demonstrated to modify the abiotic/biotic interface via efficient insertion in the plasma membrane (Figure 4.5a,b) [39]. The COE chromophore mainly undergoes radiative decay via emission or nonradiative decay via heat generation or energy/electron transfer to acceptors (such as dyes and/or oxygen) upon light excitation. This molecular unit is ultimately responsible for some important bioelectronic properties of COEs, *i.e.* the photoinduced production of reactive oxygen species, [40] increase of the local temperature, and the facilitation of extracellular electron transport to abiotic electrode surface via direct electron transfer and/or mediated electron transfer. In addition, emission enables facile tracking of the chromophore via simple fluorescence microscopies. On the other hand, the ionic side chains confer water solubility and enable specific interaction with targets via electrostatic interactions, leading to the disruption or stabilization of the plasma membrane, depending on the COE molecular size. For instance, disruption can occur via membrane thinning, as the lipid phosphate head groups are drawn toward the center of the bilayer. For all these reasons, COE have been employed for a plethora of applications, including in microbial fuel cells, as light-driven antibacterial agent, as biosensors and in photodynamic and photothermal therapy [39,41].

4.4.2 Organic Dyes and Pigments

Historically, dyes and pigments have been used as electronic materials. One of the most famous examples is perhaps Tang's photovoltaic cell, consisting of a bilayer of copper

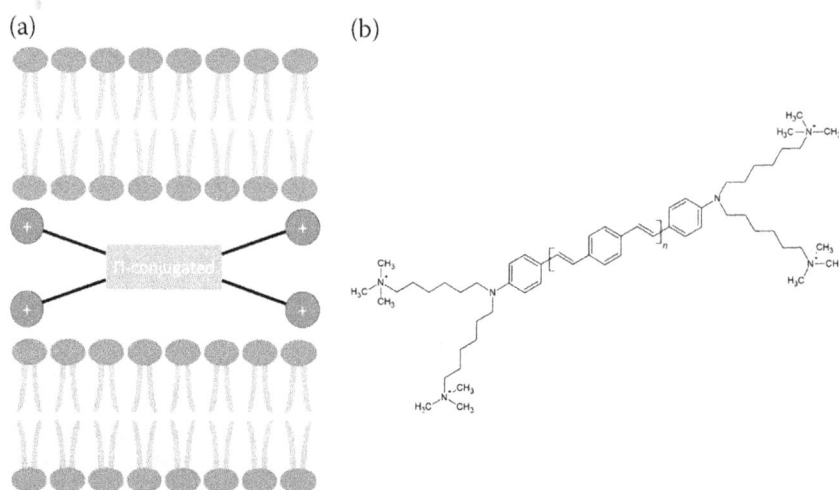

FIGURE 4.5
(a) Schematic of the COE structure with a π-conjugated internal region (rectangle) and polar pendant group terminals (circle) intercalating into a lipid bilayer. b) Typical COE chemical structure.

phthalocyanine and a perylene tetracarboxylic derivative [42]. This, and a plethora of other works, have certainly inspired the use of organic dyes and pigments in bioelectronics. A recent example is a study reported by Rand et al., in which the authors used a p-n junction consisting of nontoxic and commercially available pigments (phthalocyanine and N,N'-dimethyl perylene-3,4:9,10-tetracar-boxylic diimide) to photostimulate neurons through photocapacitive effects [43]. By exploiting the same stimulation approach, this research group has also built up organic electrolytic photocapacitors to generate capacitive current for *X. laevis* oocyte stimulation [44].

Apart from synthetic systems, nowadays there is a growing interest in naturally occurring organic electronic materials. For instance, melanin derivatives represent a popular class of naturally occurring organic pigments for bioelectronic and optoelectronic devices, owing to their water-dependent conductivity and excellent biocompatibility [45]. However, one of the most important issues displayed by these materials is connected to the relatively low solubility and, hence, processability. Currently, this problem has been overcome by employing different strategies, and now it is possible to commercially obtain soluble eumelanin samples synthesized from tyrosine with hydrogen peroxide [45]. From the application point of view, the affinity of eumelanin to metal ions has been exploited to fabricate bioelectronic devices. For example, it has been shown that the addition of copper ions can modulate the eumelanin conductivity up to four orders of magnitude. A solid-state OECT based on this eumelanin/copper composite also demonstrated a performance enhancement with metal chelation [45].

4.4.3 Photoswitches

Another important class of optical transducers is represented by molecular photoswitches that permit modulate cell signaling via a photomechanical effect. In this case, the transduction mechanism originates from the spatial rearrangement of the conformational state upon photoexcitation, which translates into a marked change of the absorption spectrum. It is important to note that such a mechanism is inherently biomimetic as it reproduces the initial fate of the retinal, the chromophore in the retina photoreceptors that is responsible for light sensitivities. Photoswitches are largely employed in several technologies. Beyond classical applications in optoelectronics and data storage, the use of photoswitches to regulate physiological signaling attracted a lot of attention in the last couple of decades. For instance, tethered azobenzenes have been covalently linked to the plasma membrane or ion channels, allowing modulation of the cell potential dynamics in a light-dependent fashion [46]. Alternatively, the non-covalent affinity of the molecules can be exploited to selected bio-target. In the seminal works of Fujiwara and Yonezawa, an aliphatic amphiphilic azobenzene derivative was employed to change the capacitance of black lipid membranes in response to prolonged ultraviolet illumination [47,48]. However, non-covalent optostimulation of neurons with photoswitches has not been achieved until recently. In this regard, our group has proposed new amphiphilic azobenzenes that dwell in the plasma membrane without the need for covalent attachment, inducing light-evoked action potential firing both *in vitro* and *in vivo* [49]. The optomechanical stimulation mechanism stems from the *trans* → *cis* photoreaction of azobenzenes: in the dark, the *trans* isomer can undergo dimerization causing a thinning of the membrane and an increase of its electrical capacitance, while illumination triggers the formation of a stable population of *cis* isomers and, thus, to the disruption of the dimers leading to a restoration of membrane thickness and capacitance (Figure 4.6) [50–52].

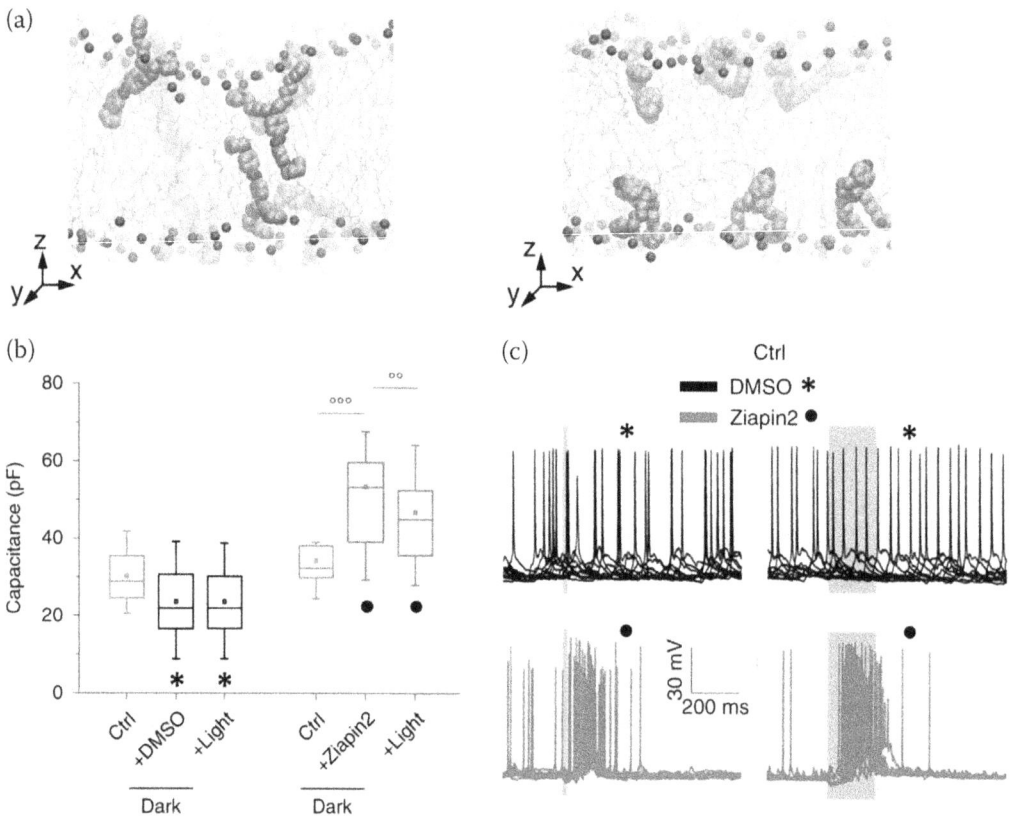

(a)

(b)

(c)

FIGURE 4.6
(a) Snapshots from molecular dynamics simulations of the azobenzene molecules (Ziapin 2) in the trans (left) and cis (right) conformations, respectively. Dimerization causes in the dark causes a thinning of the bilayer, while illumination leads to the *trans* → *cis* photoreaction, the disruption of dimers, and restoration of the initial membrane thickness. (b) Modulation of the membrane capacitance due to the insertion of the amphiphilic azobenzene and its photoreaction. (c) Representative traces showing light-induced neuronal firing. The data on cells treated either with DMSO (vehicle solvent) or with Ziapin 2 reported in (b) and (c) are highlighted by asterisks and full circles, respectively. Adapted with permission [49]. Copyright (2020) Springer Nature.

4.5 Carbon-Based Nanomaterials

Carbon-based materials, such as graphene and its micro and nanostructures, are suitable systems for bioelectronics, owing to their stability, biocompatibility, high mechanical flexibility (especially for thin films), high tunability of their optoelectronics features via chemical doping, and a variety of fabrication methods [20]. In this section, we will be reviewing the use of graphene and relative mico/nanostructures in bioelectronics.

4.5.1 Graphene

Graphene is perhaps one of the most studied materials in the last couple of decades. It displays an extraordinary charge carrier mobility (close to 10,000 $cm^2/V.s$) and a relatively high surface-to-volume ratio. These features make graphene an ideal material for metal electrode coating, usually leading to better charge injection, higher surface area, and lower electrode impedance than the separate constituents. For example, gold-doped graphene has been employed as an electrode in a wearable patch for diabetes monitoring and therapy [53]. Such a combination showed improved electrochemical properties than graphene, as well as stable operation under various mechanical deformations. Graphene has been also widely employed as bioelectronic material for building up devices. For instance, Masvidal-Codina fabricated a graphene solution-gated field-effect transistor that could map out ultraslow (< 0.1 Hz) cortical brain activity that is typical of neurological diseases [54]. In addition, graphene 3D foams can be used as conductive platforms for neuron electrostimulation. In this regard, one relevant work is reported by Liu et al. where high-density micro-electrode arrays of 3D porous graphene were employed for efficient cortical neuromodulation and sensing with minimum invasiveness (Figure 4.7). The excellent broadband optical transparency of graphene (> 90%) has enabled a range of applications, such as simultaneous optical imaging, optogenetic stimulation, and electrophysiology [20]. For instance, Duan and collaborators reported the fabrication of soft graphene contact lens electrodes (GRACEs) with broad-spectrum optical transparency, and their application in conformal, full-cornea recording of electroretinography (ERG) from cynomolgus monkeys [55]. The authors found that the GRACEs give higher signal amplitude than conventional ERG electrodes in recordings of various full-field ERG responses, as well as high-quality topographic mapping of multifocal ERG under simultaneous fundus monitoring.

Furthermore, graphene displays excellent biocompatibility. In particular, it has been reported that graphene can support neural growth without other biocompatible materials. Moreover, its biocompatibility and adhesion to cells and tissues can be further enhanced via material post-processing, such as oxygen plasma treatment or functionalization with poly-L-lysine [20].

4.5.2 Graphene Micro/Nanostructures

Graphene micro/nanostructures can be precisely synthesized for size and density, and hold promise as an approach for next-generation bioelectronic materials [57]. The most important advantage connected to the use of micro/nanostructure lies in the possibility to implement complex device interfaces and establishing close contact with biological systems. One of the most relevant examples is represented by graphene flakes. For example, Cohen-Karni et al. recorded extracellular field potentials from spontaneously beating embryonic chicken cardiomyocytes using a graphene flakes-based field-effect transistor (FET) [58]. The functioning rationale lies in the fact that extracellular field potentials generated during electrical activity induce a change in the conductance of the FET

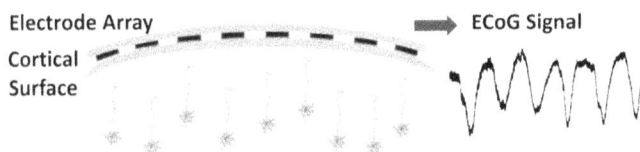

FIGURE 4.7
Schematic of the electrode array placed on top of the cortical surface during the recording. Adapted with permission [56]. Copyright (2018) Springer Nature. Distributed under a Creative Commons Attribution License 4.0 (CC BY) https://creativecommons.org/licenses/by/4.0/.

channel, which enabled electrophysiology recordings when measured as a function of time. By exploiting a similar approach, Hess et al. fabricated graphene-FET arrays for simultaneous multiplexed extracellular field potential recordings from electrogenic cells from up to eight transistors [57]. Another important field of application of graphene structures is intracellular recording, due to the fact that monitoring intracellular action potentials is critical for in-depth electrophysiological and toxicological investigations. In these regards, Dipalo et al. presented a microelectrode platform consisting of out-of-plane grown three-dimensional fuzzy graphene (3DFG) that enables recording of intracellular cardiac action potentials with high signal-to-noise ratio. The authors exploited the generation of hot carriers by ultrafast pulsed laser for opto-porating the cell membrane and creating an intimate contact between the 3DFG electrodes and the intracellular domain [59], enabling the detection of the effects of drugs on the action potential shape of human-derived cardiomyocytes (Figure 4.8). Fuzzy graphene has been also employed for stimulation, recently. Specifically, Cohen-Karni and collaborators reported a hybrid nanomaterial for remote, nongenetic, photothermal stimulation of 2D and 3D neural cellular systems [60]. The authors combined one-dimensional (1D) nanowires (NWs) and 2D graphene flakes grew out-of-plane for highly controlled photothermal stimulation at subcellular precision without the need for genetic modification, with laser energies lower

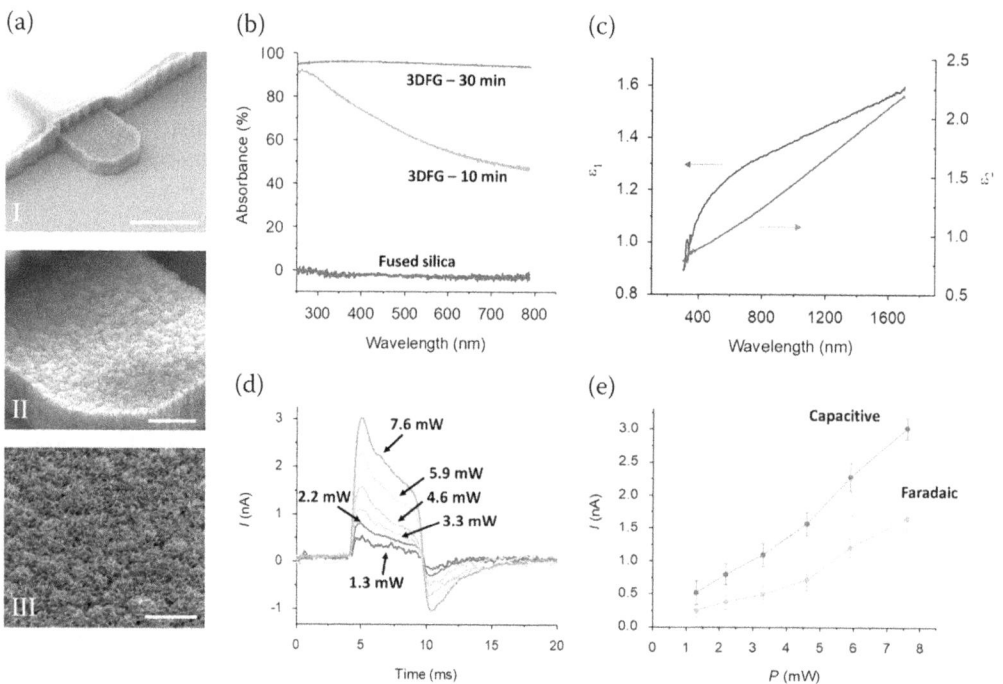

FIGURE 4.8
(a) SEM images of the fuzzy graphene electrode. Scale bars, 5 μm (I), 1 μm (II), and 0.5 μm (III). (b) UV-vis absorption spectrum of the 3DFG. (c) Real and imaginary parts of the dielectric constant of 3DFG. (d) Photocurrent generated at the interface between 3DFG electrodes and PBS under excitation with ultrafast (picosecond) pulsed laser at 1064 nm at different excitation powers. (e) Capacitive and faradaic current components of the photocurrent generated by laser excitation. Adapted with permission [59]. Copyright (2021) American Association for the Advancement of Science. Distributed under a Creative Commons Attribution License 4.0 (CC BY) https://creativecommons.org/licenses/by/4.0/.

than a hundred nanojoules, one to two orders of magnitude lower than Au-, C-, and Si-based nanomaterials. The main advantage connected to such an approach is that photothermal stimulation using NW-templated 3D fuzzy graphene (NT-3DFG) is flexible due to its broadband absorption and does not generate cellular stress.

Another important class of carbon-based and nanostructured material for bioelectronics is represented by carbon nanotubes (CNTs). Similar to graphene, CNTs display the ability to reinforce cell adhesion and growth. The large surface area of CNTs promotes neuron adhesion and the formation of tight junctions between CNTs and neural cell membranes, facilitating sensitive recording or efficient stimulation [20]. Within the context of cell stimulation, Hanein and collaborators reported the development of a CdS/CdSe nanorod-carbon nanotube-based platform for wire-free, light-induced retina stimulation [61]. The authors exploited the high absorption cross-section of the CdS/CdSe nanorods to capture light. The energy absorbed is then transferred to the carbon nanotubes via a charge transfer mechanism, which in turn elicits a response in explanted retinas. Interestingly, such a device has been shown to work with intensities not far from the one needed for real-life applications.

4.6 Perspectives

Materials technology has essentially played a paramount role in the evolution and development of bioelectronics, while organic electronics has certainly inspired new possibilities in the field. Specifically, we believe that these aspects drive not only important breakthroughs but also shape the way how we think about bioelectronics. For instance, the choice of material in-fact governs the following features: i) length scale of interaction with the bio-target, *i.e.* from the molecular scale to the organism; ii) the degree of interaction, *i.e.* from passive components (*i.e.* substrates) to active stimulating/probing elements; iii) the time-scale of interaction, from milliseconds to seconds and minutes. Given these considerations, we expect that research on bioelectronic materials will still fuel future advancements in the field.

For instance, one intriguing approach can be the development of living organic composites that are intrinsically biocompatible, in which two or more material elements are combined to provide properties unattainable by single components. In this regard, Bazan and collaborators have reported on the use of living bioelectronic composites, consisting of living electroactive bacteria and conjugated polymers [62]. These biocomposites spontaneously assemble from solution into an intricate arrangement of cells within a conductive polymer matrix and show almost an order-of-magnitude lower charge transfer resistance than the conjugated polymer alone. According to the authors, this supports the idea that the electroactive bacteria and the conjugated polymers can work synergistically toward an effective bioelectronic composite. Another interesting example is the one reported by Tortiglione and collaborators [63]. Here, the authors reported that a fluorescent semiconducting thiophene dye promotes, *in vivo*, the synthesis of fluorescent conductive protein microfibers via metabolic pathways. By feeding *Hydra vulgaris* with the dye, they demonstrated the stable incorporation of the dye into supramolecular protein-dye co-assembled microfibers. In addition, the appreciable electrical conductivity of such hybrid microfibers can open the door to new opportunities for augmenting electronic functionalities within living tissue, which may be exploited to modulate bioelectrical signaling.

As a final remark, we reckon that although materials aspects are essential in bioelectronics, a bottleneck for this multidisciplinary area is the lack of communication among scientists with different backgrounds. This issue can be overcome by creating a fertile environment based on collaborations between many different groups and institutions, in which this community can grow. Bioelectronics is an outstanding challenge of the 21st century that can provide new tools for translational medicine.

References

1. J. Rivnay, R.M. Owens, G.G. Malliaras, The rise of organic bioelectronics, *Chem. Mater.* 26 (2014) 679–685.
2. C. Pitsalidis, A.-M. Pappa, A.J. Boys, Y. Fu, C.-M. Moysidou, D. van Niekerk, J. Saez, A. Savva, D. Iandolo, R.M. Owens, Organic bioelectronics for in vitro systems, *Chem. Rev* 122 (2022) 4700–4790.
3. G. Lanzani, Materials for bioelectronics: Organic electronics meets biology, *Nat. Mater.* 13 (2014) 775–776.
4. J.L. Carvalho-de-Souza, J.S. Treger, B. Dang, S.B.H. Kent, D.R. Pepperberg, F. Bezanilla, Photosensitivity of neurons enabled by cell-targeted gold nanoparticles, *Neuron.* 86 (2015) 207–217.
5. Y. Jiang, R. Parameswaran, X. Li, J.L. Carvalho-de-Souza, X. Gao, L. Meng, F. Bezanilla, G.M.G. Shepherd, B. Tian, Nongenetic optical neuromodulation with silicon-based materials, *Nat. Protoc.* 14 (2019) 1339–1376.
6. J.H. Burroughes, D.D.C. Bradley, A.R. Brown, R.N. Marks, K. Mackay, R.H. Friend, P.L. Burns, A.B. Holmes, Light-emitting diodes based on conjugated polymers, *Nature.* 347 (1990) 539–541.
7. G.M. Paternò, M.W.A. Skoda, R. Dalgliesh, F. Cacialli, V.G. Sakai, Tuning fullerene intercalation in a Poly (thiophene) derivative by controlling the polymer degree of self-organisation, *Sci. Rep.* 6 (2016) 34609.
8. G.M. Paternò, J.R. Stewart, A. Wildes, F. Cacialli, V.G. Sakai, Neutron polarisation analysis of Polymer:Fullerene blends for organic photovoltaics, *Polymer (Guildf).* 105 (2016) 407–413.
9. H. Sirringhaus, P.J. Brown, R.H. Friend, M.M. Nielsen, K. Bechgaard, B.M.W. Langeveld-Voss, A.J.H. Spiering, R.A.J. Janssen, E.W. Meijer, P. Herwig, D.M. De Leeuw, Two-dimensional charge transport in self-organized, high-mobility conjugated polymers, *Nature.* 401 (1999) 685–688.
10. M. Berggren, A. Richter-Dahlfors, Organic bioelectronics, *Adv. Mater.* 19 (2007) 3201–3213.
11. T.J. Rivers, T.W. Hudson, C.E. Schmidt, Synthesis of a novel, biodegradable electrically conducting polymer for biomedical applications, *Adv. Funct. Mater.* 12 (2002) 33–37.
12. M.D. Angione, S. Cotrone, M. Magliulo, A. Mallardi, D. Altamura, C. Giannini, N. Cioffi, L. Sabbatini, E. Fratini, P. Baglioni, G. Scamarcio, G. Palazzo, L. Torsi, Interfacial electronic effects in functional biolayers integrated into organic field-effect transistors, *Proc. Natl. Acad. Sci. U. S. A.* 109 (2012) 6429–6434.
13. J. Isaksson, P. Kjäll, D. Nilsson, N. Robinson, M. Berggren, A. Richter-Dahlfors, Electronic control of Ca2+ signalling in neuronal cells using an organic electronic ion pump, *Nat. Mater.* 6 (2007) 673–679.
14. C. Pitsalidis, A.M. Pappa, M. Porel, C.M. Artim, G.C. Faria, D.D. Duong, C.A. Alabi, S. Daniel, A. Salleo, R.M. Owens, Biomimetic electronic devices for measuring bacterial membrane disruption, *Adv. Mater.* 30 (2018) 1–8.
15. G.P. Kittlesen, H.S. White, M.S. Wrighton, Chemical derivatization of microelectrode arrays by oxidation of pyrrole and n-methylpyrrole: Fabrication of molecule-based electronic devices, *J. Am. Chem. Soc.* 106 (1984) 7389–7396.

16. D. Khodagholy, T. Doublet, P. Quilichini, M. Gurfinkel, P. Leleux, A. Ghestem, E. Ismailova, T. Hervé, S. Sanaur, C. Bernard, G.G. Malliaras, In vivo recordings of brain activity using organic transistors, *Nat. Commun.* 4 (2013) 1575.

17. A.M.D. Wan, R.M. Schur, C.K. Ober, C. Fischbach, D. Gourdon, G.G. Malliaras, Electrical control of protein conformation, *Adv. Mater.* 24 (2012) 2501–2505.

18. R.L. Razalli, M.M. Abdi, P.M. Tahir, A. Moradbak, Y. Sulaiman, L.Y. Heng, Polyaniline-modified nanocellulose prepared from Semantan bamboo by chemical polymerization: Preparation and characterization, *RSC Adv.* 7 (2017) 25191–25198.

19. J. Liu, Y.S. Kim, C.E. Richardson, A. Tom, C. Ramakrishnan, F. Birey, T. Katsumata, S. Chen, C. Wang, X. Wang, L.-M. Joubert, Y. Jiang, H. Wang, L.E. Fenno, J.B.H. Tok, S.P. Paşca, K. Shen, Z. Bao, K. Deisseroth, Genetically targeted chemical assembly of functional materials in living cells, tissues, and animals, *Science.* 367(80) (2020) 1372–1376.

20. Y. Fang, L. Meng, A. Prominski, E.N. Schaumann, M. Seebald, B. Tian, Recent advances in bioelectronics chemistry, *Chem. Soc. Rev* 49 (2020) 7978–8035.

21. S. Hara, T. Zama, W. Takashima, K. Kaneto, Artificial muscles based on polypyrrole actuators with large strain and stress induced electrically, *Polym. J.* 36 (2004) 151–161.

22. M. Golabi, A.P.F. Turner, E.W.H. Jager, Tunable conjugated polymers for bacterial differentiation, *Sensors Actuators, B Chem.* 222 (2016) 839–848.

23. Y. Wei, X. Mo, P. Zhang, Y. Li, J. Liao, Y. Li, J. Zhang, C. Ning, S. Wang, X. Deng, L. Jiang, Directing stem cell differentiation via electrochemical reversible switching between nanotubes and nanotips of polypyrrole array, *ACS Nano.* 11 (2017) 5915–5924.

24. J. Huang, P.F. Miller, J.S. Wilson, A.J. de Mello, J.C. de Mello, D.D.C. Bradley, Investigation of the effects of doping and post-deposition treatments on the conductivity, morphology, and work function of poly(3,4- ethylenedioxythiophene)/poly(styrene sulfonate) films, *Adv. Funct. Mater.* 15 (2005) 290–296.

25. C. Yeon, G. Kim, J.W. Lim, S.J. Yun, Highly conductive PEDOT:PSS treated by sodium dodecyl sulfate for stretchable fabric heaters, *RSC Adv.* 7 (2017) 5888–5897.

26. D. Pani, A. Dessi, J.F. Saenz-Cogollo, G. Barabino, B. Fraboni, A. Bonfiglio, Fully textile, PEDOT:PSS based electrodes for wearable ECG monitoring systems, *IEEE Trans. Biomed. Eng.* 63 (2016) 540–549.

27. D. Gan, Z. Huang, X. Wang, L. Jiang, C. Wang, M. Zhu, F. Ren, L. Fang, K. Wang, C. Xie, X. Lu, Graphene oxide-templated conductive and redox-active nanosheets incorporated hydrogels for adhesive bioelectronics, *Adv. Funct. Mater.* 30 (2020) 1907678.

28. R.A. Green, N.H. Lovell, G.G. Wallace, L.A. Poole-Warren, Conducting polymers for neural interfaces: Challenges in developing an effective long-term implant, *Biomaterials.* 29 (2008) 3393–3399.

29. C. Tortiglione, M.R. Antognazza, A. Tino, C. Bossio, V. Marchesano, A. Bauduin, M. Zangoli, S.V. Morata, G. Lanzani, Semiconducting polymers are light nanotransducers in eyeless animals, *Sci. Adv.* 3 (2017) e1601699.

30. G. Bondelli, S. Sardar, G. Chiaravalli, V. Vurro, G.M. Paternò, G. Lanzani, C. D'Andrea, Shedding light on thermally induced optocapacitance at the organic biointerface, *J. Phys. Chem. B.* 125 (2021) 10748–10758.

31. F. Lodola, V. Vurro, S. Crasto, E. Di Pasquale, G. Lanzani, Optical pacing of human-induced pluripotent stem cell-derived cardiomyocytes mediated by a conjugated polymer interface, *Adv. Healthc. Mater.* 8 (2019) 1–7.

32. D. Ghezzi, M.R. Antognazza, R. MacCarone, S. Bellani, E. Lanzarini, N. Martino, M. Mete, G. Pertile, S. Bisti, G. Lanzani, F. Benfenati, A polymer optoelectronic interface restores light sensitivity in blind rat retinas, *Nat. Photonics.* 7 (2013) 400–406.

33. P. Feyen, E. Colombo, D. Endeman, M. Nova, L. Laudato, N. Martino, M.R. Antognazza, G. Lanzani, F. Benfenati, D. Ghezzi, Light-evoked hyperpolarization and silencing of neurons by conjugated polymers, *Sci. Rep.* 6 (2016) 22718.

34. J.F. Maya-Vetencourt, D. Ghezzi, M.R. Antognazza, E. Colombo, M. Mete, P. Feyen, A. Desii, A. Buschiazzo, M. Di Paolo, S. Di Marco, F. Ticconi, L. Emionite, D. Shmal, C. Marini,

I. Donelli, G. Freddi, R. Maccarone, S. Bisti, G. Sambuceti, G. Pertile, G. Lanzani, F. Benfenati, A fully organic retinal prosthesis restores vision in a rat model of degenerative blindness, *Nat. Mater.* 16 (2017) 681–689.

35. J.F. Maya-Vetencourt, G. Manfredi, M. Mete, E. Colombo, M. Bramini, S. Di Marco, D. Shmal, G. Mantero, M. Dipalo, A. Rocchi, M.L. DiFrancesco, E.D. Papaleo, A. Russo, J. Barsotti, C. Eleftheriou, F. Di Maria, V. Cossu, F. Piazza, L. Emionite, F. Ticconi, C. Marini, G. Sambuceti, G. Pertile, G. Lanzani, F. Benfenati, Subretinally injected semiconducting polymer nanoparticles rescue vision in a rat model of retinal dystrophy, *Nat. Nanotechnol.* 15 (2020) 698–708.

36. L. Ferlauto, M.J.I. Airaghi Leccardi, N.A.L. Chenais, S.C.A. Gilliéron, P. Vagni, M. Bevilacqua, T.J. Wolfensberger, K. Sivula, D. Ghezzi, Design and validation of a foldable and photovoltaic wide-field epiretinal prosthesis, *Nat. Commun.* 9 (2018) 1–15.

37. J. Du, C. Catania, G.C. Bazan, Modification of Abiotic–Biotic Interfaces with Small Molecules and Nanomaterials for Improved Bioelectronics, *Chem. Mater.* 26 (2014) 686–697.

38. S. Cheng, B.E. Logan, Ammonia treatment of carbon cloth anodes to enhance power generation of microbial fuel cells, *Electrochem. Commun.* 9 (2007) 492–496.

39. H. Yan, C. Catania, G.C. Bazan, Membrane-intercalating conjugated oligoelectrolytes: Impact on bioelectrochemical systems, *Adv. Mater.* 27 (2015) 2958–2973.

40. B. Wang, M. Wang, A. Mikhailovsky, S. Wang, G.C. Bazan, A. Membrane-Intercalating, Conjugated oligoelectrolyte with high-efficiency photodynamic antimicrobial activity, *Angew. Chemie – Int. Ed.* 56 (2017) 5031–5034.

41. B. Wang, B.N. Queenan, S. Wang, K.P.R. Nilsson, G.C. Bazan, Precisely defined conjugated oligoelectrolytes for biosensing and therapeutics, *Adv. Mater.* 31 (2019) 1–21.

42. C.W. Tang, Two-layer organic photovoltaic cell, *Appl. Phys. Lett.* 48 (1986) 183–185.

43. D. Rand, M. Jake ová, G. Lubin, I. Vėbraitė, M. David-Pur, V. Ðerek, T. Cramer, N.S. Sariciftci, Y. Hanein, E.D. Głowacki, Direct electrical neurostimulation with organic pigment photocapacitors, *Adv. Mater.* 30 (2018) 1707292.

44. M. Jake ová, M. Silverå Ejneby, V. Ðerek, T. Schmidt, M. Gryszel, J. Brask, R. Schindl, D.T. Simon, M. Berggren, F. Elinder, E.D. Głowacki, Optoelectronic control of single cells using organic photocapacitors, *Sci. Adv.* 5 (2019) eaav5265.

45. J.V. Paulin, C.F.O. Graeff, From nature to organic (bio)electronics: a review on melanin-inspired materials, *J. Mater. Chem. C.* 9 (2021) 14514–14531.

46. J. Zhang, J. Wang, H. Tian, Taking orders from light: Progress in photochromic bio-materials, *Mater. Horizons.* 1 (2014) 169–184.

47. H. Fujiwara, Y. Yonezawa, Photoelectric response of a black lipid membrane containing an amphiphilic azobenzene derivative, *Nature.* 351 (1991) 724–726.

48. Y. Yonezawa, H. Fujiwara, T. Sato, Photoelectric response of black lipid membranes incorporating an amphiphilic azobenzene derivative, *Thin Solid Films.* 210–211 (1992) 736–738.

49. M.L. DiFrancesco, F. Lodola, E. Colombo, L. Maragliano, M. Bramini, G.M. Paternò, P. Baldelli, M.D. Serra, L. Lunelli, M. Marchioretto, G. Grasselli, S. Cimò, L. Colella, D. Fazzi, F. Ortica, V. Vurro, C.G. Eleftheriou, D. Shmal, J.F. Maya-Vetencourt, C. Bertarelli, G. Lanzani, F. Benfenati, Neuronal firing modulation by a membrane-targeted photoswitch, *Nat. Nanotechnol.* 15 (2020) 296–306.

50. G.M. Paternò, E. Colombo, V. Vurro, F. Lodola, S. Cimò, V. Sesti, E. Molotokaite, M. Bramini, L. Ganzer, D. Fazzi, C. D'Andrea, F. Benfenati, C. Bertarelli, G. Lanzani, Membrane environment enables ultrafast isomerization of amphiphilic azobenzene, *Adv. Sci.* 7 (2020) 1903241.

51. G.M. Paterno, G. Lanzani, G. Bondelli, V.G. Sakai, V. Sesti, C. Bertarelli, The effect of an intramembrane light-actuator on the dynamics of phospholipids in model membranes and intact cells, *Langmuir.* 36 (2020) 11517–11527.

52. V. Vurro, G. Bondelli, V. Sesti, F. Lodola, G.M. Paternò, G. Lanzani, C. Bertarelli, Molecular design of amphiphilic plasma membrane-targeted azobenzenes for nongenetic optical stimulation, *Front. Mater.* 7 (2021) 472.

53. H. Lee, T.K. Choi, Y.B. Lee, H.R. Cho, R. Ghaffari, L. Wang, H.J. Choi, T.D. Chung, N. Lu, T. Hyeon, S.H. Choi, D.H. Kim, A graphene-based electrochemical device with thermo-responsive microneedles for diabetes monitoring and therapy, *Nat. Nanotechnol.* 11 (2016) 566–572.
54. E. Masvidal-Codina, X. Illa, M. Dasilva, A.B. Calia, T. Dragojević, E.E. Vidal-Rosas, E. Prats-Alfonso, J. Martínez-Aguilar, J.M. De la Cruz, R. Garcia-Cortadella, P. Godignon, G. Rius, A. Camassa, E. Del Corro, J. Bousquet, C. Hébert, T. Durduran, R. Villa, M.V. Sanchez-Vives, J.A. Garrido, A. Guimerà-Brunet, High-resolution mapping of infraslow cortical brain activity enabled by graphene microtransistors, *Nat. Mater.* 18 (2019) 280–288.
55. R. Yin, Z. Xu, M. Mei, Z. Chen, K. Wang, Y. Liu, T. Tang, M.K. Priydarshi, X. Meng, S. Zhao, B. Deng, H. Peng, Z. Liu, X. Duan, Soft transparent graphene contact lens electrodes for conformal full-cornea recording of electroretinogram, *Nat. Commun.* 9 (2018) 2334.
56. X. Liu, Y. Lu, D. Kuzum, High-density porous graphene arrays enable detection and analysis of propagating cortical waves and spirals, *Sci. Rep.* 8 (2018) 17089.
57. R. Garg, D.S. Roman, Y. Wang, D. Cohen-Karni, T. Cohen-Karni, Graphene nanostructures for input–output bioelectronics, *Biophys. Rev.* 2 (2021) 041304. 10.1063/5.0073870.
58. T. Cohen-Karni, Q. Qing, Q. Li, Y. Fang, C.M. Lieber, Graphene and nanowire transistors for cellular interfaces and electrical recording, *Nano Lett.* 10 (2010) 1098–1102.
59. M. Dipalo, S.K. Rastogi, L. Matino, R. Garg, J. Bliley, G. Iachetta, G. Melle, R. Shrestha, S. Shen, F. Santoro, A.W. Feinberg, A. Barbaglia, T. Cohen-Karni, F. De Angelis, Intracellular action potential recordings from cardiomyocytes by ultrafast pulsed laser irradiation of fuzzy graphene microelectrodes, *Sci. Adv.* 7 (2021) 5175.
60. S.K. Rastogi, R. Garg, M.G. Scopelliti, B.I. Pinto, J.E. Hartung, S. Kim, C.G.E. Murphey, N. Johnson, D. San Roman, F. Bezanilla, J.F. Cahoon, M.S. Gold, M. Chamanzar, T. Cohen-Karni, Remote nongenetic optical modulation of neuronal activity using fuzzy graphene, *Proc. Natl. Acad. Sci.* 117 (2020) 13339–13349.
61. L. Bareket, N. Waiskopf, D. Rand, G. Lubin, M. David-Pur, J. Ben-Dov, S. Roy, C. Eleftheriou, E. Sernagor, O. Cheshnovsky, U. Banin, Y. Hanein, Semiconductor nanorod-carbon nanotube biomimetic films for wire-free photostimulation of blind retinas, *Nano Lett.* 14 (2014) 6685–6692.
62. S.R. McCuskey, Y. Su, D. Leifert, A.S. Moreland, G.C. Bazan, Living bioelectrochemical composites, *Adv. Mater.* 1908178 (2020) 1908178.
63. M. Moros, F. Di Maria, P. Dardano, G. Tommasini, H. Castillo-Michel, A. Kovtun, M. Zangoli, M. Blasio, L. De Stefano, A. Tino, G. Barbarella, C. Tortiglione, In vivo bioengineering of fluorescent conductive protein-dye microfibers, *IScience.* 23 (2020) 101022.

5

Nanomaterials and Lab-on-a-Chip Technologies

Noorhashimah Mohamad Nor and Nurul Hidayah Ramli

School of Materials and Mineral Resources Engineering, Universiti Sains Malaysia, Nibong Tebal, Penang, Malaysia

Nor Dyana Zakaria

NanoBiotechnology Research & Innovation (NanoBRI), INFORMM, Universiti Sains Malaysia, Penang, Malaysia

Khairunisak Abdul Razak

School of Materials and Mineral Resources Engineering, Universiti Sains Malaysia, Nibong Tebal, Penang, Malaysia

NanoBiotechnology Research & Innovation (NanoBRI), INFORMM, Universiti Sains Malaysia, Penang, Malaysia

CONTENTS

5.1 Introduction to LOC

The integration of nanomaterials in lab-on-a-chip (LOC) technologies has received wide attention from researchers to develop a LOC device for a wide range of applications including clinical diagnostic, environmental analysis, food safety, and therapeutic analysis [1,2]. LOC is a miniaturized version of multi-component parts in laboratory analysis. The miniaturization of LOC devices allows a simple, low sample volume, and portable and mobile chemical analysis. LOC devices are also classified as the point of care (POC), microfluidic, microfluidic immunoarray device (µID), miniaturized total analysis system (µTAS), and microfluidic paper-based analytical devices (µPADs).

LOC devices integrate several parts including sample input, recognition element or sensor, transducer, and signal processing parts, as shown in Figure 5.1. The sample input

DOI: 10.1201/9781003263265-5

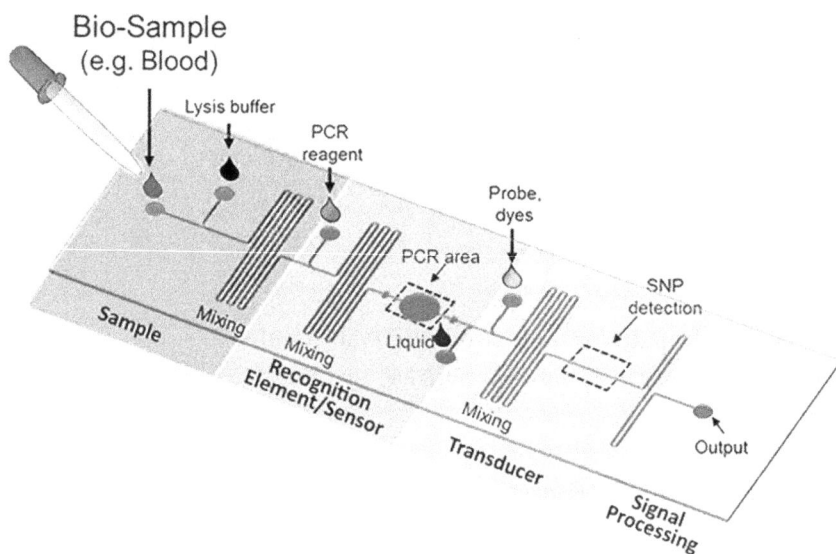

FIGURE 5.1
General components of LOC devices. Adapted with permission [4]. Copyright (2015). The Authors, some rights reserved; exclusive licensee [MDPI]. Distributed under a Creative Commons Attribution License 4.0 (CC BY) https://creativecommons.org/licenses/by/4.0/.

is the part where a multichannel or microfluidic component is placed for the analyte fluid transport and mixing into the LOC device. Various sample analytes including pathogen, pesticide, wastewater, blood, food, and urine are developed for the LOC devices. The recognition element or sensor part in LOC devices consists of components that provide selectivity to the target analyte and place where detection takes place. The selection of recognition elements is depending on the type of target analyte. An antibody or aptamer recognition element is commonly applied for diagnostic, bacteria, and pathogen detection, whereas the enzymes are commonly applied for the catalytic reaction. A transducer consists of a component that translates the interaction of analyte and recognition elements into a measurable and quantifiable signal. The measurable signal can be in the form of an optical, electrochemical, and electrical signal. Commonly the type of transducer is designated based on the physicochemical reaction that takes place at the sensing platform [3]. Both transducers and recognition elements are important for enhancing the sensitivity and detection limit of the LOC devices. A signal processing unit in LOC devices consists of electronic components that are responsible to translate and analyze data from the transducer into a visualized sensing result.

Most importantly, the LOC devices must be able to provide high sensitivity, accuracy, rapid, reliable, and real-time quantification for the analyte sample. Nanomaterials that have a large surface area and excellent electrical and chemical properties may improve the optical, electrochemical, and electrical performance of the sensor part in LOC devices [4]. A range of nanomaterials including metal, metal oxide, and carbon-based nanomaterials are widely investigated for improvement in the sensor part of the LOC devices [2,5]. Metallic nanomaterials such as gold (Au), silver (Ag), platinum (Pt), and nickel (Ni) have been used as a modifier of sensor surface due to their advantages in amplifying the signal of the sensor. Metallic nanomaterials such as Au and Ag have unique optical and electronic properties due to the close position of their conduction and valence band. Electrons can easily move to form the surface plasmon resonance (SPR) that is useful in providing sensitive detection for optical sensors [6].

Metal oxide nanoparticles such as zinc oxide (ZnO), iron oxide (Fe_3O_4), manganese oxide (MnO_2), copper oxide (CuO), cerium oxide (CeO_2), and titanium oxide (TiO_2) are applied as the signal enhancement for electrochemical sensors, biosensors, and electrical devices. Metal oxide nanomaterials have excellent chemical, electrical, and physical properties. The carbon-based nanomaterials, especially carbon nanotubes (CNT) and graphene nanomaterials, show excellent properties in improving the sensing capability in LOC devices owing to their changeable optical properties and bandgap energy, excellent conductivity for electron transfer, and the novel structure. In this chapter, the authors aim to provide an overview of the LOC design, detection techniques, and the role of nanomaterials in LOC devices applications. Additionally, the fabrication strategies, properties, and sensing applications of nanomaterials in LOC technologies are discussed based on excellent published works in recent research and future trends.

5.2 Lab-on-a-Chip Detection Technique

The transducers of the LOC devices can be classified into optical, electrochemical, and electrical types. In optical-based LOC devices, the optical changes caused by the interaction of sample analyte with recognition element are analyzed in the form of color, absorption, transmission, or emission of light. Commonly, the optical LOC devices are categorized based on optical detection techniques such as calorimetry, surface plasmon resonance (SPR), fluorescence, and chemiluminescence (CL). The optical detection in LOC devices offers advantages of low LOD, suitable for various types of analytes, nondestructive and rapid detection techniques. However, optical detection LOC devices suffer limitations in the form of bulky and expensive optical equipment and interference from the surrounding condition. The working principle of various transducers types, detection techniques, and types of nanomaterials applied are summarized in Table 5.1.

As for the electrochemical-based LOC devices, the changes in the electrochemical response caused by the interaction of sample analyte with recognition element are measured in the form of amperometric (current), voltammetric (current), and impedance (impedimetric). In an electrochemical LOC device, the device is commonly fabricated with the integration of a three-electrode system consisting of a working electrode (WE) as the sensing platform, reference electrode (RE) acts as a reference in measuring the WE potential, counter electrode (CE) to complete the current circuit, and a potentiostat to control the potential difference between WE and RE. The function of nanomaterials in this type of measurement is not limited to analyte labeling but also acts as a catalyst for the chemical reaction. The advantages of electrochemical LOC devices are high sensitivity, low LOD, high specificity, and low power requirement, which are suitable for miniaturization of the LOC devices. However, the limitations of electrochemical LOC devices are the requirement of redox elements to enhance the signal and interference from the surrounding condition.

In field-effect transistor (FET)–based LOC devices, the changes in conductance caused by the interaction between analyte and recognition element are measured. The FET detection technique is commonly composed of a semiconducting channel as the sensor platform that connects the source and the drain electrodes. Any reaction that occurs on the channel surface causes changes in the electric field that control the potential of a gate

TABLE 5.1

The LOC Detection Techniques, Principles, and Nanomaterials Applied

Transducer	Detection technique	Principles	Nanomaterials
Optical	Colorimetric	• The color changes are caused by a reaction between the analyte sample and the recognition element. • Evaluate qualitatively (by the naked eye) or quantitatively (by smartphones or flatbed scanners)	Aggregation of AuNPs or AgNPs nanoparticles
	Surface Plasmon Resonance (SPR)	• Observe and measure the changes in the refractive index of metal nanoparticles causes by the reaction between the analyte sample and the recognition element. • Aggregation of metal nanoparticles causes shifting in the SPR peak to a longer wavelength	Aggregation of AuNPs or AgNPs nanoparticles
	Fluorescence	• Measure the fluorescence property of the reaction between analyte and recognition element to absorb light at a specific wavelength and emit it at a longer wavelength	Fluorescence signal enhancement by AuNPs, AgNPs, Graphene QDs, Carbon QDs, SiNPs
	Chemiluminescence (CL)	• Measure the electromagnetic radiation caused by a reaction of analyte and recognition element in the visible or near IR region resulting by a redox reaction between two CL regents	CL signal enhancement by Graphene NPs, AuNPs, PtNPs, IONPs, and NiNPs
Electrochemical	Amperometric	• Measure an oxidation or reduction current caused by the chemical reaction of analyte and recognition element under a constant potential supplied over a period of time	Amperometric signal enhancement by AuNPs, AgNPs, PtNPs, Graphene NPs. MWCNT, GO NPs
	Voltammetric	• Measure the current dependence on potential changes caused by chemical reaction of analyte and recognition element • Potential changes in various ways; potential scan, potential step, and stripping voltammetry	Current signal enhancement by AuNPs, AgNPs, PtNPs, Graphene NPs. MWCNT, GO NPs, MnO$_2$
	Impedimetric	• Measure the electrical impedance signal caused by chemical reaction of analyte and recognition element	Signal enhancement by AuNPs, PtNPs MWCNT, GO NS, IONPs, SnO$_2$
Electrical	Field-effect transistor	Measure the change of conductance caused by the reaction of analyte and recognition element	Conductivity enhancement is caused by AuNPs, AgNPs, Graphene NPs. ZnO, IONPs, MnO$_2$ NP, SnO$_2$ NP

Abbreviation: QDs: quantum dots; SiNPs: silicone nanoparticles; PtNPs: platinum nanoparticles; IONPs: iron oxide nanoparticles; NiNPs: nickel nanoparticles; MWCNT: multiwalled carbon nanotube; GO NPs: graphene oxide nanoparticles; MnO$_2$: manganese dioxide nanoparticles; SnO$_2$ NPs: tin oxide nanoparticles.

electrode and change the drain current value. The change in the drain current value acts as the detection mechanism of the LOC devices. The FET-based LOC devices have advantages such as being small in size, suitable for mass production, and low cost.

5.3 Nanomaterials and Lab-on-a-Chip Technologies

The application of nanomaterials in the development of LOC devices is important for miniaturization, improving the sensor performance, enhancing electrical conductivity, maintaining chemical stability, and offering biocompatibility. In LOC devices, nanomaterials based on metal, metal oxide, and carbon are applied for modification of sensor platform to enhance the optical, electrochemical, and electrical performance. In the following section, the functions and capabilities of various types of nanomaterials for the modification of sensor parts of the LOC devices are discussed.

5.3.1 Metal Nanomaterials

Metallic nanomaterials such as gold (Au), silver (Ag), platinum (Pt), and nickel (Ni) have been used as a modifier of sensor platform in LOC devices owing to their advantages in amplifying the signal of sensors. Among all types of metal nanomaterials, Au nanomaterials are the most commonly applied in various sensor applications. Au nanomaterials are simple to make in a variety of sizes and shapes, easy to functionalize, compatible with biomolecules, have great electrical conductivity, and excellent optical properties. Besides that, Au nanomaterials are inert and stable against oxidation. The Au nanomaterials can be synthesized via numerous physio-chemical and biological routes to vary the size, shape, concentration, and surface chemistry [5]. The size and shape of Au nanomaterials may greatly influence their optical properties.

The most common applications of Au nanomaterials are in labeling and colorimetric assay in POC and LOC devices. Besides that, Au nanomaterials are commonly applied in electrode modification for electrochemical sensors. Au nanomaterials have a large surface-to-volume ratio that results in higher sensitivity and selectivity as well as enhancing the sensor response. The basic mechanism of Au nanomaterials in colorimetric detection is based on the binding of target analyte with Au nanomaterials, which cause aggregation. Generally, the Au nanomaterials are in red or pink color and change to purple and blue when aggregated. The Au nanomaterials aggregation also is associated with SPR peak shifts. This phenomenon occurs due to the enlargement of particle size of Au nanomaterials, which alters the local electron confinement and causes the SPR peak shifts [6]. Table 5.2 lists metal nanomaterials applied in LOC devices for various applications and detection techniques.

Zheng et al. [7] established a novel colorimetric biosensor for microfluidic LOC that uses AuNPs as a labeling agent to detect different *E. coli* O157:H7 concentrations. Then, the colorimetric biosensor is integrated with a smartphone imaging application (app) to observe the AuNPs color changes. The colorimetric biosensor for microfluidic LOC has been developed using 3D printing to fabricate the mold of the channel, silicone elastomer kit to produce poly(dimethoxy)silane (PDMS) channel, and glass slide to bond with PDMS channel. As shown in Figure 5.2a, the colorimetric biosensor for microfluidic LOC consists of three components, the first component is the mixing channel for the

TABLE 5.2

Metal Nanomaterials Applied in LOC Devices for Various Applications and Detection Techniques

Nanomaterials-electrode/LOC	Applications/analyte	Types of sensors	Detection technique	Linear range	LOD	Reference
AuNP/glass-PDMS microfluidic	Foodborne pathogens (E. coli O157:H7)	Optical Biosensor	Colorimetric of AuNPs aggregation and smartphone imaging	5.0×10^1–5.0×10^8 CFU/mL	50 CFU/mL	[7]
AuNPs-MWCNT/Aptamer/microwell plate	Foodborne pathogens (E. coli O157:H7)	Optical Biosensor	Colorimetric of AuNPs aggregation and smartphone imaging	–	524 cfu/mL	[8]
AuNPs-anti AB1 antibody/Au chip	Food Content (Aflatoxin B1)	Optical Biosensor	Surface Plasmon Resonance	0.01–50 nM	0.003 nM	[9]
AuNPs/glass-PDMS microwell plate	Heavy Metal (Pb(II) & Al(III))	Optical Sensor	Surface Plasmon Resonance	0–500 ppb / 0–400 ppb	30 ppb / 89 ppb	[10]
AuNPs/ITO/Sandwich glass slide	Heavy Metal (Hg(II))	Electrochemical Sensor	DPASV	0.63–80 ppb	0.11 ppb	[11]
AuNPs/Glass microchip	DNA	Optical Biosensor	Laser-induced fluorescence (LIF)	50–500 nM	2.6 zepto mole	[12]
AgNPs-aptamer/glass-PDMS microfluidic	Protein (Thrombin)	Optical Sensor	Colorimetric of AgNPs	20–5000 pM	20 pM	[13]
AgNPs/Chitosan/PGE microfluidic	H_2O_2	Electrochemical Sensor	Cyclic Voltammetry	1–10 µM	0.52 µM	[14]
AgNPs-PDDA/glass-PDMS microfluidic	Foodborne pathogens (E. coli O157:H7)	Electrochemical Biosensor	Impedimetric	2×10^3–2×10^5 cfu/mL	500 cfu·mL	[15]
PtNPs/PDMS microfluidic	Vitamin B	Optical Sensor	Chemilluminescence	1.0×10^{-7}–4.0×10^{-5} mol/L	4.8×10^{-9} mol/L	[16]
PtNPs-HRP/BDD/PDMS microfluidic	Pesticide (Atrazine)	Electrochemical Sensor	Chronoamperometry	0.9–4.5 nM	3 pM	[17]
AuNPs-PtNCs	Salmonella Typhimurium	Optical Biosensor	Microplate reader	1.8×10^1–1.8×10^7 25 CFU/mL	17 CFU/mL	[18]

Abbreviation: DPASV: differential pulse anodic stripping voltammetry.

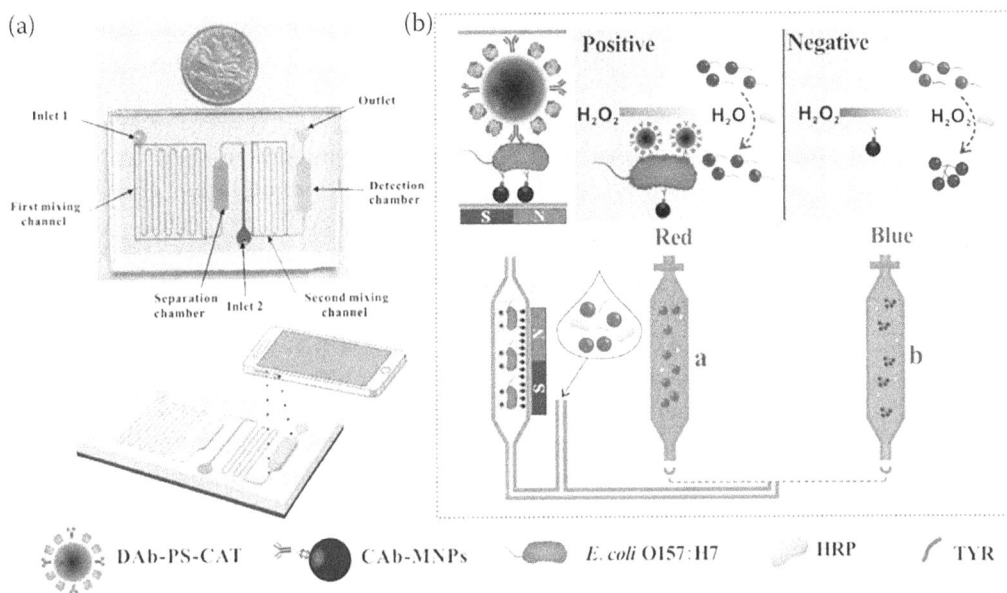

FIGURE 5.2
(a) The colorimetric biosensor microfluidic LOC components, and (b) mechanism of the colorimetric biosensor microfluidic LOC based on AuNPs aggregation and smartphone imaging for rapid detection of *E. coli* O157:H7. Adapted with permission [7]. Copyright (2019) Elsevier.

bacterial and magnetic nanoparticles (MNP) – polystyrene (PS) microsphere, the second component is for the catalyst and AuNPs cross-linking mixing channel, and the third component is for the detection chamber. The detection mechanism of the colorimetric biosensor for microfluidic LOC was based on the aggregation of AuNPs, which were then evaluated using a smartphone for imaging (Figure 5.2b). In the presence of *E. coli* O157:H7, aggregation of AuNPs was avoided, and the solution color remained red. Without *E. coli*, AuNPs aggregation occurred due to the MNP-bacteria-PS complexes not forming thus causing H_2O_2 not to catalyze. The AuNPs solution changed color from red to blue. The color changes from the reaction were evaluated using a Hue-Saturation-Lightness–based imaging app using an Android smartphone imaging to quantify the concentration of the target bacteria. The colorimetric biosensor for microfluidic LOC showed the linear detection of 5.0×10^1 to 5.0×10^8 cfu/mL, and lower LOD of 50 cfu/mL for detection of *E. coli* O157:H7 in chicken samples.

Recently, the application of AuNPs and multi-walled carbon nanotubes (MWCNT) as a label for *E. coli* O157:H7 detection was developed and evaluated using the smartphone-based colorimetric device [8]. The colorimetric device was made of acrylic plates, a light-emitting diode, and a mobile power box. With the presence of *E. coli* O157:H7, the AuNP-Aptamer that binds with *E. coli* O157:H7 remained red because of no aggregation of AuNPs. However, without *E. coli* O157:H7, the AuNP-Aptamer aggregated and appeared in blue. The colorimetric aptasensor showed LOD of 430 cfu/mL and 524 cfu/mL of *E. coli* O157:H7 when tested in pure culture and artificially contaminated milk, respectively.

Another important application of AuNPs is in the SPR biosensor application. AuNPs act as signal amplification and provide a large biocompatible surface area for binding with high-affinity biomolecules (such as an antibody, aptamer, and enzyme), which are specific towards analyte molecules to be detected. The isotropic structure of AuNPs permits strong optical coupling in every direction of the incident light, thus enhancing the sensitivity of AuNPs in SPR. The AuNPs integrated sensor chip for the detection of Aflatoxin B1 (AFB1) detection using SPR equipment has been developed by Bhardwaj et al. [9]. The AuNPs acted as SPR signal amplifiers and provided a larger area for immobilization of anti-AFB1 antibodies. The Au chips were integrated with AuNPs conjugated with anti-AFB1 antibodies (AuNPs- anti-AFB1 Ab) as the target and analyzed using the flow cell of the SPR-2 system. The AuNPs/anti-AFB1 antibodies/Au sensor chips response linearly for AFB1 detection from 0.01 to 50 nM, and LOD of 0.003 nM.

Colorimetric and SPR sensor detection are also employed in heavy metal detection. The portable heavy metal detection has been developed using AuNPs-based colorimetric technique integrated into the LOC device for Pb(II) and Al(III) ions detection [10]. The mechanism of detection is based on an aggregation of AuNPs caused by the chemically functionalized AuNPs coordinate with metal ions, resulting in shifting of the AuNPs SPR absorbance. The LOC device was developed by integrating the custom-made PDMS and glass microwell plate for sample analysis with a hand-held colorimetric reader for quantifying the absorbance shifting of the AuNPs solutions after reaction with heavy metal ions. The hand-held colorimetric reader is made of a narrow-band light-emitting diode (LED), photodiodes, printed circuit board, and microcontroller. The microcontroller functions as a LED controller, measuring the voltage output of the photodiode and transmitting measurement data to a computer. The developed portable LOC device can detect the Pb(II) and Al(III) with LOD of 30 ppb and 89 ppb, respectively.

The LOC of ITO electrode modified with electrodeposited AuNPs as the modified WE, Ag/AgCl as the RE, and ITO as the CE has been developed for online Hg(II) detection using electrochemical technique [11]. The ITO electrode was patterned with a three-electrode electrochemical system attached with a low volume cell. The AuNP/ITO on a chip was developed by the sandwich method linked to automatic sample injection systems, potentiostat, computer, and container for sample waste. The benefits of the AuNP/ITO on-chip for heavy metal detection are the small size and portability of the device for on-site measurement, one-step procedure due to automatic sample input using flow cell, and accuracy of measurement due to undiluted sample. The AuNP/ITO on-chip showed good electrochemical Hg(II) detection with a linearity of 0.63–80 ppb and LOD of 0.11 ppb.

Another metal nanomaterial that is widely applied in LOC devices is AgNPs. AgNPs have excellent optical, electrical, and biological properties to improve the sensor performance of the LOC device. AgNPs exhibits enhanced color visualization and high sensitivity, especially in optical sensor applications. However, AgNPs require stabilization or functionalization to provide colloidal stability, prevent aggregation and oxidation. Commonly, AgNPs are functionalized with polymeric molecules such as polyvinyl alcohol (PVA), polyethylene glycol (PEG), and polyvinylpyrrolidone (PVP) or surfactants such as citrate and cetyltrimethylammonium bromide (CTAB). A microfluidic LOC device for protein biomarker thrombin detection was developed by Zhao et al. [13]. The AgNPs-aptasensor was used as the labeling agent for specifically detecting the thrombin protein on a glass/PDMS microfluidic LOC. The AgNPs calorimetric color changes were quantified based on color shade grading or converted into grayscale value using a flatbed scanner. The AgNPs yellow color faded as the concentration of thrombin decreased. This happened because of the low AgNPs-aptamer complex present. The developed calorimetric LOC was able to detect the thrombin protein with LOD of 20 pM.

Salve et al. [14] reported on 3D microfluidic LOC for the supercapacitor and electrochemical sensor for H_2O_2 detection. A pencil graphite electrode (PGE) has been used as the electrode and was modified with AgNPs and chitosan. The microfluidic device contained a microchannel, reservoir, and inlet hole. The transparent glass slide was used to attach the channel. The AgNPs could enhance the storage capacity, electrical conductivity, and electrocatalytic properties, while chitosan may provide hydrophilicity and functional group for hydrogen binding with amine and hydroxyl group. The AgNPs/Chitosan/PGE electrode showed high storage capacity of 367.16 mF/cm^2 and a current density of 1 mA/cm^2 with high cyclic stability of more than 1,500 charge-discharge cycles. As for electrochemical sensors in H_2O_2 detection, the microfluidic AgNPs/Chitosan/PGE had linear detection of 1-10M and LOD of 0.52M.

PtNPs have also been utilized for the development of LOC devices. The microfluidic LOC for vitamin B detection was developed based on chemiluminescence (CL) of luminol [16]. In their work, PtNPs acted as a catalyst to enhance the luminol CL signal caused by the oxidation of $AgNO_3$. With the presence of vitamin B, the CL of luminol signal intensity increased. The microfluidic LOC was fabricated using soft lithography of the PDMS with four sample inlets and one sample outlet. The microfluidic LOC for vitamin B detection has the linear detection in the range of 1.0×10^{7} to 4.0×10^{5} mol/L and LOD of 4.8×10^{9} mol/L. In addition, an interesting LOC device which consists of two platforms for pesticide atrazine (Atz) detection and degradation was developed by Sánchez et al. [17]. The enzymatic activity of the boron-doped diamond (BDD) electrodes modified with PtNPs and horseradish peroxidase (HRP) in Atz detection was evaluated using the chronoamperometry technique. The PtNPs had improved the catalytic activity of the HRP enzymatic reaction. The magnetic beads were integrated into the LOC device to preconcentrate and direct the sample into the microchannel. Meanwhile, the degradation of the Atz pesticide was conducted using anodic electrochemical oxidation where the unmodified BDD electrode acted as the anode, carbon electrode as the cathode, and Ag/AgCl as the reference electrode. In the anodic electrochemical oxidation, the oxidation of water produced hydroxyls radicals (HO·) on the BDD anode surface. The produced HO· radicals subsequently reacted with the Atz pesticide and caused degradation. The Atz LOC chip showed a linear response in the range of 0.9–4.5 nM and a very low LOD of 3.5 pM.

5.3.2 Metal Oxide Nanomaterials in Lab on Chip

Metal oxide (MO) nanomaterials have been explored for modification of sensor platforms in LOC devices. The MO nanomaterials exhibit high surface area, excellent electron-transfer kinetics, inexpensive to produce, and have effective catalytic properties, making them an excellent choice for signal enhancing in optical, electrochemical, and electrical-based LOC devices. Metal oxides such as ZnO, CuO, Fe_3O_4, SnO_2, MnO_2, ZrO_2, TiO_2, and MgO have been applied as sensor modifiers of the LOC devices for various applications. Table 5.3 lists the metal oxide nanomaterials applied in LOC devices for various applications and detection techniques. Among all MO nanomaterials, ZnO nanomaterial is of interest for a range of sensors such as gas, biological, and electrochemical sensors. ZnO has excellent electrical, catalytic, and optical properties. ZnO is classified as a semiconductor in groups II–VI, which exhibits a direct bandgap ~3.37 eV. In principle, one-dimensional (1-D) ZnO nanostructures (nanorods, nanowires, and nanotubes) are more favorable because the structures may facilitate efficient carrier transport. This happens because of 1-D ZnO nanomaterial has decreased grain boundaries, surface defects, disorders, and discontinuous interface [19].

Most commonly, ZnO nanorods (ZnO NR) have been extensively studied for gas sensor applications. The reason is that ZnO NR is an excellent chemiresistive material. The

TABLE 5.3

The Metal Oxide Nanomaterials Applied in LOC Devices for Various Applications and Detection Techniques

Nanomaterial/electrode	Applications	Types of sensors	Detection technique	Linear range	LOD	Reference
ZnO NR/Si/SiO$_2$ Chip	Vapor Gas Sensor	Chemiresistor	Chemiresistive performance	0.2–5 ppm	–	[20]
ZnO nanocombs/Si chip-CMOS	CO Gas Sensor	FET Sensor	Resistance different	250–500 ppm	250 ppm	[21]
ZnO nanowires/Si/SiO$_2$ Chip	H$_2$S Gas Sensor	Chemiresistor	Chemiresistive performance	5–200 ppb	5 ppb	[22]
CoZn-FeONPs/microfluidic immunoarray device	Cancer Biomarker Detection	Electrochemical Immunoassay	Amperometry	3.9–5 $\times$ 10^2	0.19 fgm/L	[23]
AuNPs@Fe$_3$O$_4$- CMK-8/glass-PDMS microfluidic	IgG anti-T. canis Immunosensor	Electrochemical Immunosensor	Amperometry	0.1–100 ng/mL	0.10 ng/mL	[24]
MNPs-Antibodies/MnO$_2$ NFs/glass-PDMS microfluidic	Salmonella Biosensor	Colorimetric Salmonella Biosensor	Colorimetric and smartphone device	4.4 $\times$ 10^1–4.4 $\times$ 10^6 CFU/mL	44 CFU/mL	[25]
Microporous manganese-Reduced graphene oxide nanocomposite	Cardiac Biomarker	Electrochemical Biosensor	Impedance	0.008–20 ng/mL	8.0 pg/mL	[26]
QD-pAb- MnO$_2$ NFs/glass-PDMS microfluidic	Salmonella Biosensor	Fluorescent Biosensor	Fluorescent probes	1.0 $\times$ 102–1.0 $\times$ 10^7 CFU/mL	43 CFU/mL	[27]

alcohol vapor multisensory array was developed based on ZnO NR grown directly on a multielectrode chip via a hydrothermal method [20]. The type of alcohol vapors studied is ethanol, isopropanol, and butanol. The multisensory array chip was fabricated using Si/SiO_2 substrate, co-planar Pt/Ti sputtered cathode electrode, and connected using Au wire. The working principle of the ZnO NR gas sensor is through a reaction of gas with the ZnO surface, resulting in the change in resistance. The sign of reaction is dependent on whether the chemisorbed species undergo a reduction or oxidation process. The process may then cause electron exchange between the conductance band and the surface local energy states in the gap. Theoretically, the morphology of the transducer may greatly influence their gas sensing properties. The directly grown ZnO NR on a multi-electrode chip with a diameter of 10–20 nm and length 90–150 nm show linear range detection for alcohol vapor in the range of 0.2 to 5 ppm.

Pan and Zhao [21] have reported on the gas sensor LOC devices based on modification with ZnO nanocombs for carbon monoxide (CO) detection. The LOC device was developed on a single Si chip integrated with a complementary-metal-oxide-semiconductor (CMOS) microsensor. The ZnO nanocombs were grown on top of a silicon substrate. ZnO nanocombs were synthesized via chemical vapor deposition (CVD) based on a vapor-liquid-solid mechanism. ZnO nanocombs were employed as signal enhancers by providing a larger effective sensing area that exhibited high-sensitivity detection even at room temperature. The detection mechanism was based on the reaction of CO target gas with the generated oxygen ions, which released the combined electrons back to the conduction band. This led to a significantly narrowed depletion region and a decrease in resistance. Therefore, by measuring the overall resistance of the semiconductor metal oxide in real-time, the CO gas concentration could be quantitatively measured. The developed ZnO nanocomb gas sensor exhibited high sensitivity of 7.22 and 8.93 for CO concentrations of 250 ppm and 500 ppm at room temperature. This proved that the proposed ZnO nanocomb greatly enhanced sensitivity even at room temperature and promising nanoparticles used for CO gas sensors. The reason is that nanocomb structure with a length of 58.7 μm and width of 4.35 μm have promoted a larger surface sensing area by providing multiple conducting channels for gas detection.

Other types of MO nanomaterials commonly used for sensor signal enhancement is iron oxide nanoparticle (IONPs) or also called magnetic materials. IONPs exist in various phases such as $MnFe_2O_4$, Fe_2O_3, and Fe_3O_4. IONPs exhibit superparamagnetic properties, biocompatible, high catalytic properties, and unique physicochemical properties. Another important function of the magnetic properties of IONPs in LOC devices is the ability to be integrated into transaction systems for efficient detection of the target analytes under the influence of an external magnetic field. IONPs have been employed in numerous applications such as biological separation, immunoassay, target delivery, and biosensor.

Recently, core-shell of $AuNPs@Fe_3O_4$ and ordered mesoporous carbon (CMK-8) in chitosan were employed for signal enhancement in the electrochemical determination of IgG antibodies anti-*Toxocara canis* (IgG anti-T. canis) for Toxocariosis disease [24]. The microfluidic electrochemical immunosensor device was fabricated on PDMS/glass using the photolithography process and sputtering of Ag/Au electrode acted as the transducer. The IgG anti-T canis antibody was detected through a non-competitive immunoassay. The combination of metal and metal oxide nanoparticles in forming core-shell of $AuNPs@Fe_3O_4$ features improved the electrochemical performance, good biocompatibility, and prepare a larger surface area for binding with the recognition element, which is an antigen from *T. canis* second-stage larvae. The sensor showed outstanding performance for IgG anti-*T. canis* detection with LOD of 0.10 ng mL $^{-1}$ and linearity of 0.1–100 ng/mL.

The magnetic nanoparticles also play important role in biomarker immunocapture and detection application. The other work reported the deposition of Fe_2O_4 with cobalt (Co) and Zn (CoZn-Fe_2O_4) nanoparticles applied in a disposable enzyme-free microfluidic immunoarray device (μID) [23]. The CoZn- Fe_2O_4 nanoparticles acted as enzyme mimics of peroxidase-like catalysis. The produced sensor was tested for detection protein CYFRA 21-1 exhibited good linear response in range 3.9 to 1,000 fg/mL and ultralow LOD of 0.19 fg/mL. The CoZnFeONPs in combination with a disposable μID provided a simple and efficient biomarker detection method that could satisfy the requirements for a low-cost and speedy test for early cancer detection.

Apart from it, manganese oxide (MnO) also receives much attention as they feature outstanding physical and chemical properties, high surface area, tunable size, good biocompatibility, and stable peroxidase-mimic characteristics. A colorimetric microfluidic LOC biosensor for rapid and sensitive detection of Salmonella using MnO_2 nanoflower (MnO_2 NFs) for amplifying the biological signal, magnetic nanoparticles as recognition element, and microfluidic chip for conducting automation operation was fabricated as shown in Figure 5.3 [25]. The colorimetric microfluidic LOC biosensor was integrated with a convergence-divergence spiral micromixer for sample mixing and incubation. The colorimetric microfluidic LOC biosensor employed the magnetic nanoparticle (MNPs) conjugated with antibodies as the Salmonella recognition element and MnO_2 NF as the nanomimetic enzyme in catalyzed the MNPs-Salmonella-MnO2 NFs complex, forming yellow catalysate. The yellow catalysate was then transported into a detection chamber and its image was analyzed and processed using the smartphone app to determine the concentration of Salmonella bacteria. The colorimetric LOC biosensor was able to detect Salmonella in the range of 4.4×10^1 to 4.4×10^6 CFU/mL in 45 min detection time, and LOD of 44 CFU/mL.

Hao et al. [27] also reported on the detection of Salmonella Typhimurium using quantum dots (QDs) as fluorescent probes for recognition elements and MnO_2 NFs as the signal amplifier. The proposed detection mechanism is based on MnO_2 NFs conjugated with carboxyl-modified QDs and functionalized with polyclonal antibodies (pAbs) to form MnO_2-QD-pAb-MnO_2 NFs complex. The complex flow through the microfluidic chip and was captured at the detection chamber. In the detection chamber, glutathione was introduced to dissolve MnO_2 on the complexes into Mn^{2+}, thus resulting in the release of QDs. The fluorescent intensity of the released QDs was quantified using the fluorescent detector to determine the concentration of Salmonella. The sensor exhibited a linear relationship from 1.0×10^2 to 1.0×10^7 CFU/mL with a low LOD of 43 CFU/mL.

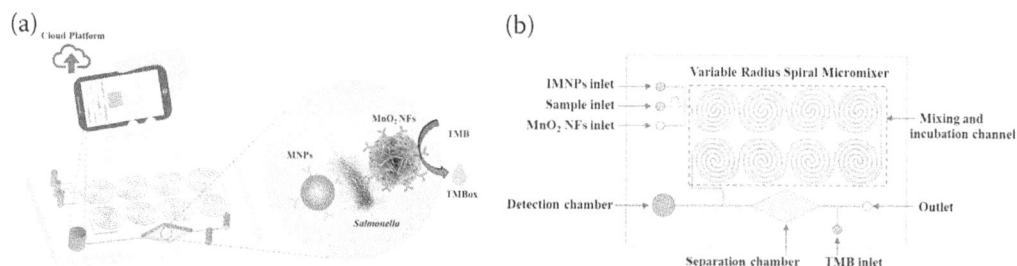

FIGURE 5.3
The schematic image of (a) colorimetric microfluidic LOC biosensor and the proposed mechanism for Salmonella detection, (b) components and operation flow in the colorimetric microfluidic LOC biosensor for Salmonella detection. Adapted with permission [25]. Copyright (2021) American Chemical Society.

The high specific surface area of MnO_2 NFs prepared a high loading area for QDs, which amplified the signal and enhanced the sensitivity of the microfluidic biosensor.

5.3.3 Carbon-Based Nanomaterials in a Lab-on-Chip

Carbon-based nanomaterials have received a lot of attention for the modification of transducer platforms in LOC devices. Carbon-based nanomaterials are abundant and low in cost materials, which feature excellent chemical and physical properties. Electrodes prepared or modified with carbon nanomaterials showed an excellent low background current, broad potential window, high surface area for entrapment of different compounds, renewability, and low cost to incorporate with different substances during fabrication. The carbon-based nanomaterials have unique and diverse allotropes like graphite, diamonds, carbon nanotubes (CNTs), graphene oxide (GO), graphene quantum dots (GQDs), and fullerene [28]. Table 5.4 lists carbon-based nanomaterials applied in LOC devices for various applications and detection techniques.

Carbon-based nanomaterials have been extensively applied in the LOC device sensor for signal enhancement of the modified sensor. Most commonly, carbon-based nanomaterials were combined with other types of nanomaterial to further enhance the property of the sensor part in the LOC device. Zhang et al. [29] reported the synergetic effect of carbon-based nanomaterials and AuNPs employed for signal enhancement in electrochemical LOC for saliva glucose detection. The electrochemical LOC was developed by integrating three electrodes consisting of WE, CE, and RE on a single chip through a micro-fabrication process. The Si wafer was pre-cleaned, oxidized with wet atmosphere, and undergo a photolithography process to create the microelectrodes desired pattern. The WE of the LOC was modified with single-walled carbon nanotubes (SWNTs), AuNPs, chitosan, and glucose oxidase (GOx) through the layer-by-layer assembly. The multilayer of SWNTs/AuNPs/chitosan can increase active surface area and promote direct electron transfer between GOx and the WE. Therefore, high sensitivity and low LOD of glucose sensor has been developed. This happens because of the high electrocatalytic properties and high electrical conductivity of the SWNTs and AuNPs. The developed electrochemical LOC chip for saliva glucose detection exhibits the linearity of 0.017–0.81 mM, and LOD of 5.6 µM, which in the future is able to be applied in a non-invasive, pain-free, and easy glucose monitoring.

Chand and Neethirajan [30] have developed a microfluidic LOC device integrated with SPCE electrode for electrochemical detection of norovirus. As shown in Figure 5.4, the PDMS microfluidic chip was equipped with silica microbeads to pre-concentrate the sample and the SPCE was modified with graphene-AuNPs composite as the sensor and norovirus specific aptamer as the recognition element components on the microfluidic LOC device. The graphene-AuNPs composite offers dual advantages in terms of increasing the surface area for an aptamer to immobilize, improve electrical conductivity and accelerate the electron transfer process. Additionally, the modification of SPCE with graphene-AuNPs composite can be easily done by a simple process such as drop casting, spin casting, or ink-jet printing. The detection principle of the aptamer norovirus microfluidic LOC device is based on the interaction of redox-aptamer and norovirus resulting in increasing the impedance thus decreasing the electrochemical signal obtained (Figure 5.4). The differential pulse voltammetry (DPV) technique has been employed in the norovirus microfluidic LOC device with a linearity of 100 pM to 3.5 nM and LOD of 100 pM.

The electrochemical microfluidic LOC for the detection of nitrate ions in a soil solution has been developed by Ali et al. [31]. The graphene foam and titanium nitrate nanofibers

TABLE 5.4

Carbon-Based Nanomaterials Used for Signal Enhancement for Lab-on-Chip Devices in Various Applications

Nanomaterial/Electrode	Applications	Types of sensors	Detection technique	Linear range	LOD	Reference
SWCNT/AuNPs/Chitosan/Si Chip	Glucose biosensor	Electrochemical Biosensor	Amperometric	0.017–0.81 mM	5.6 μM	[29]
Graphene/AuNPs/chitosan/ Aptamer/PDMS microfluidic	Aptamer Biosensor	Electrochemical Biosensor	DPV	100 pM–3.5 nM	100 pM	[30]
Graphene-TiN NF/NaR enzyme/ Si chip	Nitrite ions Enviromental sensor	Electrochemical Biosensor	Amperometric	0.01–442 mg/L	0.01 mg/L	[31]
Graphene-nTiO$_2$/anti- ErbB2 antibodied/glass PDMS microfluidic	Breast cancer Immunosensor	Electrochemical Biosensor	Impedance and Voltammetric	1 fM–0.1 μM; 1 pM–0.1 μM	–	[32]
MWCNTs-thionine-AuNP composites/paper microfluidic	17β-estradiol Hormone Immunosensor	Electrochemical Immunosensor	DPV	0.01–100 ng mL 1	10 pg mL 1	[33]
CNT NiO/ANtibody/ PDMS microfluidic	Low-density lipoprotein detection	Electrochemical Biosensor	Impedance spectroscopic	5 120 mg/dL	0.63 mg/dL	[34]
SWNCTs-FET/Si Chip	Coronavirus 2 (SARS-CoV-2)	Field effect transistor Biosensor	Source-drain current	0.1 fg/mL–5.0 pg/mL	4.12 fg/mL	[35]
CNT-FET	Detecting SARS-CoV-2	Field effect transistor Biosensor	Field effect transistor	–	10 fM	[36]

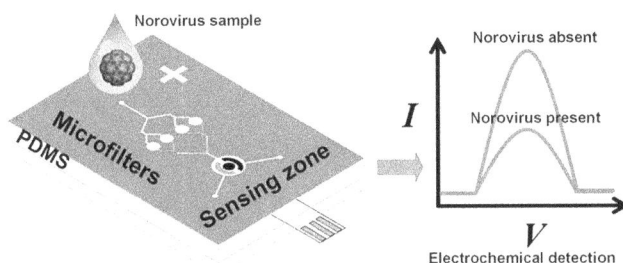

FIGURE 5.4
The schematic of the microfluidic electrochemical LOC aptasensor for norovirus detection and the electro-chemical signal obtained in the absence and presence of norovirus. Adapted with permission [30]. Copyright (2017) Elsevier.

(TiN NF) composite immobilized with nitrate reductase (NaR) enzyme has been used as the sensor platform in nitrate detection. In this work, the electrochemical microfluidic LOC was developed on the Si wafer where the Au was patterned as the CE, Ag/AgCl as the RE, and the graphene-TiN NF composite as the WE. The graphene-TiN NF composite was embedded into the channel using the liquid phase photopolymerization technique to produce flow through a microfluidic electrochemical sensor. The combination of the graphene and TiN NF composite creates three-dimensional structure nanomaterials, which increases the electrochemically active surface area and provides high loading capacity for the NaR enzyme immobilization. In the detection of nitrate ions, the graphene-TiN NF composite porous structure allows the sample analytes to flow through and react with immobilized NaR enzymes which resulted in catalytic reduction. This reaction led to increases in the amperometric current response. The fabricated electrochemical microfluidic LOC can detect the nitrite ions in agricultural soil solution samples in a linear range of 0.01 to 442 mg/L and LOD of 0.01 mg/L.

A similar research group reported on the electrochemical microfluidic immunosensor LOC for breast cancer biomarker detection [32]. This time, the combination of porous graphene and carbon-doped titanium dioxide nanofibers ($nTiO_2$) composite immobilized with functionalized anti-ErbB2 were used as the electrochemical WE. The combination of the excellent properties $nTiO_2$ embedded into the porous structure of graphene, resulted in a larger electrochemical surface area and high charge transfer resistance in the electrochemical breast cancer biomarker detection. In this LOC device, the sensor was connected to two types of detection techniques, which are impedance and DPV techniques. The impedance value increased and voltammetric peak current values decreased with the presence of high concentration ErbB2 antibodies. This happened because more ErbB2 antibodies bound to the WE thus increased the thickness of the insulating layer. The impedance and voltammetric electrochemical performance of the microfluidic immunosensor LOC display high sensitivities of 0.585 $\mu A/\mu Mcm^2$ and 43.7 $k\Omega/\mu Mcm^2$, respectively, for wide linearity concentration of 1.0 fM to 0.1 μM for impedance technique and 0.1 pM to 0.1 μM for voltammetric technique.

The reliable properties of carbon-based materials have made it a possible nanomaterial to be applied in the detection of SARS-CoV-2 (COVID-19) surface spike protein S1. Recently, Zamzami et al. [35] fabricated a high selectivity and sensitive carbon nanotubes field-effect transistor (CNT/FET) sensor that allows digital detection of the SARS-CoV-2 S1 in saliva samples. As shown in Figure 5.5, the sensor was fabricated on a Si/SiO_2 surface by deposited single-wall carbon nanotube (SWCNTs) and

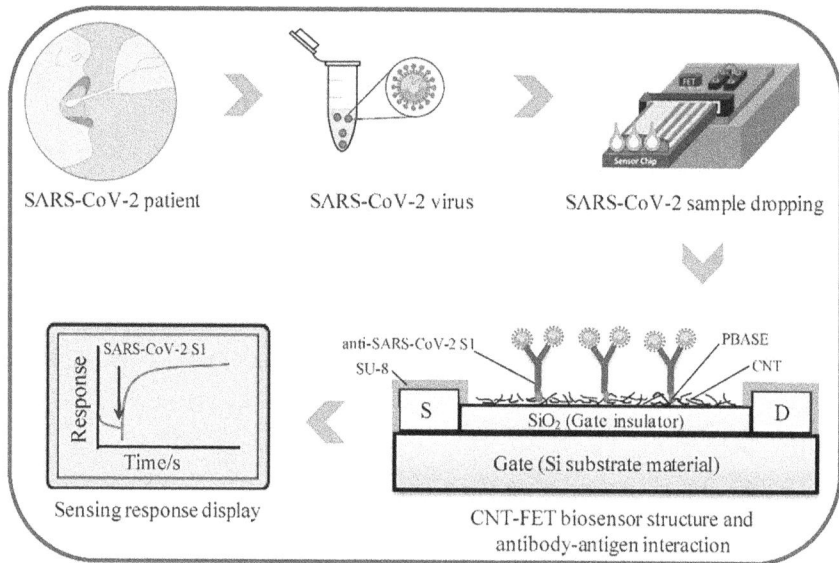

FIGURE 5.5
The schematic of SARS-CoV-2 S1 sample testing steps including the CNT-FET biosensor design and components. Adapted with permission [35] Copyright (2020) The Authors, some rights reserved; exclusive licensee [Elsevier]. Distributed under a Creative Commons Attribution License 4.0 (CC BY) https://creativecommons.org/licenses/by/4.0/.

immobilized the anti-SARS-CoV-2 S1 antibodies in between the source and drain channel as the sensing materials and recognition element. The anti-SARS-CoV-2 S1 antibodies were immobilized through a non-covalent interaction with the linker 1-pyrenebutanoic acid succinimidyl ester (PBASE). The CNT/FET operated under the p-type channel depletion principle. When there is binding in between SARS-CoV-2 spike protein and immobilized anti-SARS CoV-2 S1 antibodies, the source-drain current is depleted. The CNT-FET sensor is able to detect the SARS-CoV-2 infection in a linear range of 0.1 fg/mL to 5.0 pg/mL and LOD of 4.12 fg/mL. In this work, the large surface area and high electrical conductivity of SWCNT ensure the high loading capacity of the anti-SARS-CoV-2 S1 antibodies as the recognition element and enhance the electrical signal of the sensor.

5.4 Conclusion and Future Look

This chapter discusses metal, metal oxide, and carbon-based nanomaterials' roles and applications in sensor platforms for LOC devices. A wide range of LOC device applications has been developed including immunosensor, environmental, pathogen, protein, therapeutic, and gas analysis. Well-known nanomaterials properties such as large surface area and excellent electrical and chemical properties enhance the optical, electrochemical, and electrical performance of the sensor part in the LOC devices. Most importantly, the nanomaterials can enhance the sensitivity, allow miniaturization, and provide versatility to the LOC devices.

Even though numerous reported works on LOC devices have been published, however, the transition of the LOC devices from lab prototyping to commercialization is still challenging. The main challenges are to develop LOC devices that are cost-efficient, simple to operate, and robust. In the future, the development of LOC devices based on paper, cloth, flexible substrates, or biopolymer materials as the substrate is an interesting field to explore. The reasons are that those substrates are cost-efficient and able to control fluid flow. New trends in LOC devices also should focus on the integration of LOC devices with the Internet of Things (IoT) and through a smartphone connection and big data for simple readouts and data storage.

References

1. M. Medina-Sánchez, S. Miserere and A. Merkoçi, Nanomaterials and lab-on-a-chip technologies, *Lab on a Chip* 12 (2012), pp. 1932–1943.
2. N. Wongkaew, M. Simsek, C. Griesche and A.J. Baeumner, Functional nanomaterials and nanostructures enhancing electrochemical biosensors and Lab-on-a-Chip performances: recent progress, applications, and future perspective, *Chemical Reviews* 119 (2019), pp. 120–194.
3. A. Francesko, V.F. Cardoso and S. Lanceros-Méndez, *Lab-on-a-chip technology and microfluidics*, in *Microfluidics for Pharmaceutical Applications*, H.A. Santos, D. Liu and H. Zhang, eds., William Andrew Publishing (2019) pp. 3–36.
4. C.-W. Huang, Y.-T. Lin, S.-T. Ding, L.-L. Lo, P.-H. Wang, E.-C. Lin et al., Efficient SNP discovery by combining microarray and Lab-on-a-Chip data for animal breeding and selection, *Microarrays* 4 (2015), pp. 570–595.
5. E. Priyadarshini and N. Pradhan, Gold nanoparticles as efficient sensors in colorimetric detection of toxic metal ions: A review, *Sensors and Actuators B: Chemical* 238 (2017), pp. 888–902.
6. P.K. Jain, K.S. Lee, I.H. El-Sayed and M.A. El-Sayed, Calculated absorption and scattering properties of gold nanoparticles of different size, shape, and composition: applications in biological imaging and biomedicine, *The Journal of Physical Chemistry. B* 110 (2006), pp. 7238–7248.
7. L. Zheng, G. Cai, S. Wang, M. Liao, Y. Li and J. Lin, A microfluidic colorimetric biosensor for rapid detection of Escherichia coli O157:H7 using gold nanoparticle aggregation and smart phone imaging, *Biosensors and Bioelectronics* 124–125 (2019), pp. 143–149.
8. T. Yang, Z. Wang, Y. Song, X. Yang, S. Chen, S. Fu et al., A novel smartphone-based colorimetric aptasensor for on-site detection of Escherichia coli O157:H7 in milk, *Journal of Dairy Science* 104 (2021), pp. 8506–8516.
9. H. Bhardwaj, G. Sumana and C.A. Marquette, A label-free ultrasensitive microfluidic surface Plasmon resonance biosensor for Aflatoxin B1 detection using nanoparticles integrated gold chip, *Food Chemistry* 307 (2020). DOI: 10.1016/j.foodchem.2019.125530.
10. C. Zhao, G. Zhong, D.-E. Kim, J. Liu and X. Liu, A portable lab-on-a-chip system for gold-nanoparticle-based colorimetric detection of metal ions in water, *Biomicrofluidics* 8 (2014), pp. 052107.
11. A. Huang, H. Li and D. Xu, An on-chip electrochemical sensor by integrating ITO three-electrode with low-volume cell for on-line determination of trace Hg(II), *Journal of Electroanalytical Chemistry* 848 (2019), pp. 113189.
12. N. Shokoufi, B. Abbasgholi, Nejad Asbaghi and A. Abbasi-Ahd, Microfluidic chip-photothermal lens microscopy for DNA hybridization assay using gold nanoparticles, *Analytical and Bioanalytical Chemistry* 411 (2019), pp. 6119–6128.
13. Y. Zhao, X. Liu, J. Li, W. Qiang, L. Sun, H. Li et al., Microfluidic chip-based silver nanoparticles aptasensor for colorimetric detection of thrombin, *Talanta* 150 (2016), pp. 81–87.

14. M. Salve, A. Mandal, K. Amreen, P.K. Pattnaik and S. Goel, Greenly synthesized silver nanoparticles for supercapacitor and electrochemical sensing applications in a 3D printed microfluidic platform, *Microchemical Journal* 157 (2020). DOI: 10.1016/j.microc.2020.104973.

15. R. Wang, Y. Xu, T. Sors, J. Irudayaraj, W. Ren and R. Wang, Impedimetric detection of bacteria by using a microfluidic chip and silver nanoparticle based signal enhancement, *Microchimica Acta* 185 (2018), p. 184.

16. M. Kamruzzaman, A.M. Alam, S.H. Lee and T.D. Dang, Chemiluminescence microfluidic system on a chip to determine vitamin B1 using platinum nanoparticles triggered luminol-AgNO3 reaction, *Sensors and Actuators, B: Chemical* 185 (2013), pp. 301–308.

17. M. Medina-Sánchez, C.C. Mayorga-Martinez, T. Watanabe, T.A. Ivandini, Y. Honda, F. Pino et al., Microfluidic platform for environmental contaminants sensing and degradation based on boron-doped diamond electrodes, *Biosensors and Bioelectronics* 75 (2016), pp. 365–374.

18. J. Zheng, M. Zhu, J. Kong, Z. Li, J. Jiang, Y. Xi et al., Microfluidic paper-based analytical device by using Pt nanoparticles as highly active peroxidase mimic for simultaneous detection of glucose and uric acid with use of a smartphone, *Talanta* 237 (2022), pp. 122954.

19. N.S. Ridhuan, K. Abdul Razak, Z. Lockman and A. Abdul Aziz, Structural and morphology of ZnO nanorods synthesized using ZnO seeded growth hydrothermal method and its properties as UV sensing, *Plos One* 7 (2012), pp. e50405.

20. A. Bobkov, A. Varezhnikov, I. Plugin, F.S. Fedorov, V. Trouillet, U. Geckle et al., The multisensor array based on grown-on-chip zinc oxide nanorod network for selective discrimination of alcohol vapors at sub-ppm range, *Sensors (Switzerland)* 19 (2019).

21. X. Pan and X. Zhao, Ultra-high sensitivity zinc oxide nanocombs for On-Chip room temperature carbon monoxide sensing, *Sensors* 15 (2015), pp. 8919–8930.

22. Y. Chen, P. Xu, T. Xu, D. Zheng and X. Li, ZnO-nanowire size effect induced ultra-high sensing response to ppb-level H2S, *Sensors and Actuators B: Chemical* 240 (2017), pp. 264–272.

23. C.A. Proença, T.A. Baldo, T.A. Freitas, E.M. Materón, A. Wong, A.A. Durán et al., Novel enzyme-free immunomagnetic microfluidic device based on Co0.25Zn0.75Fe2O4 for cancer biomarker detection, *Analytica Chimica Acta* 1071 (2019), pp. 59–69.

24. C.F. Jofre, M. Regiart, M.A. Fernández-Baldo, M. Bertotti, J. Raba and G.A. Messina, Electrochemical microfluidic immunosensor based on TES-AuNPs@Fe3O4 and CMK-8 for IgG anti-Toxocara canis determination, *Analytica Chimica Acta* 1096 (2020), pp. 120–129.

25. L. Xue, N. Jin, R. Guo, S. Wang, W. Qi, Y. Liu et al., Microfluidic colorimetric biosensors based on MnO2Nanozymes and convergence-divergence spiral micromixers for rapid and sensitive detection of salmonella, *ACS Sensors* 6 (2021), pp. 2883–2892.

26. N. Singh, M.A. Ali, P. Rai, A. Sharma, B.D. Malhotra and R. John, Microporous nanocomposite enabled microfluidic biochip for cardiac biomarker detection, *ACS Applied Materials and Interfaces* 9 (2017), pp. 33576–33588.

27. L. Hao, L. Xue, F. Huang, G. Cai, W. Qi, M. Zhang et al., A microfluidic biosensor based on magnetic nanoparticle separation, quantum dots labeling and mno2 nanoflower amplification for rapid and sensitive detection of salmonella typhimurium, *Micromachines* 11 (2020), p. 281.

28. D. Maiti, X. Tong, X. Mou and K. Yang, Carbon-based nanomaterials for biomedical applications: A recent study, *Frontiers in Pharmacology* 9 (2018), p. 1401.

29. W. Zhang, Y. Du and M.L. Wang, On-chip highly sensitive saliva glucose sensing using multilayer films composed of single-walled carbon nanotubes, gold nanoparticles, and glucose oxidase, *Sensing and Bio-Sensing Research* 4 (2015), pp. 96–102.

30. R. Chand and S. Neethirajan, Microfluidic platform integrated with graphene-gold nanocomposite aptasensor for one-step detection of norovirus, *Biosensors and Bioelectronics* 98 (2017), pp. 47–53.

31. M.A. Ali, K. Mondal, Y. Wang, H. Jiang, N.K. Mahal, M.J. Castellano et al., In situ integration of graphene foam-titanium nitride based bio-scaffolds and microfluidic structures for soil nutrient sensors, *Lab on a Chip* 17 (2017), pp. 274–285.

32. M.A. Ali, K. Mondal, Y. Jiao, S. Oren, Z. Xu, A. Sharma et al., Microfluidic immuno-biochip for detection of breast cancer biomarkers using hierarchical composite of porous graphene and titanium dioxide nanofibers, *ACS Applied Materials and Interfaces* 8 (2016), pp. 20570–20582.

33. Y. Wang, J. Luo, J. Liu, X. Li, Z. Kong, H. Jin et al., Electrochemical integrated paper-based immunosensor modified with multi-walled carbon nanotubes nanocomposites for point-of-care testing of 17β-estradiol, *Biosensors and Bioelectronics* 107 (2018), pp. 47–53.
34. M.A. Ali, P.R. Solanki, S. Srivastava, S. Singh, V.V. Agrawal, R. John et al., Protein functionalized carbon nanotubes-based smart lab-on-a-chip, *ACS applied materials & interfaces* 7 (2015), pp. 5837–5846.
35. M.A. Zamzami, G. Rabbani, A. Ahmad, A.A. Basalah, W.H. Al-Sabban, S. Nate Ahn et al., Carbon nanotube field-effect transistor (CNT-FET)-based biosensor for rapid detection of SARS-CoV-2 (COVID-19) surface spike protein S1, *Bioelectrochemistry* 143 (2022), pp. 107982.
36. M. Thanihaichelvan, S.N. Surendran, T. Kumanan, U. Sutharsini, P. Ravirajan, R. Valluvan et al., Selective and electronic detection of COVID-19 (Coronavirus) using carbon nanotube field effect transistor-based biosensor: A proof-of-concept study, *Materials Today. Proceedings* 49 (2022), pp. 2546.

6

CMOS Bioelectronics: Current and Future Trends

Ching-Yi Lin, Md. Sakibur Sajal, Yann Gilpin, and Fahimeh Dehghandehnavi
Department of Electrical and Computer Engineering, Carnegie Mellon University, Pittsburgh, USA

Anna Batueva
Natural Sciences Department, Udmurt State University, Izhevsk, Udmurt Republic, Russia

Kai-Chun Lin
Department of Electrical and Computer Engineering, Carnegie Mellon University, Pittsburgh, USA

Nicole McFarlane
Min H. Kao Department of Electrical Engineering and Computer Science, University of Tennessee, Knoxville, USA

Marc Dandin
Department of Electrical and Computer Engineering, Carnegie Mellon University, Pittsburgh, USA

CONTENTS

DOI: 10.1201/9781003263265-6

6.1 Introduction

The modern era has witnessed explosive growth in the field of electronics. Indeed, there is an enormous technological gap between the first solid-state devices introduced in the early 1900s for radio communication and the modern smartphone. Silicon technologies have undeniably been at the center of this progress. And, despite a plethora of electronics applications that now require other semiconductors (e.g., silicon carbide, gallium arsenide, indium phosphide), silicon remains the most important industrial material for microchip technology. Particularly, silicon chips containing billions of transistors can now be manufactured for mass-market applications. Furthermore, recent progress in transistor fabrication capabilities is pushing transistor gate lengths further to around 5 nm, enabling additional performance gains and increased integration densities.

One particular silicon technology that is used in most consumer, military, industrial, and medical microchips is the complementary metal-oxide-semiconductor (CMOS) process. It is used to manufacture, on the same substrate, two types of transistors that are complementary from the point of view of the carriers responsible for transport. Specifically, one transistor relies on electrons to carry current, whereas the other relies on holes. This duality has enabled the creation of digital circuits that are the building blocks of microprocessors that are utilized today. It has also enabled a wide variety of sensing applications using analog circuits. Most importantly, one of the main advantages of CMOS processes is that they allow the designer to combine digital and analog circuit cores to create mixed-signal circuits that achieve sensing and digital processing on the same chip.

This chapter reviews the constitutive technologies and current trends in the development of CMOS circuits for microsystems used in bioelectronics. Here, we define the field of bioelectronics broadly to include all electronic devices and systems that are configured to interface with one or more biological species. Nevertheless, we restrict our discussion only to a subset of these systems. Namely, we discuss CMOS circuit architectures and microsystems configured for neural interfacing, electrochemical sensing, interfacial capacitance sensing, electric cell-substrate impedance spectroscopy, and image sensing. Our discussion is not an exhaustive review of the many architectures and devices that currently exist in this subset of applications; rather, it serves to introduce the unacquainted reader to the design approaches and challenges that are prevalent in the field. As such, we curate our discussion to include example systems reported by numerous colleagues and by our research groups.

6.2 CMOS Sensors for Neural Interfaces

This section provides an overview of bioelectronic CMOS chips that are configured to interface with neurons or bundles of neurons (i.e., nerves) that form neural tissue. These *neural* chips have a wide variety of uses in regenerative health applications but also in bioelectronic medicine applications where the peripheral nervous system is stimulated to trigger biochemical responses that have a therapeutic effect (see, for example, ref. [1], which describes the potential of vagus nerve stimulation as a therapeutic approach). As example technologies, we discuss the basic infrastructure for stimulating neural tissue and for recording neural signals using CMOS devices.

6.2.1 Neurostimulation

The purpose of neural stimulation is to deliver the electric charge to a nerve bundle, a neuron, or generally, to neural tissue. For example, in patients suffering from epilepsy, upon detecting the onset of a seizure via a neural recording front end, a neurostimulator is used to deliver charge to the brain tissue via a set of electrodes [2]. When enough charges are delivered, the tissue's membrane depolarizes to below its threshold; this produces a unidirectional action potential that prevents the seizure. The neurostimulator accomplishing this task must be designed such that it delivers enough charges to cause the depolarization. Secondly, the neurostimulator must deliver the stimulation such that there is no charge imbalance or residual average direct current (DC) at the membrane.

Charge imbalance can cause tissue damage [2]. For instance, Aran et al. reported tissue damage occurring in guinea pig cochleae at residual average DC levels in the range of 20–40 µA [3]. Similarly, Hurlbert et al. reported that when the average residual DC was maintained at 1.5 µA for rat spinal cords, there was no pathological change around the electrodes even after prolonged stimulation. This indicated that such an amount of average residual DC was safe for the tissue. Therefore, achieving charge balance, in addition to achieving the correct current amplitude and temporal characteristics, is a central aspect of neurostimulator design [4]. Current-mode stimulation is used to achieve biphasic stimulation and ensures that charge balance is maintained.

Figure 6.1 illustrates a general configuration for charge balanced-neurostimulation along with its associated stimulation regimen. A cathodic pulse with pre-defined amplitude I_{cath} and duration t_{cath} is applied to the nerve to deliver the required electric charge on the tissue membrane. This pulse is maintained until the threshold membrane potential is reached and the action potential is elicited. With a brief delay, the anodic pulse (I_{anod}, t_{anod}) is initiated to offset the previously supplied charge to maintain charge balance. To guarantee a complete charge balance or at least a safe average residual DC after each cycle, the current source and current sink arms of the circuit need to be accurately matched. Unfortunately, achieving such matching is not feasible in practice due

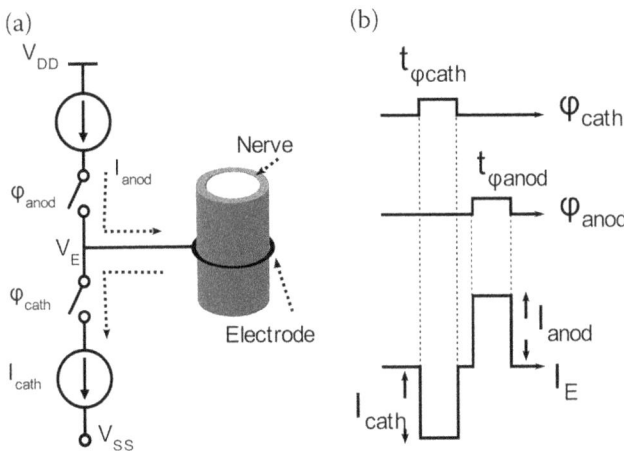

FIGURE 6.1
Schematic of an electrical stimulation scheme of a nerve. (a) Switched current sources are connected to the nerve via an electrode. (b) Typical biphasic pattern showing switch operation and the current delivered to the nerve as a function of time.

to the inherent mismatches that exist in CMOS devices. Hence, modern stimulators incorporate different charge balancing schemes to ensure safe operation [5,6].

An example neurostimulator with precise charge balance control was reported by Luo and Ker [2]. They demonstrated a neurostimulator architecture implemented in a 0.18 µm CMOS process. One particular design challenge that was overcome in this work is the incorporation of high-voltage supplies (V_{DD} and V_{SS} in Figure 6.1) in a low-voltage CMOS process. These high-voltage supplies are needed to deliver the correct amount of charge to the tissue. The authors showed a self-adaptation bias technique and stacked MOS configurations that were able to reach the desired high voltage needed for stimulation. This was achieved in the low-voltage CMOS process without compromising the devices' oxide integrity. Furthermore, they showed precise charge balancing utilizing current memory cells and dedicated calibration loops as well as leakage current compensation. The authors reported less than 6.6 nA of average residual DC after the operation.

6.2.2 Neural Recording

The counterpart of neural stimulation is neural recording. This may also be achieved utilizing CMOS chips. The goal of neural recording is to sense action potentials with a high signal-to-noise ratio (SNR) and to condition the sensed signal for further processing. Different types of neural signals exist. For instance, they can be low frequency (1 to 100 Hz) electroencephalogram (EEG) signals, local field potentials (LPF), or high frequency (100 Hz to 10 kHz) action potentials, and they may span over a wide range of amplitudes (10 µV to 10 mV).

Neural recording design is thus an intricate exercise in amplifier design. Furthermore, high-fidelity recording can be quite difficult to achieve experimentally because the weaker the signal of interest, the more likely it is to be compromised by intrinsic device noise sources (e.g., thermal noise and flicker noise) and by extrinsic noise sources like noise from power lines or EMG signals from nearby muscle tissue. To achieve high-SNR detection and mitigate intrinsic noise sources, a commonly used strategy includes employing differential signal recording schemes with low-noise and high-gain amplifiers. This approach minimizes the input-referred noise at the recording front end.

In order to mitigate extrinsic noise sources, Stein et al. demonstrated how a tripolar recording electrode configuration enables EMG cancellation when recording from peripheral nervous system tissue before and after nearby muscle denervation [7]. Figure 6.2a and Figure 6.2b show typical monopolar and bipolar recording configurations, respectively; with these configurations, the signal of interest can be heavily corrupted by nearby EMG

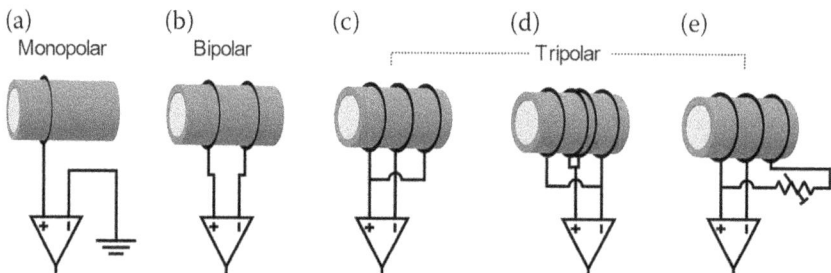

FIGURE 6.2
Typical electrode configurations used in neural recordings: (a) monopolar, (b) bipolar, and (c–e) tripolar configurations.

signals. In contrast, the tripolar configurations in Figures 6.2c–e provide the neural signal while suppressing EMG signals almost completely, but only when the input impedances on the differential inputs of the recording amplifier are matched.

In a typical tripolar configuration, at the amplifier's front end, one input sees two electrodes while the other input sees only one electrode. As such, there is an inherent mismatch in input impedances, and this must be taken into account during the design of the electrodes to ensure proper matching. One way to circumvent this problem is to employ two electrically shorted, identical, and closely placed electrodes instead of a single central electrode (Figure 6.2d). Furthermore, even when the electrode impedances are initially matched at the time of interfacing with the tissue, the tissue impedance will vary over time. This causes further impedance mismatch at the input. This issue is circumvented using a tunable resistor in series with one of the amplifier inputs (Figure 6.2e). This resistor can be varied to match the impedance as the need arises.

As an example CMOS neural amplifier, we refer here to the approach taken by Ashayeri and Yavari [8]. They showed a tunable neural amplifier suitable for implantation. This amplifier was implemented in a 0.18 µm commercial CMOS process, and it achieved input-referred noise of about 2.1 µV-rms and 1.7 µV-rms, depending on the bandwidth of the recording. One interesting feature of this amplifier is that it was tunable, i.e., the bandwidth could be altered to accommodate the recording of signals at different nominal frequencies. The differential input and amplification functions were achieved with an operational transconductance amplifier.

6.3 Electrochemical Sensors

We turn now to another type of bioelectronic circuit, namely to biosensor circuits that are configured to sense biochemical events and provide insights in the form of electrical signals. In this section, we particularly cover electrochemical biosensors. These sensors are widely used in the diagnosis of diseases due to their ability to measure target molecules with high specificity. They offer several advantages in terms of performance and utility. Notably, they can detect substances without labeling, which reduces the time, cost, and complexity of an assay.

Electrochemical biosensors can be miniaturized using CMOS technologies. Specifically, the seamless integration of electronics hardware that processes electrical signals such as current, voltage, and impedance confers the ability to directly monitor electrochemical processes in a small form factor CMOS sensor. Below, we briefly review the techniques used in electrochemical transduction, and we discuss an exemplary CMOS electrochemical sensor.

6.3.1 Electrochemical Sensing Techniques

One of several methods may be used to study the behavior of an analyte in an electrochemical environment. These methods include voltammetry, amperometry, potentiometry, or impedance spectroscopy, and they each require an electrochemical cell.

An electrochemical cell may be formed using a three-electrode system (a reference electrode, an auxiliary electrode, and a working electrode). The reference electrode provides a stable reference potential for a solution in which no reaction occurs. The auxiliary electrode and the working electrode create a potential difference in the solution, and a current flows from the auxiliary electrode to the working electrode. In voltammetry, the potential difference between the auxiliary and working electrodes is varied, and the current between the two electrodes is examined. In impedance spectroscopy, the potential of the working electrode is kept constant, and a sinusoidal voltage of fixed amplitude is applied to the auxiliary electrode. The frequency of the sinusoidal signal is varied, and the output signal frequency is examined rather than its amplitude. In potentiometric methods, the electrochemical cell's potential may be measured relative to a known reference potential, with very little current flow. In amperometric methods, the intensity of the current flowing through the electrochemical cell can be measured for a specific fixed potential.

An electrochemical biosensor consists of four functional components: an analyte, a biorecognition element, a transducer, and an instrument. These components are needed, independently of the method of analysis used. An analyte is a target of interest, such as a protein or DNA. The biorecognition element is capable of selectively recognizing the analyte. The transducer translates the interactions between the analyte and the biorecognition element into an electrical signal. A typical transducer for electrochemical biosensors is an electrode that converts an ionic current into an electrical current or a voltage, depending on the method used. The instrument usually consists of electronic circuitry that captures, amplifies, and records biorecognition signals from the transducer. The analyte is typically in a liquid medium that consists of an electrolyte solution that maintains the analyte's biological activity and transports it to the transducer.

6.3.2 Miniaturization of Electrochemical Biosensors and Example CMOS Electrochemical Biosensors

The miniaturization of electrochemical biosensors is slated to increase their role in the diagnosis of various diseases, particularly in resource-limited settings. There are two main approaches towards the miniaturization of electrochemical biosensors. A noteworthy strategy is to use pre-existing hand-held instruments and modify them such that they recognize biological components of interest that are different from those for which they were originally intended. An example of such a biosensor is a glucometer that is originally designed to detect blood glucose based on electrochemical signals generated by redox reactions but that is retrofitted to recognize other analytes of interest. For instance, the detection of non-glucose targets with a traditional miniaturized glucometer was pioneered by Lu et al. [9]. They showed that by binding aptamers to targets with an enzyme called invertase they could catalyze the hydrolysis of sucrose to glucose. Through the generation of glucose catalyzed by invertase, a series of glucometer-based biosensors were developed for a variety of analytical purposes such as the detection of disease markers and the detection of DNA [10,11].

Another strategy, in scope with the present chapter, is to create miniature biosensor systems based on CMOS sensors. Such an approach requires the integration of the instrumentation circuitry and the biorecognition element on the same CMOS chip. Furthermore, an often overlooked but necessary component is the hardware necessary for delivering the analyte to the sensor sites. Such hardware typically includes microfluidic networks, and their integration with CMOS chips has been covered extensively, for example by Huang et al. [12]. Below, we review a representative device that illustrates the integration of electrochemical sensing into a CMOS platform.

The exemplary sensor was developed by Jafari et al. [13], and it was able to detect synthetic DNA sequences consistent with biomarkers for prostate cancer (Figure 6.3). Unlike

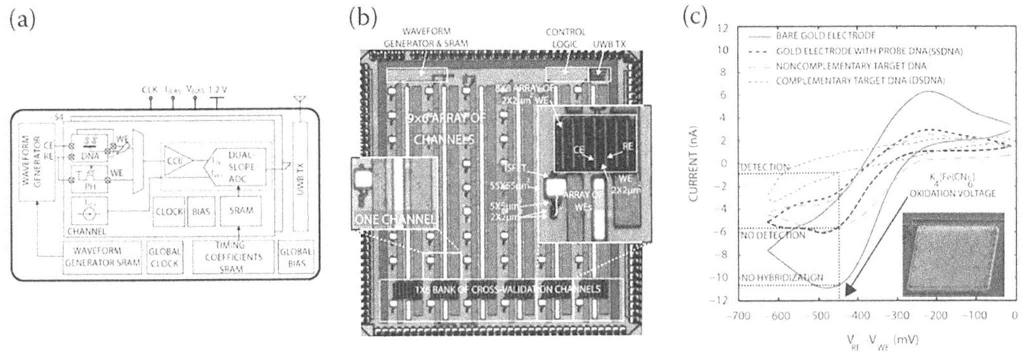

(a)

(b)

(c)

FIGURE 6.3
(a) Block diagram of a wireless DNA analysis microsystem implemented in a 0.13 µm standard CMOS process. (b) Die photomicrograph. The chip is 3 mm x 3 mm in size. (c) Experimental cyclic voltammogram showing the detection of 5 µM synthetic prostate cancer DNA. Reprinted with permission from [13]. Copyright (2014) IEEE.

typical DNA detection methods, the sensor did not require the use of polymerase chain reaction (PCR). Rather, the system featured a 54-channel, label-free, and fast-scan voltammetric DNA analysis platform. The sensor was implemented in a 0.13 µm CMOS process, and it exemplified the "system-on-a-chip" paradigm in chip design as it contained various components necessary for accomplishing a set of different tasks (e.g., sensing, signal conditioning, transmission, data storage, and signal generation).

The principle of operation of the sensor was based on the label-free detection of DNA using a potassium ferricyanide reporter $K_4[Fe(CN)_6]$. This reporter is a negatively charged redox complex, and it has a well-defined electrochemical signature that has oxidation and reduction currents at reference-to-working electrode potentials of 450 mV and 250 mV, respectively. Maximum electron transfer from the transduction electrode and the reporter occurs when there are no DNA targets and DNA probes present. When a single-stranded DNA probe molecule is present at the electrode, electron transfer is decreased; this reduces the redox current, resulting in smaller redox peaks in the cyclic voltammogram. When a target DNA strand hybridizes with the probe DNA strand on the electrode, these peaks are further reduced as a result of an additional decrease in the redox current.

The transduction electrode was implemented with nano-structured metal deposits on the aluminum sensing pads of the CMOS chip. This process involved the deposition of nickel, palladium, and gold using an autocatalytic deposition process. Further nano-structuring was achieved with electrostatic gold deposition by placing the chip in a solution containing gold and deionized water. The system achieved label-free and PCR-free DNA detection with a detection limit of 10 aM.

6.4 Interfacial Capacitance Sensors and Electric Cell-Substrate Impedance Spectroscopy

We turn now to the review of capacitance as a biosensing modality. Capacitance is a measure of the ability of a system formed from two conductors separated by an insulator to store charge. When an electric potential is applied to this two-electrode system, one electrode (the cathode) attracts positive charges and the other electrode (the anode) attracts negative charges. As these charges separate, they create an electric field across the insulator. The capacitance of this system is established by the degree to which the charges remain stored, and this depends on the permittivity of the insulator, the separation distance between the two conductors (i.e., the insulator's thickness), and the area of the electrodes.

In capacitance biosensing, this two-electrode system is interfaced with cells, biomolecules, and/or liquid samples. Introducing these species within the system leads to local perturbations in effective permittivity at the interface due to the species' dielectric properties. These perturbations manifest themselves as a change in capacitance, and this change is the basis for detecting events at the interface between the electrodes. For this reason, we term this method "interfacial capacitance sensing."

Capacitance sensing has been shown in a variety of bioassays ranging from pH measurement [14], DNA detection, biological cell sensing [15], particle migration [16], and length estimation of artificial muscles [17]. When implemented in CMOS processes, capacitance biosensing provides a compact means for label-free sensing. In the following subsections, we introduce several constitutive elements of a CMOS interfacial capacitance sensor, and we discuss an example architecture from our work.

6.4.1 Transducers for Interfacial Capacitance Sensing

In integrated circuit settings, capacitance transducers are typically implemented as interdigitated electrodes formed using the chip's top metal layer. The electrodes are passivated, i.e., they remain covered by the final insulating coating applied to the silicon wafer during the CMOS fabrication process [18,19]. This geometry results in a significant fringe field that passes through the sample when the electrodes are energized. Perturbations at the interface are thus mapped directly to the capacitance of the electrode system, and an underlying circuit in the CMOS substrate senses the induced change in capacitance. Figure 6.4 illustrates this example configuration. The electrodes can transduce cell activity by monitoring the *coupled* interfacial capacitance which is modeled as a

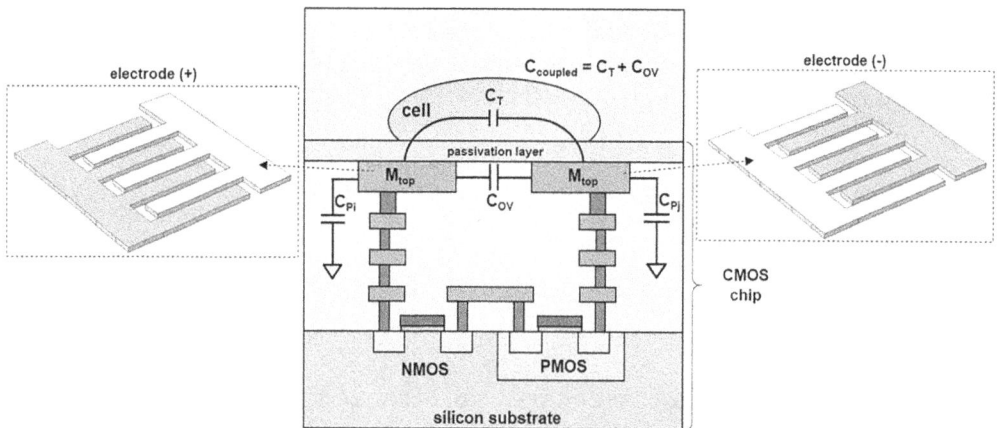

FIGURE 6.4
Schematic of a CMOS capacitance sensor configured for cell analysis. The electrodes form an interdigitated pair of conductors. The capacitance at the interface may be read by a circuit in the silicon substrate (denoted NMOS and PMOS for simplicity). The capacitors C_{Pi} and C_{Pj} are parasitic capacitances.

variable sense capacitance denoted C_T and the fixed intrinsic capacitance of the electrode denoted C_{OV}; the latter corresponds to the overlap capacitance between the two conductors M_{TOP} that form the electrodes.

6.4.2 Examples of Applications of CMOS Capacitance Sensors

Figure 6.5 shows an example CMOS capacitance-to-frequency sensor for studying the proliferation of ovarian cancer cells. In this work, we used two human ovarian cancer cell lines (CP70 and A2780). The sensor was implemented in a 0.35 µm CMOS process, and it included a 4 × 4 array of capacitance sensing pixels. Each pixel included an interdigitated set of electrodes connected to a free-running NMOS oscillator. The output from the oscillator in each pixel was fed to a counter via a multiplexer, thereby allowing the pixels to share the counter. The counter was read via an I²C serial interface.

During operation, the pixels were able to measure the activity of overlying ovarian cancer cells with a front-end conversion of 590 kHz/fF. The sensor was able to detect single-cell binding events as well as changes in morphology and cell migration. With concurrent optical imaging as a means to obtain ground truth data, we demonstrated that such a sensor could also be used to estimate cell coverage, thereby providing an easy means to perform cell counting. The sensor only needed a microcontroller for readout, which made it easy to interface with a personal computer. In addition to studying cell coverage, this sensor was used to show how different concentrations of cisplatin, a chemotherapeutic agent, affected cancer cells. Specifically, the data showed that time of death could be estimated with the sensor following exposure to different concentrations of cisplatin [21–26].

6.4.3 Electric Cell-Substrate Impedance Sensing

Interfacial capacitance sensors are unable to provide information on the complex impedance of biological materials such as DNA and whole cells. To that end, electric

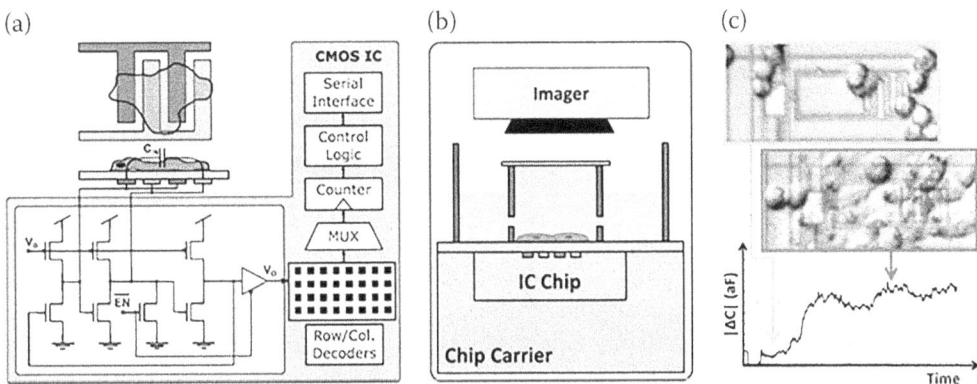

FIGURE 6.5
Overview of a CTF capacitance sensor configured for studying cell proliferation via substrate coupling monitoring. (a) Pixel and readout chain schematic. (b) Schematic of a packaged CTF capacitance sensor chip (see ref. [20] for packaging methods). (c) Example images of cells growing on top of the sensor along with the corresponding measured time-series data. The measured change in capacitance increases as cell coverage increases. Reprinted with permission from [21]. Copyright (2019) IEEE.

cell-substrate impedance spectroscopy (ECIS) has been widely used to monitor cells in real time and without the use of labels. The technique relies on the basic application of Ohm's law to a two-electrode system [27–29]. The cells in impedance sensors can be in contact with the electrodes by adhering directly to the electrodes or they can be in suspension. The presence or absence of a cell, the location of the cell, and the shape and size of the cell all affect the electric field lines between two electrodes. The cells' interactions with the field lines are recorded as a change in current, and the relationship between this change in current and the applied voltage is recorded as the impedance.

Although impedance sensing has a significant advantage of being label-free and affording real-time monitoring, the technique lacks specificity. For example, cells moving farther away in the vertical direction from an electrode may give a similar impedance measurement compared to cells that are shrinking (smaller impedance) but are near the electrode. Despite this, impedance sensing is useful for monitoring populations of cells over time, and it provides another method for label-free imaging of cells. Furthermore, since the internal cellular environment affects cell morphology, impedance sensing is useful for monitoring, for example, the effects of external stimuli on cells and overall cell viability. Cell types can also be differentiated, and this capability can be useful in applications such as differentiating cancer cells from healthy cells. Potentially, even identifying different stages of the disease, such as early-stage versus metastasized cancer cells can be performed using impedance sensing.

6.4.4 Examples of Applications of CMOS ECIS Sensors

An example application of an impedance sensor was demonstrated by Jung et al. [30]. They showed a multi-modal array for simultaneous extracellular potential, impedance, and optical sensing. The chip used a 4-point impedance measurement based on the swept frequency approach over a 15 kHz to 500 kHz range. The design used SAR ADCs and four pixels were selected from a bank of pixels for each differential mode measurement of the complex impedance. The design was implemented in a 0.13 μm CMOS process and contained 21,592 pixels with a 16 μm × 16 μm pitch and gold-plated electrodes. The chip was able to produce an impedance image of neonatal rat ventricular myocytes.

6.5 Image Sensors

CMOS image sensors are ubiquitous in consumer electronics products, notably in cell phones. High-performance CMOS image sensors are now increasingly being considered for biosensing applications. Compared to charge-coupled devices (CCDs), CMOS image sensors have lower power consumption and can be implemented using a system-on-a-chip framework. These features offer the possibility for integrating them in biosensing platforms as a means for optical sensing via fluorescence sensing, direct contact imaging, or luminescence imaging [31–40]. These imagers typically use active pixel sensors [41] as the pixel configuration for intensity-based detection or single-photon avalanche diodes for time-resolved detection [39], [40], [42–48]. In this section, we discuss the basic architecture of CMOS image sensors and their design, and we discuss several example applications.

6.5.1 CMOS Image Sensor Architecture

A CMOS image sensor is a mixed-signal circuit that typically includes at least four main blocks. These blocks are the pixel array (typically disposed of in a 2D configuration), analog signal processors, row and column selectors, and timing/control units.

Each pixel in the array typically consists of a photodiode that is configured to sense impinging photons by converting them into photo-generated carriers. These free carriers are collected by the field across the reverse-biased photodiode, thus creating a photo-current that is proportional to the light intensity, notwithstanding losses at the interface due to reflection and the non-unity quantum efficiency of the photodiode. Each pixel in the array is subjected to a different amount of light, consistent with the scene that is being imaged by the device. The pixel array is then scanned to reproduce the image based on the number of carriers that are collected at each pixel.

The row and column selector circuits may be implemented using programmable logic elements to select any pixel in the array. With this hardware, the array may be rasterized and reset to produce an image. The timing and control units generate bus access and pixel readout control signals, and the analog signal processors generally can include circuits for fixed pattern noise (FPN) mitigation, reset noise mitigation, and other front-end processing (e.g., correlated-double sampling, difference double sampling, histogram equalization, etc.). Additionally, the peripheral circuitry can include digital signal processing modules for on-chip image conditioning. Lastly, an array of microlenses and color filters may be applied on top of the passivation to increase external quantum efficiency and to provide color information, respectively.

6.5.2 CMOS Image Sensors in Fluorescence Imaging

In many biomedical and environmental applications, the presence of a target substance, i.e., a specific molecule or nucleic acid sequence, is detected through fluorescence sensing. Since CMOS image sensors offer lower power consumption, on-chip functionality, and high temporal resolution, they have been used in integrated fluorescence sensors for point-of-care settings. For instance, Manickam et al. [38] implemented a biochip for DNA and RNA testing employing a CMOS image sensor. This biochip module is shown in Figure 6.6; it was

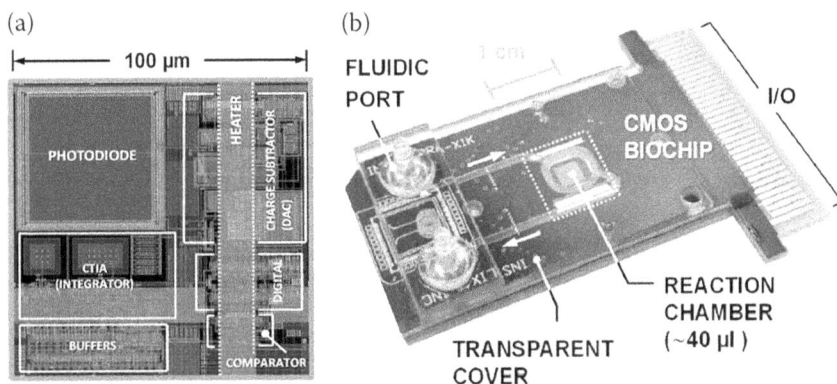

FIGURE 6.6
(a) Layout view of a pixel from a CMOS biochip configured for fluorescence-based bioassays. (b) System integration, showing the readout board, the chip, and the fluidic layer for sample delivery to the analysis sites. Reprinted with permission from ref. [38] Copyright (2017) IEEE.

composed of a CMOS chip, an integrated emission filter (see refs. [49,50] for example integrated filters for CMOS fluorescence sensors), DNA probes, and a fluidic cap. The CMOS integrated circuit itself included an array of 32 × 32 fluorescence detection biosensing elements.

Each sensing element included an n-well/p-sub photodiode, a first-order current sensing modulator and all its required electronics, and a heater for DNA amplification procedures such as PCR. Each biosensing element was 100 μm × 100 μm, and the photodetector was 50 μm × 50 μm. The current sensing modulator was a ΣΔ operator that enhanced the noise performance significantly. As a proof of concept, the authors demonstrated the successful detection of a panel of human upper respiratory viruses.

6.6 Conclusions

In this chapter, we discussed several trends in the development of microsystems for bioelectronics. Specifically, we reviewed CMOS circuits and some of their salient design aspects as they pertain to the development of neural interfaces, electrochemical sensors, interfacial capacitance, cell impedance sensors, and image sensors. The devices we discussed all had a common denominator: their engineering featured the confluence of several fields (e.g., biochemistry, microsystems engineering, cell biology, to name a few). This illustrates the multi-disciplinary nature of the bioelectronics field and the need for a co-design approach that leverages insights from various technological and scientific domains to provide viable solutions to the many problems addressed.

In closing, we will point the reader to two additional trends in bioelectronics. The first, which is apparent from some of the exemplary devices we discussed, is the drive towards multi-modal systems that can support two or more sensing modalities on the same platform. Such multi-modal devices will enable new capabilities in biospecies analysis by providing orthogonal sensing capabilities that offer a more complete view of the microenvironments under study. The second trend is the increasing use of big data and machine learning techniques to gain additional insights from measured sensor data. We envision that bioelectronics hardware will be rendered more effective when combined with the power of machine learning algorithms capable of identifying and classifying signal patterns that are consistent with biophysical or biochemical cues of interest.

References

1. B. Bonaz, V. Sinniger, and S. Pellissier, "Therapeutic potential of vagus nerve stimulation for inflammatory bowel diseases." *Frontiers in Neuroscience*, vol. 15, 2021, pp. 1–16.
2. Z. Luo and M.D. Ker. "A high-voltage-tolerant and precise charge-balanced neuro-stimulator in low voltage CMOS process." *IEEE Transactions on Biomedical Circuits and Systems*, vol. 10, no. 6, 2016, pp. 1087–1099.
3. J.M. Aran, Z. Y. wu, Y. Cazals, R.C. de Sauvage, and M. Portmann, "Electrical stimulation of the ear: Experimental studies." *Annals of Ontology, Rhinology & Laryngology*, vol. 92, no. 6, 1983, pp. 614–620.

4. R.J. Hurlbert, C.H. Tator, and E. Theriault, "Dose-response study of the pathological effects of chronically applied direct current stimulation on the normal rat spinal cord." *Journal of Neurosurgery*, vol. 79, no. 6, 1993, pp. 905–916.
5. M.J. Lei Yao, Peng Li, "A pulse-width-adaptive active charge balancing circuit with pulse-insertion based residual charge compensation and quantization for electrical stimulation applications." *IEEE Asian Solid-State Circuits Conference*, 2015, pp. 1–4.
6. Z. Chen, X. Liu, and Z. Wang, "A charge balancing technique for neurostimulators." *Analog Integrated Circuits and Signal Processing*, vol. 105, no. 3, 2020, pp. 483–496.
7. R.B. Stein, T.R. Nichols, J. Jhamandas, L. Davis, and D. Charles, "Stable long-term recordings from cat peripheral nerves." *Brain Research*, vol. 128, no. 1, 1977, pp. 21–38.
8. M. Ashayeri and M. Yavari. "A front-end amplifier with tunable bandwidth and high value pseudo resistor for neural recording implants." *Microelectronics Journal*, vol. 119, 2022, p. 105333.
9. Y. Xiang and Y. Lu, "Using personal glucose meters and functional DNA sensors to quantify a variety of analytical targets." *Nature Chemistry*, vol. 3, no. 9, 2011, pp. 697–703.
10. Y. Xiang and Y. Lu, "Portable and quantitative detection of protein biomarkers and small molecular toxins using antibodies and ubiquitous personal glucose meters." *Analytical Chemistry*, vol. 84, no. 9, 2012, pp. 4174–4178.
11. Y. Xiang and Y. Lu, "Using commercially available personal glucose meters for portable quantification of DNA." *Analytical Chemistry*, vol. 84, no. 4, 2012, pp. 1975–1980.
12. Y. Huang and A.J. Mason, "Lab-on-CMOS integration of microfluidics and electrochemical sensors." *Lab on a Chip*, vol. 13, no. 19, 2013, pp. 3929–3934.
13. H.M. Jafari, K. Abdelhalim, L. Soleymani, E.H. Sargent, S.O. Kelley, and R. Genov, "Nanostructured CMOS wireless ultra-wideband label-free PCR-free DNA analysis SoC." *IEEE Journal of Solid-State Circuits*, vol. 49, no. 5, 2014, pp. 1223–1241.
14. K.B. Parizi, A.J. Yeh, A.S.Y. Poon, and H.-S.P. Wong, "Exceeding Nernst limit (59mV/pH): CMOS-based pH sensor for autonomous applications." *International Electron Devices Meeting*, 2012, pp. 24.7.1–24.7.4.
15. G. Nabovati, E. Ghafar-Zadeh, A. Letourneau, and M. Sawan, "Towards high throughput cell growth screening: A new CMOS 8x8 biosensor array for life science applications." *IEEE Transactions on Biomedical Circuits and Systems*, vol. 11, no. 2, 2017, pp. 380–391.
16. N.T. Ali Othman, H. Obara, A. Sapkota, and M. Takei, "Measurement of particle migration in micro-channel by multi-capacitance sensing method." *Flow Measurement and Instrumentation*, vol. 45, 2015, pp. 162–169.
17. J. Legrand, B. Loenders, A. Vos, L. Schoevaerdts, and E. vander Poorten, "Integrated capacitance sensing for miniature artificial muscle actuators." *IEEE Sensors Journal*, vol. 20, no. 3, 2019, pp. 1363–1372.
18. S.B. Prakash and P. Abshire, "A fully differential rail-to-rail capacitance measurement circuit for integrated cell sensing." *IEEE Sensors Conference*, 2007, pp. 1444–1447.
19. S. Forouhi, R. Dehghani, and E. Ghafar-Zade, "Toward high throughput core-CBCM CMOS capacitive sensors for life science applications: A novel current-mode for high dynamic range circuitry." *Sensors*, vol. 18, no. 10, 2018, article 3370.
20. M. Dandin, Im Deok Jung, Menake Piyasena, James Gallagher, Nicole Nelson, Mario Urdaneta, Chantelle Artis, Pamela Abshire, and Elisabeth Smela. "Post-CMOS packaging methods for integrated biosensors." *IEEE Sensors Conference*, 2009, pp. 795–798.
21. B.P. Senevirathna, S. Lu, M. Dandin, E. Smela, and P.A. Abshire. "Correlation of capacitance and microscopy measurements using image processing for a Lab-on-CMOS microsystem." *IEEE Transactions on Biomedical Circuits and Systems*, vol. 13, no. 6, 2019, pp. 1214–1225.
22. B.P. Senevirathna, S. Lu, M. Dandin, E. Smela, and P. Abshire. "Lab-on-CMOS capacitance sensor array for real-time cell viability measurements with I2C readout." *IEEE International Symposium on Circuits and Systems*, 2016, pp. 2863–2866.

23. S. Lu, B. Senevirathna, M. Dandin, E. Smela, and P. Abshire, "System integration of IC chips for lab-on-CMOS applications." IEEE International Symposium on Circuits and Systems, 2018, pp. 1–5.

24. B. Senevirathna, S. Lu, M. Dandin, J. Basile, E. Smela, and P. Abshir, "High resolution monitoring of chemotherapeutic agent potency in cancer cells using a CMOS capacitance biosensor." *Biosensors and Bioelectronics*, vol. 142, 2019, p. 111501.

25. B. Senevirathna, S. Lu, N. Renegar, M. Dandin, E. Smela, and P. Abshire, "System on a chip for automated cell assays using a Lab-on-CMOS platform." IEEE International Symposium on Circuits and Systems, 2019, pp. 1–5.

26. B.P. Senevirathna, S. Lu, M. Dandin, J. Basile, E. Smela, and P.A. Abshire, "Real-time measurements of cell proliferation using a lab-on-CMOS capacitance sensor array." *IEEE Transactions on Biomedical Circuits and Systems*, vol. 12, no. 3, 2018, pp. 510–520.

27. A. Hedayatipour, S. Aslanzadeh, and N. McFarlane, "CMOS integrated impedance to frequency converter for biomedical applications." IEEE International Symposium on Circuits and Systems, 2020, pp. 1–5.

28. S. Aslanzadeh, A. Hedayatipour, M. Smalley, and N. McFarlane, "A combined pH-impedance system suitable for portable continuous sensing." *IEEE Transactions on Biomedical Circuits and Systems*, vol. 15, no. 3, 2021, pp. 390–401.

29. A. Hedayatipour, S. Aslanzadeh, and N. McFarlane, "CMOS based whole cell impedance sensing: Challenges and future outlook." *Biosensors and Bioelectronics*, vol. 143, 2019, article 111600.

30. D. Jung, J.S. Park, G.V. Junek, S.I. Grijalva, S.R. Kumashi, A. Wang, S. Li, H.C. Cho, and H. Wang. "A 21952-pixel multi-modal CMOS cellular sensor array with 1568-pixel parallel recording and 4-point impedance sensing." Symposium on VLSI Circuits, 2019, C62–C63.

31. N. Nelson, D. Sander, M. Dandin, S.B. Prakash, A. Sarje, and P. Abshire, "Handheld fluorometers for lab-on-a-chip applications." *IEEE Transactions on Biomedical Circuits and Systems*, vol. 3, no. 2, 2009, pp. 97–107.

32. N. Nelson, D. Sander, M. Dandin, A. Sarje, S. Prakash, H. Ji, and P. Abshire. "A handheld fluorometer for measuring cellular metabolism." IEEE International Symposium on Circuits and Systems, 2018, pp. 1080–1083.

33. N. Nelson, S. Prakash, D. Sander, M. Dandin, A. Sarje, H. Ji, and P. Abshire. "A handheld fluorometer for UV excitable fluorescence assays." IEEE Biomedical Circuits and Systems Conference, 2007, pp. 111–114.

34. D. Sander, M. Dandin, H. Ji, N. Nelson, and P. Abshire, "Low-noise CMOS fluorescence sensor." IEEE International Symposium on Circuits and Systems, 2007, pp. 2007–2010.

35. H. Ji, D. Sander, A. Haas and P.A. Abshire, "Contact imaging: Simulation and experiment." *IEEE Transactions on Circuits and Systems I*, vol. 54, no. 8, 2007, pp. 1698–1710.

36. R.R. Singh, D. Ho, A. Nilchi, G. Gulak, P. Yau and R. Genov, "A CMOS/Thin-Film fluorescence contact imaging microsystem for DNA analysis." *IEEE Transactions on Circuits and Systems I*, vol. 57, no. 5, 2010, pp. 1029–1038.

37. A.K. Mudraboyina, L. Blockstein, C.C. Luk, N.I. Syed and O. Yadid-Pecht, "A novel lensless miniature contact imaging system for monitoring calcium changes in live neurons." *IEEE Photonics Journal*, vol. 6, no. 1, 2014, pp. 1–15.

38. A. Manickam, R. Singh, M.W. McDermott, N. Wood, S. Bolouki, P. Naraghi-Arani, K.A. Johnson, R.G. Kuimelis, G. Schoolnik, and A. Hassibi. "A fully integrated CMOS fluorescence biochip for DNA and RNA testing." *IEEE Journal of Solid-State Circuits*, vol. 52, no. 11, 2017, pp. 2857–2870.

39. A. Usai, N. Finlayson, C.D. Gregory, C. Campbell, and R.K. Henderson. "Separating fluorescence from Raman spectra using a CMOS SPAD TCSPC line sensor for biomedical applications." *Optical Biopsy XVII: Toward Real-Time Spectroscopic Imaging and Diagnosis*, vol. 10873, 2019, pp. 75–90.

40. F.M. della Rocca, F. Mattioli, J. Nedbal, D. Tyndall, N. Krstajić, D.D. Li, S.M. Ameer-Beg, and R.K. Henderson. "Real-time fluorescence lifetime actuation for cell sorting using a CMOS SPAD silicon photomultiplier." *Optics Letters*, vol. 41, no. 4, 2016, pp. 673–676.
41. P.J.W. Noble, "Self-scanned silicon image detector arrays." *IEEE Transactions on Electron Devices*, vol. 15, no. 4, 1968, pp. 202–209.
42. M. Dandin, A. Akturk, B. Nouri, N. Goldsman, and P. Abshire, "Characterization of single-photon avalanche diodes in a 0.5 μm standard CMOS process—Part 1: Perimeter breakdown suppression." *IEEE Sensors Journal*, vol. 10, no. 11, 2010, pp. 1682–1690.
43. M. Dandin, M. Habib, B. Nouri, P. Abshire, and N. McFarlane, "Characterization of single-photon avalanche diodes in a 0.5 μm standard CMOS process—Part 2: Equivalent circuit model and Geiger mode readout." *IEEE Sensors Journal*, vol. 16, no. 9, 2016, pp. 3075–3083.
44. M. Dandin and P. Abshire, "High signal-to-noise ratio avalanche photodiodes with perimeter field gate and active readout." *IEEE Electron Device Letters*, vol. 33, no. 4, 2012, pp. 570–572.
45. M. Dandin and P. Abshire, "Near breakdown spectral responsivity of perimeter-gated single-photon avalanche diodes." International Midwest Symposium on Circuits and Systems, 2017, pp. 867–870.
46. M. Dandin, A. Akturk, A. Vert, S. Soloviev, P. Sandvik, S. Potbhare, N. Goldsman, P. Abshire, and K.P. Cheung, "Optoelectronic characterization of 4H-SiC avalanche photodiodes operated in DC and in Geiger mode." International Semiconductor Device Research Symposium, 2011, pp. 1–2.
47. M. Dandin, N. Nelson, V. Saveliev, H. Ji, P. Abshire, and I. Weinberg, "Single photon avalanche detectors in standard CMOS." IEEE Sensors Conference, 2007, pp. 585–588.
48. A. Akturk, M. Dandin, N. Goldsman, and P. Abshire, "Modeling of perimeter-gated silicon avalanche diodes fabricated in a standard single-well CMOS process." International Semiconductor Device Research Symposium, 2009, pp. 1–2.
49. M. Dandin, P. Abshire, and E. Smela. "Polymer filters for ultraviolet-excited integrated fluorescence sensing." *Journal of Micromechanics and Microengineering*, vol. 22, no. 9, 2012, p. 095018.
50. M. Dandin, P. Abshire, and E. Smela. "Optical filtering technologies for integrated fluorescence sensors." *Lab on a Chip*, vol. 7, no. 8, 2007, pp. 955–977.

7

Identification of the Scientific and Technological Trajectory in the Area of Bioelectronics: A Patent and Networks Analysis

Alejandro Barragán-Ocaña and Paz Silva-Borjas

Center for Economic, Administrative and Social Research (CIECAS), National Polytechnic Institute (IPN), Mexico City, Mexico

María de los Ángeles Olvera-Treviño

Faculty of Chemistry, National Autonomous University of Mexico (UNAM), Metrology Unit, Mexico City, Mexico

CONTENTS

7.1 Introduction

The application of electric current to a biological system (frog legs) by Luigi Galvani is considered to be the birth of bioelectronics. Nowadays, progress in this discipline is remarkable, and it has multiple health care and environmental protection applications. Besides electronics and biology, bioelectronics integrates elements of other fields, such as small-scale technologies and bionanotechnology applications. This context favors the integration of biomaterials with electronic or electrical applications that can be materialized into useful devices. Among these developments are biosensors used to measure glucose; devices intended to restore physiological functions, such as cochlear implants; as well as other instruments that allow for insights into the communication between living cells and the environment [1,2]. Other contemporary bioelectronic applications are implantable cardioverter defibrillators and human-machine interfaces for the disabled [3].

Bioelectronics is a relatively young discipline, but its evolution has already produced complex devices for application in multiple types of tissues [4]. Interdisciplinarity is an essential characteristic of this field of knowledge. Examples of this characteristic are new biomaterials necessary for the operation of some electronic transducers [5]. Biomolecules and ions constitute the communication mechanism within biological systems at the intra- and inter-cellular level; this mechanism is the basis of bioelectronics; it opens possibilities for lifesaving future therapeutic applications and integrates other types of applications, including those envisioned by synthetic biology [6]. Thus, this discipline provides different alternatives; some of them are already feasible while others have promising technological development potential. Plastic bioelectronics stands out among these developments: it combines polymers with the principles of soft organic electronics to produce applications or materials that allow for adequate interfaces to achieve efficient implementation within biological systems. [7].

Other relevant research includes bio-inspired adhesive architectures used in the health sector on human body surfaces [8]; self-adhesive bioelectronics that can use hydrogels to enhance the use of implants and wearable devices [9]; implantable bioelectronics, an emerging and widely useful biomedical field whose applications could be used in diagnostic tasks and therapeutic procedures [10]; and miniaturized devices, whose adequate operation will require new power storage and supply technologies such as wireless transfer to increase their useful life with compact designs [11]. Although bioelectronics has already produced important advances, its challenges ahead are enormous. Therefore, supporting science and technology is an essential activity, as well as developing mechanisms to promote innovation in this sector.

7.2 Scientific and Technological Advances in Bioelectronics

Concerning living tissue, bioelectronics relies on a signal transduction mechanism that, via different devices, creates an interface that allows for the measurement and regulation of different biological functions to improve health and interventions against diseases [12]. Bioelectronic interfaces can be used on the skin or inside the organism [13]. An attractive feature of organic electronic materials is their ability to conduct electronic and ionic signals, which allows for adequate processing. On the other hand, organic electronic polymers based on ad-hoc designs provide opportunities for specific answers regarding the chemical and physical properties necessary for creating bioelectronic systems and developing devices that combine mouldability, flexibility, and elasticity with stable and biocompatible surface chemistry [14].

An interesting case is conjugated polymers, which can play the role of bridges for multiple and potential applications combining biology and electronics thanks to the versatile nature of their electronic and ionic conductivity profiles [15]. However, these types of polymers are limited in terms of biodegradability, and for long-term use, very few studies have focused on their biocompatibility, which has delayed their adoption and the development of clinical applications [16]. Graphene is another suitable material for bionic applications due to its physical and chemical properties and characteristics, idoneous for constructing bioelectronic platforms [17,18]. For its part, ionic and electronic (or mixed) transport offers valuable and feasible possibilities for organic bioelectronics, and its uses can already be observed in applications such as electrolyte-based organic electrochemical transistor activation [19,20]. These transistors can be used to detect ions, hormones, and even pathogens, and they are idoneous for *in-vivo* applications capable of capturing electrophysiological registers or detecting neurotransmitters, among other functions [21,22].

The development of hybrid systems is undoubtedly feasible because, at a nanometric scale, biomolecules such as enzymes or antibodies are comparable to metallic/semiconductor nanoparticles, which makes it possible to integrate the properties of nanoparticles with functions of biomolecules to make way for novel material functions in nanometric circuits and devices, as well as biosensors [23]. There is also substantial progress in neuroscience and cardiology, which will allow this field to address future challenges posed by the electrophysiology of cells and excitable tissues; the goal is to increasingly understand the dynamics of healthy and diseased cellular circuits and networks [18]. Neurological disorder treatment can expect many new alternatives from bioelectronics [24,25].

Nanobioelectronics is heading toward specialized studies focused on brain activity, such as neural circuits that require the use of both cellular and subcellular resolutions for an adequate approach [26]. Likewise, neuroprosthetics and neuroscience have seized the opportunities of bioelectronics to devise numerous new technologies [27]. Bioelectronics is a complex field, requiring multiple elements to implement solutions. Among these elements is the study of hydrogels, a fundamental and promising operation interface between biological and electronic systems [28]. For its part, smartphone technology has promising areas of opportunity; for example, its integration with sensors capable of providing rapid and inexpensive biochemical detections relevant for health, environmental, and food-related issues [29].

Concerning the environment, microbial electronic devices provide energy production solutions and options for wastewater treatment, contaminant detection, and obtaining chemical products [30]. In medicine, bioelectronic devices show great versatility, which will probably increase in the future thanks to flexible materials that provide more options for the design of new applications [31,32], for instance, organic electronic devices will be more flexible and softer to better mimic original biological structures [33], so one of the main purposes of this discipline is to create interfaces for these developments to be properly merged with biological tissue [34]. Similarly, the potential of nanomedicine will increase thanks to the advantages of organic bioelectronics [35].

In this context, it is essential to describe the scientific and technological trajectory of bioelectronics in terms of academic research and developed applications. In this regard, bibliometric studies reveal relevant information on the progress of basic science in the field, and the analysis of patent documents represents a supply of important technical and economic information because it allows to determine trends in technological fields, to understand these trends, and to help to define and establish strategies and policies at the country level to stimulate technological progress and competitiveness [36–38]. Furthermore, these analysis techniques can be complemented by network analysis to better understand the analyzed cases. Research has already demonstrated this point; studies have used bibliometrics to explore biomedicine, clinical research, and public health [39,40], as well as nanotechnology and bionanotechnology [41], which shows the feasibility of outlining the evolution of basic research in different scientific areas.

Research and development (R&D) programs have often been approached using patent documents analysis [42]. Examples include research efforts that integrate more than one of these tools (bibliometric studies, patent document search, and network analysis) on topics such as emerging technologies related to optical storage [43], microbial fuel cells [44], enzyme immobilization [45], biomaterials oriented to the development of health applications [46], and electrical conducting polymer nanocomposite [47]. In the present research, the study of scientific trajectories used bibliometric and network analyses. In contrast, the study of technological trajectories used patent application analysis, including indicators such as main technological classes, principal applicants, and jurisdictions, and a network-based study (co-occurrence analysis).

7.3 Methodology

The research process to identify the scientific and technological trajectory was carried out in two phases. The first phase used the Scopus database [48] to obtain bibliographic data to conduct the bibliometric and network analyses. The terms *bioelectronics* and *bioelectronic* were entered into the search field (article title, abstract, keywords) under the following criteria: ((TITLE-ABS-KEY(bioelectronics) OR TITLE-ABS-KEY (bioelectronic))). A total of 4,384 documents published between 1963 and 2022 were obtained from the query. The documents were analyzed to show the top ten positions on the following indicators: 1. Country or territory; 2. Affiliation; 3. Subject area; and 4. Source. Subsequently, the bibliographic information of the 2,000 most-cited documents was downloaded and, based on these data, we carried out the co-occurrence analysis using authors' keywords and the full counting method. This analysis produced 4,045 keywords, which were filtered by an occurrence for each word (equal to or greater than five), for a total of 196 terms that met this condition; 195 presented some type of connection. This information was used to create a normalized network map using the fractionalization method, which included 195 nodes distributed in 12 clusters, with 1,476 links and a total link strength of 2,403.

The second phase of the methodological development used the Lens [49] database, which includes different patent document databases (World Intellectual Property Organization-WIPO; the U.S. Patent and Trademark Office-USPTO; European Patent Office-EPO; and IP Australia). As in the previous case, the terms *bioelectronics* and *bioelectronic* were entered for query, but in this case, in the "title, abstract, or claims" field, using the following search criteria: (title:(bioelectronics) OR abstract:(bioelectronics) OR claim:(bioelectronics)) AND (title:(bioelectronic) OR abstract:(bioelectronic) OR claim: (bioelectronic)). The patent applications filter was added to analyze the trends of technologies that applicants want to protect. A total of 349 records were obtained for the period from 1988 to 2022, which were grouped into 192 simple families and 177 extended families. With this information, we highlighted the top ten positions for the following indicators: (i) jurisdiction, (ii) applicants, and (iii) technological sectors, according to International Patent Classification (IPC) guidelines. Subsequently, we downloaded data from the 349 patent documents. With these data, we created a network map with the following characteristics: (i) The terms to be analyzed were obtained from the title and abstract; (ii) the counting method was full counting, with which 2,915 terms were obtained; (iii) of these, 466 presented an occurrence equal to or greater than five, and these were evaluated to determine their relevance (only 60% were selected); (iv) from these, 280 items were obtained, although the largest set of related terms was 261; and (v) with this information, it was possible to create a normalized network map through the fractionalization method with 261 nodes grouped into 14 clusters, with 2,404 links and a total link strength of 28,448.

7.4 Analysis and Discussion of Results

The bibliographic data obtained from the Scopus database was used for the bibliometric analysis, which revealed relevant scientific production indicators. Table 7.1 shows the ten most important results for each of these items. China and the United States are the leading countries, and the rest of the list includes only Asian and European countries. However, in terms of affiliation, the first nine positions are occupied by institutions from Asia and Europe, and the United States appears in the tenth position, with the Northwestern University. In other words, although the United States dominates in total scientific production, Asian and European institutions are displaying remarkable progress in bioelectronics-related research.

The number of publications classified in the categories of engineering; materials science; chemistry; biochemistry, genetics and molecular biology; and physics was over 1,000. Although in the case of physics the category is shared with astronomy, the documents are related to bioelectronics. Nevertheless, there is significant progress in areas such as chemical engineering, medicine, computer science, multidisciplinary studies, and energy. In other words, progress is being made in the study and understanding of the

TABLE 7.1

Main Bibliometric Indicators for Bioelectronics

No.	Country	Documents	Affiliation	Documents
1	United States	1,419	Chinese Academy of Sciences	135
2	China	725	Linköpings Universitet	122
3	South Korea	356	Ministry of Education China	116
4	United Kingdom	345	Seoul National University	94
5	Italy	323	Consiglio Nazionale delle Ricerche	92
6	Germany	293	Sogang University	73
7	France	214	École des Mines de Saint-Étienne	71
8	Sweden	192	Imperial College London	71
9	Japan	174	Istituto Italiano di Tecnologia	66
10	India	165	Northwestern University	64

No.	Subject area	Documents	Source	Documents
1	Engineering	2,082	Biosensors and Bioelectronics	286
2	Materials Science	1,948	Advanced Materials	132
3	Chemistry	1,655	Advanced Functional Materials	119
4	Biochemistry, Genetics and Molecular Biology	1,050	ACS Applied Materials and Interfaces	112
5	Physics and Astronomy	1,050	Proceedings of SPIE The International Society for Optical Engineering	61
6	Chemical Engineering	734	Sensors and Actuators B Chemical	54
7	Medicine	337	ACS Nano	52
8	Computer Science	302	Advanced Materials Technologies	46
9	Multidisciplinary	164	Journal of Materials Chemistry B	44
10	Energy	132	Langmuir	44

Source: Authors' elaboration based on Scopus [48].

principles that govern bioelectronics, but at the same time, all these disciplines are bound to transform this knowledge into tangible technological solutions. In addition, several journals specialize in the field. According to Scopus, these journals held important positions in the 2020 SJR [50] ranking, and some classifications, their best position made the Q1 quartile, for example, (i) biosensors and bioelectronics: 2.55 and Q1 in biomedical engineering; (ii) advanced materials: 10.71 and Q1 in materials science; (iii) advanced functional materials: 6.07 and Q1 in biomaterials; (iv) ACS applied materials and interfaces: 2.54 y Q1 in materials science (see Table 7.1).

The network analysis based on the bibliographic data showed the presence of high-occurrence nodes: basic research fields of knowledge that have been fundamental for the advancement of bioelectronics (Figure 7.1). For example, in cluster 3, the biosensor node stands out with 89 occurrences, 80 links, and a total link strength of 173. The term is related to other elements of interest, such as electrochemistry, glucose oxidase, biofuel cells, and carbon nanotubes, among others. Another relevant case was found in cluster 1, where graphene appears with 55 occurrences, 54 links, and a total link strength of 109, and one more in cluster 5, where organic bioelectronics presented 63 occurrences, 36 links, and a total link strength of 81. In the first case, the node is related to terms such as conductive polymers and flexible electronics, while in the second case, the node relates with interesting terms such as bioelectronic medicine and conjugated polymers.

It should be highlighted that, unlike in the bibliometric analysis, the number of patent applications is significantly lower, and their presence begins in the 1980s, which indicates that basic science is more developed than technology. In terms of patent applications, the United States is the leader. This country represents an important technology market par excellence, although a significant number of PCT applications are processed through WIPO; that is, protection for these patent applications is sought in places other than their origin. The rest of the ranking includes Asian countries, European patents, Canada, Australia, and Greece. The case of China is of particular interest because it more than doubles European patents. Regarding patent documents by the applicant, U.S. companies stand out, and European companies and individuals to a lesser extent. The participation of the academy and individuals who file these requests is worth attention. One likely explanation is that further progress is still needed in materializing the scientific principles of bioelectronics in different devices to encourage companies to make these applications available to markets (Table 7.2).

The IPC International Patent Classification is a valuable progress indicator for different technological sectors, as becomes evident when grouping these patent applications into different categories. In this case, many patent documents were located in the C12Q 1/68 subcategory, which involves technological developments related to nucleic acids. This subcategory belongs to another subcategory integrating essential elements for the development of bioelectronics, such as enzymes. The following classification also considers elements that cannot be integrated into any other group in this subclass; in other words, bioelectronic technologies are difficult to categorize due to their nature, complexity, and novelty. This ranking also shows other elements related to immunoassays, immunochemical immobilization, diagnosis, processes (chemical, physical, and physical-chemical), and stimulation electrotherapy. The discipline of bioelectronics is creating inventions within related emerging fields of knowledge, but they will take time to materialize in complete technological developments. Consequently, specific applications derived from the progress of basic science will take on greater strength in the medium and long terms (Table 7.3).

Regarding the network analysis, a fairly populated map was created from the downloaded records and the analysis criteria. The map shows many clusters and nodes

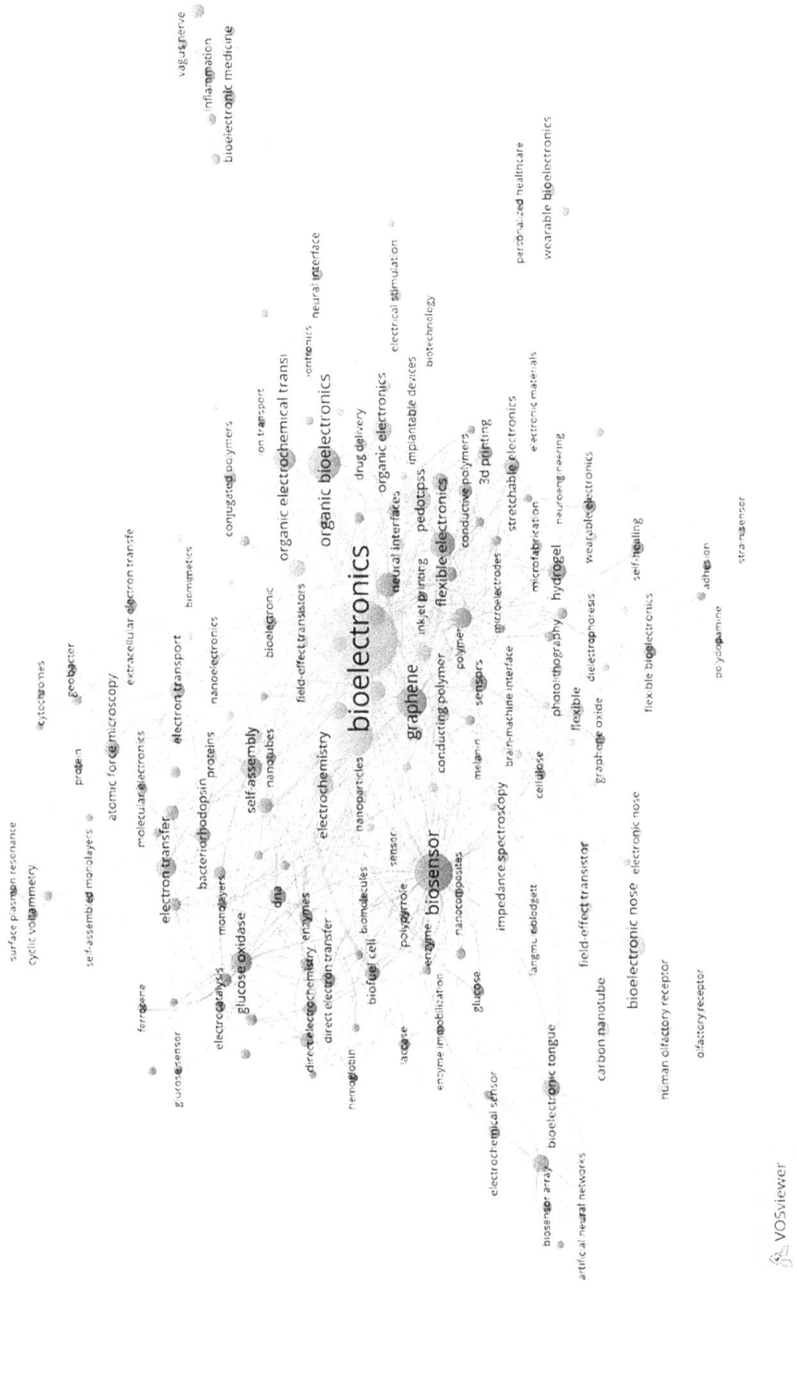

FIGURE 7.1

Co-occurrence analysis of keywords (author) – full counting (bioelectronics and bioelectronic).

Source: Authors' elaboration based on Scopus [48] and VOSviewer [51].

TABLE 7.2

Main Indicators of Patent Applications in the Field of Bioelectronics

No.	Jurisdiction	Documents	Applicants	Documents
1	United States	121	Nanogen INC	24
2	WO – WIPO	87	University of Arizona State	17
3	China	47	Edman Carl F	11
4	European Patents	22	Nanogen Becton Dickinson Partn	11
5	Canada	16	Nerenberg Michael I	11
6	Korea, Republic of	13	Orthogonal INC	11
7	Australia	12	Univ Texas	10
8	Japan	11	Tyco Healthcare	8
9	Greece	5	Ab Medica Spa	7
10	Israel	5	Max Planck Gesellschaft	7

Source: Authors' elaboration based on Lens [49].

TABLE 7.3

Main Technology Sectors According to the IPC Classification

No.	IPC classification	Description	Documents
1	C12Q1/68	"**C12Q 1/00**-Measuring or testing processes involving enzymes, nucleic acids or microorganisms (measuring or testing apparatus with condition measuring or sensing means, e.g. colony counters, C12M 1/34); Compositions therefor; Processes of preparing such compositions. **C12Q 1/68**-involving nucleic acids."	49
2	G01N37/00	"**G01N**-Investigating or analysing materials by determining their chemical or physical properties (measuring or testing processes other than immunoassay, involving enzymes or microorganisms C12M, C12Q). **G01N 37/00**-Details not covered by any other group of this subclass."	27
3	G01N33/53	"**G01N 33/00**-Investigating or analysing materials by specific methods not covered by groups G01N 1/00-G01N 31/00. **G01N 33/53**-Immunoassay; biospecific binding assay; materials therefor."	23
4	G01N33/543	"**G01N 33/00**-Investigating or analysing materials by specific methods not covered by groups G01N 1/00-G01N 31/00. **G01N 33/543**-With an insoluble carrier for immobilising immunochemicals."	23
5	A61B5/00	"Measuring for diagnostic purposes (radiation diagnosis A61B 6/00; diagnosis by ultrasonic, sonic or infrasonic waves A61B 8/00); Identification of persons."	21
6	B01J19/00	"Chemical, physical or physico-chemical processes in general; Their relevant apparatus."	20
7	A61N1/36	"**A61N 1/00**-Electrotherapy; Circuits therefor (A61N 2/00 takes precedence; electrically conductive preparations for use in therapy or testing in vivo A61K 50/00). **A61N 1/36**-For stimulation, e.g. heart pace-makers."	18

TABLE 7.3 (Continued)
Main Technology Sectors According to the IPC Classification

No.	IPC classification	Description	Documents
8	B01L3/00	"Containers or dishes for laboratory use, e.g. laboratory glassware (bottles B65D; apparatus for enzymology or microbiology C12M 1/00); Droppers (receptacles for volumetric purposes G01F)."	17
9	C12Q1/6837	"**C12Q 1/00**-Measuring or testing processes involving enzymes, nucleic acids or microorganisms (measuring or testing apparatus with condition measuring or sensing means, e.g. colony counters, C12M 1/34); Compositions therefor; Processes of preparing such compositions. **C12Q 1/6837**-Using probe arrays or probe chips (C12Q 1/6874 takes precedence)."	17
10	C12N15/09	"**C12N 15/00**-Mutation or genetic engineering; DNA or RNA concerning genetic engineering, vectors, e.g. plasmids, or their isolation, preparation or purification; Use of hosts therefor (mutants or genetically engineered microorganisms C12N 1/00, C12N 5/00, C12N 7/00; new plants A01H; plant reproduction by tissue culture techniques A01H 4/00; new animals A01K 67/00; use of medicinal preparations containing genetic material which is inserted into cells of the living body to treat genetic diseases, gene therapy A61K 48/00; peptides in general C07K). **C12N 15/09**-Recombinant DNA-technology."	16

Source: Authors' elaboration based on Lens [49] and WIPO [52].

associated with technological development in bioelectronics. Several interesting nodes stand out, such as determination, located in cluster 1, with 22 occurrences (O), 33 links (L), and a total link strength (TLS) of 637; its links connect with disease diagnostic, genetic target, and microchip systems, among others. Another example is the biopolymer node, in cluster 7, with the following results O:19/L:14/TLS:131; it is connected with the following five nodes: 1. alloy; 2. heater; 3. drug patch; 4. polymer film; and 5. bioelectronic patch device. Finally, another representative case is the stage node in cluster 3, with the following attributes: O:24/L:25/TLS:648. It connects with the terms *medical device, energy storage, low-frequency signal, signal transmission,* and *bioelectronic stimulator* (see Figure 7.2).

Finally, to illustrate the types of inventions for which protection is being sought, we present five examples of the most relevant patent applications. When considering these applications, one of the first aspects that come to mind is that four belong to academic institutions and the remainder application to individuals, which confirms the preponderant role of educational institutions and that the United States is a target market for this technological field. These inventions, shown in Table 7.4, have to do with interface development, and they approach elements related to systems, devices, circuits, and methods. They are fundamental technologies for the field's advancement, and they address the challenges of bioelectronics. Undoubtedly, the development of more efficient interfaces, the miniaturization of devices, and the construction of other cutting-edge elements will speed up the potential solutions that basic science envisions in its current state.

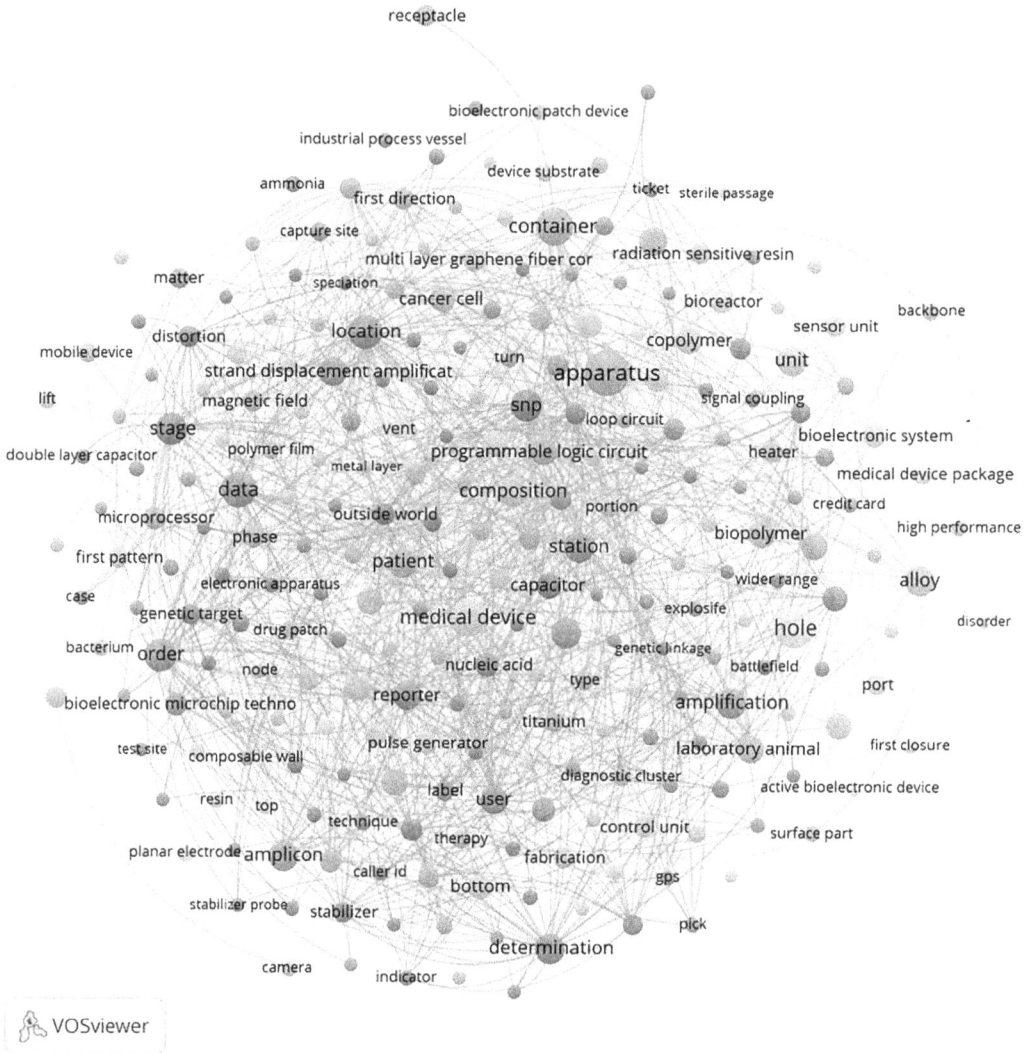

FIGURE 7.2

Co-occurrence analysis – full counting (bioelectronics and bioelectronic).

Source: Authors' elaboration based on Lens [49] and VOSviewer [51].

7.5 Conclusions

Although the birth of bioelectronics dates back to the 18th century, it is considered a relatively young discipline because the most significant applications and advances are recent. Consequently, its evolution still poses with many challenges; for instance, generating implantable devices and human-machine interfaces, bringing current technologies to a smaller scale, obtaining new biomaterials, designing novel devices focused on diagnostics and restoration of physiological functions, and developing laboratory instrumentation to augment the theoretical framework of bioelectronics. The advancement of this discipline

TABLE 7.4

Examples of Patent Applications According to Relevance

No.	Title	Published	Applicants	Identifier
1	Renewable bioelectronic interface for electrobiocatalytic reactor	10/11/2016	University of Michigan State	US 2016/0326658 A1
2	Live bioelectronic cell-gated nanodevice	30/09/2010	University of Nebraska	US 2010/0243984 A1
3	Electronic conductance in bioelectronic devices and systems	19/08/2021	University of Arizona State	WO 2021/163275 A1
4	Bioelectronic circuits, systems, and methods for preparing and using them	06/08/2020	Lindsay Stuart; Zhang Bintian; Deng Hanqing	WO 2020/160300 A2
5	S-Layer protein 2D lattice coupled detergent-Free GPCR bioelectronic interfaces, devices, and methods for the use thereof	21/11/2019	Massachusetts Institute of Technology	US 2019/0353654 A1

Source: Authors' elaboration based on Lens [49].

promises a wide range of therapeutic and synthetic biology applications, among other types. Work on potentially promising areas such as plastic bioelectronics, bio-inspired adhesive architectures, implants, and energy supply and storage must continue.

Interface development will also be essential to address health problems, and future solutions include both skin-based and internal applications, although the implications of this type of technology will have to be addressed efficiently and collaboratively. Consequently, materials-related fields must continue to evolve to achieve these objectives, where organic electronic polymers and conjugated polymers present two viable alternatives with pending challenges to address. In addition, organic electrochemical transistors will play a relevant role in detecting elements such as hormones or neurotransmitters, as well as different electrophysiological records. Thus, cardiology and neuroscience (for example, neuroprosthetics) are among the areas that will continue moving forward faster soon, both in basic research and technological development. Nevertheless, given their dependence on the progress of other discoveries and disciplines, experimental technologies will certainly take time to consolidate until they can materialize and be commercially available.

The contributions of bioelectronics to the environment will continue developing around energy generation, chemical production, contaminant detection, and wastewater treatment. New areas will continue to emerge, and as bioelectronics converges with other fields of knowledge and solutions that used to be deemed impossible will become a reality. According to the results obtained in the present study, it is evident that, in terms of documents produced and historical records, basic science is more developed than patent applications. Therefore, the materialization of findings from basic research has a slow dynamism. However, the analysis and mapping revealed highly developed areas, and others that show significant future potential. Finally, generating public policies, training human resources, investing in infrastructure, formulating collaboration agreements, and supporting bioelectronics programs are fundamental actions to accomplish these goals, and all of these actions must be carried out under a perfectly regulated framework based on strict surveillance of security, technical, economic, and ethical matters.

Acknowledgments

We wish to acknowledge the support provided by the National Polytechnic Institute (Instituto Politécnico Nacional) and the Secretariat for Research and Postgraduate Studies (Secretaría de Investigación y Posgrado), grant numbers 20220729 and 20220275.

References

1. J. Rivnay, R.M. Owens, G.G. Malliaras (2014) The rise of organic bioelectronics. *Chem. Mater.* 26 (1): 679–685.
2. D. Pankratov, E. González-Arribas, Z. Blum, S. Shleev (2016) Tear based bioelectronics. *Electroanal.* 28 (6): 1250–1266.
3. G.G. Malliaras (2013) Organic bioelectronics: A new era for organic electronics. *Biochim. Biophys. Acta.* 1830 (9): 4286–4287.
4. F. Vitale, B. Litt (2018) Bioelectronics: The promise of leveraging the body's circuitry to treat disease. *Bioelectronics in Medicine.* 1 (1): 3–7.
5. I. Willner, B. Willner (2001) Biomaterials integrated with electronic elements: en route to bioelectronics. *Trends Biotechnol.* 19 (6): 222–230.
6. M. Jia, S. Ray, R. Breault, M. Rolandi (2020) Control of pH in bioelectronics and applications. *APL Materials.* 8, 120704: 1–8.
7. T. Someya, Z. Bao, G.G. Malliaras (2016) The rise of plastic bioelectronics. *Nature.* 540: 379–385.
8. S. Baik, H.J. Lee, D.W. Kim, J.W. Kim, Y. Lee, C. Pang (2019) Bioinspired adhesive architectures: From skin patch to integrated bioelectronics. *Adv. Mater.* 31 (34), 1803309: 1–18.
9. C. Xie, X. Wang, H. He, Y. Ding, X. Lu (2020) Mussel-inspired hydrogels for self-adhesive bioelectronics. *Adv. Funct. Mater.* 30 (25), 1909954: 1–30.
10. X. Huang, L. Wang, H. Wang, B. Zhang, X. Wang, R.Y.Z. Stening, X. Sheng, L. Yin (2020) Materials strategies and device architectures of emerging power supply devices for implantable bioelectronics. *Small.* 16 (15), 1902827: 1–21.
11. A. Ma, A. Poon (2015) Midfield wireless power transfer for bioelectronics. *IEEE Circ. Syst. Mag.* 15 (2): 54–60.
12. P. Chen, X. Sun, H. Peng (2020) Emerging soft bioelectronics. *Adv. Funct. Mater.* 30 (29), 2001827: 1–2.
13. D. Gao, K. Parida, P.S. Lee (2020) Emerging soft conductors for bioelectronic interfaces. *Adv. Funct. Mater.* 30 (29), 1907184 1–30.
14. D.T. Simon, E.O. Gabrielsson, K. Tybrandt, M. Berggren (2016) Organic bioelectronics: Bridging the signaling gap between biology and technology. *Chem. Rev.* 116 (21): 13009–13041.
15. D. Ohayon, S. Inal (2020) Organic bioelectronics: From functional materials to next-generation devices and power sources. *Adv. Mater.* 32 (36, 2001439): 1–29.
16. J. Tropp, J. Rivnay (2021) Design of biodegradable and biocompatible conjugated polymers for bioelectronics. *J. Mater. Chem. C.* 9 (39): 13543–13556.
17. C. Schmidt (2012) Bioelectronics: The bionic material. *Nature* 483: S37.
18. S.K. Rastogi, A. Kalmykov, N. Johnson, T. Cohen-Karni (2018) Bioelectronics with nano-carbons. *J. Mater. Chem. B*, 6: 7159–7178.
19. G. Tarabella, F.M. Mohammadi, N. Coppedè, F. Barbero, S. Iannotta, C. Santato, F. Cicoira (2013) New opportunities for organic electronics and bioelectronics: Ions in action. *Chem. Sci.* 4: 1395–1409.

20. C. Pitsalidis, M.P. Ferro, D. Iandolo, L. Tzounis, S. Inal, R.M. Owens (2018) Transistor in a tube: A route to three-dimensional bioelectronics. *Sci. Adv.* 4 (10), eaat4253: 1–9.
21. J. Rivnay, P. Leleux, M. Ferro, M. Sessolo, A. Williamson, D.A. Koutsouras, D. Khodagholy, M. Ramuz, X. Strakosas, R.M. Owens, C. Benar, J.M. Badier, C. Bernard, G.G. Malliaras (2015) High-performance transistors for bioelectronics through tuning of channel thickness. *Sci. Adv.* 1 (4), e1400251: 1–5.
22. A. Nawaz, Q. Liu, W.L. Leong, K.E. Fairfull-Smith, P. Sonar (2021) Organic electrochemical transistors for in vivo bioelectronics. *Adv. Mater.* 33 (49), 2101874: 1–51.
23. I. Willner, R. Baron, B. Willner (2007) Integrated nanoparticle-biomolecule systems for biosensing and bioelectronics. *Biosens. Bioelectron.* 22 (9–10): 1841–1852.
24. Y. Liu, A. Urso, R.M. Da Ponte, T. Costa, V. Valente, V. Giagka, W.A. Serdijn, T.G. Constandinou, T. Denison (2020) Bidirectional bioelectronic interfaces: System design and circuit implications. *IEEE Solid-State Circuits Magazine.* 12 (2): 30–46.
25. A.H. Sunwoo, S.I. Han, H. Joo, G.D. Cha, D. Kim, S.H. Choi, T. Hyeon, D.H. Kim (2020) Advances in soft bioelectronics for brain research and clinical neuroengineering. *Matter.* 3 (6): 1923–1947.
26. X. Duan, C.M. Lieber (2015) Nanoscience and the nano-bioelectronics frontier. *Nano Res.* 8 (1): 1–22.
27. T.D.Y. Kozai, A. Vazquez (2015) Photoelectric artefact from optogenetics and imaging on microelectrodes and bioelectronics: new challenges and opportunities. *J. Mat. Chem. B.* 3 (25): 4965–4978.
28. H. Yuk, B. Lu, X. Zhao (2019) Hydrogel bioelectronics. *Chem. Soc. Rev.* 48: 1642–1667.
29. D. Zhang, Q. Liu (2016) Biosensors and bioelectronics on smart phone for portable biochemical detection. *Biosens. Bioelectron.* 75: 273–284.
30. C.P. Tseng, J.J. Silberg, G.N. Bennett, R. Verduzco (2020) 100th anniversary of macromolecular science viewpoint: Soft materials for microbial bioelectronics. *ACS Macro Letters.* 9 (11): 1590–1603.
31. K. Feron, R. Lim, C. Sherwood, A. Keynes, A. Brichta, P.C. Dastoor (2018) Organic bioelectronics: Materials and biocompatibility. *Int. J. Mol. Sci.* 19, 2382: 2–21.
32. Y. Yu, H.Y.Y. Nyein, W. Gao, A. Javey (2020) Flexible electrochemical bioelectronics: The rise of in situ bioanalysis. *Adv. Mater.* 32 (15), 1902083: 1–25.
33. Berggren M., Richter-Dahlfors A. (2007) Organic bioelectronics. *Adv. Mater.* 19 (20): 3201–3213.
34. S. Löffler, K. Melican, K.P.R. Nilsson, A. Richter-Dahlfors (2017) Organic bioelectronics in medicine. *J. Intern. Med.* 282 (1): 24–36.
35. K. Svennersten, K.C. Larsson, M. Berggren, A. Richter-Dahlfors (2011) Organic bioelectronics in nanomedicine. *Biochim. Biophys. Acta* 1810 (3): 276–285.
36. B. Yoon, Y. Park (2004) A text-mining-based patent network: Analytical tool for high-technology trend. *The Journal of High Technology Management Research.* 15 (1): 37–50.
37. T.S. Cho, H.Y. Shih (2011) Patent citation network analysis of core and emerging technologies in Taiwan: 1997–2008. *Scientometrics.* 89 (3):795–811.
38. M. Kim, Y. Park, J. Yoon (2016) Generating patent development maps for technology monitoring using semantic patent-topic analysis. *Comput. Ind. Eng.* 98: 289–299.
39. Y. Liu, S. Zhu, Z. Gu, Y. Zhao (2021) A bibliometric analysis: Research progress and prospects on transition metal dichalcogenides in the biomedical field. *Chinese Chem. Lett.* In press.
40. P. Mansoori (2018) 50 years of Iranian clinical, biomedical, and public health research: a bibliometric analysis of the web of science core collection (1965–2014). *J. Glob. Health.* 8 (2): 020701.
41. L.F. Borisova, N.S. Bogacheva, V.A. Markusova, E.E. Suetina (2007) Bionanotechnhology: A bibliometric analysis using science citation index database (1995–2006). *Scientific and Technical Information Processing.* 34 (4): 212–218.
42. T. Hayashi (2003) Bibliometric analysis on additionality of Japanese R&D programmes. *Scientometrics.* 56 (3): 301–316.

43. T.U. Daim, G. Rueda, H. Martin, P. Gerdsri (2006) Forecasting emerging technologies: Use of bibliometrics and patent analysis. *Technol. Forecast. Soc.* 73 (8): 981–1012.

44. B. Ji, Y. Zhao, J. Vymazal, Ü. Mander, R. Lust, C. Tang (2021) Mapping the field of constructed wetland-microbial fuel cell: A review and bibliometric analysis. *Chemosphere.* 262, 128366: 1–12.

45. M.C.P. Gonçalves, T.G. Kieckbusch, R.F. Perna, J.T. Fujimoto, S.A.V. Morales, J.P. Romanelli (2019) Trends on enzyme immobilization researches based on bibliometric analysis. *Process Biochem.* 76: 95–110.

46. S. Zhu, Y. Liu, Z. Gu, Y. Zhao (2021) A bibliometric analysis of advanced healthcare materials: Research trends of biomaterials in healthcare application. *Adv. Healthc. Mater.* 10 (10), 200222: 1–9.

47. P.C. Lee, H.N. Su, F.S. Wu (2010) Quantitative mapping of patented technology—The case of electrical conducting polymer nanocomposite. *Technol. Forecast. Soc.* 77 (3): 466–478.

48. Scopus (2022). Abstract and citation database. Available in: https://www.scopus.com (accessed January 15, 2022).

49. Lens (2022) Search, analyze and manage patent and scholarly data. Available in: https://www.lens.org/ (accessed January 22, 2022).

50. SJR (2022) Scimago journal & country rank. Avaible in: https://www.scimagojr.com/ (accessed January 20, 2022).

51. VOSviewer (2022). Vosviewer (Software). Version 1.6.17.

52. WIPO (2022). International patent classification (IPC). https://www.wipo.int/classifications/ipc/en/, (accessed January 27, 2022).

8

Innovative Electronic Approaches for Biomarker Detection

Ummama Saeed and Batool Fatima

Department of Biochemistry, Bahauddin Zakariya University, Multan, Pakistan

Muhammad Najam-ul-Haq

Institute of Chemical Sciences, Bahauddin Zakariya University, Multan, Pakistan

CONTENTS

8.1 Introduction

The term "biomarker" dates back to 1970. It is also known as "surrogate marker" and "surrogate end point." Biomarkers are the indicators of biological processes and represent the alterations linked to cellular, molecular, and biochemical processes by which the diseased conditions can be recognized or monitored. Biomarkers are also considered signaling molecules and their levels can be quantified through biofluid analysis. Clinical analysis of biomarkers includes their detection and quantification and can be repeatedly analyzed in short periods. Biomarkers can be used in disease screening, diagnosis, prognosis, prediction of adverse drug reactions, and identification of cell types. According to the World Health Organization (WHO), a biomarker can be a quantifiable

DOI: 10.1201/9781003263265-8

substance, and its metabolites, structure, or process reflect the interaction between biological systems. According to the Food and Drug Administration (FDA), biomarkers can be the results of pathogenic processes or any response towards the therapeutic interventions and exposures [1], [1–3].

Biomarkers are the indicators for distinguishing normal state from diseased and need specific, sensitive, repeatable, and reliable methods for their detection and quantification. The detection of biomarkers from biofluids can particularly assist in the early diagnosis which is the key to timely treatment. Biomarkers are often present in lower concentrations and the presence of interfering substances makes their identification difficult. Antigens, DNA, mRNA, enzymes, and proteins are the common types of biomarkers used in medical diagnosis. Biomarkers can be the diagnostic and prognostic markers that help in assessing the risk, disease severity, and therapeutic efficacy. High throughput technologies provide information about the disease genotype and phenotype in dynamic ways which enhance the utility of the biomarker in both theoretical and clinical perspectives [4–6].

Various diseases are tracked through the quantification of biomarkers such as cardiovascular, diabetes, Alzheimer, cancer, osteoporosis, osteoarthritis, age-related diseases, anti-inflammatory diseases, etc. [7]. In cancer, biomarkers are used to assess the cancer risk, tumor burden, and cellular functions [3]. Chronic inflammation mainly contributes to cancer occurrence and its progression. Inflammatory biomarkers quantify the low-grade chronic inflammation and are a potential predictor of cancer survival [8]. Clinical biomarkers are useful in avoiding the ethical problems associated with the clinical end points quantifications. The overdosage of paracetamol leads to liver damage and its identification in biofluids is more authentic and less time-consuming than the institute therapy. The plasma concentration of paracetamol is thus the pharmaceutical biomarker and is used to predict whether the treatment is required or not. Various detection methods have been employed for the identification and quantification of biomarkers from biological fluids which include enzyme-linked immunosorbent assay (ELISA), gel electrophoresis, surface plasmon resonance, surface-enhanced Raman spectroscopy, calorimetric assay, electrochemical assay, and fluorescence method [6].

In this chapter, the electronic detection methods are encompassed for the sensing and quantification of biomarkers used in disease diagnosis and disease monitoring. The effect of nano-based materials in the tools of biomarkers detection and their respective characteristics like the limit of detection, stability, and reliability are discussed in innovative electronic approaches.

8.2 Two-Dimensional Gel Electrophoresis

Two-dimensional gel electrophoresis (2DE) is a principal technique for separating proteins from complex mixtures. It is the combination of two electrophoretic methods i.e., isoelectric focusing (IEF) where proteins are separated according to their isoelectric points (pI) and sodium dodecyl sulfate polyacrylamide gel electrophoresis (SDS-PAGE) in which proteins are separated based on the molecular weights. This technique can separate multiple proteins leading to the biomarker's identifications. 2DE provides information on protein modifications and changes in protein levels. It can isolate proteins and analyze them for the discovery of biomarkers using matrix-assisted laser desorption ionization-time of flight mass spectrometry (MALDI-TOF-MS), and liquid chromatography-electrospray ionization mass spectrometry (LC-ESI-MS) [9–11].

The common gynecological malignancy is endometrial cancer (ECa). It affects 6% of women worldwide. The early-stage diagnosis of endometrial cancer is difficult. The non-invasive and efficient diagnosis of ECa is through the detection of urinary proteins of ECa patients. Urine is one of the important biofluids for screening protein biomarkers. The kidney, prostate, and bladder cancers are also quantified by the urinary proteins. Urinary proteins separated through 2DE can be analyzed by densitometry, mass spectrometry, and database search. In a study conducted by Mu, Alan Kang-Wai, et al., urinary proteins of ECa were analyzed by 2DE where Zn-α-2-glycoprotein, α-1-acid glycoprotein, and C59 were present in the urine of patients and the lower levels of nebulin proteins were marked when compared with the control [12].

Huang, Hong-Lei, et al. in their work analyzed the protein biomarkers of breast cancer using 2DE. They identified a link between the proteins of breast cancer and tumor-igenesis. They distinguished the normal cells from non-invasive and invasive cancerous cells. They quantified the extracellular secreted proteins and the total cellular proteins from normal and cancerous breast cancer cells. They identified 133 differentially ex-pressed proteins and concluded that unreported proteins identified in their study have a positive correlation with two-dimensional difference gel electrophoresis (2D-DIGE) data. The novel proteins in their study can be used as diagnostic and therapeutic markers for cancer [13].

8.3 Enzyme-Linked Immunosorbent Assay (ELISA)

ELISA is a diagnostic tool in clinical investigations. It provides selective, sensitive, quantitative, and reproducible results in analyzing the analytes. It is a kind of gold standard technique for detecting biomarkers. It detects antibodies, antigens, proteins, glycoproteins, and hormones. It is used to test human immunodeficiency virus (HIV) infections, pregnancy, and blood typing. ELISA is unable to detect the disease at an early stage as biomarkers concentration is lower than the limit of detection of ELISA. Oligonucleotide-based immunosorbent assay is being used nowadays for achieving more sensitive results [14–16].

ELISA identifies one kind of biomarker at a time. In clinical diagnosis, a single bio-marker hardly meets the clinical demand. The identification of multiple biomarkers may enhance the accuracy of the diagnosis of various diseases. Semiconductor quantum dots-based fluorescent immunosorbent assay is more sensitive, simultaneous, and multiplexed in identifying the multiple biomarkers. Inflammatory biomarkers are the indicators of many diseases. Low levels of C-reactive protein (CRP) indicate the pa-thogenesis of cardiovascular disease while serum amyloid A (SAA) marks bacterial in-fections. A dual quantum dot-based fluorescence-linked immunosorbent assay (FLISA) was performed for detecting CRP and SAA. The as-fabricated assay has a broad linear range and lower limits of detection for both proteins. The assay results showed good specificity and efficiency and can thus be utilized for the simultaneous identification and quantification of other disease biomarkers in *in-vitro* diagnostics and are described in Figure 8.1 [17].

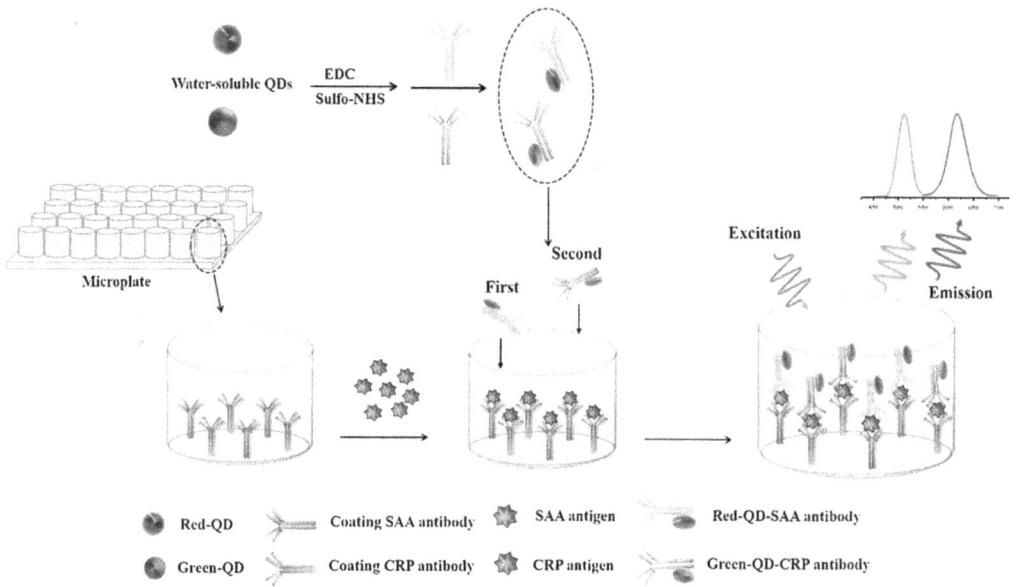

FIGURE 8.1
Dual QD-based FLISA detection of C-reactive protein and serum amyloid A. Adapted with permission [17], Copyright (2019), Elsevier.

8.4 Surface Plasmon Resonance (SPR)

SPR spectroscopy is a quantitative technique for studying antigen-antibody, DNA-DNA, DNA-protein, protein-protein, receptor-ligand, peptide-membrane, and protein-membrane interactions. SPR is a real-time label-free technique for disease diagnosis on a molecular basis, monitoring of disease development and therapy [18]. In SPR, electron charges oscillate at the metal-dielectric interface and are termed surface plasmons [19]. It quantifies the adsorption strength and determines the biological content adsorbed on the gold surface. It is thus a multiplexed sensing technique used to analyze hundreds to thousands of interactions on the metal surface [20].

Alzheimer's disease (AD) is an age-related neurodegenerative disorder leading to dementia and reducing the life expectancy to 50%. Cognitive tests, magnetic resonance imaging (MRI), and computed tomography (CT) scan are the tools used in diagnosing AD. Cerebrospinal fluid (CSF) indicates changes in biochemical parameters of AD patients and thus discriminates the patients from healthy individuals. Amyloid beta-peptide and tau protein are the AD biomarkers. Amyloid beta-peptide causes mitochondrial dysfunction and neuronal death by binding with 17β-HSD10 enzyme present in the mitochondria. In a study conducted by Hegnerová, K. et al., a SPR-based sensor was developed to clinically diagnose AD. The authors immobilized the polyclonal antibody against 17β-HSD10 through alkyl-thiolates and amino coupling chemistry. SPR-based biosensor detected 17β-HSD10 enzyme in ng/mL quantity [18,21].

Carcinoma antigen 125 (CA-125) is the ovarian cancer biomarker used in epithelial ovarian carcinoma. It affects the female reproductive system. This tumor marker has hydrophilic and lubricating properties. In ovarian cancer, it is expressed in units/mL, unlike

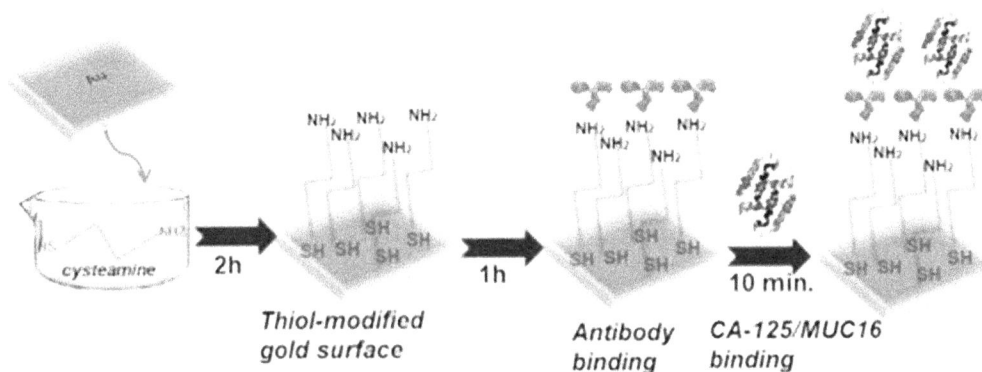

FIGURE 8.2
SPR-based detection of CA-125, which is considered an ovarian cancer biomarker. Adapted with permission [22], Copyright (2020), Elsevier.

other carcinoma markers. The CA-125 levels in the blood, serum, and plasma of patients are higher than that of healthy individuals. CA-125 is also used for the evaluation of ovarian malignancy risk and is also considered as the biomarker of endometrial cancer. Chemiluminescence immunoassay, ELISA, and nanoparticles-modified microfluidic systems are used for the quantification of this tumor marker. SPR-based imaging diagnoses epithelial ovarian carcinoma. Szymanski, B. et al. fabricated SPR-based imaging for diagnosing circulating CA-125, as shown in Figure 8.2. The developed biosensor is specific with good recovery and precision for real sample analysis of normal and cancerous samples [22].

8.5 Surface-Enhanced Raman Spectroscopy (SERS)

It is an ultrasensitive vibrational spectroscopic technique utilized for trace biomarker analysis. This technique can simultaneously detect multiple analytes due to the combination of molecular fingerprint specificity and single-molecule sensitivity [23]. It is the method for various cancer biomarker detections. The technique analyzes nucleic acid biomarkers without the limitations of time consumption, tediousness, and expensive extrinsic labeling. In SERS, adsorption of nucleic acid occurs on the nano-structured metallic surface for generating the selective sequence-dependent Raman spectral signatures [24,25].

Prostate cancer (PCa) is the most diagnosed cancer in men and its diagnosis is based on the quantification of prostate-specific antigen (PSA) for early-stage treatment and survival. In PCa, molecular variations take place in PSA which leads to unreliable diagnostic accuracy with side effects of unnecessary biopsies. Koo, Kevin M., et al. in their study applied SERS-based nano-diagnostic design for verifying PCa through PSA [24].

Liver cancer is the common malignancy of the digestive tract and its diagnosis at early stages of hepatocellular carcinoma (HCC) enhances clinical efficiency and alleviates the patients' suffering. Alpha-fetoprotein (AFP) is the liver cancer biomarker. AFP levels are low at the early stages of HCC. Lens culinaris agglutinin (LCA) is the reactive fraction of AFP taken as a specific biomarker of liver cancer. Zhu, Aonan, et al. fabricated the nano-honeycomb SERS-based active chip for determining LCA from HCC patients. SERS-active chips have a large surface area for AFP and AFP-L3 specific detection. The as-fabricated chip accurately performs in the linear range of 0.003–3 ng/mL and has potential in the clinical diagnosis of HCC [26].

8.6 Colorimetric Assay

The colorimetric assay detects biomarkers based on color. Substrates convert to colored molecules via the interaction of the enzyme with antibodies. Enzyme brings specificity while sensitivity is controlled by the signal amplification [27,28].

Dietary macronutrients are linked to health and their imbalance leads to diseases including obesity, diabetes, cardiovascular disease, metabolic disease, and cancer. Volatile compounds released from the human body provide information on metabolic processes. Volatile biomarkers are correlated to dietary macronutrients intake. Volatile biomarkers are selectively and sensitively identified through the calorimetric assay of biofluids. Calorimetric assays/sensors are low cost and detect the color change after the chemical reaction of the analyte with the sensing molecule. This assay is capable of multiplexed analysis with qualitative and semi-quantitative detection. In a study, a transdermal volatile biomarker detection system was built for the calorimetric sensing of dietary macronutrients explained in Figure 8.3. The study finds that the transdermal acetone levels increase after the usage of keto-acids while levels decrease after the carb-rich-diet intake. The calorimetric sensor exhibits a linear range from 0 to 40 ppm. The as-fabricated calorimetric sensor can be used in laboratories and hospital settings for nutrient-related disease monitoring and disease management [29].

8.7 Electrochemical Assay

The electrochemical assay is based on the electrode potential, interfacial capacitance, impedance, and oxidation-reduction current. Electrochemical assays have fast response, low cost, high sensitivity, selectivity, accuracy, and reliable properties for the detection and quantification of biomarkers [30]. Micro-RNAs (miRNA) are the endogenous non-coding short RNAs and regulate gene expression. miRNA in cancer cells act as diagnostic

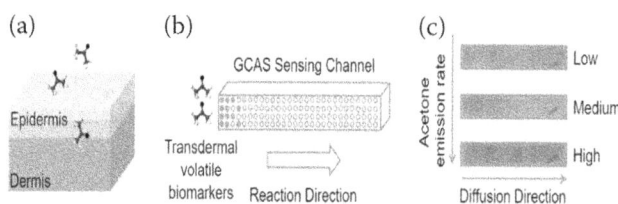

FIGURE 8.3
Calorimetric detection of macronutrients by the use of a transdermal volatile biomarker detection system. Adapted with permission [29], Copyright (2022), Elsevier.

biomarkers or therapeutic targets for disease progressive stage monitoring. Over- and under-regulation of miRNA leads to either inhibition of tumor suppressor genes or activation of oncogenes in cancer cells. miRNAs are more stable than mRNA and act as invasive and robust biomarkers. The quantification of miRNA is made either as label-free or label-based electrochemical assays. Oligonucleotide miRNA microarray analysis is used as a high throughput technique for analyzing cancer-specific expression levels of hundreds of miRNAs in cancer samples. In a study, an osmium-based nitrogenous ligand was synthesized onto which hybridization occurs between DNA probe and miRNA. Through this hybridization, a sequence of specific miRNA is detected in femtomolar levels from the mixture of other non-complementary miRNAs. This osmium-based electroanalytical sensor can be used in cancer stage diagnosis and monitoring the therapeutic systems [31].

DNA methylation is an epigenetic event of DNA repair and coordination of gene expression in higher eukaryotes. Changes in DNA methylation lead to changes in normal cellular functions and generate biomarkers of cancer and other diseases. In normal cells, DNA methylation occurs in the presence of DNA methyltransferase (MTase) and abnormality in MTase activity leads to acute monocytic leukemia. Therefore, DNA MTase activity analysis is critical in understanding the regulation of genetic information, early-stage cancer diagnosis, and quantification of disease pathogenesis. Electrochemical assays detect the DNA MTase activity. These assays are low-cost, sensitive, selective, and offer ease of miniaturization. In a study, gold nanoparticles (Au NPs) were used for the detection of DNA MTase. Au NPs were modified with single-strand DNA hybrid and a complementary sequence of DNA hybrid was assembled with modified Au NPs at a specific recognition sequence. The modified electrochemical assay for MTase activity exhibited the limit of detection of about 0.12 U/mL with a linear range of 0.2 U/mL to 10 U/mL. The mechanism of electrode fabrication for detecting DNA MTase is explained in Figure 8.4 [32].

Escherichia coli (E. coli) is the versatile bacteria found in the digestive tract as beneficial probiotics and act as a poisonous pathogen in food and environment and cause food poisoning, urinary tract infections, and meningitis. In a study, a microfluidic electrochemical sensor was used for the detection and quantification of *E. coli*. The as-fabricated microfluidic sensor detected and quantified the bacteria as 24 CFU/mL and 8.6 fg/μL DNA in 60 minutes. The fabricated microfluidic sensor can be used as a point of care diagnostic device in clinical and hospital applications [33].

Obesity is a physiological state characterized by high amounts of fats in the body. Obesity is linked to diabetes, hypertension, respiratory system disease, and cerebrovascular diseases. Adiponectin is an anti-inflammatory adipokine and has a role in lipids and glucose metabolism. It is the biomarker of metabolic syndrome. In obesity, adiponectin is dysregulated. Adiponectin has a role in vascular healing and angiogenesis and is the clinical biomarker of cardiovascular disease. It is observed that the adiponectin levels are lower in the plasma of obese people than the non-obese ones. In the early diagnosis of obesity, biosensing systems were employed in the form of electrochemical impedance spectroscopy. In a study, a graphite paper (GP) electrode was used as a working electrode for the detection of adiponectin. GP electrode has electrical conductivity with usability in a wide linear range and stable physical and electrochemical properties. GP electrode was used to analyze the interaction between anti-adiponectin and adiponectin through impedimetric and cyclic voltammetric studies. The as-fabricated sensor detected adiponectin with a limit of detection of 0.003 pg/mL in a linear range of 0.05–25 pg/mL. The as-fabricated immunosensor was also tested for the detection of other proteins (leptin, creatine kinase, parathyroid hormone, etc.) in the presence of adiponectin. The sensor exhibited long storage life with usability in detecting proteins from real samples [34].

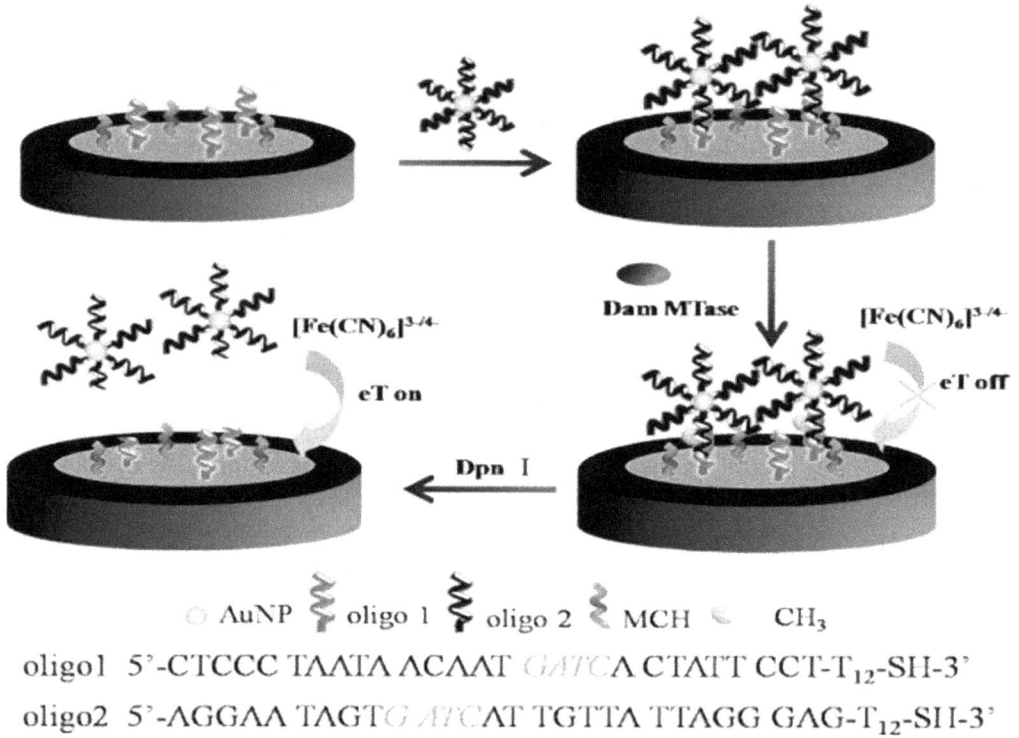

○ AuNP 〰 oligo 1 〰 oligo 2 〰 MCH ～ CH₃

oligo1 5'-CTCCC TAATA ACAAT GATCA CTATT CCT-T$_{12}$-SH-3'

oligo2 5'-AGGAA TAGTG ATCAT TGTTA TTAGG GAG-T$_{12}$-SH-3'

FIGURE 8.4
Electrochemical-based sensing of DNA methyltransferase (MTase) as a biomarker of monocytic leukemia. Adapted with permission [32], Copyright (2011), Elsevier.

8.7.1 Electromagnetic Sensors

Electromagnetic sensors are non-destructive and used in disease monitoring and biomarker analysis. Biological tissues possess specific dielectric properties and electromagnetic materials interact with biological tissues to generate the response. Electromagnetic materials are classified into diamagnetic, ferromagnetic, antiferromagnetic, ferrimagnetic, and paramagnetic. Electromagnetic sensors are designed to identify and monitor the physiological changes in normal cells/tissues and diseased cells/tissues or act as therapeutic tools for the affected tissues [35,36]. Detection of disease-specific molecular targets is significant for understanding the physiological and biological functions in disease diagnosis and prognosis. Nano-based magnetic materials are used in analytical sensing and biomedicine fields due to modular structure, low toxicity, enzyme mimicking activity, supramagnetic behavior, and biocompatibility [37].

In cardiovascular patients, point of care testing of coagulation protein and monitoring of anti-coagulation protein is required during the intensive care before surgery. The coagulation process in cardiovascular disease (CVD) requires analysis of 12 factors done by wet chemical method for reflecting the platelet functions of coagulation-related disorders. In electromagnetic induction, the elastic sensor probe is utilized for detecting biological analytes. In a study, the coagulation process was analyzed in blood by the electromagnetic sensor. The sensor detected changes in blood viscosity and density before and after coagulation based on the damped vibration principle. The as-synthesized electromagnetic sensor is a reproducible and accurate clinical detection system. The sensor also exhibits the property of dynamic testing of the coagulation process [38].

Testosterone, a male sex hormone, is linked to high-grade prostate cancer. Low testosterone levels are linked to high-risk mortality and death by CVD. Monitoring of testosterone is significant in clinical, biochemical, and sports endocrinology research [39]. Testosterone doping in sports through illegal consumption is a matter of concern. Magnetic nanoparticles (MNPs), due to their magnetic behavior, have gotten attention in biomedical diagnosis. They have electrochemical conductivity and the desired physicochemical properties for sensing devices. In a study, magnetic iron oxide nanoparticles were synthesized for the estimation of testosterone. The MNPs were employed to fabricate the screen-printed electrode. The fabricated sensor was used to capture anti-testosterone antibodies for detecting testosterone. Testosterone sense was confirmed by cyclic voltammetry, differential pulse voltammetry, and electrical impedance spectroscopy (EIS). The proposed sensor showed a LOD of 23.68 ng/mL with a linear range of 50–1,000 ng/mL. The sensor detected testosterone from urine and serum in the presence of interferants. The authors proposed that the sensor be used in the clinical diagnosis of testosterone and the sensor fabrication, as shown in Figure 8.5 [40].

8.7.2 Optical Sensors

Optical sensors are used in the biotechnological industry, ecological science, and health care. Optical sensors are classified into catalytic and affinity-based and are in wider use than electrochemical or piezoelectric sensors. Surface plasmon resonance sensors are also optical sensors [41]. Pathogenic bacteria cause infectious diseases leading to life-threatening conditions. Bacterial counts of less than 10 CFU/mL of blood are not detected

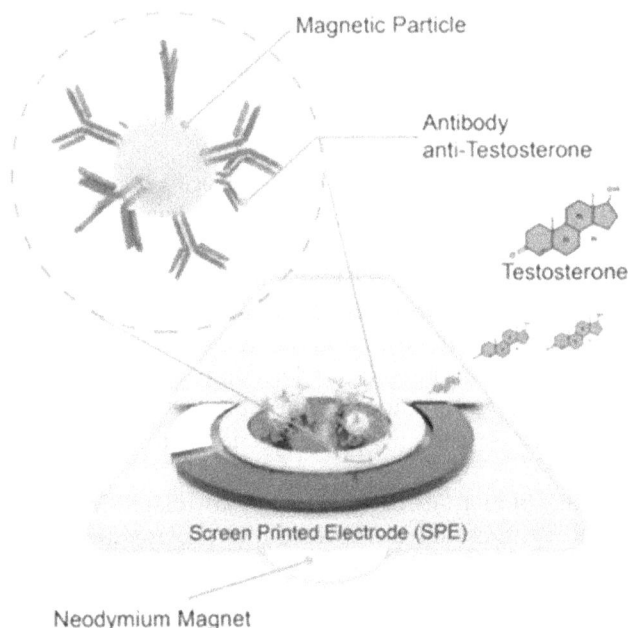

FIGURE 8.5
Illustration of MNPs-modified SPE for the detection of testosterone. Adapted with permission [40], Copyright (2020), Elsevier.

by non-DNA-based detection techniques. These pathogenic disease-related biomarkers can be detected by methods involving nanostructures. Nanomaterials modified sensors require minute sample concentrations and provide accurate results with high sensitivity. Nanoparticles-based sensors possess magnetic and optical properties for detecting pathogenic bacteria in real samples. Bimetallic gold-silver nanocluster was synthesized for detecting *Campylobacter jejuni*. Bimetallic NPs possess optical properties and enhance the optical intensity, color perception, and sensitivity for *Campylobacter jejuni*. The detection of the bacterium was also done by immunoassay. The sensor exhibited an acceptable linear range with a LOD of 10 CFU/mL [42].

8.7.3 Acoustic Sensor

An acoustic wave sensor, also known as quartz crystal microbalance quantify thin film by identifying the resonance frequency. These sensors simultaneously detect changes in electrical and mechanical properties. They are used in biomarker detection, especially the malignant tumor-related biomarkers for early-stage disease screening [43].

Glial-fibrillary-acidic protein is expressed by astrocytes in the central nervous system. This protein acts as a biomarker in brain-related diseases. The presence of glial-fibrillary-acidic protein in circulating blood is the indicator of diseases such as glioblastoma multiforme (GBM) and multiple sclerosis etc., In a study, an acoustic wave sensor was used for the detection of glial-fibrillary-acidic protein. They fabricated an ultra-high frequency wave sensor based on lab on a chip and detected the protein from clinical samples with 35 pM concentrations. The authors suggested that this point of care lab-on-a-chip can be used for multiple brain pathologies in detecting biomarkers [44].

8.8 Fluorescence (FL) Methods

Fluorescent probes are used in analytical sensing and optical imaging. Fluorescent probes specifically interact with the target analyte under optimized conditions. In ratiometric fluorescent sensors, fluorescent probes cause target-induced FL-intensity which results in emission bands at different wavelengths. Dual emission ratiometric FL methods influence the detection systems and background signals by improving the accuracy and reliability during the detection process. In FL detection methods, naked-eye identification of target reflects content changes of biomarkers in the detection system [45]. Fluorescent detection of biomarkers comes under the photonic techniques in which detection of target biomolecule occurs in the form of changes in absorbance, transmittance, luminescence, and reflectance properties [46].

Norepinephrine is the biomarker of depression correlated with potassium ion concentration. Zhou et al. synthesized a fluorescent probe for detecting K^+-induced norepinephrine transduction signal in neuroendocrine PC12 cells [47]. Alkaline phosphatase is the indicator of signal transduction and tumor metabolism. Alkaline phosphatase is the combination of cysteine residues, Mg and Zn. In a study, a fluorescent probe was synthesized by the combination of quinoline malononitrile core decorated with a hydrophilic phosphate group. The as-synthesized probe causes fluorescent detection of ALP by DQM-OH aggregates in the presence of alkaline phosphatase. The FL probe can differentiate tumor cells from normal cells both in *ex-vivo* and *in-vivo* imaging. The authors suggested that the FL probe can assist surgeons during tumor resection [48].

The detection of chloride ions in biofluids is necessary as their abnormal levels lead to multiple diseases including cystic fibrosis. Cystic fibrosis is diagnosed by monitoring the chloride ions levels in sweat. A fluorescence sensor was used for detecting chloride ions because of its high sensitivity and rapid response kinetics. A citrate-based fluorescent sensor was fabricated for chloride ions detection in the sweat of cystic fibrosis patients. The fabricated sensor exhibited characteristics of a low-cost multi-analysis system and can be used in the point-of-care diagnosis of cystic fibrosis in clinical applications [49].

8.9 Nuclear Magnetic Resonance (NMR) Spectroscopy

NMR spectroscopy is a multivariate metabolic profiling technique in disease diagnosis. It requires one internal standard for biochemical alteration investigation. It is a rapid and single-step technique with high specificity for identifying multiple analytes in a single run. In NMR spectroscopy, a minute quantity of targeted sample is required for the quantification of metabolites in micromolar concentrations. NMR spectroscopy provides insight about tumor biomarkers for early diagnosis of disease, biochemical changes linked to disease progression, and provides information about disease biology [50].

Chronic inflammatory bowel disease (IBD) exists in two subtypes i.e., Crohn's disease (CD) and ulcerative colitis (UC). The diagnosis of IBD depends on the histologic, endoscopic, and radiologic techniques, which are expensive and time-consuming. Clinical diagnosis of IBD is less invasive and useful for primary diagnosis and early-stage detection of disease. In a study, NMR-based metabolic profiles of serum, plasma, and urine of IBD patients were examined. The authors concluded that the levels of methanol, mannose, isoleucine, formate, and 3-methyl-2-oxovalerate were high in serum and plasma while levels of creatinine, xylose, allantoin, and mannitol were high in the urine. These clinical results can be used as biomarkers in early-stage diagnosis of IBD [51].

Pancreatic ductal adenocarcinoma (PDAC) is an aggressive disease that develops without prior symptoms. In pancreatic ductal carcinoma, genetic mutations occur in KRAS, TP53, SMAD4, and CDKN2A genes which lead to alterations in metabolic pathways with aggressive phenotypes. Identification of non-invasive biomarkers indicates the aggressive subtypes and therapeutic targets to improve the patient's survival. NMR spectroscopic study was designed on patients' derived-PDAC xenograft models to investigate the association between glycolytic metabolism and tumor aggressiveness. The authors found pyruvate conversion to lactate, which enhances the levels of lactate dehydrogenase (LDH) enzyme in aggressive patients' derived-PDAC xenografts [52].

8.10 Microfluidic Devices

Microfluidic devices have dimensions less than 1 mm and are used in molecular biology and cell separations for disease diagnosis [53]. Microfluidics is also known as lab on chip technology and is used in a variety of biological assays due to minimal reagent consumption. These devices can be used in point-of-care testing and medical screening for early-stage disease diagnosis. Microfluidic devices are classified into paper-based, continuous-flow and digital. These devices are portable, cost effective, and easy to fabricate. Microfluidic devices transport fluid samples (target materials) and store chemical reagents for electrochemical and calorimetric sensing [54].

Neurodegenerative disease results in loss of neuronal function due to oxidative stress, aggregation of proteins, and misfolding in the central and peripheral nervous systems. Catecholamine neurotransmitter such as dopamine is the precursor for quinones and semi-quinones. Dopamine-based quinones form protein adducts and depurinating DNA adducts which are the risk factors of neurodegenerative diseases including Parkinson's disease (PD). In PD, loss of dopaminergic neurons in nigrostrial pathway of the brain occurs. In a study, a microfluidic device with an electrochemical system was fabricated for protein identification and depurinating DNA adducts in Parkinson's disease patients. The system was efficient, required minute targeted sample and chemical reagents, portable, high speed, integrable, enhanced parallelism, and automatable. The as-fabricated sensor exhibited reproducible results with LOD of DA-6-*N7*Gua adducts in femtomolar concentration and linear range between 2 and 300 μM [55,56].

Melatonin exhibits antioxidant activity and regulates body hormones. In several studies, it is observed that melatonin is linked with the risk of breast cancer, prostate cancer, and type II diabetes. Melatonin quantification in urine is useful for monitoring its levels in serum. Melatonin was imprinted on the working electrode as an electrochemical sensing chip. The as-fabricated chip exhibited a limit of detection in pM and can be used in clinical applications for diagnosing prostate and breast cancers [57].

8.11 High Throughput Technologies

High throughput technologies speed up the discovery and development process. These technologies are also known as next-generation sequencing techniques and are applied to DNA, RNA, and proteomics. The approaches can be used in disease diagnosis and prognosis after the detection of disease-related biomarkers from complex biological samples [58]. Genome sequencing provides information of individual variants known as single nucleotide polymorphism to predict the disease through analyzing genetic diversity and population genomics [59].

DNA repair deficiency causes cancer susceptibility and carcinogenesis and drives the malignant transformations with genomic alterations in cancer cells. In high-grade, severe ovarian cancer, defected double-stranded DNA break occurs, which leads to inactivation of homologous recombination (HR) pathway genes by germline and somatic mutations. Genomic sequencing of HR-related genes of BRCA1/2 was recognized in HR deficiency-related ovarian cancer while CDK-12 mutated tumors were associated with the loss of heterozygosity-based scores having distinct patterns of genomic alterations. These genomic variations can be used as predicting models for targeted treatments [60].

Mass spectrometry is the developed tool for analyzing biomolecules leading to biomarker discovery procedures. The MS-based sensor was fabricated for the identification of acetylcholine. Acetylcholine being a neurotransmitter is associated with biological functions in the brain and dysregulation of this neurotransmitter leads to neurological disorders. In a study, microfluidic sampling was coupled with MALDI-MS for *in-vivo* imaging of acetylcholine in a rat's brain. The versatility of the MS-based sensor was explained by simultaneous monitoring of metabolites and other targeted analytes [61].

8.12 Conclusion

Biomarkers are the indicators of physiological processes in the human body and discriminate the normal physiological state from the diseased state. Diverse types of electronic techniques are in use nowadays for early-stage diagnosis and monitoring of disease states after therapy. The detection techniques have their specific characteristics for detecting biomarkers. Some techniques are non-destructive and require minute sample amounts to analyze biomarkers. It is a global concern to utilize smaller sample quantities for analysis and decrease the limit of detection of biological analytes to sense biomarkers. Among the sensing techniques, microfluidic electrochemical sensors can be used in point-of-care diagnosis due to portability and simplicity. The above-mentioned techniques are high-throughput technologies for the detection of biomarkers and can be used in personalized medicine in the future.

References

1. I.T. Gug, M. Tertis, O. Hosu & C. Cristea (2019) Salivary biomarkers detection: Analytical and immunological methods overview. *TrAC Trends in Analytical Chemistry, 113*, 301–316.
2. P.D. Wagner, M. Verma & S. Srivastava (2004) Challenges for biomarkers in cancer detection. *Annals of the New York Academy of Sciences, 1022*, 9–16.
3. J.K. Aronson & R.E. Ferner (2017) Biomarkers—A general review. *Current Protocols in Pharmacology, 76*, 9.23.1–9.23.17.
4. R. Liu, X. Wang, K. Aihara & L. Chen (2014) Early diagnosis of complex diseases by molecular biomarkers, network biomarkers, and dynamical network biomarkers. *Medicinal Research Reviews, 34*, 455–478.
5. A. Nsabimana, X. Ma, F. Yuan, F. Du, A. Abdussalam, B. Lou & G. Xu (2019) Nanomaterials-based electrochemical sensing of cardiac biomarkers for acute myocardial infarction: Recent progress. *Electroanalysis, 31*, 177–187.
6. S.B. Nimse, M.D. Sonawane, K.S. Song & T. Kim (2016) Biomarker detection technologies and future directions. *Analyst, 141*, 740–755.
7. S. Ren, P. Lin, J. Wang, H. Yu, T. Lv, L. Sun & G. Du (2020) Circular RNAs: Promising molecular biomarkers of human aging-related diseases via functioning as an miRNA sponge. *Molecular Therapy-Methods & Clinical Development, 18*, 215–229.
8. B.L. Pierce, R. Ballard-Barbash, L. Bernstein, R.N. Baumgartner, M.L. Neuhouser, M.H. Wener, K.B. Baumgartner, F.D. Gilliland, B.E. Sorensen, A. McTiernan & C.M. Ulrich (2009) Elevated biomarkers of inflammation are associated with reduced survival among breast cancer patients. *Journal of Clinical Oncology, 27*, 3437.
9. M.R. Kim & C.W. Kim (2007) Human blood plasma preparation for two-dimensional gel electrophoresis. *Journal of Chromatography B, 849*, 203–210.
10. Y. Ahmad & N. Sharma (2009) An effective method for the analysis of human plasma proteome using two-dimensional gel electrophoresis. *Journal of Proteomics & Bioinformatics, 2*, 495–499.

11. W. Liu, B. Liu, Q. Cai, J. Li, X. Chen & Z. Zhu (2012) Proteomic identification of serum biomarkers for gastric cancer using multi-dimensional liquid chromatography and 2D differential gel electrophoresis. *Clinica Chimica Acta, 413,* 1098–1106.

12. A.K.-W. Mu, B.-K. Lim, O.H. Hashim & A.S. Shuib (2012) Detection of differential levels of proteins in the urine of patients with endometrial cancer: Analysis using two-dimensional gel electrophoresis and O-glycan binding lectin. *International Journal of Molecular Sciences, 13,* 9489–9501.

13. T.-C. Lai, H.-C. Chou, Y.-W. Chen, T.-R. Lee, H.-T. Chan, H.-H. Shen, W.-T. Lee, S.-T. Lin, Y.-C. Lu, C.-L. Wu & H.-L. Chan (2010) Secretomic and proteomic analysis of potential breast cancer markers by two-dimensional differential gel electrophoresis. *Journal of Proteome Research, 9,* 1302–1322.

14. S.D. Gan & K.R. Patel (2013) Enzyme immunoassay and enzyme-linked immunosorbent assay. *Journal of Investigative Dermatology, 133,* e12.

15. M. Alhajj & A. Farhana. *Enzyme linked immunosorbent assay.* StatPearls [Internet], 2021.

16. K.-C. Han, E.-G. Yang & D.-R. Ahn (2013) Elongated oligonucleotide-linked immunosorbent assay for sensitive detection of a biomarker in a microwell plate-based platform. *Biosensors and Bioelectronics, 50,* 421–424.

17. Y. Lv, F. Wang, N. Li, R. Wu, J. Li, H. Shen, L.S. Li & F. Guo (2019) Development of dual quantum dots-based fluorescence-linked immunosorbent assay for simultaneous detection on inflammation biomarkers. *Sensors and Actuators B: Chemical, 301,* 127118.

18. K. Hegnerová, M. Bockova, H. Vaisocherová, Z. Krištofiková, J. Říčný, D. Řípová & J. Homola (2009) Surface plasmon resonance biosensors for detection of Alzheimer disease biomarker. *Sensors and Actuators B: Chemical, 139,* 69–73.

19. P. Bhatia & B.D. Gupta (2012) Fabrication and characterization of a surface plasmon resonance based fiber optic urea sensor for biomedical applications. *Sensors and Actuators B: Chemical, 161,* 434–438.

20. H.J. Lee, D. Nedelkov & R.M. Corn (2006) Surface plasmon resonance imaging measurements of antibody arrays for the multiplexed detection of low molecular weight protein biomarkers. *Analytical Chemistry, 78,* 6504–6510.

21. A. Rezabakhsh, R. Rahbarghazi & F. Fathi (2020) Surface plasmon resonance biosensors for detection of Alzheimer's biomarkers; an effective step in early and accurate diagnosis. *Biosensors and Bioelectronics, 167,* 112511.

22. B. Szymańska, Z. Lukaszewski, K. Hermanowicz-Szamatowicz & E. Gorodkiewicz (2020) A biosensor for determination of the circulating biomarker CA125/MUC16 by Surface Plasmon Resonance Imaging. *Talanta, 206,* 120187.

23. W. Zhou, Y.F. Tian, B.C. Yin & B.C. Ye (2017) Simultaneous surface-enhanced Raman spectroscopy detection of multiplexed microRNA biomarkers. *Analytical Chemistry, 89,* 6120–6128.

24. K.M. Koo, J. Wang, R.S. Richards, A. Farrell, J.W. Yaxley, H. Samaratunga, P.E. Teloken, M.J. Roberts, G.D. Coughlin, M.F. Lavin, P.N. Mainwaring, Y. Wang, R.A. Gardiner & M. Trau (2018) Design and clinical verification of surface-enhanced Raman spectroscopy diagnostic technology for individual cancer risk prediction. *ACS Nano, 12,* 8362–8371.

25. X. Lin, Y. Wang, L. Wang, Y. Lu, J. Li, D. Lu, T. Zhou, Z. Huang, J. Huang, H. Huang, S. Qiu, R. Chen, D. Lin & S. Feng (2019) Interference-free and high precision biosensor based on surface enhanced Raman spectroscopy integrated with surface molecularly imprinted polymer technology for tumor biomarker detection in human blood. *Biosensors and Bioelectronics, 143,* 111599.

26. A. Zhu, X. Zhao, M. Cheng, L. Chen, Y. Wang, X. Zhang, Y. Zhang & X. Zhang (2019) Nanohoneycomb surface-enhanced Raman spectroscopy-active chip for the determination of biomarkers of hepatocellular carcinoma. *ACS Applied Materials & Interfaces, 11,* 44617–44623.

27. H. Ye, K. Yang, J. Tao, Y. Liu, Q. Zhang, S. Habibi, Z. Nie & X. Xia (2017) An enzyme-free signal amplification technique for ultrasensitive colorimetric assay of disease biomarkers. *ACS Nano, 11,* 2052–2059.

28. S. Krumova, R. Balansky, A. Danailova, G. Ganchev, L. Djongov, L. Gartcheva, S.G. Taneva & S. Todinova (2020) Calorimetric assay to follow colorectal cancer development in experimental rat models. *Thermochimica Acta, 691*, 178723.

29. J. Yu, D. Wang, V.V. Tipparaju, W. Jung & X. Xian (2022) Detection of transdermal biomarkers using gradient-based colorimetric array sensor. *Biosensors and Bioelectronics, 195*, 113650.

30. J. Wu & H.X. Ju. Clinical immunoassays and immunosensing, in *Comprehensive Sampling and Sample Preparation*, J. Pawliszyn, Editor. 2012, Academic Press: Oxford. pp. 143–167.

31. M. Bartosik, M. Trefulka, R. Hrstka, B. Vojtesek & E. Palecek (2013) Os (VI) bipy-based electrochemical assay for detection of specific microRNAs as potential cancer biomarkers. *Electrochemistry Communications, 33*, 55–58.

32. X. He, J. Su, Y. Wang, K. Wang, X. Ni & Z. Chen (2011) A sensitive signal-on electrochemical assay for MTase activity using AuNPs amplification. *Biosensors and Bioelectronics, 28*, 298–303.

33. M. Safavieh, M.U. Ahmed, M. Tolba & M. Zourob (2012) Microfluidic electrochemical assay for rapid detection and quantification of Escherichia coli. *Biosensors and Bioelectronics, 31*, 523–528.

34. B. Ozcan & M.K. Sezginturk (2021) Highly sensitive and single-use biosensing system based on a GP electrode for analysis of adiponectin, an obesity biomarker. *ACS Biomaterials Science & Engineering, 7*, 3658–3668.

35. A. Abbosh (2019) Electromagnetic medical sensing. *Sensors (Basel, Switzerland), 19*, 1662.

36. M. Wang & G. Wang. Electromagnetic sensors for assessing and monitoring civil infrastructures, in *Sensor Technologies for Civil Infrastructures*, Wang, M. L., Lynch, J. P., & Sohn, H. 2014, Elsevier: Amsterdam. pp. 238–264.

37. M.K. Masud, J. Na, M. Younus, M.S.A. Hossain, Y. Bando, M.J.A. Shiddiky & Y. Yamauchi (2019) Superparamagnetic nanoarchitectures for disease-specific biomarker detection. *Chemical Society Reviews, 48*, 5717–5751.

38. Z. Wang, Y. Yu, Z. Yu & Q. Chen (2018) Electromagnetic induction sensor for dynamic testing of coagulation process. *Australasian Physical & Engineering Sciences in Medicine, 41*, 105–115.

39. W. Liu, Y. Ma, G. Sun, S. Wang, J. Deng & H. Wei (2017) Molecularly imprinted polymers on graphene oxide surface for EIS sensing of testosterone. *Biosensors and Bioelectronics, 92*, 305–312.

40. S. Sanli, H. Moulahoum, F. Ghorbanizamani, Z.P. Gumus & S. Timur (2020) On-site testosterone biosensing for doping detection: Electrochemical immunosensing via functionalized magnetic nanoparticles and screen-printed electrodes. *ChemistrySelect, 5*, 14911–14916.

41. M. Pirzada & Z. Altintas (2020) Recent progress in optical sensors for biomedical diagnostics. *Micromachines, 11*, 356.

42. C. Cao, L.C. Gontard, L.L. Thuy Tram, A. Wolff & D.D. Bang (2011) Dual enlargement of gold nanoparticles: from mechanism to scanometric detection of pathogenic bacteria. *Small, 7*, 1701–1708.

43. J. Zhang, X. Zhang, X. Wei, Y. Xue, H. Wan & P. Wang (2021) Recent advances in acoustic wave biosensors for the detection of disease-related biomarkers: A review. *Analytica Chimica Acta, 1164*, 338321.

44. M. Agostini, F. Amato, M.L. Vieri, G. Greco, I. Tonazzini, L. Baroncelli, M. Caleo, E. Vannini, M. Santi, G. Signore & M. Cecchini (2021) Glial-fibrillary-acidic-protein (GFAP) biomarker detection in serum-matrix: Functionalization strategies and detection by an ultra-high-frequency surface-acoustic-wave (UHF-SAW) lab-on-chip. *Biosensors and Bioelectronics, 172*, 112774.

45. R. Gui, H. Jin, X. Bu, Y. Fu, Z. Wang & Q. Liu (2019) Recent advances in dual-emission ratiometric fluorescence probes for chemo/biosensing and bioimaging of biomarkers. *Coordination Chemistry Reviews, 383*, 82–103.

46. O. Tagit & N. Hildebrandt (2017) Fluorescence sensing of circulating diagnostic biomarkers using molecular probes and nanoparticles. *ACS Sensors, 2*, 31–45.

47. N. Zhou, F. Huo, Y. Yue & C. Yin (2020) Specific fluorescent probe based on "protect–deprotect" to visualize the norepinephrine signaling pathway and drug intervention tracers. *Journal of the American Chemical Society, 142*, 17751–17755.

48. H. Li, Q. Yao, F. Xu, Y. Li, D. Kim, J. Chung, G. Baek, X. Wu, P.F. Hillman, E.Y. Lee, H. Ge, J. Fan, J. Wang, S.-J. Nam, X. Peng & J. Yoon (2020) An activatable aiegen probe for high-fidelity monitoring of overexpressed tumor enzyme activity and its application to surgical tumor excision. *Angewandte Chemie, 132,* 10272–10281.

49. J.P. Kim, Z. Xie, M. Creer, Z. Liu & J. Yang (2017) Citrate-based fluorescent materials for low-cost chloride sensing in the diagnosis of cystic fibrosis. *Chemical Science, 8,* 550–558.

50. V. Kumar, D.K. Dwivedi & N.R. Jagannathan (2014) High-resolution NMR spectroscopy of human body fluids and tissues in relation to prostate cancer. *NMR in Biomedicine, 27,* 80–89.

51. R. Schicho, R. Shaykhutdinov, J. Ngo, A. Nazyrova, C. Schneider, R. Panaccione, G.G. Kaplan, H.J. Vogel & M. Storr (2012) Quantitative metabolomic profiling of serum, plasma, and urine by 1H NMR spectroscopy discriminates between patients with inflammatory bowel disease and healthy individuals. *Journal of Proteome Research, 11,* 3344–3357.

52. P. Dutta, M.R. Perez, J. Lee, Y. Kang, M. Pratt, T.C. Salzillo, J. Weygand, N.M. Zacharias, S.T. Gammon, E.J. Koay, M. Kim, F. McAllister, S. Sen, A. Maitra, D. Piwnica-Worms, J.B. Fleming & P.K. Bhattacharya (2019) Combining hyperpolarized real-time metabolic imaging and NMR spectroscopy to identify metabolic biomarkers in pancreatic cancer. *Journal of Proteome Research, 18,* 2826–2834.

53. B.K. Gale, A.R. Jafek, C.J. Lambert, B.L. Goenner, H. Moghimifam, U.C. Nze & S.K. Kamarapu (2018) A review of current methods in microfluidic device fabrication and future commercialization prospects. *Inventions, 3,* 60.

54. V. Soum, S. Park, A.I. Brilian, O.S. Kwon & K. Shin (2019) Programmable paper-based microfluidic devices for biomarker detections. *Micromachines, 10,* 516.

55. T. Osaki, Y. Shin, V. Sivathanu, M. Campisi & R.D. Kamm (2018) In vitro microfluidic models for neurodegenerative disorders. *Advanced Healthcare Materials, 7,* 1700489.

56. A.A. Dawoud, T. Kawaguchi, Y. Markushin, M.D. Porter & R. Jankowiak (2006) Separation of catecholamines and dopamine-derived DNA adduct using a microfluidic device with electrochemical detection. *Sensors and Actuators B: Chemical, 120,* 42–50.

57. M.H. Lee, D. O'Hare, Y.L. Chen, Y.C. Chang, C.H. Yang, B.D. Liu & H.Y. Lin (2014) Molecularly imprinted electrochemical sensing of urinary melatonin in a microfluidic system. *Biomicrofluidics, 8,* 054115.

58. X. Yang, R. Jiao, L. Yang, L.P. Wu, Y.R. Li & J. Wang (2011) New-generation high-throughput technologies based'omics' research strategy in human disease. *Yi Chuan Hereditas, 33,* 829–846.

59. S. Oh, Y. Jo, S. Jung, S. Yoon & K.H. Yoo (2020) From genome sequencing to the discovery of potential biomarkers in liver disease. *BMB Reports, 53,* 299.

60. A. Vanderstichele, P. Busschaert, S. Olbrecht, D. Lambrechts & I. Vergote (2017) Genomic signatures as predictive biomarkers of homologous recombination deficiency in ovarian cancer. *European Journal of Cancer, 86,* 5–14.

61. P. Song, N.D. Hershey, O.S. Mabrouk, T.R. Slaney & R.T. Kennedy (2012) Mass spectrometry "sensor" for in vivo acetylcholine monitoring. *Analytical Chemistry, 84,* 4659–4664.

9

Bioinspired Prosthetic Interfaces for Bioelectronics

Saadat Majeed, Muhammad Umer Farooq, and Sayed Tayyab Raza Naqvi
Division of Analytical Chemistry, Bahauddin Zakariya University, Multan, Punjab, Pakistan

Naeem Akhtar Khan
IRCBM, COMSAT University Islamabad, Lahore, Punjab, Pakistan

Batool Fatima
Department of Biochemistry, Bahauddin Zakariya University, Multan, Pakistan

Dilshad Hussain
International Centre for Chemical and Biological Sciences, HEJ Research Institute of Chemistry, University of Karachi, Pakistan

Fahad Ali
Division of Analytical Chemistry, Bahauddin Zakariya University, Multan, Punjab, Pakistan

Muhammad Najam-ul-Haq
Institute of Chemical Sciences, Bahauddin Zakariya University, Multan, Pakistan

CONTENTS

DOI: 10.1201/9781003263265-9

9.1 Introduction

Prosthetics have played an important role in the fields of information technology, biology, materials, and mechanics. These are lowering the barriers in the life of those people who have lost part/parts of the body due to disease, injury, or aging [1]. A high barrier in the development of prosthetics is the computing hardware. However, the decrease in the size of electronic devices made it sophisticated. Signal analysis and digital computing provided the advancements in prosthetics that are seen in the trials taken on human and non-human models [2]. In the early days, the versatility of the amputees was limited due to the poor performance of the prosthetic limb. However, neural interfaces have provided possible solutions to restore the tactile solution. Specific areas of the somatosensory cortex in hand can be stimulated to evoke tactile sensations of pressure and pain. Periphery nerves are helpful for the better movement of the prosthetics. Key nerves can be rerouted to provide the required motions in the chest muscles. Instead of the advancements in prosthetics, their wide use has been limited due to invasive surgery, neural plasticity from repeated stimulations, and complexity of intent. Human skin provides the inspiration of touch for these prosthetics [3].

    Action potentials generated from the neurons enable the somatosensory feedback. These electrical signals are transmitted through neurons to the brain and analyzed. A combination of any of the five senses can generate neural activity through the stimulation of receptor cells. Encoded information in the form of shape, quantity, frequency, and pattern in action potentials are transferred with the speed of 1–100 m/s from distances of 0.1 mm to 2 m [4]. Neurotransmitters and chemical substances are released from the cells at the terminal of the axon and bind to the receptors after diffusing across the synaptic cleft. There are three main parts of sensory feedback: (1) transduction of stimuli into electrical signals, (2) signal transmissions through neurons, and (3) neural stimulation of neurons in the brain. This chapter discusses the materials as well as technological interfaces that create the artificial sense of touch. Skin-inspired multifunctional interfaces make the bridge with external stimuli for prosthetic limbs. The multifunctionality, sensory components, and stretchability of the artificial interfaces are evaluated and reviewed. Accessing methods for artificial signals, signal encoding, and transmission will be summarized along with the implantable neural interfaces of the materials. These methods are inspired by analog to the digital

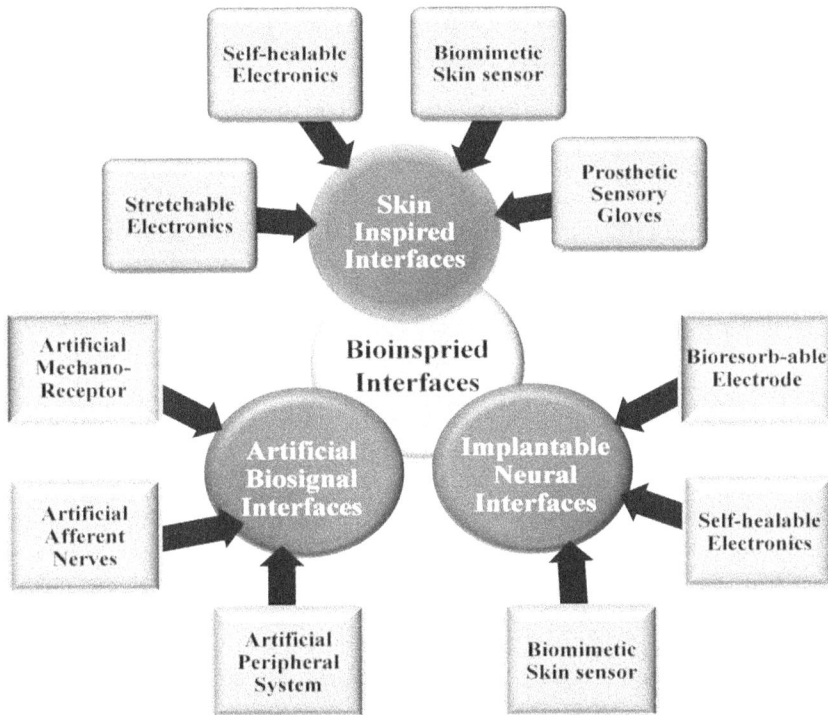

FIGURE 9.1
Interfaces bioinspired by the human body.

conversion process and synaptic transmission of action potentials. A brief look into the interfaces on the materials and techniques that stimulate the neurons in the brain and record the input signals has been included in the chapter as well. These interfaces (Figure 9.1) offer a well-established system of prosthetics with sensory feedback. This chapter concludes with the current and future perspectives of the interfaces.

9.2 Skin-Inspired Multifunctional Interfaces

The human skin has versatile functionalities along with its complex structure. It acts as a physical barrier that protects the internal systems. It integrates conductibility, sensibility, self-healing, and stretchability. Human skin inspired the researchers to develop interfaces and robotic hands along with augmented skin for human beings as well as animals.

9.2.1 Artificial Mechanoreceptors

A variety of mechanoreceptors transduce the signals into action potentials in human skin [1]. The slowly adapting (SA) receptors are responsible for measuring the static forces. SA-I have high resolution, sensitivity for normal forces while SA–II responds more evidently to the stretching in the skin. Rapid adapting of these mechanoreceptors provides vibrational sensitivity and dynamic force.

9.2.1.1 Mimicking the SA Receptors – Static Force Transduction

Sensors are made up of a variety of materials such as polyurethane, polydimethylsiloxane (PDMS), and poly (styrene-butadiene-styrene). The working of these sensors is based on two phenomena, piezocapacitive, and piezoresistive. In capacitance sensors, a change in capacitance occurs under the pressure because of the compression of the dielectric film. The films can be the air gap, elastomer, and microfluidic channel [5]. The sensitivity of a sensor has been reportedly improved by using the array of PDMS film as a dielectric layer. The shaped and structured layer deformed under the pressure as compared to its shapeless design. The structured film detected the pressure up to 3 Pa with enhanced sensitivity of 0.55–1 kPa. The microstructuring of the biocompatible materials as sensor show quick response time and excellent sensitivity. In piezoelectric sensors, resistance change under pressure takes place due to two mechanisms. In the first, the gap between conductive fillers changes by applying the pressure that results from the increase of the number of conductive pathways. In the second mechanism, the microstructured dielectric film contains an additional deposited film of a conductive layer that interfaces the electrode. An applied pressure deforms the microstructure hence leading to the increase of contact area and decrease of contact resistance [6]. These resistive-based sensors are simple, sensitive, and require only a readout circuit. The piezoelectric sensor made up of poly(ethylene dioxythiophene)–poly(styrene sulfonate) with an aqueous polyurethane dispersion elastomer layered on the micro-pyramid array shows a sensitivity up to 4.88 kPa [1] [7]. This sensor can detect an arterial pulse. A variety of microstructures such as micropillars, microstructures, and interlocked structures has improved the sensitivity and linearity of resistive-based sensors. In piezocapacitive sensors and piezoelectric sensors, mechanical signals are transduced into electrical signals, while pressure values correspond to the capacitance and resistance, respectively [8].

9.2.1.2 Mimicking the Rapid Adapting (RA) Receptors – Dynamic Force Transduction

RA receptors are more responsive toward the stimuli to detect the vibrations and movement of the body while triboelectric and piezoelectric sensors are more sensitive to rapid dynamic motion. The piezoelectric sensor deals with the intrinsic properties of the material in which applied force changes the lattice of the materials. A variety of inorganic and soft materials has been used in energy systems and pressure sensors to enhance the response time and sensitivity. In triboelectric sensors, the loss of electrons takes place in materials through triboelectrification and electrostatic induction. In electrification, two surfaces contact and separate by periodic force; hence, charges separate after induction and current flows. The triboelectric sensor responds to the pressure, in which frequency, force, and separation distance affect the output. Electrostatic induction can be improved by the addition of ionic liquid, microstructural designs, and surface treatment of the materials [9]. Self-powered flexible devices developed by triboelectric effect can be used in wearable electronics for the next generation. Recently, various kinds of tactile sensors as flexible devices (Table 9.1) have been developed that demonstrate better sensing to human skin.

9.2.1.3 Biomimetic Sensors

Biomimetic sensors are kind of sensors that uses designated biomaterials and biomimetic approaches similar to those of biological system. These sensors consist of voltammetric, potentiometric, and impedance phenomena. The electronic skin, taste sensors (sweetness, bitterness, sourness, saltiness, umami), odor sensor, cochlear amplifier, and cochlear

TABLE 9.1

Comparisons of Different Parameters Between Human Skin and Some Sensors Type

Active material	Sensitivity	Detection range	Response time/ frequency	Mechanism	References
PVDF/ZnO	0.33 V kPa [1]	1–30 kPa	16 ms	Piezoelectric	[10]
AgNWs/Rose petal	1.54 kPa [1] (<1 kPa)	0.0006–115 kPa	–	Capactive	[11]
Human skin	–	**0–110 kPa**	**0.005–0.4 kHz**	**Biosensing**	[12]
Au/m-PDMS	15 kPa [1] (<0.1 kPa)	<4 kPa	<100 ms	Resistive	[13]
m-PDMS	150 kPa [1] (<0.2 kPa)	0.005–1 kPa	–	Triboelectric	[14]
FEP/Au	112.4 mV dB [1]	50–100 dB	0.1–50 kHz	Triboelectric	[15]
AgNWs/PU	26.07 (0.6%)	0%–80%	–	Resistive	[16]
TPU/IL	23.3 V kPa [1]	<50 kPa	–	Triboelectric	[17]
CNT-PDMS	9617 (90%–120%)	0%–120%	10 ms	Resistive	[18]
PTNWs/Graphene	9.4×10^3 (G.F)	<1.5 kPa	5–7ms	Piezoelectric	[19]

speech recognition are a few examples of biomimetic sensors. This electronic skin has been synthesized with different materials of different shapes. These sensors are fabricated from a 3D electrode at the top and bottom for the detection of multidirectional forces. The bottom electrode contains the microdermis on the bottom in the form of periodic arrays. There are 25 capacitors in a single microdome arranged in the top, surrounding, corners, and slope directions. These capacitors are used for quantitative analysis that responds to the pressure experienced by different strains. This non-uniform sensor provides a more accurate evaluation of the applied force because each sensing pixel experiences the characteristic pressure and responsive curve [20]. The electrolytes also plays important role in biomimetic sensors and measure the induced dynamic and static pressure. An applied pressure generated the piezo potential that induces the movement of ions through electrolytes. The induced flow of ions generates the piezoelectric signals. Thus, dynamic and static signals are measured simultaneously. In some biomimetic devices, piezoelectric and triboelectric effects have been induced, collectively. The electronic skin inspired by the fingerprint (Figure 9.2) contains both of these phenomena. The signals

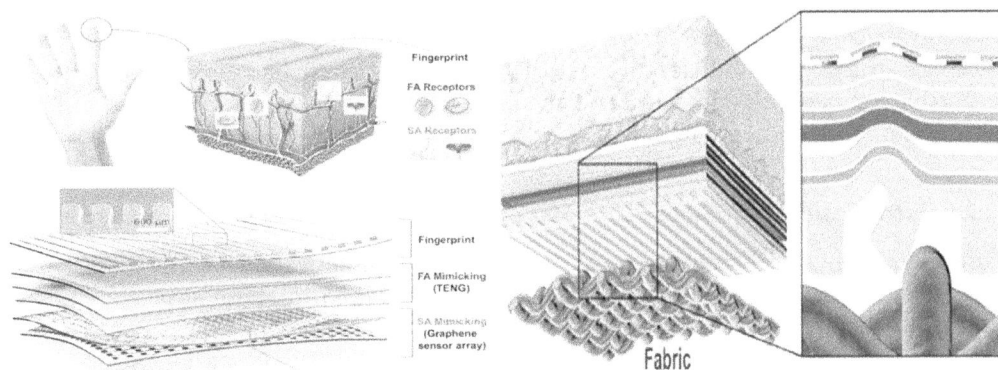

FIGURE 9.2
Biomimetic skin with triboelectric and piezoresistive layers. Adapted with permission [21]. Copyright 2019, American Chemical Society.

obtained by the combination of these effects together exhibit more accuracy as compared to the signals achieved by the separate component analysis. Current trends in the design of flexible and soft artificial hands and limbs, similar to lifelike have led to the study of the human hand motion in detail. In human hands, mechanoreceptors record the tactile motion that is processed and understood by the somatosensory cortex. For data interpretation, the neural system is replaced by artificial mechanoreceptors. Thus recorded and analyzed tactile information provides information about objects [21]. The tactile gloves are examples of these sensors. The deep convolution networks integrated into the gloves are used to check the spatial and temporal relationship for interactive maps. Thus, a tactile glove is used to distinguish the objects and measure their weights [22].

9.2.2 Skin-Like Stretchable Electronics

Human skin plays an important role to communicate with animals and objects through its mechanoreceptors. The body can move due to the flexibility and stretchability of the skin. Mechano-electronic systems bioinspired from the skin are used for robotics and prosthetics. These receptors are made up of silicon devices that can bend and stretch the body.

9.2.2.1 Intrinsically Stretchable Materials

The electronic skin requires all the components such as stretchability, flexibility, invariance, and higher conductivity in the electrode. To mimic the human skin, elastomers and polymers are used as intrinsically stretchable materials. These can elongate equally or larger (30%) as compared with human skin. Elastomer materials include polyurethane, poly (dimethylsiloxane) (PDMS), poly (styrene-butadiene-styrene), inorganic and organic materials (nickel, graphene flakes, and carbon black), and organic polymers have required intrinsic properties. The incorporation of these materials, for example graphene, as electrode material increases stretchability (70%) and resistance [23]. The conductivity and stretchability of materials are highly shaped dependent. The irregular dispersion of organic-inorganic composites causes brittleness and limits stretchability. The implementation of shape-controlled materials like 1D and 2D enhances the desired properties of biomimetic devices. These materials improve their conductivity by maintaining the percolation pathways and stretchability by reducing the percolation threshold. Silver nanowires and carbon nanotubes are examples of these materials. The longer the length of nanowires, the better is the percolation network. However, the smaller density of nanowires improves the transparency and mechanical strength of these nanowires.

9.2.2.2 Extrinsically Stretchable Platforms

Artificially designed structures are used in electronics to achieve stretchability in the circuit level for electronic skins. Inorganic materials are developed to attain stretchability and softness just like real skin. Plant tendrils possess the helix, a natural compound. Helix is more flexible just like gold and copper, due to its 3D structure. It can be wrapped into stretchable devices like robots, conductors, and smart sprigs [24]. No change in length occurs due to the stretching of the wires, thus it remains conductive even at connection points. Helix-containing systems show more conductivity as compared to intrinsically stretchable materials. The elastomer containing copper helical possesses no variant

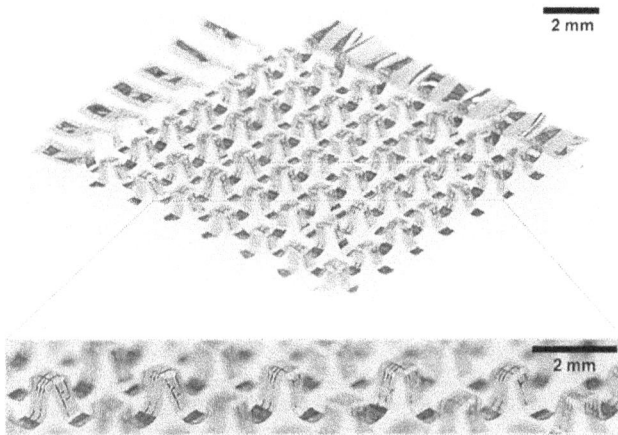

FIGURE 9.3
A network of 3D piezoresistive sensors. Adapted with permission [26]. Copyright 2019, American Chemical Society.

conductivity even at 170% stretching [25]. These elastomers are used in microelectronic systems, where conductivity is most important. Deposition of a conductive and flexible device on elastomer as substrate results in the buckled electrical conductor. The contraction in the flexible device is observed, as the strain is released at its normal phase. Flexible devices made from composite material can be stretched safely without disturbing the flexibility and conductivity of the device. Many materials like silver, gold, and graphene-based composites have attained flexibility and stretchability by buckling method that enables their use in wide applications like sensors and electrode materials. Compressing buckling can be used for the fabrication of scalable sensors array (Figure 9.3) of 3D micro/nanostructures from their 2D precursors [26].

9.2.3 Multifunctional Electronic Skin as Interactive Interfaces

The use of electronic skin in human skin and prosthetic limbs has been encouraged for past decades. In prosthetic limbs, electronic skin restores the sense of touch that needs different types of sensing functionalities integrated on the substrates. The feeling of humidity and temperature along with detection of pressure, the use of biodegradable and self-healing materials are more favored. The development of flexible electronics with human skin provides more functionalities and provide look lifelike.

9.2.3.1 Electronic Skins for Human

Electronic skin acts as a bridge between the internal organs of the human body and machines or computers. Some of the functionalities like detection of body movements, monitoring of physiological signals, and a human-machine interface can be taken by artificial interfaces. Bold pressure can be recorded by tactile sensors that provide important information for clinical and diagnosis purposes. Similarly twisting, bending, and stretching of the limb can be detected by using strain sensors. The movement of the robotic limbs is controlled by the signals transmitted from the e-skin to the various parts of the body to respond to the various stimuli. Epidermal electronics and wearable skin

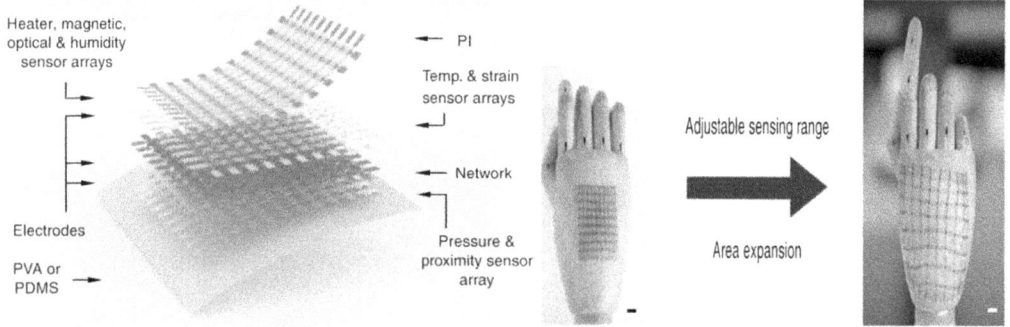

FIGURE 9.4
Multifunctional electronic skin. Adapted with permission [27]. Copyright 2018, Nature Publishing Group.

(Figure 9.4) have a network structure in their first version, integrated with the stretchable sensor circuits of multifunctionality.

9.2.3.2 Electronic Skins for Prosthesis

A sensory network is needed for the restoration of a sense of touch through the rigid prosthesis. Temperature and force sensing can be achieved by direct attachment of sensors with a prosthetic device. The attached fingertip interacts with temperature and pressure as external stimuli and grasps the information. However, a small interactive area limits this method. An increase in the number of sensors at different locations can provide better detection on a prosthetic device. Lack of softness and tactile feedback can be overcome by using a large area, multifunctional, and scalable interface. One example of prosthetic hand material is silicon nanoribbon encapsulated by PDMS. External stimuli are sensed by different sensors for stimuli like pressure, humidity, temperature, and strain. This study demonstrated that nerves were stimulated by the signals transmitted from the pressure sensor and responsive signal was recorded. In this approach, complex integrated materials and devices are needed. The semiconducting ultrathin nanomembrane is one of the materials that is easy to handle and are successfully conformed onto a hand compared to the conventional method, based on direct wrapping [28]. The gloves are another medium to incorporate the sensors. These gloves are laminated with an artificial and heated skin layer. This skin layer contains the skin tones, and fingertip textures just like the real human hand to attain all the attributes of the hand (Figure 9.5) [29].

9.2.4 Self-Healing and Biodegradability

The ability to biodegrade and self-healing makes the construction of prosthetic skins full of sensations. Recently devices with full healing have been introduced that have proprietors of self-healing even in drastic conditions. Ionic liquids and polymer matrix have ion-dipole forces that help the self-healing under acidic, wet, and basic conditions. Supramolecular gels have the ability to self-healing. Carbon nanotubes-based networks in combination with polymers provide a high self-healable system. A multifunction and integrated system of an electrocardiogram sensor, strain sensor, and a light-emitting capacitor is an example of a self-healable system. Transient electronics are an eco-friendly class of electronics for future use.

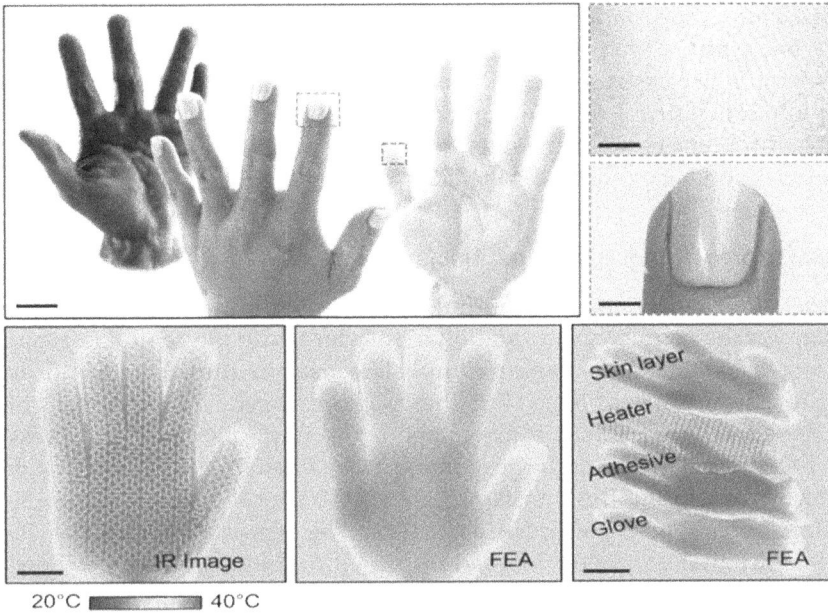

FIGURE 9.5
Artificial prosthetic hand synthesized on gloves to mimic human-like features. Adapted with permission [29]. Copyright 2019, Springer Nature.

9.3 Artificial Biosignal Interfaces

The interfaces inspired by human skin act as a bridge between prosthetic limb and nervous system. To synchronize the work of sensors present on a prosthetic limb and nervous system, an artificial path for signal transmission is needed for a prosthetic interface. The transmission of these biosignals is performed by encoding techniques. These techniques are inspired by the synaptic transmission of action potentials and analog to digital conversion.

9.3.1 Signal Encoding/Transmission in the Nervous System

Biosignals are collected, transformed, and processed by the nervous system in the human body. Different receptors like thermal receptors, mechanoreceptors, and nociceptors receive the physical stimuli that are encoded into electrical signals. Afterward, these electrical signals are converted into action potentials by sensory neurons. Different types of stimuli are sensed by various types of sensory receptors. Temperature, pressure, and smell are sensed by thermoreceptors, mechanoreceptors, and olfactory receptors, respectively. Specific receptor converts the stimulus-response into action potential with specific codes. The intensity of the signal from receptors is represented as a frequency of action potentials after conversion into digital pulses, accordingly.

9.3.2 Signal Encoding in Electronic Skin Systems

External stimuli are converted into electrical quantities like current, voltage, capacitance, and resistance in an electronic skin. A pulse-like potential that contains the information of the amplitude, duration, and frequency of encoded information of receptors is received by the nervous system. The prosthesis cannot respond to external stimuli due to the gap between readable devices and neutrally intelligible. Signal coding and transmission are converted into an electrical response by the sensor that can communicate with the nervous system. In recent years, many attempts have been taken for establishing the bridge between electrical devices and the systems of the human body.

9.3.2.1 Analog Signal Conversion and Amplification

The prosthetic device converts the output of the sensor into current and voltage. It is the first step for the coding of information to interface with the central nervous system. In most prosthetic devices, external stimuli like heat or pressure are not converted directly into current and voltage. But these devices need an additional circuit that converts the capacitive readout into voltage for example in capacitive pressure sensors [30]. Pressure changes can be responded to by changing the transistor drain current; either by integrating the transistor gate with piezocapacitive/piezoelectric senor or transistor source with a piezoresistive sensor. The transistor in these devices works like an amplifier that amplifies the readout signal for better sensitivity. Low gate capacitance and mobility limits these sensors to work at higher voltage, which requires safety concerns [31].

9.3.2.2 Biomimetic Analog to Digital Transform

Action potential, in the form of a digital signal, is transmitted in subcutaneous receptors. After the conversion of signal into current and voltage, is digitized into biological signals. Digitizing of signals is performed by transistors. Silicon-based transistors are the traditional form that is made up of elastomers. Mechanical modulus of these transistors mismatch with the human e-skin. Although scientists have explored the ways to integrate these transistors with flexible systems by converting these into wires for connection with a rigid surface. Organic transistors have more flexibility and are used in electronic skin systems. The organic transistors convert pressure signals into frequency. The ring oscillator in these systems is made up of plastic polyethylene naphthalte foils printed with organic transistors, which converts the voltage input into a periodic voltage signal. Each ring oscillator is equipped with a pair of complementary transistors. Resistance of the pressure sensor is measured with a piezoresistive sensor that determines its output frequency which later turned into pulse signals.

9.3.2.3 Synaptic Signal Processing

Synapses transfer the signal from one neuron into another neuron in the nervous system. The signal is not directly transmitted but undergoes learning and memory, i.e., time and intensity modulation occurs known as synaptic plasticity. Signal processing can bring the learning and recovery of specific functions for the disabled in electronic skin-based prosthetics. Synaptic plasticity can be well performed with ion-gated transistors. The ion-gated transistor integrated with a tensile sensing element provides synaptic plasticity in response to pressure as stimuli. Channel current of the ion-gated transistor encodes the information on the frequency, amplitude, and duration of the applied stimulus. Synaptic transistors can regulate the triboelectric and piezoelectric signals, while memristor-based systems simulate the synaptic plasticity.

9.3.3 Multiple Access Techniques for Signal Transmission

Prosthetic devices contain a somatosensory system in which large sensor arrays are integrated into the electronic skin. The origin of the signal and information that it contains are provided to the sensing systems.

9.3.3.1 Time-Divisional Access

The electronic skin sensor is structured in a crossbar of rows and columns. A 2D map is formed periodically as the sensors are sampled with divisional multiple access. These kinds of sensors measure the signals in a very short time. Time divisional multiple acess (TDMA) transmissions are organized in a frame structure and are used for measuring the performance of the device in electronic skin sensors. TDMA method is suitable for small-scale sensors. However, this approach is limited for a large number of the sensors; as the sensor increases, they are closer to the skin receptors and increases overall sampling time. This increase in sampling time creates challenges to achieving real-time feedback.

9.3.3.2 Event-Based Access

The central nervous system can receive multiple stimuli from different parts of the body simultaneously. Several studies can demonstrate the concept of the nervous system, including a data acquisition system for skin applications. The framework used in these studies triggers the readout at a constant rate. The frame attains the data from a sensor and collects this data instead of pixel by pixel. It provides the results of the real-time sampling in a short time. However, it requires a large network of wires and high power consumption. Another promising strategy is event-based signaling. It transmits the signal when the output of the sensor changes, thus saving power and bandwidth. The coded electronic skin system provides information on the transmission of real-time tactile. A tiny microcontroller, present in the asynchronously coded electronic skin system, is connected with a sensor that generates the signature signal for each sensor. The signals transmitted by a single wire are decoded and recorded as temporal skin patterns.

9.3.3.3 Biomimetic Synaptic Access

The central nervous system uses the synapses for addressing the stimuli. The potential of the system is decided by bionic synapses based on distance recognition and spatial orientation [32]. The distribution of multi-gates at different distances and directions is adopted around the channel in the in-plane gate ion-gate transistor. The postsynaptic current will be smaller as the distance between the gate and channel is increased. Postsynaptic current from different directions is provided by different gates present in that area. Gate position in transistors is decided based on the magnitude of the postsynaptic current. Synaptic transistors provide the features of pattern in combination with pressure sensors. A neuromorphic tactile processing system is made up of an ionic conductor, ion-gated transistor, and piezoelectric sensor. The sensor is attached to the fingertip; motion of the finger on different patterns of groups produces waveforms of the different currents. These patterns are identified by machine learning tools and information is indirectly used to measure tactile functions.

9.4 Implantable Neural Interfaces

Biosignals are transmitted from prosthetic limbs to the central nervous system. The signals transmitted to the brain enable the body to respond to the prosthesis. The process is simple, yet there is a need to reduce the complex interaction of chemical and electrical signals of neurons in the nervous system. The function of the human brain is complex that can be understood by invasive and non-invasive methods in which electronic skin acts as a neural interface. Traditionally, a patch-clamp has been used that records the brain signal. It contains electrodes on the surface of the head. The data obtained is used to attain the intentions of the user and stimulation external factors such as face recognition and muscle movement. Many diseases and/or conditions such as depression, dementia, and Parkinson's disease are now treated with memory implants and brain pacemakers [33]. Electrodes are placed in the target location of the brain. Then electrical signals are sent to the electrodes by the planted brain pacemaker. These devices are not biocompatible due to their limited battery life. Material technology can help us to record and stimulate the neurons to help patients with many diseases such as epilepsy, sclerosis, and tetraplegia [34]. This section covers neuroprosthetic applications of the probes and flexible electronic skin. Here we will also demonstrate stimulation methods by probes that use optical, electrical, and microfluidic delivery.

9.4.1 Stimulation Methods

Microelectrodes are the best neural interfaces that are used for bidirectional communication. These are used for listening and talking with neurons that are inserted in the brain area. Each electrode performs two functions: stimulates and records the electrical activity of a group of a neuron. There are some important factors for designing the neural interface. These include size and quantity of stimulation channel, means to use interface, biological response of cells, electrical requirements, and structure of the intended device [35]. Electrophysiological methods are used for stimulation and recording of neural activity. Penetrating multi-electrodes in the brain is one of the best electrophysiological methods. Electrically stimulated depolarized membranes of cells in the brain are used for the initiation of functional response. Microelectrodes are used for improving selectivity and resolution. Charge injection density can increase the performance of microelectrodes.

9.4.1.1 Flexible Stimulation Probes

For the development of penetration and comfortable electrodes, material chemistry has achieved great intentions. The material includes the polymers such as polyimide, parylene, and polydimethylsiloxane. These materials are used with metal electrodes as insulation layers and substrates. Conducting polymers as the outermost layer provides the electrical insulation and these do not need any additional coating. The probe based on polyimide performs the stimulation and recording in the deep brain. The device record the neural spike signal at the depth of 7 mm in the brain of a rat [36]. However, the insertion of a soft tungsten guide stick is needed in the brain to record the signal. Extraction of the neural probe can damage the tissues surrounding the brain. To minimize this risk, electrodes of soft stimulation and freestanding materials like conducting polymers and elastomers have been synthesized. These electrodes are constructed with two layers; the outer layer of parylene and the inner layer of poly (ethylene dioxythiophene) poly (ethylene glycol) and silicone. The electrodes can perform the stimulation and recording with the help of a counter electrode made up of stainless steel. These microwires show enhanced properties like biocompatibility and a high level of electrode integration. Polymers with flexible and transparent properties allow the stimulation of electrical signals at high curvature surfaces like the retina and spinal cord.

9.4.1.2 Multifunctional Stimulation Probes

Recently, optogenetics and biochemical drug delivery including many other neural transmission methods have emerged as an attractive multifunctional probes. In optogenetics, neurons are stimulated by using visible light of a specific wavelength. Opsins, also called transmembranes, change the response as these are exposed to specific visible light that excites them or inherent neural activity [37]. In optrodes, silicon microelectrodes are combined with optical fibers for stimulation and recording of the signal. In microfluidics, chemicals or analytes of interest are delivered to the specific area to check their response at that area. This method can be used for the treatment of diseases like brain disorders. Various multifunctional probes can facilitate the drug delivery, recording of neurons, and stimulation of signals. These functionalities are achieved through silicon probes. Microfabrication helps to concentrate the active metals in probes [38].

A probe designed for drug delivery consisting of micro-electro-mechanical systems of 40 µm thickness combined with microelectrode arrays and a microfluidic channel of optical guide records the signal from different areas [39]. The probe successfully delivers the drug in mice. The probes can be synthesized with different spacing, widths, and depths having less cross-sectional area. These probes can be used for multifunctional purposes. Metal electrodes and electrical wiring can be integrated with optical guides and microfluidic channels into one device [37]. Neurons present near the electrode are stimulated by light and response is recorded. Optical fibers used for telecommunication over a long distance can also inspire this design. For rerecording and drug delivery, fibers based on polymers are well preferred. Human hair-like thickness containing fibers made up of polymers and metals is another attractive material [40].

9.4.2 Recording Methods

Electrodes can be implanted into the neuron or at the surface of the neuron to obtain the best action potential. These electrodes receive the recording and provide the control of prosthesis to patients for communication. These microelectrodes have a surface area lower the 200 µm. Action potential has the amplitude of 100 µV. Impedance of electrodes plays an important role for the noisy signal that depends on the distance between electrode and neuron as well as the distance of tissue. Neural recordings of large scale can be obtained by uniformity and low impedance. Various attempts have been made for improving the signal-to-noise ratio through electronics and nano-electrodes by addressing the issue of hemocompatibility, mechanical integrity, and biocompatibility [41].

9.4.2.1 Epidermal Recording Devices

The most widespread non-invasive technique for signal recording in bioelectronics is the epidermal recording electrodes. In electroencephalography, a set of electrodes is kept on the scalp of the subject and electrical rhythms are recorded. Brain waves have different ranges and these define the functions of the brain and its state. These ranges are converted into cognitive action after their detection in neuroprosthetic devices. Brain activity can be sensed by sensors or the flexible electronic skin. While playing games, brain simulators are used for attaining the attention of common people. These simulators are non-invasive and simple; many companies like Neurosky and Focus are selling these simulators. Long-term stability and high performance can be achieved by using different fabrication processes and a variety of materials. Conductive polymers provide lower impedance as contacted with tissues; thus, a high-quality signal is achieved compared to metal-based electrodes [42].

9.4.2.2 Implantable Recording Devices

Electrodes can record the neural signal when placed in the brain cortex through a technique called electrocorticography. The resolution of this method is very high as compared to other methods. Gamma rhythms of higher frequency can decode the sound, speech, and motor movements from their stored information. Stretchable electrode grids can detect the signal more conveniently. These grids can record the signals for many months. The brain area decides the stretchability and number of inserted electrodes. Nanoelctrodes can increase the electrode area and decrease the impedance for capturing a signal [43]. A neural device is directly connected with neural tissues to lower the signal-to-noise ratio with better quality. Microscale devices can provide high performance when integrated with biocompatible systems.

9.5 Summary and Perspectives

The tremendous efforts for the development of sensory feedback systems lead the skin-like electronics interface to the implantable human-machine interface. Bioinspiration has provided the facilities to merge the artificial electronic system with biological systems and prosthetics. Implementation of artificial sensory networks to prosthetic hands and human skin is useful to achieve better human-machine interaction.

At the start of this chapter, it was discussed that artificial sensory networks contain properties similar to the skin; thus, applicable for prosthetic hands and human skin. Then, the signal transmission process through conditioning, encoding, and conveying from receptors to the interface of the neural system has been highlighted. Finally, progress in electrodes has been demonstrated. Advancement in sensing materials features great promises towards the high level of devices integration, multifunctionality, and softness of the interfaces. But there are still challenges for the integration of interfaces with full functionality such as achievement of recording of humidity, pressure, and heat simultaneously through intrinsically stretchable designs due to their high density. In the future, research will focus on the integration of artificial skin in a self-healing system and biodegradability for prosthetic hands. In the artificial biosignal interface, an output signal is encoded and conditioned along with it is accessed and processed in between the brain and artificial skin sensing system. Easy access of output signal to the nervous system, conversion, amplification, digitization, and coding of a signal is an important aspect to be explained.

Ring oscillators are the best tools for the digitization and coding of signals [44]. However, the integration of small-scale devices is still under discussion. Flexible transistors are larger compared to silicon-based transistors. Their integration is still changing in a smaller portion of space like in multilayer logic circuits. Low mobility of electrons in semiconductors, high operating voltage, and stability of transistors are still problematic. In the future, advanced materials may solve these problems. Low mobility of ions in an artificial synaptic transistor helps them to make a high degree of mimicry. In dielectric layer output, signals are in the form of time information, yet the process of decoupling of information is still unclear. There are various methods for reading and processing signals to cope with the situation. In all of these methods, electronic skin sensors are distributed and mixed with skin in a prosthesis. Event-based coding is an efficient method that is closest to the nervous system. The asynchronously coded electronic skin technique allows the terminal to access the 10,000 sensors simultaneously. In this technique, low constant latency of 1 ms and a power supply of high precision is required that make these receptors larger compared to the receptors of human subcutaneous.

MCUs in combination with wiring signals can achieve the arrays sensor of high density. However, numerous wires required for this technology make its implementation challenging. Mismatched integration of rigid chips with flexible electronic skin is still a difficult task. The size of the receptors can be decreased with the application of specific integrated circuits. New methods and devices that work on new mechanisms enable in-situ coding in further investigation. The transmission of signals through digitized electronic skin still needs to be explored. Some electronic skin implements optical technology or wireless methods for signal transmission while most of the electronic skin uses direct signal transmission. Sensor arrays are frozen in wireless technology by bound wires. Traditional wireless networks for electronic skin rely on radio-wave communication. These networks provide inefficient energy and are vulnerable to eavesdropping. A wireless network of body sensors is an alternative to fill the above shortcoming. This network is propagated at the surface of textile made of metal material. It is connected through radio surface plasmons. This metal-based material is used to improve the security and efficiency of transmission of the signal. These transmit the signal from different parts of the body from different multiple sensors in a wireless way. This may be fruitful in the prosthesis. Associated receivers and receptors rely on the chips. These are still compared with the sensory units of humans. There will be a new trending way for developing the new methods of signal transmission to decrease the difficulties created by numerous wiring.

Polymers materials are stretchable and flexible. These are used for manufacturing the new designs of bioinspired devices. These materials can stimulate the neurons. Then, these record the signals and activate the prosthetic action or body. Implantable neural interfaces that are early discussed can represent the mesh electronics and implantable probes that are deeply embedded. This embedding helps accurate stimulation and recording at a specific region of the brain. These probes and electronics are biocompatible, small, and have a minimal immune response to glial infections. Actuators in combination with sensors respond to light, heat, and electricity. These provide multifunctionality in these probes and are used to monitor the pH, glucose, and oxygen in the blood.

Mesh electronic interface, together with optical waveguides based on polymer materials, can pursue the stimulation in deeper tissues of the brain matter. Until now, a large variety of sophisticated bioelectronics has been developed. However, these devices still face many challenges. A highly functional prosthetic system is required that corresponds to the sensory feedback. The dexterity of human skins can be achieved by integrating the higher level of devices. These high levels of devices provide a variety of a large number of mechanoreceptors. These devices are embedded in the human skin. In addition, wire-bond transmission is embedded in the electronic skin of a human. These wire-bond transmissions are replaced by wireless transmissiones, as these provide better energy efficiency. Mesh electrodes are the neural interrogation systems that are compatible with human skin. These provide high chronic performance and show high efficiency when applied to the rodents. However, with these advancements to achieve a complete vision of neuroprosthetic, there will be a need for interdisciplinary cooperation to address the critical issues.

References

1. A. Chortos, J. Liu, and Z. Bao, *Pursuing prosthetic electronic skin*. Nature Materials, 2016. **15**(9): pp. 937–950.
2. J.E. O'Doherty, et al., *Active tactile exploration using a brain–machine–brain interface*. Journal of Nature, 2011. **479**(7372): pp. 228–231.
3. E.C. Leuthardt, J.L. Roland, and W.Z. Ray, *Neuroprosthetics*. Journal of Scientist, 2014. **28**(11).
4. B.P. Bean, *The action potential in mammalian central neurons*. Journal of Nature Reviews Neuroscience, 2007. **8**(6): pp. 451–465.
5. S.G. Yoon and S.T. Chang, *Microfluidic capacitive sensors with ionic liquid electrodes and CNT/ PDMS nanocomposites for simultaneous sensing of pressure and temperature*. Journal of Materials Chemistry C, 2017. **5**(8): pp. 1910–1919.
6. S.C. Mannsfeld, et al., *Highly sensitive flexible pressure sensors with microstructured rubber dielectric layers*. Journal of Nature Materials, 2010. **9**(10): pp. 859–864.
7. C.L. Choong, et al., *Highly stretchable resistive pressure sensors using a conductive elastomeric composite on a micropyramid array*. Journal of Advanced Materials, 2014. **26**(21): pp. 3451–3458.
8. C. Pang, et al., *A flexible and highly sensitive strain-gauge sensor using reversible interlocking of nanofibres*. Journal of Nature Materials, 2012. **11**(9): pp. 795–801.
9. S. Wang, et al., *Molecular surface functionalization to enhance the power output of triboelectric nanogenerators*. Journal of Materials Chemistry A, 2016. **4**(10): pp. 3728–3734.
10. W. Deng, et al., *Cowpea-structured PVDF/ZnO nanofibers based flexible self-powered piezoelectric bending motion sensor towards remote control of gestures*. Journal of Nano Energy, 2019. **55**: pp. 516–525.
11. Y. Wan, et al., *Natural plant materials as dielectric layer for highly sensitive flexible electronic skin*. Journal of Small, 2018. **14**(35): pp. 1801657.
12. R.S. Johansson and J.R. Flanagan, *Coding and use of tactile signals from the fingertips in object manipulation tasks*. Journal of Nature Reviews Neuroscience, 2009. **10**(5): pp. 345–359.
13. Y. Zhang, et al., *Flexible and highly sensitive pressure sensor based on microdome-patterned PDMS forming with assistance of colloid self-assembly and replica technique for wearable electronics*. Journal of ACS Applied Materials & Interfaces, 2017. **9**(41): pp. 35968–35976.
14. Z. Liu, et al., *Expandable microsphere-based triboelectric nanogenerators as ultrasensitive pressure sensors for respiratory and pulse monitoring*. Journal of Nano Energy, 2019. **59**: pp. 295–301.
15. X. Pu, et al., *Rotation sensing and gesture control of a robot joint via triboelectric quantization sensor*. Journal of Nano Energy, 2018. **54**: pp. 453–460.
16. S. Zhang, et al., *Ultrasensitive and highly compressible piezoresistive sensor based on polyurethane sponge coated with a cracked cellulose nanofibril/silver nanowire layer*. Journal of ACS Applied Materials & Interfaces, 2019. **11**(11): pp. 10922–10932.
17. H.J. Hwang, et al., *An ultra-mechanosensitive visco-poroelastic polymer ion pump for continuous self-powering kinematic triboelectric nanogenerators*. Journal of Advanced Energy Materials, 2019. **9**(17): pp. 1803786.

18. J. Park, et al., *Tactile-direction-sensitive and stretchable electronic skins based on human-skin-inspired interlocked microstructures.* Journal of ACS Nano, 2014. **8**(12): pp. 12020–12029.
19. Z. Chen, et al., *Flexible piezoelectric-induced pressure sensors for static measurements based on nanowires/graphene heterostructures.* Journal of ACS Nano, 2017. **11**(5): pp. 4507–4513.
20. Z. Pei, et al., *A fully 3D printed electronic skin with bionic high resolution and air permeable porous structure.* Journal of Colloid & Interface Science, 2021. **602**: pp. 452–458.
21. S. Chun, et al., *Self-powered pressure-and vibration-sensitive tactile sensors for learning technique-based neural finger skin.* Journal of Nano Letters, 2019. **19**(5): pp. 3305–3312.
22. S. Sundaram, et al., *Learning the signatures of the human grasp using a scalable tactile glove.* Journal of Nature, 2019. **569**(7758): pp. 698–702.
23. Y.R. Jeong, et al., *Highly stretchable and sensitive strain sensors using fragmentized graphene foam.* Journal of Advanced Functional Materials, 2015. **25**(27): pp. 4228–4236.
24. S.J. Gerbode, et al., *How the cucumber tendril coils and overwinds.* Journal of Science, 2012. **337**(6098): pp. 1087–1091.
25. Y. Zhao, et al., *Highly conductive 3D metal-rubber composites for stretchable electronic applications.* Journal of APL Materials, 2019. **7**(3): pp. 031508.
26. S.M. Won, et al., *Multimodal sensing with a three-dimensional piezoresistive structure.* Journal of ACS Nano, 2019. **13**(10): pp. 10972–10979.
27. Q. Hua, et al., *Skin-inspired highly stretchable and conformable matrix networks for multifunctional sensing.* Journal of Nature Communications, 2018. **9**(1): pp. 1–11.
28. K. Sim, et al., *Metal oxide semiconductor nanomembrane–based soft unnoticeable multifunctional electronics for wearable human-machine interfaces.* Journal of Science Advances, 2019. **5**(8): pp. eaav9653.
29. M.K. Kim, et al., *Soft-packaged sensory glove system for human-like natural interaction and control of prosthetic hands.* Journal of NPG Asia Materials , 2019. **11**(1): pp. 1–12.
30. J.C. Lotters, et al., *A sensitive differential capacitance to voltage converter for sensor applications.* IEEE Transactions on Instrumentation; Measurement, 1999. **48**(1): pp. 89–96.
31. M.-J. Kim, et al., *Controlling the gate dielectric properties of vinyl-addition polynorbornene copolymers via thiol–ene click chemistry for organic field-effect transistors.* Journal of Materials Chemistry C, 2021. **9**(14): pp. 4742–4747.
32. C. Qian, et al., *Multi-gate organic neuron transistors for spatiotemporal information processing.* Journal of Applied Physics Letters, 2017. **110**(8): pp. 083302.
33. D. Wu, et al., *The effects of motif net charge and amphiphilicity on the self-assembly of functionally designer RADA16-I peptides.* Journal of Biomedical Materials, 2018. **13**(3): pp. 035011.
34. L.R. Hochberg, et al., *Reach and grasp by people with tetraplegia using a neurally controlled robotic arm.* Journal of Nature, 2012. **485**(7398): pp. 372–375.
35. D.J. Weber, R. Friesen, and L.E. Miller, *Interfacing the somatosensory system to restore touch and proprioception: Essential considerations.* Journal of Motor Behavior, 2012. **44**(6): pp. 403–418.
36. G. Hong and C.M. Lieber, *Novel electrode technologies for neural recordings.* Nature Reviews Neuroscience, 2019. **20**(6): pp. 330–345.
37. E.S. Boyden, et al., *Millisecond-timescale, genetically targeted optical control of neural activity.* 2005. Journal of Nature Neuroscience, **8**(9): pp. 1263–1268.
38. T.-I. Kim, et al., *Injectable, cellular-scale optoelectronics with applications for wireless optogenetics.* Journal of Science, 2013. **340**(6129): pp. 211–216.
39. H. Shin, et al., *Multifunctional multi-shank neural probe for investigating and modulating long-range neural circuits in vivo.* Journal of Nature Communications, 2019. **10**(1): pp. 1–11.
40. A. Canales, et al., *Multifunctional fibers for simultaneous optical, electrical and chemical interrogation of neural circuits in vivo.* Journal of Nature Biotechnology, 2015. **33**(3): pp. 277–284.
41. M. Dipalo, et al., *Intracellular and extracellular recording of spontaneous action potentials in mammalian neurons and cardiac cells with 3D plasmonic nanoelectrodes.* Journal of Nanoletters, 2017. **17**(6): pp. 3932–3939.

42. T. Sekitani, et al., *Invited Paper: A Sheet-type Wireless electroencephalogram (EEG) Sensor System using Flexible and Stretchable Electronics.* in *SID Symposium Digest of Technical Papers.* 2017. Wiley Online Library, pp. 143–146.
43. Y. Qiang, et al., *Transparent arrays of bilayer-nanomesh microelectrodes for simultaneous electrophysiology and two-photon imaging in the brain.* Journal of Science Advances, 2018. **4**(9): pp. eaat0626.
44. B.C.-K. Tee, et al., *A skin-inspired organic digital mechanoreceptor.* Journal of Science, 2015. **350**(6258): pp. 313–316.

10

Biocompatible and Biodegradable Organic Transistors

Selcan Karakuş

Department of Chemistry, Faculty of Engineering, Istanbul University-Cerrahpasa, Avcılar, Istanbul, Turkey

Nazlı Albayrak

School of Medicine, Acibadem M. A. Aydınlar University, Avcılar, Istanbul, Turkey

Sinem Özlem Enginler

Department of Obstetrics and Gynecology, Faculty of Veterinary Medicine, Istanbul University-Cerrahpasa, Avcılar, Istanbul, Turkey

CONTENTS

10.1 Bio-organic Transistors

Nowadays, biocompatible and biodegradable organic transistors for stretchable and flexible electronic devices have gained attractive attention due to their ability to exhibit unique performances by implementing new technological solutions in biomedical and sensor applications. With the emergence of smart nano-micro platforms for human-digital technologies, new applications based on stretchable electronics, flexible bioelectronics, and wearable biosensors have been developed. Biopolymer-based organic transistors are especially highly stable, mobile, biocompatible, biodegradable, solvent-processable for a wide variety of consumer products at a low cost. In the literature, the new-generation organic transistors are fabricated fibrous, thin-film, porous nanocrystalline, and fullerene-rich morphologies in the nanoscale range. According to recent advances and developments on integrating nanotechnology with implantable or wearable bioelectronic devices, these systems change biochemical and microenvironmental signals to digital readouts and enable biosensing with high spatial resolution, high temporal resolution, and rapid.

The sensitive and selective detection of different types of biomarkers (molecular, histologic, radiographic, and physiologic types of biomarkers) are for the basic application of bioanalytical chemistry. Advanced sensor technologies have been mostly developed in mobile healthcare systems and wearable bioelectronic devices, while in target analytes biosensing is based on green methods that exhibit real-time monitoring. In addition to the bioelectronic devices, many studies have reported the performance effects of green organic transistors with natural materials, experimental conditions, morphological, and structural properties. When compared to other materials, green organic transistors have many advantages in the presence of biopolymer and biopolymer blends such as egg albumen, starch, gelatine, silk, polysaccharides, collagen, algal, chitosan, polyvinyl alcohol, gum arabic, polylactic acid, poly-lactic-go-glycolacid, polycaprolactone, poly(1,8-octanediol-co-citrate), polypropylene carbonate, polyvinylpyrrolidone, polyhydroxyalkanoates, poly(3-hydroxybutyrate), poly(3-hydroxyvalerate), and poly(3,4-ethylenedioxythiophene) polystyrene sulfonate (PEDOT:PSS). Lai et al. prepared a novel gelatin-hydrogel-based organic synaptic transistor for the application of environment-friendly neuromorphic electronics to understand the neuromorphological computing system of learning and memory in the human brain using the principle of sustainable development [1].

Therefore, to expand the applications of polymers in green transistors, Rullyani et al. developed eco-friendly 3,4,9,10-perylene-tetracarboxylic-diimide (PTCDI)–based organic thin-film transistors (OTFTs) using natural rubber, chitosan, and cis-polyisoprene extract. The green OTFTs were characterized by the tapping-mode atomic force microscopy (AFM) technique to investigate the surface properties of the gate dielectric electrode and the formation of the organic semiconductor on the surface. Experimental results revealed that chitosan (biopolymer) and natural rubber are some of the most promising materials for use as gate dielectric materials in biomedical applications with their high dielectric strength and insulation properties [2]. Ji et al., in 2020, discussed flexible, sensitive, and selective carbonized silk fabric-based electrochemical transistors that remarkably elevated the sensor performance on the detection of dopamine. The sensor exhibited an effective performance parameter with an ultra-low detection limit of 1 nM in a wide concentration range from 1 nM to 30 μM [3]. In literature, Lee et al. prepared a fully stretchable, wearable, and lab-on-a-patch impedimetric biosensor for immunodetection of cortisol biomarkers in a wide concentration range from 1 pg/mL to 1 μg/mL with a high correlation (relative difference of ∼14.7%) [4]. These experimental results showed that the proposed biosensor had great potential for medical diagnostics and monitoring in biomedical applications. With this approach, Wang et al. prepared a novel wearable and stretchable textile gold fiber-based electrochemical biosensor for the detection of on-body sweat lactate and sensing of soft robotic glove lactate with a high sensitivity of 19.13 μA/mMcm^2 and 14.6 μA/mMcm^2 in artificial sweat solutions [5]. Hashemi et al. developed a green polyrhodanine/graphene oxide/Fe_3O_4 nanocomposite based ultrasensitive biosensor with a natural kombucha extract as a biomaterial for the determination of doxorubicin hydrochloride in human body fluids. Electrochemical results showed that the ultrasensitivity, low limit of detection (LOD), and quantification limit of the proposed polyrhodanine/graphene oxide/Fe_3O_4 nanocomposite-based biosensor were calculated 167.62 μA μM^{-1} cm^{-2}, 0.008 μM, and 0.056 μM, respectively, due to the electrochemical redox in the human blood plasma [6].

Several studies have reported that the most frequently used forms of the high-performance fully printed OTFT-based devices with very higher carrier mobility (up to 10 cm^2/V·s) [7–9]. Singh et al. prepared a novel printed high-performance OTFT using a polymer blend of 2,7-dihexyl-dithieno[2,3-d;2′,3′-d′]benzo[1,2-b;4,5-b′]dithiophene (DTBDT-C6) and polystyrene (PS) [10]. Previous studies highlighted that it's a major strategy to prepare a uniform material on a substrate by simple and low-cost solution-process methods using a solution with a low viscosity. To overcome the dewetting limitation and prepare high-performance nanostructures with unique surface properties and large surface areas enhancing electrochemical properties of materials for efficient charge transport. In literature, Shen et al. developed green high-performance OFET using a blend of 2,7-dioctyl[1]benzothieno[3,2-b][1]benzothiophene (C8-BTBT) and polymer binder based thin films for flexible and printed electronic devices. Experimental results showed that the proposed bio-based transistors use a blend of C8-BTBT and PS with a high stability and mobility up to 6.80 cm^2/Vs. It was clear that these excellent properties were related to large domain sizes, smooth grain boundaries, and phase-separated [11]. Furthermore, OFETs have been categorized into two types of approaches. Accordingly, they are grouped into top-down and bottom-up methods, depending on either the bulk or nanomaterial structure of the initial material [12]. As known, the typical design of an OFETs consists of the drain, gate, metallic source, organic semiconductor, and electrolyte [13]. In Figure 10.1, schematic diagrams of the bottom gate bottom contact, bottom gate top contact, top gate bottom contact, and top gate top contact of OFETs are presented.

Three-dimensional (3D) printing is a low-cost and simple technique based on the cumulation of thin layers of structures with a 3D digital type of material. As known, green organic materials have a high solubility, high-quality support, and ease of use for un-masked patterns in a single 3D application for advanced device fabrication. In the research study of Fan et al. in 2019 [14], they developed a novel 3D-printed functional organic electrochemical transistors by a polymer blend of PEDOT:PSS as a channel material and silver as a source/drain for wearable and stand-alone biosensing applications. The prepared organic electrochemical transistors based device showed good stability, high electrical conductivity, high transconductance, low operating voltage, and high current ON/OFF ratio in the voltage range of 0.66 ± 0.01 V. In another study, Majak et al. in 2019 [15], fabricated a fully 3D-printed inverter logic gate sensor-based using a

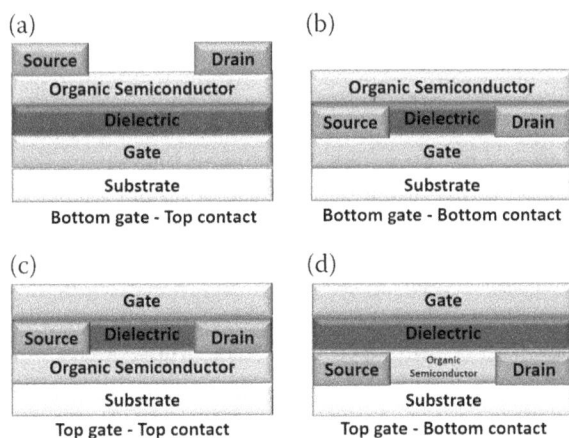

FIGURE 10.1
Schematic diagrams of (a) bottom gate top contact, (b) bottom gate bottom contact, (c) top gate top contact, and (d) top gate bottom contact of OFETs.

polymer blend of PEDOT:PSS-based electrochemical transistors as ions (NaCl, KCl, and $CaCl_2$) level detector. In this study, they demonstrated highly sensitive organic electrochemical transistors sensors with a low LOD of 1 mM for different soluble ionic compound-based electrolytes and high sensitivities 650 and 200 mV/dec for Na^+ ions in the electrolyte range of 1–100 mM and 100–1,000 mM.

In addition, in 2017, Damiati et al. presented the fabrication of anti-CD133 antibody/ S-layer fusion protein (rSbpA/ZZ lattice)/Au-based electrodes and electrochemical properties of efficient acoustic 3D-printed electrochemical biosensors for the real-time immunodetection of liver cancer cells (HepG2) for the detection of the tumor biomarker CD133 [16]. Moreover, in 2018, Zhang et al. fabricated a novel ultrasensitive and selective biosensor for the detection of ascorbic acid using a combination of an organic transistor and a molecularly imprinted polymer (MIP)–modified gate in a wide ascorbic acid concentration range from 1 µM to 100 µM [17]. The electrochemical results showed that the novel MIP-OECT biosensor had a low LOD of 10 nM (S/N > 3) and high sensitivity of 75.3 µA for target analyte (ascorbic acid) in the presences of different analytes such as glucose, aspartic acid, uric acid, glutathione, glycine, metal ions (K^+, Na^+, Ca^{2+}, Mg^{2+}, and Fe^{2+}), and H_2O_2.

10.2 Electrochemical Properties of Bio-Organic Transistors

The use of bio-based nanostructures in preparation of enzymatic/non-enzymatic electrochemical biosensors act as new types of medical devices for detecting and quantifying cancer biomarkers and are advantageous with sensitive early detection, high selectivity, accurate, rapid, and low LOD. To improve the sensitivity and selectivity of biosensors, a variety of green signal amplification strategies have been studied, such as the use of metal/metal oxide nanoparticles (NPs), graphene/graphene oxide (GO), carbon nanotubes (CNTs), fullerenes, and biopolymers. Depending on the synergistic effects of targeted analytes and bio-nanostructures used, different electrochemical biosensors can be examined using different detection measurement strategies such as potentiometric, amperometric, conductometric, voltammetric, and colorimetric change. These bio-based electrochemical sensors have been shown very low LODs for targeted biomarkers and molecules such as drugs, dyes, toxic substances, pathogens, viruses, heavy metals, DNA, RNA, pesticides, antibodies, small molecules, cancer cells, and human proteins over a wide concentration range. However, electrochemical biosensors must have still specific limitations such as industrial production, the integration of a biosensor's components and deficiency of multi-step strategies, insufficient clinical trial data, an insufficient number of experts on nanotechnology applications.

To overcome these issues, several scientists and researchers have studied the preparation and experimental research of advanced electrochemical biosensors and nanobiosensors with high affinity targeted molecules, high-performance electrodes, and efficient signal transferring in recent studies. Among several types of nanostructures used in the modification of the surface of electrodes, Zheng et al. in 2021 produced a novel effective peptide–antibody sandwich electrochemical biosensor using metallic AuPt nanoparticle and manganese dioxide (MnO_2) – functionalized covalent organic frameworks (AuPt@MnO_2@COF) for the detection of prostate-specific antigen (PSA). The biosensing mechanism was based on the redox signal of methylene blue (MB) and experimental parameters were calculated with a linear response (0.00005–10 ng/mL) and a low LOD of 16.7 fg/mL in the presence of the PSA [18]. In the past decades, Xies et al. [19] developed a novel multi-residue electrochemical biosensor based on a composite of graphene/ chitosan/parathion, which supported the sensitivity of working electrodes for organo-phosphorus pesticides. The detection of organophosphorus pesticides had a linear range from 1 to 1500 ng/mL with low LODs of 0.012–0.23 ng/mL in the presence of different organophosphorus. Furthermore, the proposed biosensor was examined for the detection of chlorpyrifos and dichlorvos in real food samples (apple samples), and the recovery rate of the proposed biosensor was found to be 87.24%–110.20%.

While the COVID-19 pandemic threatens human and animal health, the progress of the detection of coronavirus disease (COVID-19) using green and sensitive methodologies are vital issues for medical diagnosis at an early stage. In 2021, Tran et al. [20] did a literature review about conducting polymer and COVID-19 virus and discussed a critical issue of green strategies for the detection of COVID-19 using polymer-based biosensors. This green detection method reflects the use of green methods to improve the bio-based surface properties and affect the development of the affinity-based surface modification strategy of the electrochemical biosensor under physiological conditions as well. To understand the detection mechanism of COVID-19 electrochemical biosensors, the scientists focused on the interactions of the virus, antigen, viral RNA, and antibody [20]. Bio-organic/compatible transistors are one of the most emerging technologies for the medical diagnosis of cancer and COVID-19 at an early stage with clinical advantages. For this purpose, Tian et al. fabricated a novel electrochemical enzymatic biosensor using metal-organic frameworks MIL-53 – Au@Pt nanoparticles for the detection of SARS-CoV-2 nucleocapsid protein (2019-nCoV-NP) using horseradish peroxidase (HRP) and hemin/ G-quadruplex DNAzyme [21].

10.3 Organic Transistors or Biosensors for Cancer Detection

Cancer is a disease that has a terrifying sound to all human beings. In definition, it might be new for us regarding the recent decades; however, findings are showing that it has been among us for millions of years. Throughout the history of humanity, there are major causes of death to balance the population. Unlike infectious diseases, parasites, and environmental diseases, cancer is not an organism causing the disease, but the tumor cell itself as a part of the body creating the disease. There are over 11 million people who are diagnosed with some kind of cancer every year, and it is expected to increase every year. Since it is a serious health issue of human beings, understanding the nature of the disease, assessing the risks, prevention, and early diagnosis take an important place for scientists who are focusing on this specific subject [22].

A tumor by definition is an abnormal growth of cells where they have no functional purpose and spread to other parts of the body; however, when it becomes cancerous, the cells become different than the organ or the body part they locate which is called un-differentiation showing the aggressiveness of the tumor cells. The morphological and functional resemblance of the tumor to the cell that it is originated is called differentiation. Tumor with benign character is usually well differentiated and resemble the cells that are originated. Endocrine cancer cell synthesizing hormone, squamous cell cancers synthesizing keratin, and bile synthesis by hepatocellular carcinoma are several samples of good differentiation [23].

Loss of differentiation is called anaplasia, and the tumors originating from these cells are called anaplastic tumors. Morphological findings belong to anaplastic tumors: pleomorphism (tumor cells, nucleus, and shapes, dying parameters are different), anomalies in nucleus morphologies (increase in active RNA synthesis), increase in mitosis frequency, and loss of polarity and orientation. Irregular proliferation in epithelial cells characterized with pleomorphism, hyperchromasia, nucleomegaly, abnormal mitosis, is called dysplasia. Dysplasia is usually formed on a metaplasia basis and could disappear if the predisposing factor is removed, and in case it is not affecting all the epithet layers. If it is affecting all layers of the epithelium without basal membrane invasion, it is named grade 3 dysplasia or in situ carcinoma. Whenever the basal membrane invasion is seen, it is called invasive carcinoma [23].

There are roles of inheritance as well as environmental factors in the basis of tumorigenesis. The role of inheritance is well known for several tumors. Cancers with genetic predispositions usually appear at younger ages, with multi-centric retention, and bilateral foci with worse prognoses.

Geographical conditions are blamed for some types of cancer etiologies such as gastric carcinoma, seen more in Japan, whereas Burkitt lymphoma is mostly diagnosed in Africa [24]. Besides geographical factors, chronic alcohol use and smoking increase some types of cancers in particular. There are also occupational carcinogens such as asbestosis, arsenic, benzene, beryllium, cadmium, and vinyl chloride that are causing cancer in the patients who have regular exposure due to their working conditions [23].

Early diagnosis is sometimes lifesaving for several cancers. Therefore, screening strategies come along with these purposes. Some screening tests are designed for all the population, whereas some are specified for the increased risk group. Colorectal cancer, cervical cancer, and mammary cancer are the cancer types with screening protocols for all the population. Patients applying to physicians receive a physical examination at first. The most important finding would be lymphadenopathies. Besides lumps, symptoms such as major weight loss, tiredness, or night sweats could be a clue, and changes in skin color and palpable organs may also give an idea for further investigations.

Laboratory experimental results such as urine and blood analysis may give an idea about the causes of the symptoms. Sometimes, specific tumor markers might be requested due to the suspicion of the physician according to the performed physical examination. Calcitonin, catecholamine, and human chorionic gonadotropin are hormones that may be used as tumor markers in medullary thyroid cancer, pheochromocytoma, related tumors, and trophoblastic tumors, respectively. Carsino-embryogenic antigen and alpha feta protein are oncofetal antigens that are also used as tumor markers on colon, pancreas, gastric, lung carcinoma, and hepatocellular carcinoma, respectively [25]. Another tool that is used for the diagnosis is imaging tests, such as computerized tomography, positron emission tomography scan, bone scan, magnetic resonance imaging (MRI), and ultrasound. For the treatment of diagnosed cancer, if there is a presence of a solid tumor, surgery may come up as an option of treatment to decompress the organs near the tumor. Chemotherapy and radiation therapy are the other options of treatment according to the tumor's sensitivity to those treatment modalities. In some cases, before the planned tumor surgery, chemotherapy may be used to decrease the tumor burden before the surgery, which is called neoadjuvant chemotherapy. Immunotherapy is another method of cancer therapy that makes the patient's cells fight the cancer cells. In immunotherapy, monoclonal antibodies are very popular by blocking the specific protein functions on the cancer cells causes the immune system to recognize the diseased cells easier. Throughout the developments in technology, new cancer therapy modalities emerged with the increased knowledge of tumor biology, and the underlying patho-physiology [25].

Sensors of nanotechnology enable an increase in the detection of sensitivity, specificity, and capability rates in chemical and biological ways in a variety of areas. The biosensor, specifically, as a feature of nanotechnology, is used to detect a biological substance that has an environmental or biological origin. Proteins, nucleic acids, or any other biological or metabolic components can be analyzed by biosensors. There is a variety of application areas of biosensors in medicine. Detection of microbes in the air or food and monitoring blood glucose levels are examples of the use of biosensor technology in the field of medicine.

As mentioned earlier in the chapter, one of the traditional ways to diagnose cancer is to measure the levels of tumor markers in the peripheric blood. In the field of cancer, bio-sensors are used to detect specific proteins that are secreted by cancer cells. Since there might be multiple tumor markers specific to certain cancer, biosensors are specialized in detecting more than one substance at once, which helps save time for the diagnosis. As biosensors can measure the protein expression in tumor cells and can differentiate the healthy cells from the cancerous cells by the expressed protein levels, it is possible to state whether the tumor cells are present or not. It is even possible to declare whether the tumor cell has benign properties or has a malignant structure by the levels of expressed proteins. Biosensor technology can also have the feature to determine if the treatment that the patient is going to receive will be effective on the tumor or not [26].

Simply, a biosensor consists of a recognition element, a signal transducer, and a signal processor that interpret the results. Receptor recognition elements are for drugs and are used to follow up the response to the cancer therapeutics. As the second component of the biosensors, the "biosensor transducer" is to interpret the knowledge obtained into a digital signal [26].

Nanotechnology is an emerging technology in the field of medicine, and has an im-portant role in biosensors, by this way of monitoring the diseases, prognosis, and diag-nosis of cancer. Since cancer is a life-threatening disease as the reason for deaths all over the world in the second place, there is a high interest in this field to reduce the numbers. Because cancer is usually a disease diagnosed at the late stages, there is a huge demand for detecting it in earlier phases which could make it easier to manipulate the disease and the prognosis. In future practice, there is a lot of space in the field to fill out related to biomarkers and biosensors. There is a great need for biosensors to detect more than one tumor marker and have them be more precise to catch the tumor cells in the early onset [27]. However, the most important part to achieve this technology is to understand the underlying pathophysiology and the progression strategy of cancer.

10.4 The Mechanism of Green Organic Transistors/Biosensors in the Cancer Therapy

Recently, the fabrication and evaluation of high-performance and sustainable bio-devices for the detection and measurement of bio-sourced organic materials have received great attention. The basic principle of the mechanism of green organic transistors/biosensors in cancer applications is based on the chemical changes due to the electric and optical

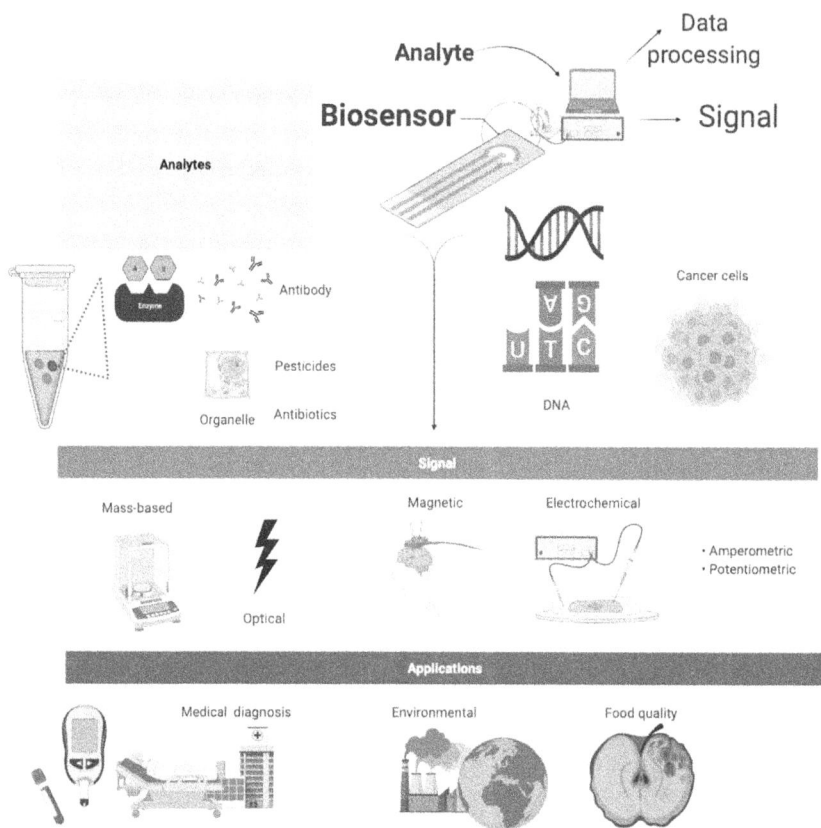

FIGURE 10.2
Schematic diagrams of classification and application of biosensors.

signals with biomarker sensing strategies. Chemical changes are the measurement of optical and electrical properties such as electron, charge, energy, mass, and signal using different techniques such as fluorescence spectroscopy, UV–visible spectroscopy, and cyclic voltammetric due to different kinds of noncovalent interactions. In Figure 10.2, schematic diagrams of the classification and application of biosensors were given.

In literature, it is reported that the basic principle of biosensing of cancer biomarkers is related to the chemical and structural changes in the chemical signal transduction using their spectral results. These observed electronic, structural, and chemical changes in signals show the efficiency of the biosensor on the determination of the biochemical events for electron and energy transfers from orbitals. The chemical interactions between biosensors and target analytes can result in chemical interaction owing to the electro-active sites in the medium and dual electrochemical signal outputs. Especially, the cancer biomarkers have a major role in the electrochemical signal changes between the active surface of the sensor and target analyte by the electron transfer process in the electro-chemical redox mechanism for rapid and early medical diagnostics. Furthermore, as it is known, different factors such as affinity, adsorption process, covalent bonding, and cross-linking are significant for the development of the biosensor by an effective immobiliza-tion method.

Several studies have been reported on green biosensors for early-stage cancer diagnostics in sensor technology. Bondancia et al. developed a high-performance bacterial nanocellulose-based biosensor for the immunosensing of the p53 cancer biomarker in concentration range from 0.01 to 1,000 Ucell. mL ^{1} with a low LOD of 0.16 Ucell mL ^{1} [28]. Pothipor et al. fabricated a novel Au NPs-dye/poly(3-aminobenzylamine)/two-dimensional (2D) MoSe2/graphene oxide (GO)–based electrochemical biosensor for the cancer antigen 15-3 and microRNA-21 detection [29]. Results showed that the proposed biosensor exhibited a good linear response with low LOD values of 0.14 U mL 1 for CA 15-3 and 1.2 fM for miRNA-21 for point-of-care medical diagnostic applications [29]. Giang et al. highlighted the performance of the visible and pyrophosphates (PPi) responsive TiO_2/Cu^{2+}-carbon dots-based biosensor for wireless electrochemical cancer detection [30]. Chen et al. investigated the electrochemical performance of the polydopamine-Au composite-based biosensor for the detection of the pancreatic cancer-associated microRNA in human biological fluids with a low LOD of 0.26 pM [31]. The mechanism electrochemical of the proposed biosensor was based on the single polymerase-boosted dual amplification reaction of DNA [31]. Esmaeili et al. developed a novel mesoporous silica@chitosan@Au NPs-based "on/off" optical biosensor for the targeted cancer imaging with remarkable ability in the stable structure with the target analyte. The mechanism was based on the electrostatic interactions between silanol groups of the nanostructure and positively charged membrane of cancer cells [32]. Javar et al. fabricated a novel electrochemical DNA biosensor using Eu^{3+}-doped NiO for the detection of the anti-cancer drug (amsacrine) [24]. Electrochemical measurements proved that the prepared electrochemical DNA biosensor had significant potential for cancer detection in a wide concentration range from 0.1 μM to 100.0 μM with a low LOD of 0.05 μM due to the intercalations of amsacrine with ds-DNA. In another study, Amethiya et al. reported the evaluation of the performance of different biosensors such as a field-effect transistor (FET), electrochemical, and sandwich electrochemical for the determination of different types of target analytes such as cancer biomarkers, DNA, cancer cells, and biological fluids. In addition, they focused on the ability to characterize the tumor size using different types of machine learning algorithms in sensor applications [33].

10.5 Biosensors in Canine Mammary Tumors

Mammary tumors are neoplasms frequently encountered in female dogs. Mammary tumors are the most common type of neoplasm in female dogs. The malignancy prevalence differs from 26–73% [34,35]. The primary and the most cost-effective treatment choice is mastectomy, but the overall survival rate after surgery is low due to local recurrence and early metastasis. Therefore, there is a need in veterinary medicine for following up on the tumor development and treatment consequences [34,35]. Since canine mammary tissue and human mammary tissue are mostly similar, biomarkers used for diagnosis, treatment options, and determination of prognosis are common. Tumor markers are products of normal cell metabolism and their production increases due to malignant transformation [36]. These; are biomarkers that play a role in intracellular adhesion, such as integrins, selectins, immunoglobulin-like particles, cadherins, cancer antigen 15-3 (CA 15-3), and carcinoembryonic antigen (CEA) [37]. These indicators reflect the malignancy and are characterized by substances found in the tumor, blood, or other body fluids that are primarily produced by the tumor or secondary in response to the presence of the tumor [38]. These biomarkers can be produced by cancer cells and they can be distinguished in tumoral tissues or biological fluids (serum, blood, urine, stool, plasma, and sputum). The use of potential biomarkers in canine mammary tumors can lead to early diagnosis, tumor grading, prognosis, and monitoring of response to treatment. Biosensors are known analytical bio-based devices which can recognize the target bio-origin integrated [39]. The biological action creates measurable changes in a medium, and the transducer transforms them into measurable electrical signals. Biosensor applications are portable, miniaturized, and more effective than analytical techniques such as immunohistochemistry or enzyme-linked immunosorbent assay (ELISA). Biosensor recognition parameters are enzymes, immunogenetics, DNA, RNA, small biomolecules, and cells. The transmission method consists of several strategies, including

a. Electrochemical
b. Optical
   i. Noble metal NPs-based platforms
   ii. Magnetic NPs-based platforms
   iii. Antibody immobilization on NPs
c. Mass measurement to detect the circulating tumor cells [40].

Generally, biosensors are medical devices that can be used outside of the hospital setting and tend to be portable, easy to assemble, flexible, rapid, and low cost. Biosensors can be identified due to their mechanism that presents biological specificity or the method of physicochemical signal transmission. According to signal transmission, biosensors can be classified as electrochemical, mass change, or optical. Electrochemical sensors are the devices that support the early detection of different public health problems [41].

Nanotechnology is a technology that incorporates innovative products that involve the exchange of matter at the atomic and molecular levels. Nanomedicine is used in nanotechnology in medical applications, diagnosis, treatment, and prevention of cancer, cardiovascular and infectious diseases. The excellent properties of nanomaterials are small size, unique morphology, uniform dispersion, large surface area, convenient functionalization, biocompatibility, preferential deposition in cancer cells, ability to bind functional portions, and reactivity. They are materials with superior abilities such as overcoming biological barriers and reaching certain tissues and cells [42]. Metal (Au, Cu, Fe, Pt, Pd, Ag, Zn, and Ni) NPs can distinguish unique features in terms of magnetic, electrochemical, optical, and electrical activities in biomedical applications such as drug/gene delivery systems, cell imaging, biosensing, and cancer monitoring.

Recently, NPs are very important for their effects in cancer therapy. In recent studies, Fe, Ni, and Co NPs have been preferred in medical biotechnology. The rising of nanotechnology in the last 20 years has opened up research horizons in the field of nanomedicine. In recent years, researchers have been discussing the prospects and challenges of electrochemical biosensors for next-generation cancer diagnosis. Combining electrochemical devices with nanoscale materials results in simultaneous measurement for multiple cancer markers. Advanced properties of electrochemical devices with a nanoapproach infrastructure are extremely valuable for increasing the effectiveness of cancer diagnosis and treatment monitoring [43]. There are several kinds of biomarkers developed to monitor breast cancer. Pacheco et al. reported an electrochemical (voltammetric) sensor for the determination of to diagnose breast cancer by direct surface imprinting of biomarker (CA 15-3) using a screen-printed gold electrode [41]. In another study, Chang et al. reported a gold/zinc oxide thin film–based biosensor to detect the CA 15-3 for breast cancer with high sensitivity [44]. Various aptasensors are used for the detection of circulating cancer cell evaluations. Electrochemical sensors can detect the current or potential changes caused by interactions at the transducer interface. Mass exchange transducers also offer options to bind and analyze cell movement as a label-free technology. This time provides a high detection speed and sensitivity with real-time results.

Fluorescence, interferometry, and spectroscopy of optical waveguides and surface plasmon resonance (SPR) are optical transducers. Some devices use fluorescent tags for detection, fluorescent reporters convert the detection of a specific biological parameter into an observable fluorescent signal. Ghosh et al. developed a novel biosensor that had a biomarker-specific layer on a transducer due to the biorecognition elements with a chemical signal [45]. It is transformed into a measurable output for further analysis of cancer diagnosis. Within the various biological recognition elements, antibodies (Abs) are very important because of their three-dimensional adhesion property. They are particularly demanding for cancer diagnosis. However, conventional biosensors cause errors at low biomarker concentrations in the early stage of cancer.

10.6 Biosensors Used in Canine Mammary Tumors

The lack of work on the use of biotransistors at the earlier stage detection of canine mammary tumors remains a mystery about their success in this area. In this respect, the importance of biosensors, which have been used in the early diagnosis of canine mammary tumors in recent years, is gradually increasing. There is limited information on this topic. A study carried out in this field by Jena et al. reported the SPR immunosensor for the determination of the Baculoviral inhibitor of apoptosis repeat containing-5 (BIRC5) protein biomarker in dog sera suffering from mammary tumors [46]. They reported that this immune-sensor can be used as a sensitive device for the BIRC5 in the diagnosis of Charcot-Marie tooth disease (CMT).

10.7 Conclusion and Future Perspectives

The development and advantages of several modern biocompatible and biodegradable organic transistors-based applications remarkably reflect in the detection of biomarker or molecule profiles and their identification-induced modifications in biomedical applications. Rapid, ultrasensitive, selective, flexible, wearable, and low-cost bio-based strategies are significantly accelerated for enzymatic/non-enzymatic electrochemical studies for personal biological data and food detection. Mostly *in-vitro* and *in-vivo* experimental results proved to be successful fully printed OTFTs, high-performance flexible electronics, biosensors, and so on which led to the scientific discovery of new bio-based nanosystems. Experimental results, especially, showed that the green approach of disposable and portable biosensors has the potential in the early-stage cancer diagnosis in medicine.

Further studies are needed to prove the success of biocompatible and biodegradable organic transistors-based sensors in early diagnosis for canine mammary tumors, especially with the biosensors which use cancer biomarkers in both serum and tissue samples.

References

1. D. Lai, E. Li, Y. Yan, Y. Liu, J. Zhong, D. Lv, Y. Ke, H. Chen, T. Guo, Gelatin-hydrogel based organic synaptic transistor, *Organic Electronics*. 75 (2019) 105409.
2. C. Rullyani, M. Ramesh, C.F. Sung, H.C. Lin, C.W. Chu, Natural polymers for disposable organic thin film transistors, *Organic Electronics*. 54 (2018) 154–160.
3. W. Ji, D. Wu, W. Tang, X. Xi, Y. Su, X. Guo, R. Liu, Carbonized silk fabric-based flexible organic electrochemical transistors for highly sensitive and selective dopamine detection, *Sensors and Actuators B: Chemical*. 304 (2020) 127414.
4. H.B. Lee, M. Meeseepong, T.Q. Trung, B.Y. Kim, N.E. Lee, A wearable lab-on-a-patch platform with stretchable nanostructured biosensor for non-invasive immunodetection of biomarker in sweat, *Biosensors and Bioelectronics*. 156 (2020) 112133.
5. R. Wang, Q. Zhai, T. An, S. Gong, W. Cheng, Stretchable gold fiber-based wearable textile electrochemical biosensor for lactate monitoring in sweat, *Talanta*. 222 (2021) 121484.
6. S.A. Hashemi, S.M. Mousavi, S. Bahrani, A. Gholami, W.-H. Chiang, K. Yousefi, N. Omidifar, N.V. Rao, S. Ramakrishna, A. Babapoor, C.W. Lai, Bio-enhanced polyrhodanine/graphene oxide/Fe3O4 nanocomposite with kombucha solvent supernatant as ultra-sensitive biosensor for detection of doxorubicin hydrochloride in biological fluids, *Materials Chemistry and Physics*. 279 (2022) 125743.
7. H. Matsui, Y. Takeda, S. Tokito, Flexible and printed organic transistors: From materials to integrated circuits, *Organic Electronics*. 75 (2019) 105432.
8. A.F. Paterson, N.D. Treat, W. Zhang, Z. Fei, G. Wyatt-Moon, H. Faber, G. Vourlias, P.A. Patsalas, O. Solomeshch, N. Tessler, M. Heeney, T.D. Anthopoulos, Small molecule/polymer blend organic transistors with hole mobility exceeding 13 cm^2 V 1 s 1, *Advanced Materials*. 28 (2016) 7791–7798.
9. P. Mittal, S. Yadav, S. Negi, Advancements for organic thin film transistors: Structures, materials, performance parameters, influencing factors, models, fabrication, reliability and applications, *Materials Science in Semiconductor Processing*. 133 (2021) 105975.
10. S. Singh, H. Matsui, S. Tokito, Flexible high-performance organic thin film transistors and PMOS inverters: Trap controlled grain boundaries and contact resistance effect in different channel length devices, *Synthetic Metals*. 278 (2021) 116808.
11. T. Shen, H. Zhou, J. Xin, Q. Fan, Z. Yang, J. Wang, T. Mei, X. Wang, N. Wang, J. Li, Controllable microstructure of polymer-small molecule blend thin films for high-performance organic field-effect transistors, *Applied Surface Science*. 498 (2019) 143822.
12. K. Zekentes, J. Choi, V. Stambouli, E. Bano, O. Karker, K. Rogdakis, Progress in SiC nanowire field-effect-transistors for integrated circuits and sensing applications, *Microelectronic Engineering*. 255 (2022) 111704.
13. L.H. Chou, Y. Na, C.H. Park, M.S. Park, I. Osaka, F.S. Kim, C.L. Liu, Semiconducting small molecule/polymer blends for organic transistors, *Polymer*. 191 (2020) 122208.
14. J. Fan, C. Montemagno, M. Gupta, 3D printed high transconductance organic electrochemical transistors on flexible substrates, *Organic Electronics*. 73 (2019) 122–129.
15. D. Majak, J. Fan, M. Gupta, Fully 3D printed OECT based logic gate for detection of cation type and concentration, *Sensors and Actuators B: Chemical*. 286 (2019) 111–118.

16. S. Damiati, S. Küpcü, M. Peacock, C. Eilenberger, M. Zamzami, I. Qadri, H. Choudhry, U.B. Sleytr, B. Schuster, Acoustic and hybrid 3D-printed electrochemical biosensors for the real-time immunodetection of liver cancer cells (HepG2), *Biosensors and Bioelectronics*. 94 (2017) 500–506.

17. L. Zhang, G. Wang, D. Wu, C. Xiong, L. Zheng, Y. Ding, H. Lu, G. Zhang, L. Qiu, Highly selective and sensitive sensor based on an organic electrochemical transistor for the detection of ascorbic acid, *Biosensors and Bioelectronics*. 100 (2018) 235–241.

18. J. Zheng, H. Zhao, G. Ning, W. Sun, L. Wang, H. Liang, H. Xu, C. He, C.P. Li, A novel affinity peptide–antibody sandwich electrochemical biosensor for PSA based on the signal amplification of MnO2-functionalized covalent organic framework, *Talanta*. 233 (2021) 122520.

19. X. Xie, B. Zhou, Y. Zhang, G. Zhao, B. Zhao, A multi-residue electrochemical biosensor based on graphene/chitosan/parathion for sensitive organophosphorus pesticides detection, *Chemical Physics Letters*. 767 (2021) 138355.

20. V. van Tran, N.H.T. Tran, H.S. Hwang, M. Chang, Development strategies of conducting polymer-based electrochemical biosensors for virus biomarkers: Potential for rapid COVID-19 detection, *Biosensors and Bioelectronics*. 182 (2021) 113192.

21. J. Tian, Z. Liang, O. Hu, Q. He, D. Sun, Z. Chen, An electrochemical dual-aptamer biosensor based on metal-organic frameworks MIL-53 decorated with au@Pt nanoparticles and enzymes for detection of COVID-19 nucleocapsid protein, *Electrochimica Acta*. 387 (2021) 138553.

22. D.M. Hausman, What is cancer?, *Perspectives in Biology and Medicine*. 62 (2019) 778–784.

23. E. Dzeng, Book review for "Values at the end of life: The logic of palliative care," *American Journal of Sociology*. 4 (2019) 163–165.

24. H. Akbari Javar, Z. Garkani-Nejad, G. Dehghannoudeh, H. Mahmoudi-Moghaddam, Development of a new electrochemical DNA biosensor based on Eu3+ doped NiO for determination of amsacrine as an anti-cancer drug: Electrochemical, spectroscopic and docking studies, *Analytica Chimica Acta*. 1133 (2020) 48–57.

25. Tumor microenvironment: Recent advances in various cancer treatments, (n.d.). https://www.europeanreview.org/article/15270 (accessed January 20, 2022).

26. B. Bohunicky, S.A. Mousa, Biosensors: The new wave in cancer diagnosis, *Nanotechnology, Science and Applications*. 4 (2011) 1.

27. V.S.P.K.S.A. Jayanthi, A.B. Das, U. Saxena, Recent advances in biosensor development for the detection of cancer biomarkers, *Biosensors and Bioelectronics*. 91 (2017) 15–23.

28. T.J. Bondancia, A.C. Soares, M. Popolin-Neto, N.O. Gomes, P.A. Raymundo-Pereira, H.S. Barud, S.A.S. Machado, S.J.L. Ribeiro, M.E. Melendez, A.L. Carvalho, R.M. Reis, F.V. Paulovich, O.N. Oliveira, Low-cost bacterial nanocellulose-based interdigitated biosensor to detect the p53 cancer biomarker, *Materials Science and Engineering: C*. 134 (2022) 112676.

29. C. Pothipor, S. Bamrungsap, J. Jakmunee, K. Ounnunkad, A gold nanoparticle-dye/poly (3-aminobenzylamine)/two dimensional MoSe2/graphene oxide electrode towards label-free electrochemical biosensor for simultaneous dual-mode detection of cancer antigen 15–3 and microRNA-21, *Colloids and Surfaces B: Biointerfaces*. 210 (2022) 112260.

30. N.N. Giang, H.J. Won, G. Lee, S.Y. Park, Cancer cells targeted visible light and alkaline Phosphatase-responsive TiO^2/Cu^2+ carbon dots-Coated wireless electrochemical biosensor, *Chemical Engineering Journal*. 417 (2021) 129196.

31. S.-C. Chen, K.T. Chen, A.F.-J. Jou, Polydopamine-gold composite-based electrochemical biosensor using dual-amplification strategy for detecting pancreatic cancer-associated microRNA, *Biosensors and Bioelectronics*. 173 (2021) 112815.

32. Y. Esmaeili, M. Khavani, A. Bigham, A. Sanati, E. Bidram, L. Shariati, A. Zarrabi, N.A. Jolfaie, M. Rafienia, Mesoporous silica@chitosan@gold nanoparticles as "on/off" optical biosensor and pH-sensitive theranostic platform against cancer, *International Journal of Biological Macromolecules*. 202 (2022) 241–255.

33. Y. Amethiya, P. Pipariya, S. Patel, M. Shah, Comparative analysis of breast cancer detection using machine learning and biosensors, *Intelligent Medicine*. 2 (2021) 69–81.

34. L.C. Campos, G.E. Lavalle, A. Estrela-Lima, J.C. Melgaço de Faria, J.E. Guimarães, Á.P. Dutra, E. Ferreira, L.P. de Sousa, É.M.L. Rabelo, A.F.D. Vieira da Costa, G.D. Cassali, CA15.3, CEA and LDH in dogs with malignant mammary tumors, *Journal of Veterinary Internal Medicine*. 26 (2012) 1383–1388.

35. J.E. Moulton, D.O.N. Taylor, C.R. Dorn, A.C. Andersen, Canine mammary tumors, *Veterinary Pathology*. 7 (1970) 289–320.

36. A.L.A. Eisenberg, S. Koifman, Câncer de mama: Marcadores Tumorais (Revisão de Literatura), *Revista Brasileira de Cancerologia*. 47 (2001) 377–388.

37. I. Kaszak, A. Ruszczak, S. Kanafa, K. Kacprzak, M. Król, P. Jurka, Current biomarkers of canine mammary tumors, *Acta Veterinaria Scandinavica*. 60: 1 (2018) 1–13.

38. E.L. Jacobs, C.M. Haskell, Clinical use of tumor markers in oncology, *Current Problems in Cancer*. 15 (1991) 301–350.

39. A. Farooq, K.A. Bhat, R.A. Mir, R. Mahajan, M. Nazir, V. Sharma, S.M. Zargar, Emerging trends in developing biosensor techniques to undertake plant phosphoproteomic analysis, *Journal of Proteomics*. 253 (2022) 104458.

40. G. Ghosh, Early detection of cancer: Focus on antibody coated metal and magnetic nanoparticle-based biosensors, *Sensors International*. 1 (2020) 100050.

41. J.P.G. Pacheco, M.S.V. Silva, M. Freitas, H.P.A. Nouws, C. Delerue-Matos, Molecularly imprinted electrochemical sensor for the point-of-care detection of a breast cancer biomarker (CA 15-3), *Sensors and Actuators B: Chemical*. 256 (2018) 905–912.

42. S. Jain, J.A. Coulter, K.T. Butterworth, A.R. Hounsell, S.J. McMahon, W.B. Hyland, M.F. Muir, G.R. Dickson, K.M. Prise, F.J. Currell, D.G. Hirst, J.M. O'Sullivan, Gold nanoparticle cellular uptake, toxicity and radiosensitisation in hypoxic conditions, *Radiotherapy and Oncology*. 110 (2014) 342–347.

43. J. Wang, Electrochemical biosensors: Towards point-of-care cancer diagnostics, *Biosensors and Bioelectronics*. 21 (2006) 1887–1892.

44. C.C. Chang, N.F. Chiu, D.S. Lin, Y. Chu-Su, Y.H. Liang, C.W. Lin, High-sensitivity detection of carbohydrate antigen 15-3 using a gold/zinc oxide thin film surface plasmon resonance-based biosensor, *Analytical Chemistry*. 82 (2010) 1207–1212.

45. G. Ghosh, Early detection of cancer: Focus on antibody coated metal and magnetic nanoparticle-based biosensors, *Sensors International*. 1 (2020) 100050.

46. S. Chandra Jena, S. Shrivastava, S. Saxena, N. Kumar, S. Kumar Maiti, B. Prasad Mishra, R. Kumar Singh, Surface plasmon resonance immunosensor for label-free detection of BIRC5 biomarker in spontaneously occurring canine mammary tumours, (n.d.). 10.1038/s41598-019-49998-x.

11

Microbial Nanowires

Ahmed Marroki

Department of Biology, Faculty of Natural and Life Sciences, University Djillali Liabes, Sidi Bel Abbès, Algeria

Laboratory of Molecular Biology and Microbial Genetic, Faculty of Natural and Life Sciences, University Oran1, Oran, Algeria

Leila Bousmaha-Marroki

Department of Biology, Faculty of Natural and Life Sciences, University Djillali Liabes, Sidi Bel Abbès, Algeria

Laboratory of Research in Environment and Health, Faculty of Medicine, University Djillali Liabes, Sidi Bel Abbès, Algeria

CONTENTS

DOI: 10.1201/9781003263265-11

11.1 Introduction

The concept of bioelectronics, proposed in 1968, means the combination between the biological system and the field of electronics. This field focuses on the different mechanisms of electron transfer in a biological system and their potential applications. However, bioelectronics, according to pioneer Göpel, aimed at the direct combination between biomolecular and electronic structures [1]. This concept is defined by the International Union of Pure and Applied Chemistry (IUPAC) as the application of biomolecular principles to microelectronics [2]. Recently, with the discovery of electrically conductive bacterial structures, termed *microbial nanowires*, new fields had emerged in bioelectronics. The bacterial nanowires structure is an extracellular appendage that has been serving as a strategy for electron transport in diverse microbes. Generally, two mechanisms can be implicated in microbes electrochemically direct and mediated electron transfer. In direct electron transfer (DET), the electron transfers between microorganisms and solid acceptors implicate on bacteria cell membrane's contact. The DET may also involve insoluble Fe (III) or an anode of microbial bioelectrochemical systems (BES). This type was first discovered and described in *Geobacter* species which are effective in the bioremediation of subsurface contaminants [3]. Recently, several studies demonstrated the electron transport along bacterial nanowires. This discovery has been observed in some *Geobacter*, *Shewanella*, and *Cyanobacterium* species [4]. The electronically conducting structure termed nanowires permits these bacteria to reach the solid electron acceptors without cell contact. The second mechanism is called mediated electron transfer (MET). The MET is facilitated by using artificial mediator compounds or by a biocatalyst and classified according to the origin and redox species. For growth, the bacteria can generate energy by using diverse strategies. The nanowires represent nano-objects produced by microbes that enable the transfer of electrons to extracellular electron acceptors. The electron transfered through the nanowires permit possibilities for cell-cell and cell-surface interaction. Through that, their potential applications in bioremediation, bioengineering, and bioelectronics have been demonstrated. In this chapter, we describe different non-flagella proteinaceous appendages such as Chaperone-Usher pili (CU pili), curli pili, and type 3 and 4 secretion system pili (T3SS and T4SSs). The diverse types of extracellular electron transfer exhibited by microbial cells were presented. A brief taxonomy, principal characteristics, and even the pili type 4 assemblage of the two types of species implicated in electron transfer via nanowires *Geobacter* and *Shewanella* were detailed. We also discuss important aspects of microbial nanowires (MNWs) including their types, roles, and mechanisms of electron transfer in *Geobacter* and *Shewanella* species. Along with that, the potential applications of both bacteria in the field of bioremediation, bioelectricity, and energy production are also reviewed.

11.2 Microbial Pilus: From Fimbriae to Nanowires

The term "pili" (Latin for *hair*), first identified by Duguid et al. [5], were non-flagellar proteinaceous appendages that occur among Gram-negative bacteria. The pili have been mostly referred to as "filaments," "bristles," "fimbriae," or "pili" by Ottow [6]. The pili, introduced in 1959 [7], were distinguished mainly based on morphology, which can be described as two distinct phases in bacteria: piliated and non-piliated. However, the term "fimbriae" was introduced in 1975, by Ottow [6]. They are filamentous surface structures of many different Gram-negative bacteria. In 1968, the pili were detected and described by Yanagawa et al. [8] on the surface of a *Corynebacterium renale* Gram-positive bacteria by using electron microscopy. These structures were employed by the bacteria for several functions such as attachment, biofilm formation, motility, and DNA transport through bacteria membranes. Bacterial pili are characterized by their uniform diameter, straightness, and fragility. Also, they can be removed by mechanical agitation in a high-speed mixer [7]. On the basis of their biosynthetic pathways, different pilus classes are characterized and described based on the assembly pathways in Gram-negative bacteria (Figure 11.1) [9]. The pili have been employed in many functions and used for attachment in host cells, a biofilm, or for the formation of an extracellular matrix. Along with that, it can function as nanowires or as a support structure for the secretion of proteins and nucleic acids.

11.2.1 Chaperone-Usher (CU) Pili

The Chaperone-Usher (CU) pili are ubiquitous appendages mainly found in Gram-negative bacteria [10]. The CU pili are typically 1–2 µm in length fibers composed with the pilin subunits arranged in a helical fashion, consisting of pilus subunits (pilins). The CU pili play a crucial role in the infection and virulence, often constituting an important factor in attachment and adhesion to host tissues. The genes involved in the assembly of pili belong to the chaperone/usher biosynthesis clustered into operons. These operons encoded can be classified into three different proteins: a major structural pili subunit,

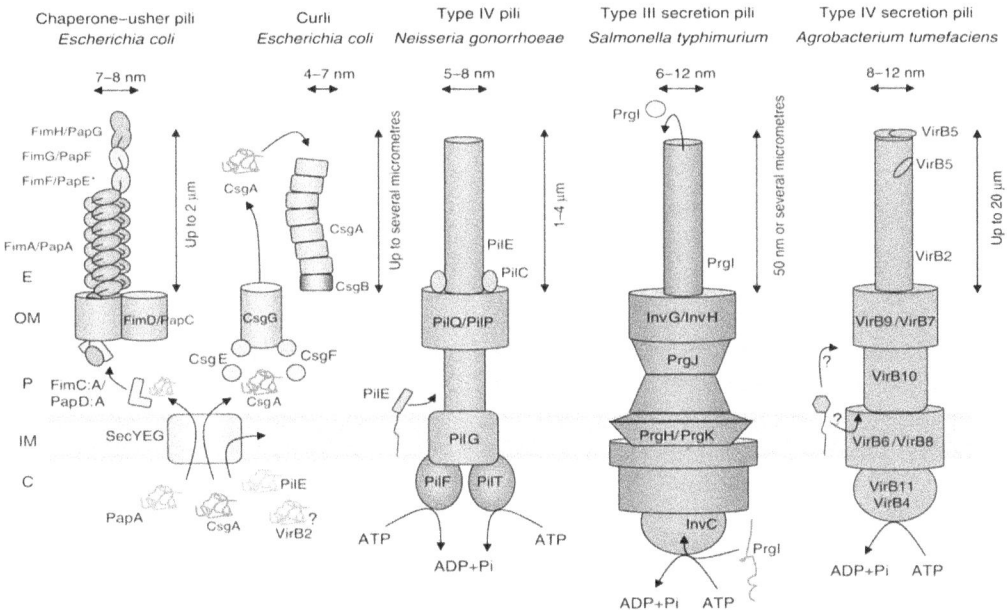

FIGURE 11.1
Schematic of different pili and biosynthesis pathways in Gram-negative. Reprinted with permission [9]. Copyright © 2008 European Molecular Biology Organization, With permission from Wiley and Sons. The article is available under the Creative Commons CC-BY-NC-ND license.

usher, and chaperone protein [11]. However, the CU pili biosynthetic pathway at the outer membrane involved two assembly proteins (i.e., chaperones and ushers) [10].

11.2.2 Curli

Curli pili are a class of thin, irregular extracellular amyloid fibers produced by *Salmonella* and *E. coli* species. Curli was first isolated and characterized in the late 1980s as it was responsible for causing bovine mastitis. Curli has been considered as another bacterial filaments class of fibers termed amyloids. They have been involved in various pathogenic patterns of many Gram-negative bacteria. The two species belonging to this group such as *E. coli* and *Salmonella* express proteinaceous appendages termed *curli pili*. The curli are implicated in cellular communication, colonization, and biofilm formation. The morphology of curli can be inspected through an electron microscope, which usually presents a coiled surface structure, thin, irregular, highly aggregated, and wired fibers, which can have a diameter of 2 nm composed of a single type of curli as a subunit [12].

11.2.3 Type III Secretion System (T3SS)

Several pathogenic bacteria like *Salmonella*, enteropathogenic *E. coli* (EPEC), *Shigella*, and *Pseudomonas* possess the ability to deliver effector proteins directly to eukaryotic host-cell via T3SS also called injectisome [13]. It has been recently discovered in Gram-positive bacteria, particularly in clostridia species. The essential part of the T3SS injectisome is a hollow needle channel used by bacteria to cause infections into the eukaryotic host cells. Some of the human pathogenic bacteria that present T3SS injectisome are *Salmonella* spp., *Shigella* spp., *Burkholderia* spp., *Yersinia pestis*, *Ps. aeruginosa*, *Chlamydia* spp., *V. cholerae*, enteropathogenic and enterohemorrhagic *E. coli*, *Xanthomonas* spp., plantlike *Ps. syringae*, *Erwinia* spp., *Xanthomonas*, *E. amylovora*, *Ps. syringae*, *Ralstonia solanacearum*, and *Xanthomonas* spp. [14]. The T3SS is composed of more than 20 different proteins that oligomerize to form three components consisting of the basal body, needle filament, and translocation. In bacteria, the mechanism of injectisome assembly is similar to flagellum assembly.

11.2.4 Type IV Secretion System (T4SS)

The T4SSs is a secretion systems type, described in Gram-negative or positive pathogenic bacteria and some of the *archaea* species. Many bacteria use T4SSs to secrete a large number of virulent protein substrates like protein–DNA complexes. Within this line, the T4SSs family can be classified into four groups: effector protein translocation into host cells; conjugative transfer of chromosomal and plasmid DNA from a cell-to-cell or transposons of *E. coli* and *Agrobacterium tumefaciens*; and some Gram-positive bacteria [15]. However, for many Gram-negative bacteria such as *Helicobacter pylori*, *Bordetella pertussis*, *L. pneumophila*, and *Brucella* spp., the T4SSs have a role in mediating the transfer of virulent proteins and transferring toxins into the host cell [16]. The architecture of T4SSs can be assembled mostly by the type IVa and IVb [17].

11.2.5 Type IV Pili

The T4P is a filamentous structure that extends from the cell's surface, usually from a cell pole. The type IV (T4P) pili were first described in the 1970s for *P. aeruginosa* [18] and afterward were characterized on many human pathogenic bacteria such as *Vibrio cholerae*,

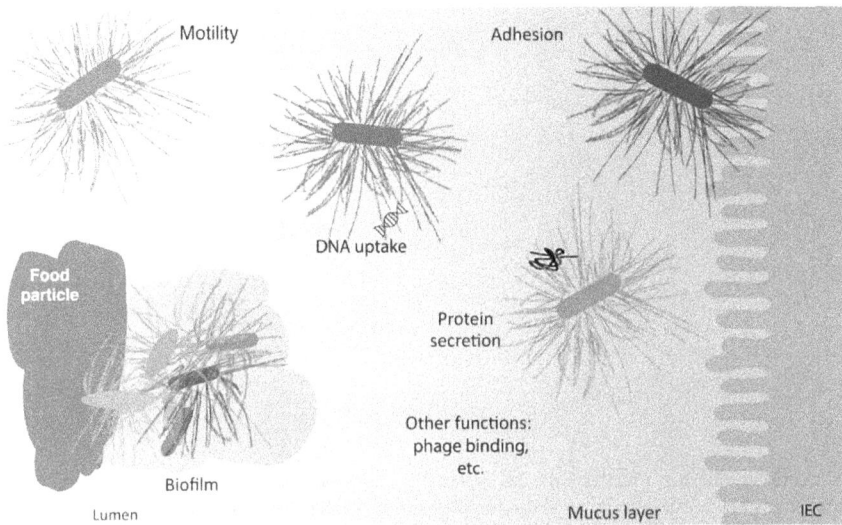

FIGURE 11.2
Schematic illustrations of the different functions of type IV pili. Reprinted with permission [19]. Copyright © 2020 Published by Elsevier, under a Creative Commons Attribution 4.0 International License (CC BY-NC-ND).

N. gonorrhoeae, Legionella pneumophila, enteropathogenic *E. coli* (EPEC), and Gram-positive species. Type IV pili can present a 6 nm diameter and up to some μm in length. The T4P are subdivided into three subtypes: T4aP, T4bP Tad pili, and T4cP designated recently based on a sequence of amino acids of pilin [19]. The type IVa pili (T4aP) are long, straight, and present polar bundles characterized by the existence of a PiT retraction ATPase and are associated with enteric pathogens [20]. The type IVbP is present in between 180–238 amino acids and has a signal peptide of 15–30 amino acids leader sequence. Many important biological functions have been attributed to the T4P in Gram-negative bacteria such as adherence to host cells, pathogenesis, formation of biofilms and microcolony, auto-aggregation, and electric transfer as nanowires (Figure 11.2) [19,21]. They are considered important virulence factors for many human and animal pathogens. In addition, the T4P carries out another function, which is related to locomotion, termed *twitching* and gliding motility in many bacterial species [22].

11.3 Microbial Nanowires and Bacterial Extracellular Electron Transfer (EET)

In 2005, Reguera et al. [23] described the "microbial nanowire," for the first time in microbiology literature. The bacterial nanowires are considered an important component in microbe-electrode and microbe-microbe electron exchange. The microbial nanowires rang up tens of μm long and facilitated long-range EET (Figure 11.3). In the field of electro-microbiology, the nanowires enabled the bacteria that has electrically conductive pili, to be considered as one of the most important discoveries. The microbial nanowires can be defined as extracellular proteins that transfer an electron from cell to extracellular substances under physiological conditions [24,25].

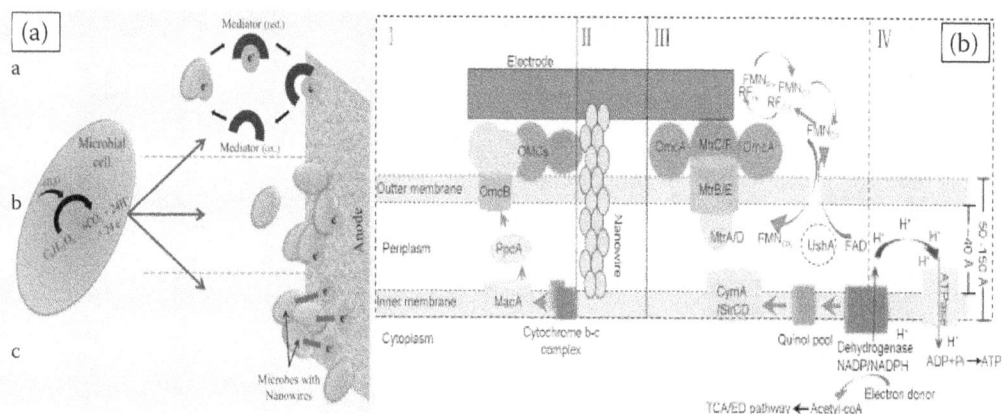

FIGURE 11.3
Bacterial extracellular electron transfer EET. (a) Schematic representation of proposed mechanisms of electron transfers from microbes to the anode: a. Mediator transfer, b. Direct transfer, c. Nanowires transfer. Reprinted with permission [3]. Copyright © 2015, Elsevier. (b) Type of bacterial EET mechanisms of *Geobacter* and *Shewanella*. (I) The OMC-based DET conduit in *Geobacter*; (II) bacterial nanowire; (III) electron transfer in *Shewanella* including flavins and CTCs; (IV) electrode respiration-coupled proton motive force and energy (ATP). Reprinted with permission [26,27]. Copyright © 2012 Elsevier.

11.4 Nanowire-Producing Bacteria: Taxonomy, Description, and nanowire Production

11.4.1 Description of the Genus *Geobacter*

The *Geobacter* species belong to the Geobacteraceae family, which are Gram-negative, rod-like, non-spore-forming, anaerobic, classified into three phylogenetic clades, and have the *G. metallireducens* strain type. The two most studied *Geobacter* species are *G. metallireducens* and *G. sulfurreducens* and play an important role in the bioremediation process. The *Geobacter* species were considered the first ones described to use hydrogen as an electron donor [28].

11.4.2 Description of the Genus *Shewanella*

The genus *Shewanella*, belonging to the Shewanellaceae family [29], was described first in 1931 by Derby [30,31]. They are Gram-negative, rod-shaped, non-spore-forming, facultatively anaerobic, and aerobic. They do not form endospores or microcysts and are chemo-organotrophic, oxidase-positive. This bacteria is commonly found in aquatic habitats. The genus includes around 70 species and the type of species is *S. putrefaciens*.

11.4.3 Nanowire Formation and Structure

Bacterial nanowires have been involved in EET. The structure and composition of bacterial nanowires are diverse depending on the species. *Geobacter* nanowires anchored in outer membrane cells are essential for the electron transfer among *G. sulfurreducens* and to Fe(III) oxides [21]. Their conductivity can be attributed to the two models of electron transfer such as hopping or a metallic-like mechanism [32]. The microbial nanowires of *S. oneidensis*

MR-1 are described as a form of conductive pilus associated with the membrane. Also, the lipids colocalized on these extracellular structures aid in performing a multistep redox hopping mechanism that contributes to electron transfer (Figure 11.4).

Recently, Subramanian et al. [32], used electron cryotomography microscopy to determine the ultrastructure of the nanowire produced by the *S. oneidensis* strain. In the outer membrane and periplasm of the strain, EET was observed on the microbial nanowires. In this study, the authors used light and electrons which revealed that these structures on *S. oneidensis* were curved and an extension tabulation form was observed. Moreover, less c-cytochrome in mutant strain compared to the wild type strain was observed. The periplasm and outer membrane proteins were consistent with cytochromes [32]. The result obtained revealed that *S. oneidensis* MR-1 nanowires were outer membrane vesicles with variable lengths [33].

11.5 Geobacter and Shewanella EET Mechanism

11.5.1 The Hopping Mechanism by *S. Oneidensis* Strain MR-1 Nanowires

Several mechanisms are used by the bacteria in electron transfer including DET, mediated electron transfer, and through nanowires, as represented in Figure 11.3. For the *S. oneidensis* strain MR-1 nanowires, the electron transfer by extracellular nanowires occurred through the hopping mechanism. The hopping mechanism is a transferred electron that can be determined between two sites in a solid specimen from one molecule to another with the acquisition of energy (Figure 11.5) [23].

This concept has been described in connection with ionic conduction in amorphous non-metallic solids and after it has been extended to electrons. The hopping transition can be determined by both the distance between the two sites and the potential. If the potential barrier width is larger than 10 Å, it causes the electrons to hop rather than tunnel from one molecule to the neighboring one. In fact, the hopping process is similar to the atomic diffusion process. However, in hopping, there is no electron transfer until the thermal motion of nuclei permits electron motion over the barrier by rearrangement of the molecule. In the electron hopping mechanism, it was suggested that the outer surface cytochromes were aligned along the filament, which enabled sufficient electronic coupling. To form the microbial nanowires, the *S. oneidensis* MR-1 strain requires cytochromes called MtrC and OmcA, which can be involved in electron transfer [4,34]. The composition analysis of the bacterial nanowires by electron microscopy imaging of *Shewanella S. oneidensis* MR-1 nanowires showed that the outer membrane extensions contained components rather than pilin-based structures, which include cytochromes that improve the electron hopping pattern. These multiheme cytochromes of the MtrC and OmcA are localized on the outer membranes. They can be associated with the nanowires of *Shewanella* and are mediators for electron transfer.

11.5.2 Tunneling Mechanism

Tunneling is a mechanical phenomenon in which the excited state electron can tunnel to the neighboring molecule in one of the multiple consecutive steps by exchanging energy through the tunneling process. In the tunneling effect, an electron moves through the

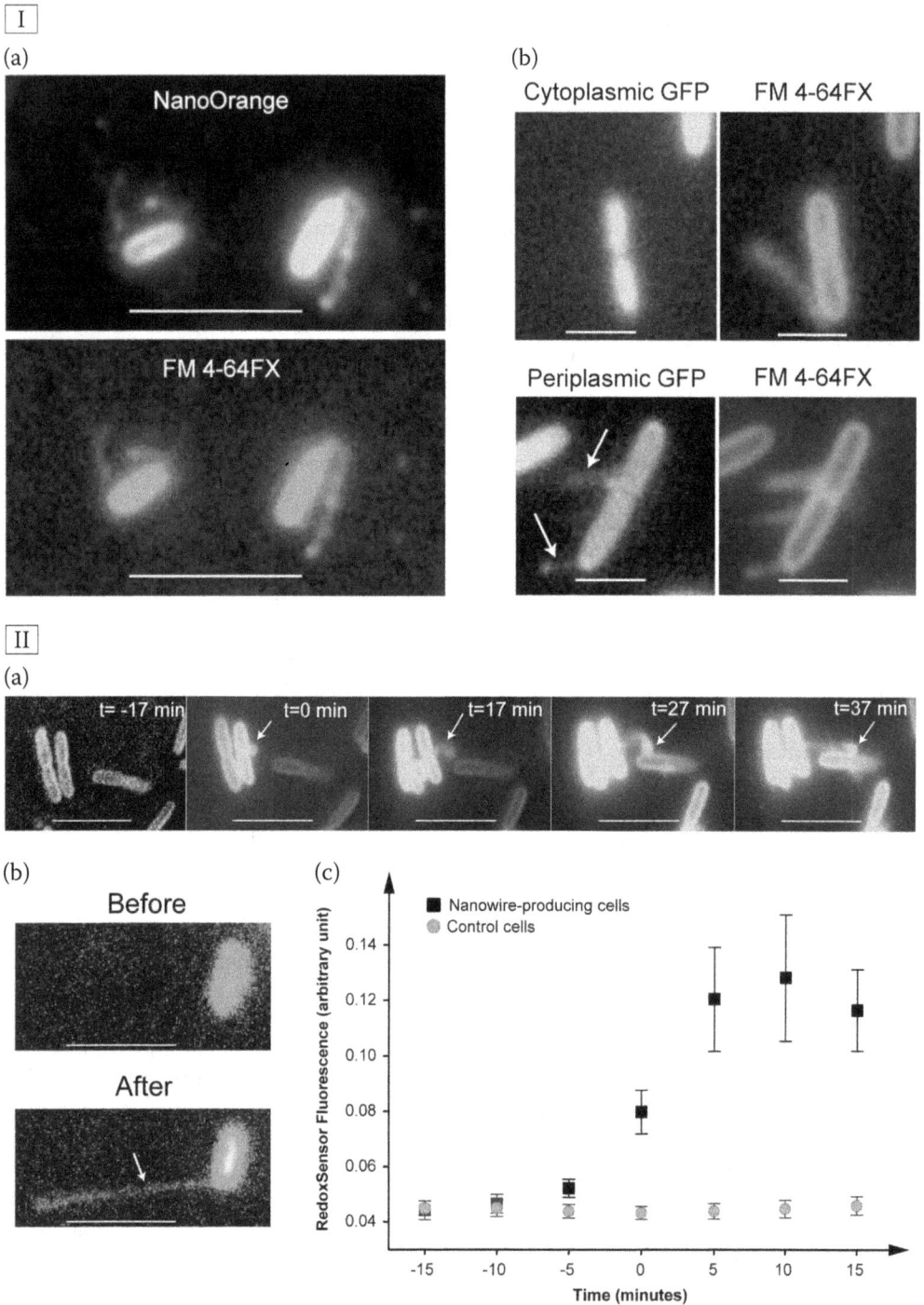

FIGURE 11.4
Structural and *in vivo* illustration of the formation of nanowires in *Shewanella oneidensis* MR-1. I. (a) Presence of proteins and membranes in MR-1 cells and nanowires. (b) Bacterial nanowires from *S. oneidensis* MR-1 strains. II. (a) Growth of a bacterial nanowire. (b) Illustration of a single cell before and after, the production of a bacterial nanowire. Reprinted with permission [33]. Copyright © 2014 PNAS. The article is available under the Creative Commons CC-BY license.

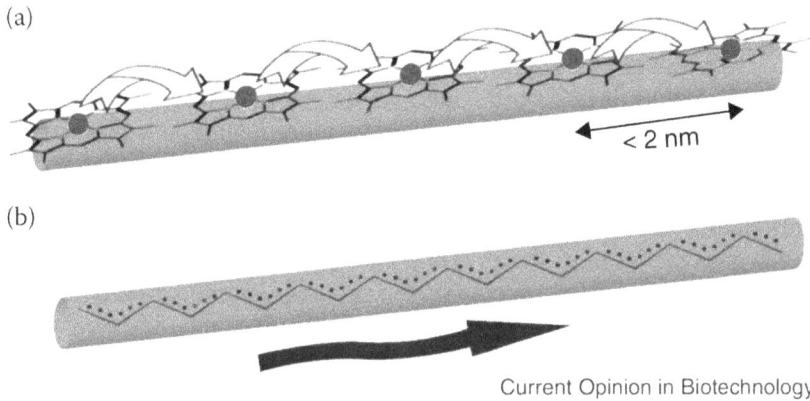

(a)

< 2 nm

(b)

Current Opinion in Biotechnology

FIGURE 11.5
Electron current model along bacterial nanowires. (a) Electron hopping and *S. oneidensis* filaments model's (b) metallic-like conduction for *G. sulfurreducens* pili. Reprinted with permission from [23]. Copyright © 2013 Elsevier.

barrier from one side to the other side without requiring nuclear movement. It is due to the formation of a complex structure with different functional groups.

11.5.3 Metal-Like Conductivity by *G. Sulfurreducens* Nanowires

Nanowire conductivity was the first discovery in *G. sulfurreducens* and some of *Geobacter* species [21]. The mechanism of transfer electron of *Geobacter* spp. nanowires are suggested by a metallic-like conductivity. In the metal-like conductivity (Figure 11.5), there is a dependence on the cytochromes, which is a condition that differs from the electron hopping mechanism. However, the nanowires of *G. sulfurreducens* can promote electron transfer to the cell that follows up to Fe (III). Yet, several components have been identified which include *c*-type cytochrome located in the inner as well as an outer membrane which are associated with the pili [35,36]. Alongside that, a study conducted by El-Naggar et al. [34] demonstrated that the electric conduction along bacterial nanowires of *S. oneidensis* MR-1 can occur through EET. The nanowires of *G. sulfurreducens* consist of PilA. Also, homology with PilA in Gram-negative bacteria is related to the production of type IV pili. This PilA subunit of pilin from *G. sulfurreducens* contains five conserved aromatic amino acids that can play a role in long-distance electron transfer [37]. Generally, the conductivity of *G. sulfurreducens* nanowires can increase exponentially upon cooling and low pH of around 2 [38]. In conclusion, the different studies published demonstrated that the electron transfers in microbial nanowires of *G. sulfurreducens* proposed the metal-type conduction instead of the electron hopping model.

11.6 Biotechnological Application of Microbial EET

The discovery of mechanisms of microorganisms with electron transfer capability has been explored in many fields of biotechnology application and bioengineering. In this part, we developed the field in which these microbes have been explored for applications such as bioremediation of environmental contaminants, bioelectricity, and bioenergy production.

11.6.1 Bioremediation

Bioremediation is a novel technology accomplished by a complex chain of biologically mediated transformation. It is a promising and inventive system that uses microorganisms to decontaminate pollutants. In another word, bioremediation is defined as a process that uses microorganisms for clearance or degradation of contaminants and hazardous substances including toxins, and other organic pollutants under controlled conditions to an innocuous state [39]. Several advances in bioremediation techniques including *ex-situ* and *in-situ* bioremediation with the microbe and organic pollutants are both present in the soil. *Ex-situ* bioremediation is considered a faster method based on: the cost of treatment, type of pollutant, and geology of the polluted site. The main goal of this technique is to effectively restore polluted environments. Several techniques include *in-situ* remediation such as bioslurping, biosparging, bioaugmentation, etc. however, in *ex-situ* the most employed techniques are biopile, windrows, composting, and bioreactors [40]. Therefore, it is highly involved in the degradation, eradication, immobilization, or detoxification of various chemicals and hazardous physical materials from the environment through microorganisms. Today, bioremediation is a permanent solution that can reduce or degrade pollutants and control dangerous substances in subsurface environments. Recently, a new strategy for the bioremediation of toxic metal contaminants has been used in agricultural soils, industrial environments, and waters reservoir by using the microorganism to decompose substances such as hydrocarbons, petroleum, heavy metals, pesticides, among others. Generally, the pollutants can be remediated through three basic levels. First, through natural attenuation, at which pollutants are reduced by native microorganisms. Second, biostimulation is employed where nutrients and oxygen are applied to accelerate biodegradation. The third level is during bioaugmentation, at which organisms are added to improve the efficiency when compared to native microorganisms to reduce the contaminants. The efficiency of bioremediation to reduce environmental pollutants is strongly related to the appropriate species employed to degrade the chemicals. In that sense, many microbes have the potential for environmental restoration by removing metals contaminated water. For example, the *Geobacter* and *S. oneidensis* MR-1 play a role in the bioremediation processes by potentially degrading a diverse number of contaminants including Cr and U [41,42]. The capacity to reduce radionuclides like U(VI) by *S. oneidensis* MR-1 strain is correlated with the presence of *c*-type cytochromes [26]. Yet, the reduced solubility of U(VI) in sedimentary environments imposes a challenge that requires novel strategies for bioremediation to properly eliminate this environmental pollutant. The capacity of these microorganisms to degrade many other compounds including radionuclides elements, minerals substances like nitrite, sulfate, chromium, dye solution contaminated wastewaters, and petroleum-contaminated by *S. oneidensis* MR-1, are described in various studies [43,44].

11.6.2 Bioelectricity and Bioenergy Production

The interaction between the microorganisms and insoluble electron donors or acceptors is an emerging field within applied microbiology. The term *electromicrobiology* is a research area of science that studies the mechanism of microbial electron exchange that has contributed to developing a branch of bioelectronics [44,45]. A considerable amount of microorganisms have metallic-like properties that provide them with electronic characteristics. There are three types of microbial EET mechanisms at the anode of microbial fuel cells (MFCs), including direct/indirect transfers and through conductive nanowires, which are provided in Figure 11.6 [44].

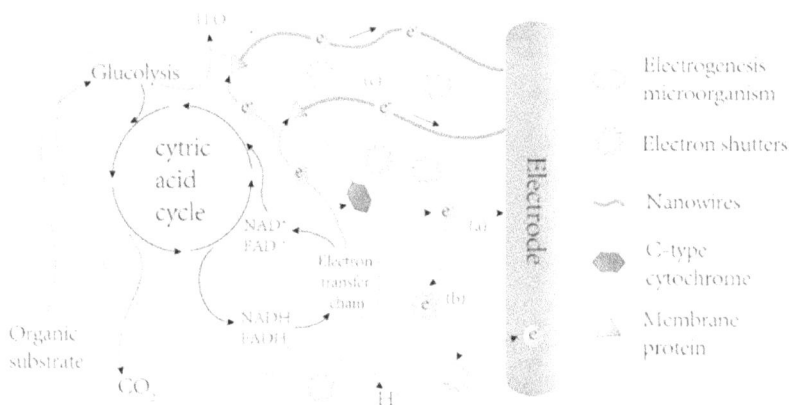

FIGURE 11.6
Types of microbial EET mechanisms at the anode of MFCs. Reprinted with permission [44]. Copyright © 2017 MDPI. The article is available under the Creative Commons CC-BY license.

Electricity harvesting from organic matter has been a topic in several studies and reviews as the recent signs of progress in MFC are being described as a promising technology to generate electricity. Alongside that, a variety of microorganisms seems to produce proteic nanowires with electrically conductive properties. In that sense, *Geobacter* pili have provided one of the most satisfactory results in terms of nanowire conductibility [37]. For EET, some bacteria have employed different mechanisms including direct or indirect/mediated EET, as provided in Figure 11.6. Within this line, microorganisms such as *G. sulfurreducens* and *S. oneidensis* have gained attention from the scientific community within the field of microbiology and bioengineering due to their promising conducting properties. Such an effect is based on the consumption of several compounds that are converted into electricity, just like MFCs.

MFC is a type of bioelectrochemical system that converts organic wastes into electricity through the catalytic action of EAMs associated with an electrode. That process can enable novel applications such as the generation of electricity, wastewater treatment, and biosensor applications. In that sense, an MFC is a bioreactor incorporated with an electrochemical system that employs bacteria to generate electricity from bioconvertible substrates directly. The concept of MFC as promising environmental biotechnology was first explored in the 1970s, which proposed power production and wastewater treatment using microorganisms. To generate current, the MFCs use bacteria as the catalysts to oxidize organic compounds [3,46]. Several studies have been conducted using UFCs inoculated with *S. oneidensis* MR-1 as a strain with potential electron transfer for generating bioelectricity along with energy production from biomass or carbon sources as electron donors [47,48]. Recently, MFC-based systems were employed as biosensors, which were employed for the identification of toxic substances in water and wastewater and therefore serving as a tool for environmental monitoring. In that sense, a biosensor is a device that can identify different analytes which can be employed for monitoring ecosystems, quality control of food and water, identification of pathogens, and drug delivery systems. It can be integrated into a bacteria or enzyme with an electronic component. In addition, biosensors can be fabricated in several sizes along with presenting extremely low detection limits to the other of around 1×10^{15}, which aids in the precise identification of pathogens microorganisms, or toxic substances [49]. Biosensors can be classified on different

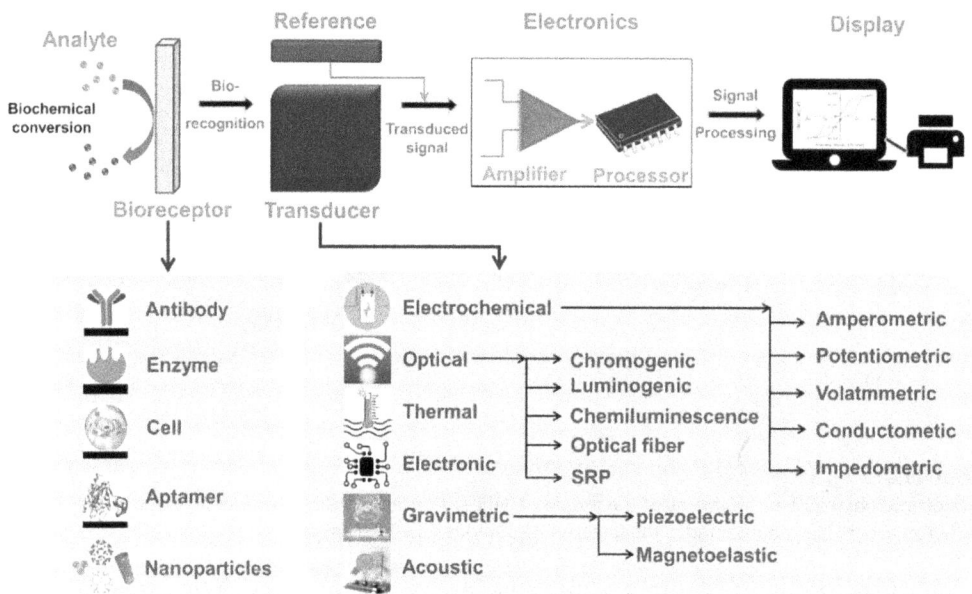

FIGURE 11.7
Schematic illustration of typical biosensors and types of bioreceptors and transducers used in the biosensors. Reprinted with permission [49]. Copyright © 2021. MDPI, Article is available under the Creative Commons CC-BYlicense.

bioreceptors which comprises an analyte along with different bioreceptors, electronic systems, transducers, among other components, as seen in Figure 11.7 [49].

Many biological materials are used in the fabrication of biosensors including microorganisms (algae, bacteria, and yeast), enzymes, and cells because they can be massively produced and easier manipulated [50]. The microbial biosensors are a close contact analytical device between microorganisms and the transducer [50]. Recently, the recovery of the high-value product of MFC such as biohydrogen and methane has increased attention towards this technology. MFC-based biosensors can be used as an analytical tool for the measurement of various analytes and parameters that include biochemical oxygen demand (BOD), chemical oxygen demand (COD), toxicants, and microbial activity [49]. The characteristics of MFC-based biosensors vary according to the substrates, solution, and can incorporate the use of both bacterial consortia and single strains. In an MFC-based biosensor device, microorganisms are capable to sense the analyte and give an equivalent response to its yielded electric current. Electrobiosensors comprise cathode and anode chambers, and both are separated by a membrane that enables proton exchange. The performance of MFC-based biosensors for toxicity detection depends on the type of electroactive microbes with special properties used in the cell.

11.7 Conclusion

The discovery of many properties of microbial nanowires, and the possibility to modulate their conductivity can offer a basis for new fields and future research between microbiology, molecular biology, biophysical chemistry, and physics. Moreover, the discovery of structures termed *microbial nanowires* are capable of reducing metal and transferring electrons to anodes, which are synthesized by *Geobacter* spp. and *S. oneidensis* MR-1 strain and offer viable alternatives for researchers that are aiming for renewable energy source technologies. In addition, the most suitable properties and functionalities of microbial nanowires demonstrated can offer promising specific applications within the areas of bioremediation of environmental contaminants, production of bioenergy and nanomaterials, applications for sensing, biotherapeutics, and bioelectronics, among many others. Thus, the studies on microbial nanowires can provide interesting research areas that are likely to shape the future of several technology sectors.

References

1. W. Gopel, "Bioelectronics and nanotechnologies," *Biosensors and Bioelectronics*, vol. 13, 1998, pp. 723–728.
2. B. Nagel, H. Dellweg, L.M. Gierasch, "Glossary for chemists of terms used in biotechnology (IUPAC recommendations 1992)," *Pure and Applied Chemistry*, vol. 64, no. 1, 1992, pp. 143–168.
3. S.K. Butti, G. Velvizhi, M.L.K. Sulonen, J.M. Haavisto, E.O. Koroglu, A.Y. Cetinkaya, S. Singh, D. Arya, J.A. Annie Modestra, K.V. Krishna, A. Verma, B. Ozkaya, A.M. Lakaniemi, J.A. Puhakka, S.V. Mohan, "Microbial electrochemical technologies with the perspective of harnessing bioenergy: Maneuvering towards upscaling," *Renewable and Sustainable Energy Reviews*, vol. 53, 2016, pp. 462–476.
4. Y.A. Gorby, S. Yanina, J.S. McLean, K.M. Rosso, D. Moyles, A. Dohnalkova, T.J. Beveridge, I.S. Chang, B.H. Kim, K.S. Kim, D.E. Culley, S.R. Reed, M.F. Romine, D.A. Saffarini, E.A. Hill, L. Shi, D.A. Elias, D.W. Kennedy, G. Pinchuk, K. Watanabe, S. Ishii, B. Logan, K.H. Nealson, J.K. Fredrickson, "Electrically conductive bacterial nanowires produced by *Shewanella oneidensis* strain MR-1 and other microorganisms," *Proceedings of the National Academy of Sciences*, vol. 103, no. 30, 2006, pp. 11358–11363.
5. J.P. Duguid, I.W. Smith, G. Dempster, P.N. Edmunds, "Non-flagellar filamentous appendages ('fimbriæ') and hæmagglutinating activity in bacterium coli," *J. Pathol.*, vol. 70, no. 2, 1955 pp. 335–348.
6. J.C. Ottow, "Ecology, physiology, and genetics of fimbriae and pili," *Annu. Rev. Microbiol.*, vol. 29, no. 1, 1975, pp. 79–108.
7. Brinton, "Non-flagellar appendage of bacteria," *Nature*, vol. 183, 1959. pp. 782–786.
8. R. Yanagawa, K. Otsuki, T. Tokui, "Electron microscopy of fine structure of *corynebacterium renale* with special reference to pili," *The Graduate School of Veterinary Medicine*, vol. 16, no. 1, 1968, pp. 31–37.
9. R. Fronzes, H. Remaut, G. Waksman, "Architectures and biogenesis of non-flagellar protein appendages in gram-negative bacteria," *EMBO J*, vol. 27, no. 17, 2008, pp. 2271–2280.
10. F.G. Sauer, H. Remaut, S.J. Hultgren, G. Waksman, "Fiber assembly by the chaperone–usher pathway," *Biochimica et Biophysica Acta (BBA) - Molecular Cell Research*, vol. 1694, no. 1–3, 2004, pp. 259–267.
11. S.P. Nuccio, A.J. Bäumler, "Evolution of the chaperone/usher assembly pathway: Fimbrial classification goes greek," *Microbiol Mol Biol Rev*, vol. 71, no. 4, 2007, pp. 551–575.
12. A. Olsén, A. Jonsson, S. Normark, "Fibronection binding mediated a novel class of surface organelles of *Escherichia coli*," *Nature*, vol. 338, 1989, pp. 652–655.
13. C.L. Tsai, B.J. Burkinshaw, N.C.J. Strynadka, J.A. Tainer, "The *salmonella* type III secretion system virulence effector forms a new Hexameric chaperone assembly for export of effector/chaperone complexes," *J Bacteriol*, vol. 197, no. 4, 2015, pp. 672–675.

14. S. Dey, A. Chakravarty, P. Guha Biswas, R.N. De Guzman, "The type III secretion system needle, tip, and translocon," *Protein Science*, p. pro.3682, vol. 28, 2019, pp. 1582–1593.
15. E. Grohmann, P.J. Christie, G. Waksman, S. Backert, "Type IV secretion in gram-negative and gram-positive bacteria: Type IV secretion," *Molecular Microbiology*, vol. 107, no. 4, 2018, pp. 455–471.
16. R. Fronzes, P.J. Christie, G. Waksman, "The structural biology of type IV secretion systems," *Nat Rev Microbiol*, vol. 7, no. 10, 2009, pp. 703–714.
17. K. Wallden, A. Rivera-Calzada, G. Waksman, "Microreview: Type IV secretion systems: Versatility and diversity in function," *Cellular Microbiology*, vol. 12, no. 9, 2010, pp. 1203–1212.
18. D.E. Bradley, "Evidence for the retraction of *Pseudomonas aeruginosa* RNA phage pili," *Biochemical and Biophysical Research Communications*, vol. 47, no. 1, 1972, pp. 142–149.
19. K. Ligthart, C. Belzer, W.M. de Vos, H.L.P. Tytgat, "Bridging bacteria and the gut: Functional aspects of type IV pili," *Trends in Microbiology*, vol. 28, no. 5, 2020, pp. 340–348.
20. D.G. Thanassi, S.P. Nuccio, S.S.K. So, A.J. Bäumler, "Fimbriae: Classification and biochemistry," *EcoSal Plus*, vol. 2, no. 2, 2007, p. ecosalplus.2.4.2.1.
21. G. Reguera, K.D. McCarthy, T. Mehta, J.S. Nicoll, M.T. Tuominen, D.R. Lovley, "Extracellular electron transfer via microbial nanowires," *Nature*, vol. 435, no. 7045, 2005, pp. 1098–1101.
22. J.S. Mattick, "Type IV pili and twitching motility," *Annu. Rev. Microbiol.*, vol. 56, no. 1, 2002, pp. 289–314.
23. N.S. Malvankar, D.R. Lovley, "Microbial nanowires for bioenergy applications," *Current Opinion in Biotechnology*, vol. 27, 2014, pp. 88–95.
24. N.S. Malvankar, D.R. Lovley, "Microbial nanowires: A new paradigm for biological electron transfer and bioelectronics," *Chem Sus Chem*, vol. 5, no. 6, 2012, pp. 1039–1046.
25. A. Ilshadsabah, T.V. Suchithra, "Bacterial nanowires: An Invigorating tale for future," in *Microbial Nanobionics*, R. Prasad, Ed., 2019, Cham: Springer International Publishing, pp. 77–88.
26. M.J. Marshall, A.S. Beliaev, A.C. Dohnalkova, D.W. Kennedy, L. Shi, Z. Wang, M.I. Boyanov, B. Lai, K.M. Kemner, J.S. McLean, S.B. Reed, D.E. Culley, V.L. Bailey, C.J. Simonson, D.A. Saffarini, M.F. Romine, J.M. Zachara, J.K. Fredrickson, "c-type cytochrome-dependent formation of U(IV) nanoparticles by *Shewanella oneidensis*," *PLoS Biol*, vol. 4, no. 8, 2006, p. e268.
27. T. Li, J.T. Guthrie, "Colour removal from aqueous solutions of metal-complex azo dyes using bacterial cells of *Shewanella* strain J18 143," *Bioresource Technology*, vol. 101, no. 12, 2010, pp. 4291–4295.
28. D.R. Lovley, E.E. Roden, E.J.P. Phillips, J.C. Woodward, "Enzymatic iron and uranium reduction by sulfate-reducing bacteria," *Marine Geology*, vol. 113, no. 1–2, 1993, pp. 41–53.
29. E.P. Ivanova, S. Flavier, R. Christen, "Phylogenetic relationships among marine Alteromonas-like proteobacteria: Emended description of the family Alteromonadaceae and proposal of Pseudoalteromonadaceae fam. nov., Colwelliaceae fam. nov., Shewanellaceae fam. nov., Moritellaceae fam. nov., Ferrimonadaceae fam. nov., Idiomarinaceae fam. nov. and Psychromonadaceae fam. nov.," *International Journal of Systematic and Evolutionary Microbiology*, vol. 54, no. 5, 2004, pp. 1773–1788.
30. H.A. Derby, "Bacteriology of butter. IV. bacteriological studies on surface taint butter," *Iowa Agr Expt Sta Research Bull*, vol. 6, 1931, p. 145.
31. H.M. Holt, B. Gahrn-Hansen, B. Bruun, "*Shewanella algae* and *Shewanella putrefaciens*: Clinical and microbiological characteristics," *Clinical Microbiology and Infection*, vol. 11, no. 5, 2005, pp. 347–352.
32. P. Subramanian, S. Pirbadian, M.Y. El-Naggar, G.J. Jensen, "Ultrastructure of *Shewanella oneidensis* MR-1 nanowires revealed by electron cryotomography," *Proc Natl Acad Sci USA*, vol. 115, no. 14, 2018, pp. E3246–E3255.
33. S. Pirbadian, S.F. Barchinger, K.M. Leung, H.S. Byun, Y. Jangir, R.A. Bouhenni, S.B. Reed, M.F. Romine, D.A. Saffarini, L. Shi, Y.A. Gorby, J.H. Golbeck, M.Y. El-Naggar MY. "*Shewanella oneidensis* MR-1 nanowires are outer membrane and periplasmic extensions of the extracellular electron transport components," *Proceedings of the National Academy of Sciences*, vol. 111, no. 35, 2014, pp. 12883–12888.

34. M.Y. El-Naggar, G. Wanger, K.M. Leung, T.D. Yuzvinsky, G. Southam, J. Yang, W.M. Lau, K.H. Nealson, Y.A. Gorby, "Electrical transport along bacterial nanowires from Shewanella oneidensis MR-1," *Proceedings of the National Academy of Sciences*, vol. 107, no. 42, 2010, pp. 18127–18131.

35. S.S. Richter, W.J. Howard, M.P. Weinstein, D.A. Bruckner, J.F. Hindler, M. Saubolle, G.V. Doern, "Multicenter Evaluation of the BD phoenix Automated microbiology system for antimicrobial susceptibility Testing of *streptococcus* species," *Journal of Clinical Microbiology*, vol. 45, no. 9, 2007, pp. 2863–2871.

36. C.L. Giltner, Y. Nguyen, L.L. Burrows, "Type IV pilin proteins: Versatile molecular modules," *Microbiol Mol Biol Rev*, vol. 76, no. 4, 2012, pp. 740–772.

37. M. Vargas, N.S. Malvankar, P.L. Tremblay, C. Leang, J.A. Smith, P. Patel, O. Snoeyenbos-West, K.P. Nevin, D.R. Lovley, "Aromatic amino acids Required for pili conductivity and long-range extracellular electron transport in *Geobacter sulfurreducens*," *mBio*, vol. 4, no. 2, 2013.

38. N.S. Malvankar, M. Vargas, K. Nevin, P.L. Tremblay, K. Evans-Lutterodt, D. Nykypanchuk, E. Martz, M.T. Tuominen, D.R. Lovley, "Structural basis for metallic-like conductivity in microbial nanowires," *mBio*, vol. 6, no. 2, 2015.

39. A.I. Zouboulis, P.A. Moussas, S.G. Psaltou, "Groundwater and soil Pollution: Bioremediation," in *Encyclopedia of Environmental Health*, Nriagu, J.O., 2019, Elsevier, pp. 369–381.

40. C.C. Azubuike, C.B. Chikere, G.C. Okpokwasili, "Bioremediation techniques–classification based on site of application: Principles, advantages, limitations and prospects," *World J Microbiol Biotechnol*, vol. 32, no. 11, 2016, p. 180.

41. R. Bencheikh-Latmani, R. Bencheikh-Latmani, S.M. Williams, L. Haucke, C.S. Criddle, L. Wu, J. Zhou, B.M. Tebo. "Global Transcriptional Profiling of *Shewanella oneidensis* MR-1 during cr (VI) and U(VI) reduction," *Appl Environ Microbiol*, vol. 71, no. 11, 2005, pp. 7453–7460.

42. J. Yun, T. Ueki, M. Miletto, D.R. Lovley, "Monitoring the Metabolic status of *Geobacter* species in contaminated groundwater by Quantifying key Metabolic proteins with *Geobacter*-specific Antibodies," *Appl. Environ. Microbiol.*, vol. 77, no. 13, 2011, pp. 4597–4602.

43. R.T. Anderson, D.R. Lovley, "Anaerobic bioremediation of benzene under sulfate-reducing conditions in a petroleum-contaminated aquifer," *Environ. Sci. Technol.*, vol. 34, no. 11, 2000, pp. 2261–2266.

44. T. Zhou, H. Han, P. Liu, J. Xiong, F. Tian, X. Li, "Microbial fuels cell-based biosensor for toxicity detection: A review," *Sensors*, vol. 17, no. 10, 2017, p. 2230.

45. D.R. Lovley, D.E. Holmes, "Electromicrobiology: The ecophysiology of phylogenetically diverse electroactive microorganisms," *Nat Rev Microbiol*, vol. 20, no. 1, 2022, pp. 5–19.

46. Z.K. Liu, T.K. Ling, A.F. Cheng, "Evaluation of the BD phoenix Automated microbiology system for identification and antimicrobial susceptibility testing of common clinical isolates," *Med Princ Pract*, vol. 14, no. 4, 2005, pp. 250–254.

47. Y.Z. Wang, Y. Shen, L. Gao, Z.-H. Liao, J.-Z. Sun, Y.-C. Yong, "Improving the extracellular electron transfer of Shewanella oneidensis MR-1 for enhanced bioelectricity production from biomass hydrolysate," *RSC Adv.*, vol. 7, no. 48, 2017, pp. 30488–30494.

48. F. Li, Y. Li, L. Sun, X. Li, C. Yin, X. An, X. Chen, Y. Tian, "Engineering *Shewanella oneidensis* enables xylose-fed microbial fuel cell," *Biotechnol Biofuels*, vol. 10, no. 1, 2017, p. 196.

49. V. Naresh, N. Lee, "A review on biosensors and recent development of Nanostructured materials-enabled biosensors," *Sensors*, vol. 21, no. 4, 2021, p. 1109.

50. Y. Lei, W. Chen, A. Mulchandani, "Microbial biosensors," *Analytica Chimica Acta*, vol. 568, no. 1–2, 2006, pp. 200–210.

12

Semiconducting Nanostructured Materials for Bioelectronics

Jayshree Khedkar

Department of Chemistry, Shri Anand College, Pathardi, Ahmednagar, India

Anil M. Palve

Department of Chemistry, Mahatma Phule ASC College, Panvel, Navi-Mumbai, India

Ram K. Gupta

Department of Chemistry, National Institute for Materials Advancement, Pittsburg State University, Pittsburg, USA

CONTENTS

12.1 Introduction

Over the last several years, electronic technologies have revolutionized biology and medicine. A variety of bio-devices have been developed to date, all of which have aided in this revolution. A multidisciplinary approach integrating material science, microelectronics, and bioengineering enabled these bioelectronics breakthroughs [1]. Due to the significant developments in materials science, notably nanomaterial-based technology, the field of bioelectronics has gained new dimensions. In biomedical studies, devices that are durable and demonstrate long-term performance in soft tissues or physiologic environments are pivotal [2]. The various biomedical applications such as monitoring,

DOI: 10.1201/9781003263265-12

tracking, and recording people's vital signs have seen advancements due to wearable and implantable devices or electronics [3]. The factors at the interfaces between biosensors and cellular membranes determine the efficacy of these kinds of devices. The electro-physiology recording and stimulating capabilities of biosensor implants integrated with electrogenic cells, on the other hand, are reliant on the electrode impedance, the revealed surfaces area, and the cell-electrode connectivity [4–7]. Smart watches, armbands, and optics are among the accessories that are bringing some of these technologies into our day-to-day lives [1,8,9]. The commercialization of these gadgets has been aided by semiconductor nanostructured bio-nanotechnology. The flexibility of nanomaterials in terms of alteration and modification of their localized structure during the synthesis, as well as their doping and functionalization capabilities, allows them to serve the specific requirements of such applications. This unique nature of the nanomaterials has made them multi-functional prerequisites for the conception of flexible and wearable electronics [10]. The downsizing of semiconductor devices is paving the way for new biomedical research and commercial medical applications. A basic way for manu-facturing very flexible electronics is to utilize inorganic materials in form of either one-dimensional (1D) or two-dimensional (2D) nanostructures [11]. Many inorganic materials, namely nanosheet, nanoribbon, and nanowire, provided tunable and dynamic features for conductor and semiconductor devices as well as dielectric materials [11].

Carbon nanotubes (CNTs), followed by several 2D materials, were among the first nano-materials to be investigated for the designing of wearable electronics [12]. With the best active electrical conductivities and higher electron mobility, flexibility in single layer form, the optical transparency of 98.7%, and extraordinarily high tensile strength, graphene materials have emerged as the most promising and extensively researched 2D materials. The graphene also demonstrates exceptional resistance to high temperatures, pressures, and highly corrosive conditions. Graphene is a suitable candidate for wearable biosensors and other biomedical applications because of its ease of fabrication and bio-compatibility [13,14]. Electronic and optical bio-interface studies mainly use inorganic semiconductors. They are needed to make high-performance devices for applications like electrical sensing, signal amplification, and transduction. Researchers have increasingly focused on semiconducting Si because of its biocompatibility and well-developed micro-fabrication technologies. Other inorganic semiconductors explored in bioelectronics and bioelectrical research include zinc sulfide (ZnS), titanium dioxide (TiO_2), and molybdenum disulfide (MoS_2), which are available as nanoparticles, nanowires, nanotubes, layered nanomaterial, and nanosheets [2]. Semiconducting oxides, in particular, are growing rapidly as silicon substitutes in active matrix display backplane thin-film transistors, as well as opaque, elastic devices and energy scavengers [15]. ZnO has a unique combination of properties such as excellent visible wa-velength transparency, rapid charge carrier mobility, and high piezoelectric susceptibility. Therefore, it has been explored in a variety of forms, including films, wires, and rods, for sensing, catalysis, optical emission, piezoelectric transduction, and actuation. ZnO is also potentially ideal for chemical sensing, biological labeling and sensing, and energy transfer at bio-interfaces due to its stability, various band gaps, and wide range of morphologies [15,16]. Transition metal dichalcogenide (MoS_2) could be used in ultrathin wearable touch sensors, owing to their outstanding photo-absorption and piezoresistivity [17].

The first functional implants, heart pacemakers, were introduced in the 1950s [18]. Since then, the emergence of implantable electronic devices has streamlined the evolution of nanoelectronics and nanofabrication technologies. Biomedical devices that help restore and manage the activities of dysfunctional parts include hearing aid, nervous system stimulators, and cardiac pacemakers [19]. These battery-operated implantable devices are made up of programmable circuitry as well as biocompatible electrodes and wires. The self-degradation of implanted devices in biofluids benefits through reducing the medical treatment cost and also risk associated with it. Flexible implanted devices achieve self-degradation by using relevant semiconducting materials. Silicon, along with Ge and ZnO, is one of the most widely utilized bioresorbable semiconductor materials for making soft electronics that are implanted temporarily [19]. Wide bandgap bioelectronics have also been applied in a versatile field, with long-lasting electronics, nano energy storage, bioresorbable machinery, printable and implantable devices, and optogenetic devices. [20].

12.2 Semiconducting Materials and Their Advantages for Bioelectronics

12.2.1 Wide Bandgap-Based Materials for Bioelectronics

Silicon has drawbacks such as degradation in biofluids, fast ion diffusion, etc. Due to these disadvantages, Si is inappropriate for wearable and implantable uses. Also, due to low piezoelectric coefficient and indirect bandgap of silicon limit itself in soft energy harvesting applications. The wide bandgap (WBG) materials have been the point of attraction due to superior chemical and physical properties over silicon [20]. Herein, we summarize alternative semiconducting materials of the class like IV–IV, III–V, and II–VI. The bandgap of these materials is greater than 2 eV and can be used for a high breakdown electric field. Also, it enhances the durability of devices due to the strong covalent bond in the atoms of WBG nanomaterials.

The II-VI class of the materials is made up of second group elements and six group chalcogen elements. This class of materials was explored for optoelectronics. One of the prominent materials in this group is zinc oxide. ZnO is popular due to its piezoelectricity, biodegradability, and direct WBG nature. Dagdeviren et al [16] reported that zinc oxide is soluble in demineralized H_2O at a normal temperature in 15 hours and shows no evidence after the method. In addition to this test, ZnO show in vitro biocompatibility cell culture assays test so it is useful for wearable and implantable uses due to its biocompatibility (Figure 12.1) [21]. SiC is another class of the WBG semiconducting material for

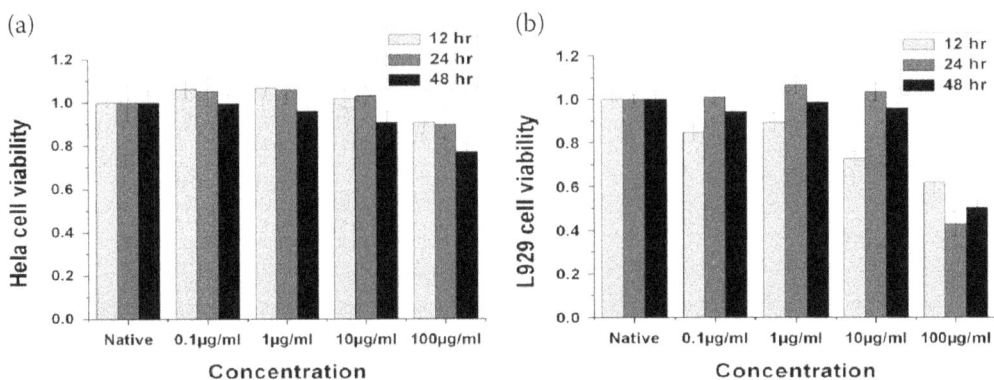

FIGURE 12.1
Biocompatibility test of ZnO nanowires at 12 hours, 24 hours, 48 hours: (a) Hela cell line in vitro viability cell (MTT) test and (b) viability of L929 cell line in MTT test. Adapted with permission [21]. Copyright 2008, American Chemical Society.

extraordinary power. SiC is naturally related as hard but liable to break easily. It can transfer SiC nano-thin film onto a soft substrate so used for stretchy energy delivery and biosignal application in recent years.

12.2.2 Conducting Polymer-Based Materials for Bioelectronics

The conducting polymer contains a conjugated system that involves alternating single (σ) and double (π) bonds. The double bond which is present in the conducting polymers allows them for electron delocalization. The electronic conduction property has been increased enormously. Therefore, the conductive polymers (CPs) have allowed direct delivery of electrical, electrochemical, and electromechanical signals at the interface concerning living systems with abiotic devices. Conventional inorganic semiconductors have few limitations so to overcome these, research has focused on evolving unique materials such as conducting polymer substrate for bioelectronics to increase electrical performance. The conducting polymers like polyaniline (PANI), polypyrrole (PPy), and polyacetylene are widely engaged polymers for electrical and antimicrobial applications. An electrochemical biosensor has been developed using bacterial cellulose (BC) made up of electron transferable polyvinylaniline/polyaniline (PVAN/PANI). The electrochemical properties through BC/PVAN/PANI nanocomposites as a potent biosensor for investigation and detection of many biotic systems are shown in Figure 12.2 [22]. The electron transporting and shielding property is attributed to the three-dimensional junction-free polyaniline networks. The use of flexible PANI paper shows applications in the shielding effect [23].

12.2.3 Carbon-Based Materials for Bioelectronics

Carbon-based nanomaterials, like graphene, graphene oxide (GO), and reduced graphene oxide (rGO) added substantial consideration because of their optical, mechanical, and electrical properties. Similar to the above, carbon-based materials carbon nanotubes (CNTs) also show electrical and optical properties. Using carbon-based bioelectronics it is possible to synthesize cheap, disposable, and low-cost sensing devices. Organic or plant-based materials can be used in a platform for flexible devices. Carbon nanotubes–based field-effect transistors (CNT-FETs) were reported by the Dekker group at Delft University [24].

In addition to the above-mentioned materials, in the last decade a new family of 2D materials, MXenes (transition metal 2D carbides, nitrides, or carbonitrides), have shown prospective applications in bioelectronics. Recently, TiO_2@MXene based nanosheet/PAA hydrophilic polymer shows good non-aggregation, electron transportation, and flexible nature [25]. During this synthesis, the author has grown *in-situ* nanoscale TiO_2 on MXene shells. This leads to overcoming the nanosheets restacking and ultrafast polymerization without heating.

12.3 Methods Used for Fabrication of Bioelectronics

Due to the applicable physical, chemical, electronic and magnetic properties, nanostructure materials have appealed their candidature in various industries. One of the most

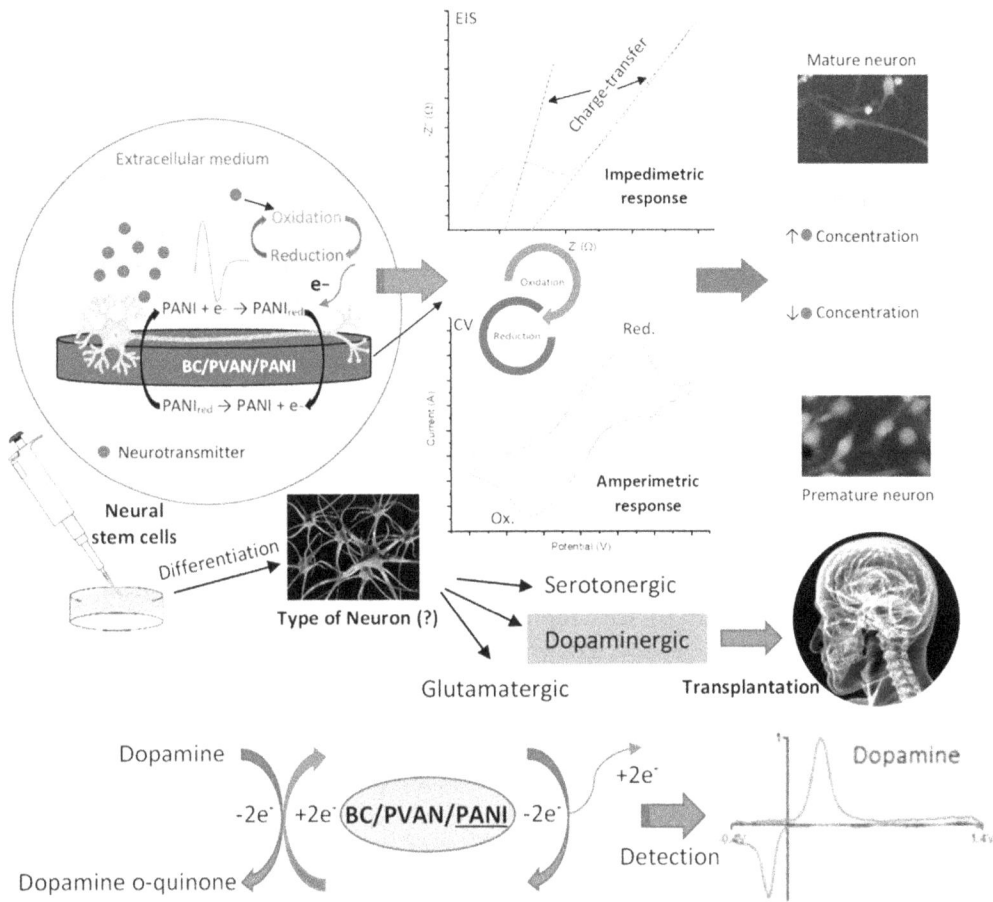

FIGURE 12.2
Dual-mode electrochemical biosensor using BC/PVAN/PANI nanocomposites Adapted with permission [22]. Copyright 2019, American Chemical Society.

important tasks for which more emphasis should be focused is the synthesis of nano-bio materials. There are many difficulties in the assembling of bio-nano materials using any process. To control the size, shapes are the main difficulties during the synthesis of the nanoscale materials. In addition, morphology, crystallinity, and distribution of the nano-scale particles are also challenges before the intellectuals.

Two harmonized methods such as top-down and bottom-up can be used for the synthesis of the nanostructured semiconductor bioelectronics. In the top-down method, bulk counterpart material is converted into nano-scale materials or by stripping down a complex entity. The top-down synthesis technique is simple and initiated with the ball milling method to obtained small-scale materials. The top-down approach is comparatively simpler than to bottom-up approach. This is indifferent to the bottom-up method, in which materials are assembled atom by atom or cluster by cluster. This approach is quite economical as it creates less waste. Some of the processes involved in the top-down approach are the thermal decomposition of organometallic precursors using the hydro-thermal and solvothermal routes. The different methods such as revere-micelle route, sol-gel, colloidal, hydrothermal, template-assisted, electrodeposition, etc. are popular.

12.3.1 Top-Down Approach

The top-down methods are popular and easy as compared to the bottom-up methods. The most common and famous top-down process used for the fabrication of the materials is a combination of photolithography and the dry/wet etching method. This method is used for the synthesis of wide bandgap (WBG) semiconducting micromaterials on a silicon substrate [20]. In addition, the electron beam lithography (EBL) or focused ion beam (FIB) is used for the nanofabrication of WBG materials. Figure 12.3 shows lift-off and negative mask surface nano-machining practices for the production the silicon carbide nanowires (NWs) and their applications in the device such as nano-electrochemical switches [26]. Another method that is similar to conventional photolithography is electron beam lithography (EBL). The drawing of the pattern with sub-10 nm resolution can be done with the help of the EBL as a top-down approach. After fabricating, the micro-nonostructures are transferred to soft platforms using the dry transfer printing process.

12.3.2 Bottom-Up Approach

In the bottom-up approach, various materials have been grown by different techniques. A few of them are listed in this section. The three-dimensional, meticulous graphene on silicon nanowire mesh pattern was reported with personalized electron transfer and absorption properties. These selected properties can be used for future applications where it is needed like sensor, energy, and bioelectronics. The growth condition during the synthesis of the graphene-like growth time and pressure of methane gives novel properties to the material [27]. Sapphire substrate has been used for the synthesis of very long self-organized GaN nano-wires with hexagonal sections. Here, the GaN was

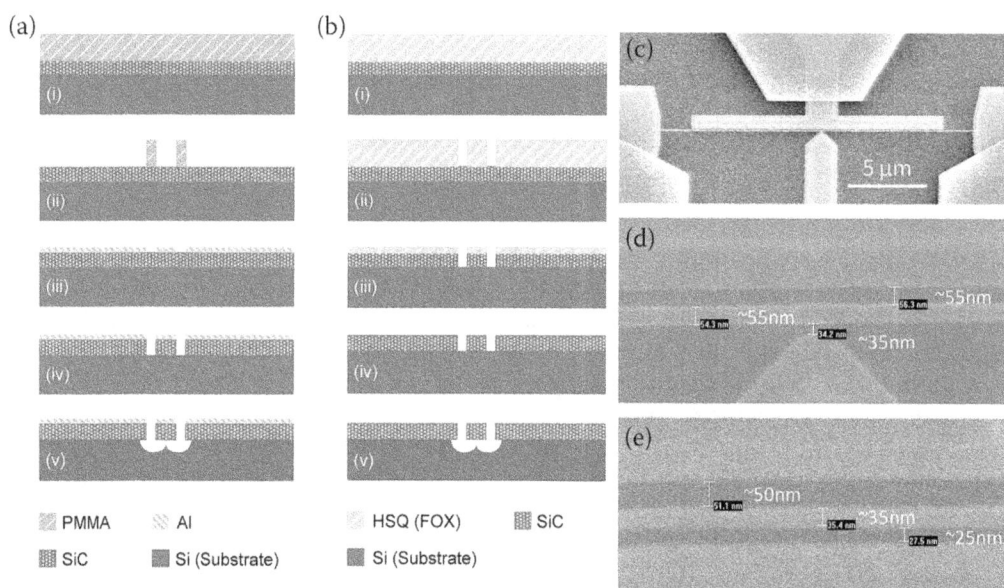

FIGURE 12.3
(a, b) SiC nanowires (NWs) lift-off and negative mask surface nano-machining processes for making the SiC NWs, (c) a 20 μm long SiC NW, (d) close-in view of the device, (e) typical nonmetallized SiC NWs and gaps achieved by the negative mask process in this work. Adapted with permission [26]. Copyright 2010. American Chemical Society.

(a) (b)

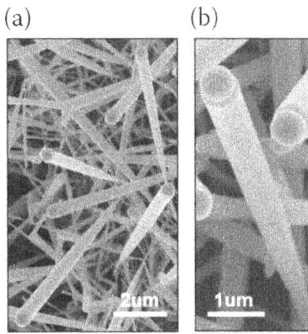

FIGURE 12.4
(a) SEM image (b) HRSEM images of the SiC nanowires obtained at 1,550°C. Adapted with permission [29]. Copyright 2008, American Chemical Society.

manufactured by the metal-organic vapor phase epitaxy (MOVPE) method [28]. Various shapes such as Eiffel-tower, spindle, and modulated nanowires have been synthesized by a new technique. This technique helps in tuning the morphology of SiC nanowires by the vapor-liquid-solid method by changing the pressure of the source species [29]. The scanning electron microscopy (SEM) and high-resolution scanning electron microscopy show uniform formation silicon carbide nanowires (Figure 12.4).

In addition to the above methods, there are several advanced methods established for the synthesis of wide bandgap semiconductor nanomaterial. The methods used like sol gel, pyrolysis, and inkjet printing are fascinating, and synthesized materials can be used for wearable and implantable bio-integrated electronics applications. Functional and geometrically complex constructions can be done with the help of 3D additive manufacturing techniques. The elementary advantages of this process are the convenience synthesis for widespread nano-crystallites, cheap, and huge manufacturing abilities. Table 12.1 lists some of the wide bandgap material, fabrication methods, properties, and their applications in bioelectronics.

12.4 Applications of Bioelectronics

12.4.1 Biosensors

Recent advancements in materials have broadened the research topics to include practical applications in clinical care, based on biology and physiology principles [8]. Wearable electronics that respond to temperature, strain, health monitoring [32,33], voice, and facial expression [34] could provide useful, real-time feedback to a centralized server [35]. A wide range of products, including smartwatches, fitness trackers, e-textiles, and even smart medical implants, have already been introduced to the market. Due to its unique capacity to detect minor stimulus changes, biological, elastic artificial skins have lately spurred interest. E-skin generates artificial tactile systems by converting physiological parameters such as stress, tension, shearing, and torque into electrical impulses [36]. Thus, e-skin could enhance wearable fitness tracking, sensory displays, prosthetics, and adaptable robotic epidermis [37,38].

Wearable sensors with low weight, outstanding mechanical and thermal capabilities, flexibility, and cost efficiency are ideal to avoid any discomfort and safeguard sensors from any damage [36]. Organic and inorganic nanomaterials with various morphologies

TABLE 12.1

Wide Bandgap Material, Fabrication Method, Properties, and Their Applications in Bioelectronics

Wide bandgap materials	Fabrication methods	Fabrication technique	Properties	Applications
II-VI	bottom-up [16].	• growth combining with transferring flexible substrates	• piezoelectric polarization • biodegradability • direct bandgap	• sensitive mechanical sensing • wearable ultraviolet (UV) photosensor
III-nitride	bottom-up [28].	• growth combining with transferring flexible substrates	• high electron mobility • chemical inertness	• sensitive mechanical sensing • long-term energy scavenger
	top-down [30].	• micro/nano- machining combined with transfer printing	• high optical transmittance	• optogenetics LED
SiC	bottom-up [29].	• growth combining with transferring flexible substrates	• chemical inertness • biocompatibility	• long-lived recording and sensing • sensitive mechanical sensing
	top-down [31].	• micro/nano- machining combined with transfer printing	• thermal and mechanical robustness	• radio frequency wireless communication devices

with elasticity and responsiveness are employed in a range of applications [39]. Biosensors based on field-effect transistors (FETs) are found useful for detecting bio-molecules. Silicon nanowires, carbon nanotubes, and graphene are examples of inorganic materials which could be used in FET substrates owing to their high surface-to-volume ratios and comparable electrical potentials of the surface and bulk [40]. One of the major challenges when using nanocomposites for FET-based biosensors is obtaining the re-quisite conformity and reproducibility. Rim et al [13]. devised a simple solution treatment approach for fabricating ultrathin, selective Indium (III) oxide (In_2O_3) semiconducting FETs with outstanding device performance and minimal mechanical stress for biological sensing applications. Two-dimensional transition metals dichalcogenides (TMDs) have attracted interest in biosensors with intriguing properties, such as a changeable bandgap and a fast heterogeneous electron-transfer (HET) rate. These materials are, under-standably, very appealing in the realm of biosensors [41].

In bioelectronics, two-dimensional ultrathin materials with softness and adaptability, like graphene, can be used. Because the graphene-based soft neural implantation has such a good elasticity, it can mitigate mechanical injury to neural cells while developing precise integration with the brain [42].

12.4.2 Wearable and Implantable Devices

As described in the preceding sections, electronics that may be worn or implanted have made significant advances in biomedical applications [1,13]. Some of these technologies are being integrated into our modern routines through gadgets such as smartwatches, bracelets, and protective clothing. In the 1960s, the first implanted cardiac pacemaker for arrhythmia patients was invented. Nevertheless, millions of patients were treated with improved pacemakers, implanted cardioverter defibrillators (ICDs), and implantable deep brain stimulators [43]. Because of the morphological disparity between those brittle, massive implanted equipment and tender muscle tissue, inadequate electrical and phy-sicochemical operations, as well as severe immunological reactions, limited their utility for extended practical purposes [10,44]. To achieve these goals, several soft-material bioelectronic devices have been proposed. Paper-thin pliable 2D composites have indeed been recognized among the materials available [20,45].

Inorganic semiconductors are a preferred option for flexible electronics because of their homogeneity, stability, exceptional electrical characteristics, and scalable manufacturing [46]. Another area of interest is to utilize the biomechanical energy of our body for self-powered wearable devices. It needs only a few electrodes that can convert the bio-mechanical energy during body moving (Figure 12.5). This technique is very simple and effective to produce biomechanical energy during the walk or exercise, which has great possibilities for being functional to self-energy wearable and implantable electronics in the forthcoming days [47].

Inorganic semiconductors could be integrated on soft and fine surfaces because of breakthroughs in transfer-printing and minimal temperature techniques, allowing structural fit between electronics and biological tissues. Initially, silicon proved to be a promising candidate for several wearable and implantable electronics, owing to their relatively minimal cost, ease of access, and conventional processing technologies [20]. Flexible silicon devices include soft wireless transmission systems based on crystalline silicons on polymeric materials with high transport mobilities [48], as well as cardiac electrophysiology recording devices [49]. The indirect bandgap, poor piezoelectric coef-ficients, rapid ionic dispersion, and biofluid disintegration of silicon, however, limit its

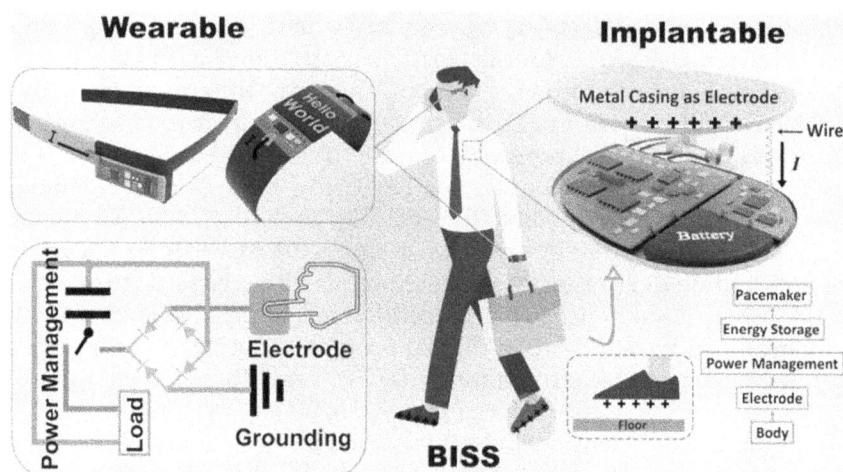

FIGURE 12.5
Self-powered system (BISS) of the human body shows the conversion of mechanical energy from the human body to electrical energy. Adapted with permission [47]. Copyright 2019, American Chemical Society.

usage in elastic photonics and soft energy scavenging component, as well as wearable and implantable technologies [50]. As a result, wide bandgap materials (with a bandgap of 2.2 electron volts (eV) or higher) have become a promising alternative for overcoming silicon's limitations. Flexible wide bandgap semiconductors for wearable and implantable electronics have outstanding features, such as chemical inertness, better electrical qualities at elevated temperatures, rapid saturation drifting velocity, and high breakdown voltages [49]. Moreover, tremendous progress has been made in micro electromechanical system (MEMS) technology for transferring wide bandgap materials onto polymer surfaces and forming functioning sensors within the last several years. These flexible wide bandgap materials are successfully used in enduring electronics, power harvesters, biodegradable wearable, and implantable devices [20]. Zinc oxide (ZnO) is among the most often explored II-VI molecules in optoelectronics with direct bandgap (3.4 eV) and large electron-hole binding energy (60 meV). This establishes the suitability of these materials as LEDs and ultra-violet photodetectors [51]. The direct energy bandgap in ZnO nanowires was paired with the significant optical absorption to create photodetectors with excellent photon efficiency. For the ultraviolet light spectrum, the photodetector based on ZnO nanowires exhibited better sensitivity and remarkable frequency specificity [52]. Wearable and implantable physiological applications demand benign materials. The ZnO nanowires were shown to be biocompatible by the Hela cells' 95% survival after 48 hours of cultivation with it [21]. III-nitrite is an area of excellence for logical circuits in biomedical applications because of its nontoxicity and biocompatibility, as well as the flexibility of its electronics [53]. Graphene's unique properties, including softness, flexibility, transparency, ease of functionalization, and biocompatibility, make it one of the most fascinating 2D materials [1,54–56]. Because of its deformability and transparency, it has been used to create innovative nervous system probes for optogenetics [57] and "smart" endoscopes for cancer detection [58]. MoS_2 has a fine thickness, excellent photoabsorption, and piezoresistivity; consequently, it might be used in a high-density curved image sensor array for a soft retinal prosthesis and very thin wearable tactile sensors [59]. GaN's long-term stability, in addition to its biocompatibility, is a great component for wearable and implanted devices [60].

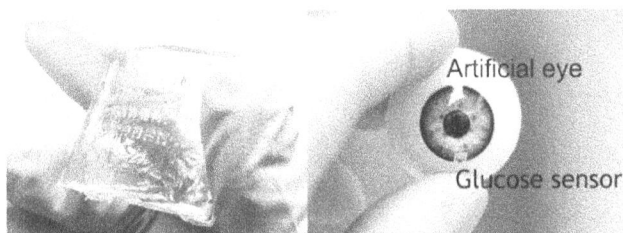

FIGURE 12.6
In$_2$O$_3$-based conformal biosensors based on field-effect transistors. Adapted with permission from [70]. Copyright 2015. American Chemical Society.

12.4.3 Printable/Flexible Bioelectronics

The production of printable electrical devices on plastic foils or paper is a rapidly expanding area of study that has contributed to improving scientific and technological curiosity in recent years. Flexible actuators provide various advantages, including light weight, foldability, and wearability. When compared to wafer-based microelectronics, the printing technique offers great ability to drastically lower fabrication costs. It also has the potential to expand the usage of bio-sensing equipment in a range of applications to enhance people's living standards. Solution processing methods or printable electronics are being used in elastic, adaptive, economical, degradable drug-delivery electronic patches, and surgical implants. Hence, printable thin-film transistors (TFTs) [61]. Recently progressed into greater sensors and biomedical implant frameworks for bio-interface research. There is a range of organic and inorganic semiconductor materials suitable for use as active channels in TFT devices that can be printed or solution treated. Pentacene, silicon nanowires, zinc oxide, and graphene are among the materials being used [62,63].

Due to its superior physical and optical properties, comparable stability in the atmosphere, and suitability with numerous printing methodologies to establish semiconducting thin films, carbon nanotubes (CNTs) demonstrated growing potential among the many printable electronic materials which are already been explored. With these appealing properties, printed CNT thin films hold promise for applications such as sensors and display backplanes [64]. Because of their enhanced electronic performances, stability, and dependability, chalcogenide compounds, nanoparticles, and a range of oxides of metals can be solution-processed or printed [46].

. The inorganic compounds can be directly printed or deposited with a precursor solution upon subsequent treatment. Inorganic materials have already been printed using an array of printing processes, including liquid embossed, inkjet, lasers, and e-beam mapping [65–69]. Another application of semiconductors, such as In$_2$O$_3$-based FET biosensors, facilitated pH and glucose detection (Figure 12.6). This could be possible in real time with linear and ultra-fast detection [70].

12.5 Conclusions and Future Perspectives

Bioelectronics research efforts involve biological sciences, physics, applied physics, chemistry, and materials science, with a focus on topics that attempt to use electronics knowledge and execution in the realms of biology and medicine for human welfare. Thus, bioelectronic research covers a broad array of topics, such as biosensors, machine intelligence in healthcare, signal receiving devices for chronic diseases, wearable gadgets, and many more applications.

Semiconductor nanostructured materials are a unique group of materials that could be used to yield high-performance electronics and optoelectronics. Bioelectronics has been transformed the technology from a hard and huge shape to a flexible and small format with astounding properties because of breakthroughs in nanocomposite materials. Aside from this progress, there are still many practical hurdles to overcome. Bioelectronics devices with material designing have high efficiency and flexibility, but the long-lasting durability of the nanoscale active layer is still missing, particularly in humid conditions. To address this issue, soft encapsulating components and coating methods are necessary.

There is still plenty of room for wide bandgap materials to be used in implanted device performances. Biocompatibility, safety, and signal-receiving and stimulating systems, on the other hand, require additional consideration. Advanced technologies for efficient and cost-effective mass manufacture are required to bring nanomaterial-based commodities, to the marketplace. Bioelectronic discoveries that include perspectives from a variety of fields have substantial opportunities. Meaningful collaborative efforts between chemists, material researchers, technology developers, and therapists would help to take nanomaterial-based bioelectronics closer to therapeutic strategies and, also ultimately, to address a range of concerns.

References

1. C. Choi, Y. Lee, K.W. Cho, J.H. Koo, D.H. Kim, Wearable and implantable soft bioelectronics using two-dimensional materials, *Acc. Chem. Res.* 52 (2019) 73–81.
2. Y. Fang, L. Meng, A. Prominski, E.N. Schaumann, M. Seebald, B. Tian, Recent advances in bioelectronics chemistry, *Chem. Soc. Rev.* 49 (2020) 7978–8035.
3. J. Ge, L. Sun, F.-R. Zhang, Y. Zhang, L. Shi, H. Zhao, H. Zhu, H.-L. Jiang, S.-H. Yu, A Stretchable electronic fabric artificial skin with pressure-, lateral strain-, and flexion-sensitive properties, *Adv. Mater.* 28 (2016) 722–728.
4. S.K. Rastogi, A. Kalmykov, N. Johnson, T. Cohen-Karni, Bioelectronics with nanocarbons, *J. Mater. Chem. B.* 6 (2018) 7159–7178.
5. M.E. Spira, A. Hai, Neuroscience and cardiology, *Nat. Nanotechnol.* 8 (2013) 83–94.
6. S.F. Cogan, Neural stimulation and recording electrodes, *Annu. Rev. Biomed. Eng.* 10 (2008) 275–309.
7. D. San Roman, R. Garg, T. Cohen-Karni, Bioelectronics with graphene nanostructures, *APL Mater.* 8 (2020) 100906.
8. G. Yao, C. Yin, Q. Wang, T. Zhang, S. Chen, C. Lu, K. Zhao, W. Xu, T. Pan, M. Gao, Y. Lin, Flexible bioelectronics for physiological signals sensing and disease treatment, *J. Mater.* 6 (2020) 397–413.
9. D. Dias, J.P.S. Cunha, Wearable health devices—Vital sign monitoring, systems and technologies, *Sensors (Switzerland).* 18 (2018) 2414.
10. W.B. Han, G.J. Ko, T.M. Jang, S.W. Hwang, Materials, devices, and applications for wearable and implantable electronics, *ACS Appl. Electron. Mater.* 3 (2021) 485–503.
11. P. Kang, M.C. Wang, S. Nam, Bioelectronics with two-dimensional materials, *Microelectron. Eng.* 161 (2016) 18–35.

12. R. Rauti, M. Musto, S. Bosi, M. Prato, L. Ballerini, Properties and behavior of carbon nano-materials when interfacing neuronal cells: How far have we come?, *Carbon N. Y.* 143 (2019) 430–446.

13. H. Lee, T.K. Choi, Y.B. Lee, H.R. Cho, R. Ghaffari, L. Wang, H.J. Choi, T.D. Chung, N. Lu, T. Hyeon, S.H. Choi, D.-H. Kim, A graphene-based electrochemical device with thermo-responsive microneedles for diabetes monitoring and therapy, *Nat. Nanotechnol.* 11 (2016) 566–572.

14. B. Cho, M.G. Hahm, M. Choi, J. Yoon, A.R. Kim, Y.J. Lee, S.G. Park, J.D. Kwon, C.S. Kim, M. Song, Y. Jeong, K.S. Nam, S. Lee, T.J. Yoo, C.G. Kang, B.H. Lee, H.C. Ko, P.M. Ajayan, D.H. Kim, Charge-transfer-based gas sensing using atomic-layer MoS2, *Sci. Rep.* 5 (2015) 8052.

15. J. Jo, S. Kang, J.S. Heo, Y. Kim, S.K. Park, Flexible metal oxide semiconductor devices made by solution methods, *Chem. – A Eur. J.* 26 (2020) 9126–9156.

16. C. Dagdeviren, S.W. Hwang, Y. Su, S. Kim, H. Cheng, O. Gur, R. Haney, F.G. Omenetto, Y. Huang, J.A. Rogers, Transient, biocompatible electronics and energy harvesters based on ZnO, *Small.* 9 (2013) 3398–3404.

17. M. Pumera, A.H. Loo, And biosensing, *Trends Anal. Chem.* 61 (2014) 49–53.

18. Y.H. Joung, Development of implantable medical devices: From an engineering perspective, *Int. Neurourol. J.* 17 (2013) 98–106.

19. H.-P. Phan, Implanted flexible electronics: Set device lifetime with smart nanomaterials, *Micromachines.* 12 (2021) 157.

20. N.K. Nguyen, T. Nguyen, T.K. Nguyen, S. Yadav, T. Dinh, M.K. Masud, P. Singha, T.N. Do, M.J. Barton, H.T. Ta, N. Kashaninejad, C.H. Ooi, N.T. Nguyen, H.P. Phan, Wide-band-gap semiconductors for biointegrated electronics: Recent advances and future directions, *ACS Appl. Electron. Mater.* 3 (2021) 1959–1981.

21. Z. Li, R. Yang, M. Yu, F. Bai, C. Li, Z.L. Wang, Cellular level biocompatibility and biosafety of ZnO nanowires, *J. Phys. Chem. C.* 112 (2008) 20114–20117.

22. A.R. Rebelo, C. Liu, K.H. Schäfer, M. Saumer, G. Yang, Y. Liu, Poly(4-vinylaniline)/polyaniline bilayer-Functionalized bacterial cellulose for flexible electrochemical bio-sensors, *Langmuir.* 35 (2019) 10354–10366.

23. Y. Zhang, T. Pan, Z. Yang, Flexible polyethylene terephthalate/polyaniline composite paper with bending durability and effective electromagnetic shielding performance, *Chem. Eng. J.* 389 (2020) 124433.

24. S.J. Tans, A.R.M. Verschueren, C. Dekker, Room-temperature transistor based on a single carbon nanotube, *Nature.* 393 (1998) 49–52.

25. Q. Wang, X. Pan, C. Lin, H. Gao, S. Cao, Y. Ni, X. Ma, Modified Ti_3C_2TX (MXene) nanosheet-catalyzed self-assembled, anti-aggregated, ultra-stretchable, conductive hydrogels for wearable bioelectronics, *Chem. Eng. J.* 401 (2020) 126129.

26. X.L. Feng, M.H. Matheny, C.A. Zorman, M. Mehregany, M.L. Roukes, Low voltage nanoe-lectromechanical switches based on silicon carbide nanowires, *Nano Lett.* 10 (2010) 2891–2896.

27. R. Garg, S.K. Rastogi, M. Lamparski, S.C. De La Barrera, G.T. Pace, N.T. Nuhfer, B.M. Hunt, V. Meunier, T. Cohen-Karni, Nanowire-mesh-templated growth of out-of-plane three-dimensional fuzzy graphene, *ACS Nano.* 11 (2017) 6301–6311.

28. S. Salomon, J. Eymery, E. Pauliac-Vaujour, GaN wire-based Langmuir–Blodgett films for self-powered flexible strain sensors, *Nanotechnology.* 25 (2014) 375502.

29. H. Wang, Z. Xie, W. Yang, J. Fang, L. An, Morphology control in the vapor-liquid-solid growth of SiC nanowires, *Cryst. Growth Des.* 8 (2008) 3893–3896.

30. J.-H. Ahn, H.-S. Kim, K.J. Lee, S. Jeon, S.J. Kang, Y. Sun, R.G. Nuzzo, J.A. Rogers, Heterogeneous three-dimensional electronics by use of printed semiconductor nanomater-ials, *Science .* 314 (80) (2006) 1754–1757.

31. H.P. Phan, T. Dinh, T. Kozeki, T.K. Nguyen, A. Qamar, T. Namazu, N.T. Nguyen, D.V. Dao, The Piezoresistive effect in top-down fabricated p-type 3C-SiC nanowires, *IEEE Electron Device Lett.* 37 (2016) 1029–1032.

32. S.Y. Hong, Y.H. Lee, H. Park, S.W. Jin, Y.R. Jeong, J. Yun, I. You, G. Zi, J.S. Ha, Stretchable active matrix temperature sensor array of polyaniline nanofibers for electronic skin, *Adv. Mater.* 28 (2016) 930–935.
33. T.Q. Trung, N.E. Lee, Flexible and stretchable physical sensor integrated platforms for wearable human-activity monitoringand personal healthcare, *Adv. Mater.* 28 (2016) 4338–4372.
34. M. Su, F. Li, S. Chen, Z. Huang, M. Qin, W. Li, X. Zhang, Y. Song, Nanoparticle based curve arrays for multirecognition flexible electronics, *Adv. Mater.* 28 (2016) 1369–1374.
35. W.A.D.M. Jayathilaka, K. Qi, Y. Qin, A. Chinnappan, W. Serrano-García, C. Baskar, H. Wang, J. He, S. Cui, S.W. Thomas, S. Ramakrishna, Significance of nanomaterials in wearables: A review on wearable actuators and sensors, *Adv. Mater.* 31 (2019) 1–21.
36. S.Y. Kim, S. Park, H.W. Park, D.H. Park, Y. Jeong, D.H. Kim, Highly sensitive and multi-modal all-carbon skin sensors capable of simultaneously detecting tactile and biological stimuli, *Adv. Mater.* 27 (2015) 4178–4185.
37. D.H. Kim, J.A. Rogers, Stretchable electronics: Materials strategies and devices, *Adv. Mater.* 20 (2008) 4887–4892.
38. S. Baek, H. Jang, S.Y. Kim, H. Jeong, S. Han, Y. Jang, D.H. Kim, H.S. Lee, Flexible piezo-capacitive sensors based on wrinkled microstructures: Toward low-cost fabrication of pressure sensors over large areas, *RSC Adv.* 7 (2017) 39420–39426.
39. M. Ha, J. Park, Y. Lee, H. Ko, Triboelectric generators and sensors for self-powered wearable electronics, *ACS Nano.* 9 (2015) 3421–3427.
40. G.L. Biosensors, D. Sarkar, W. Liu, X. Xie, A.C. Anselmo, S. Mitragotri, K. Banerjee, MoS2 field-effect transistor for next-, *ACS Nano.* 8(2014) 3992–4003.
41. E. Rahmanian, C.C. Mayorga-Martinez, R. Malekfar, J. Luxa, Z. Sofer, M. Pumera, 1T-phase tungsten chalcogenides (WS2, WSe2, WTe2) decorated with TiO2 nanoplatelets with enhanced electron transfer activity for Biosensing applications, *ACS Appl., Nano Mater.* 1 (2018) 7006–7015.
42. D.-W. Park, A.A. Schendel, S. Mikael, S.K. Brodnick, T.J. Richner, J.P. Ness, M.R. Hayat, F. Atry, S.T. Frye, R. Pashaie, S. Thongpang, Z. Ma, J.C. Williams, Graphene-based carbon-layered electrode array technology for neural imaging and optogenetic applications, *Nat. Commun.* 5 (2014) 5258.
43. M.K. Lyons, Deep brain stimulation: Current and future clinical applications, *Mayo Clin. Proc.* 86 (2011) 662–672.
44. R. Chen, A. Canales, P. Anikeeva, Neural recording and modulation technologies, *Nat. Rev. Mater.* 2 (2017) 1–16.
45. I.R. Minev, P. Musienko, A. Hirsch, Q. Barraud, N. Wenger, E.M. Moraud, J. Gandar, M. Capogrosso, T. Milekovic, L. Asboth, R.F. Torres, N. Vachicouras, Q. Liu, N. Pavlova, S. Duis, A. Larmagnac, J. Vörös, S. Micera, Z. Suo, G. Courtine, S.P. Lacour, Electronic dura mater for long-term multimodal neural interfaces, *Science.* 347(80) (2015) 159–163.
46. Y. Sun, J.A. Rogers, Inorganic semiconductors for flexible electronics, *Adv. Mater.* 19 (2007) 1897–1916.
47. B. Shi, Z. Liu, Q. Zheng, J. Meng, H. Ouyang, Y. Zou, D. Jiang, X. Qu, M. Yu, L. Zhao, Y. Fan, Z.L. Wang, Z. Li, Body-integrated self-powered system for wearable and implantable applications, *ACS Nano.* 13 (2019) 6017–6024.
48. K. Zhang, J.H. Seo, W. Zhou, Z. Ma, Fast flexible electronics using transferrable silicon nanomembranes, *J. Phys. D. Appl. Phys.* 45 (2012) 143001.
49. H.P. Phan, Y. Zhong, T.K. Nguyen, Y. Park, T. Dinh, E. Song, R.K. Vadivelu, M.K. Masud, J. Li, M.J.A. Shiddiky, D. Dao, Y. Yamauchi, J.A. Rogers, N.T. Nguyen, Long-lived, transferred crystalline silicon carbide nanomembranes for implantable flexible electronics, *ACS Nano.* 13 (2019) 11572–11581.
50. J. Millan, P. Godignon, X. Perpina, A. Perez-Tomas, J. Rebollo, A survey of wide bandgap power semiconductor devices, *IEEE Trans. Power Electron.* 29 (2014) 2155–2163.
51. D. Vogel, P. Kriiger, J. Pollmann, electronic-structure calculations for, Ab initio electronic-structure calculations for II-VI semiconductors using self-interaction-corrected pseudopotentials, *Phys. Rev.* 52 (1995) 316–319.

52. B.H. Kind, H. Yan, B. Messer, M. Law, P. Yang, Nanowire ultraviolet photodetectors and optical, 14(2002) 200–202.
53. S. Linkohr, S. Schwarz, S. Krischok, P. Lorenz, V. Cimalla, C. Nebel, O. Ambacher, DNA-sensor based on AlGaN/GaN high electron mobility transistor, 1813 (2010) 1810–1813.
54. S.J. Kim, K.W. Cho, H.R. Cho, L. Wang, S.Y. Park, S.E. Lee, T. Hyeon, N. Lu, S.H. Choi, D. Kim, Stretchable and transparent biointerface using cell-sheet – Graphene hybrid for electrophysiology and therapy of skeletal muscle, *Adv. Functional Mat.* 26(2016) 3207–3217.
55. S.J. Kim, H.R. Cho, K.W. Cho, S. Qiao, J.S. Rhim, M. Soh, T. Kim, M.K. Choi, C. Choi, I. Park, N.S. Hwang, T. Hyeon, S.H. Choi, N. Lu, D.-H. Kim, Multifunctional cell-culture platform for aligned cell sheet monitoring, transfer printing, and therapy, *ACS Nano.* 9 (2015) 2677–2688.
56. D. Kuzum, H. Takano, E. Shim, J.C. Reed, H. Juul, A.G. Richardson, J. de Vries, H. Bink, M.A. Dichter, T.H. Lucas, D.A. Coulter, E. Cubukcu, B. Litt, Transparent and flexible low noise graphene electrodes for simultaneous electrophysiology and neuroimaging, *Nat. Commun.* 5 (2014) 5259.
57. D. Park, A.A. Schendel, S. Mikael, S.K. Brodnick, T.J. Richner, J.P. Ness, M.R. Hayat, F. Atry, S.T. Frye, R. Pashaie, S. Thongpang, Z. Ma, J.C. Williams. Graphene-based carbon-layered electrode array technology for neural imaging and optogenetic application, *Nat. Commun.* 5(2014) 5258.
58. H. Lee, Y. Lee, C. Song, H.R. Cho, R. Ghaffari, T.K. Choi, K.H. Kim, Y.B. Lee, D. Ling, H. Lee, S.J. Yu, S.H. Choi, T. Hyeon, D.H. Kim, An endoscope with integrated transparent bioelectronics and theranostic nanoparticles for colon cancer treatment, *Nat. Commun.* 6 (2015) 10059.
59. C. Choi, M.K. Choi, S. Liu, M.S. Kim, O.K. Park, C. Im, J. Kim, X. Qin, G.J. Lee, K.W. Cho, M. Kim, E. Joh, J. Lee, D. Son, S.-H. Kwon, N.L. Jeon, Y.M. Song, N. Lu, D.-H. Kim, Human eye-inspired soft optoelectronic device using high-density MoS2-graphene curved image sensor array, *Nat. Commun.* 8 (2017) 1664.
60. H.E. Lee, J. Choi, S.H. Lee, M. Jeong, J.H. Shin, D.J. Joe, D. Kim, C.W. Kim, J.H. Park, J.H. Lee, D. Kim, C. Shin, K.J. Lee, Monolithic flexible vertical GaN light-emitting diodes for a transparent wireless brain optical stimulator, *Adv. Mat.* 1800649 (2018) 1–10.
61. M. Magliulo, M.Y. Mulla, M. Singh, E. Macchia, A. Tiwari, L. Torsi, K. Manoli, Printable and flexible electronics: From TFTs to bioelectronic devices, *J. Mater. Chem. C.* 3 (2015) 12347–12363.
62. A.C. Arias, J.D. MacKenzie, I. McCulloch, J. Rivnay, A. Salleo, Materials and applications for large area electronics: Solution-based approaches, *Chem. Rev.* 110 (2010) 3–24.
63. B.Z. Fan, J.C. Ho, T. Takahashi, R. Yerushalmi, K. Takei, A.C. Ford, Y. Chueh, A. Javey, Toward the development of printable nanowire electronics and sensors, *Adv. Mat.* 21 (2009) 3730–3743.
64. S. Lu, A.D. Franklin, Printed carbon nanotube thin-film transistors: Progress on printable materials and the path to applications, *Nanoscale.* 12 (2020) 23371–23390.
65. E.J. Wilhelm, J.M. Jacobson, E.J. Wilhelm, J.M. Jacobson, Direct printing of nanoparticles and spin-on-glasses by offset liquid embossing, *Appl. Phys. Lett.* 3507 (2012) 10–13.
66. E.J. Wilhelm, B.T. Neltner, J.M. Jacobson, E.J. Wilhelm, B.T. Neltner, J.M. Jacobson, Nanoparticle-based microelectromechanical systems fabricated on plastic, *Appl. Phys. Lett.* 6424 (2014) 75–78.
67. S. Griffith, M. Mondol, D.S. Kong, J.M. Jacobson, S. Griffith, M. Mondol, Nanostructure fabrication by direct electron-beam writing of nanoparticles, *J. Vac. Sci. Technol. B* 2768 (2014) 1–6.
68. F. Patolsky, G. Zheng, C.M. Lieber, Fabrication of silicon nanowire devices for ultrasensitive, label-free, real-time detection of biological and chemical species, *Nat. Protoc.* 1 (2006) 1711–1724.
69. D.-H. Kim, N. Lu, R. Ghaffari, J.A. Rogers, Inorganic semiconductor nanomaterials for flexible and stretchable bio-integrated electronics, *NPG Asia Mater.* 4 (2012) e15–e15.
70. Y.S. Rim, S.H. Bae, H. Chen, J.L. Yang, J. Kim, A.M. Andrews, P.S. Weiss, Y. Yang, H.R. Tseng, Printable ultrathin metal oxide semiconductor-based conformal biosensors, *ACS Nano.* 9 (2015) 12174–12181.

13

Wide Bandgap Semiconductors for Bioelectronics

Giovana A. Parolin, Alessandra S. Menandro, Rebeca R. Rodrigues, and Laura O. Péres
Laboratory of Hybrid Materials, Institute of Environmental, Chemical, and Pharmaceutical Sciences, Federal University of São Paulo, São Paulo, Brazil

CONTENTS

13.1 Introduction

Wide bandgap (WBG) semiconductors are defined as materials owing a bandgap substantially in excess, which is greater than 2.2 eV, emerging as efficient materials for applications in high-performance optoelectronic and electronic devices. The interest of researchers in WBG compounds has been growing since the late 1980s, resulting in the inclusion of materials with hexagonal and orthorhombic structures in the range of semiconductors. WBG semiconductors could be classified mainly into three families' compounds, the II VI materials, III nitride, and SiC, including all their alloys. Among these classes, the ZnO, GaN, 4H-SiC, 3C-SiC, and diamond are the most commonly studied materials for applications since wearable and implantable devices to high-power and high-temperature electronics.

Besides the electrical and optoelectronic properties, these materials also can show biocompatibility and biodegradability, making the WBG semiconductors convenient for applications in bioelectronics. Beyond the property of emitting short wavelengths, the wide bandgap also results in a higher electric breakdown field, allowing applications in power devices supported by a high breakdown field. Due to the direct bandgap in the green and blue wavelength range, some WBG materials are suitable for optogenetic applications and wearable UV photosensors. In the electronic context, the spontaneous and piezoelectric polarization of WBG materials results in efficient mechanical sensors, and the high electron mobility makes them affordable for logical circuits in biomedical applications. Several compounds also show chemical inertness and stability due to strong covalent bonds, being useful for long-lived recording and sensing. Additionally, these semiconductors can grow or be transferred into flexible and biocompatible substrates, making it easier for the preparation of WBG materials for wearable and implantable devices.

Understanding the structural and physical properties of WBG semiconductors is a requirement to apply them in bioelectronics. In this chapter, fundamental concepts will be presented and how the crystal structure of each family compound will define the main properties. Different methodologies for the preparation of WBG-based materials will change the properties of the final device. Therefore, choosing an adequate method to prepare these materials is essential to obtain efficient devices, depending on the application. This chapter will show diverse methodologies to grow WBG compounds and the main applications of these materials in several bioelectronics devices.

13.2 Classes of Wide Bandgap Semiconductors

The main groups of wide bandgap semiconductors are II VI, III nitride, and SiC, which have attracted the attention of several researchers for the use of these materials in bioelectronics. The crystalline structure of these compounds is an important factor for determining the physical properties of semiconductor materials. This section will provide you with the general and fundamental structural properties of each material family, which enables their implantable and wearable applications.

13.2.1 II–VI Materials

In this class of WBG semiconductors, the compounds are formed by metal from the group II_A or II_B with a chalcogenide element (group-VI) [1], and they are widely applied in several optoelectronic devices, such as light-emitting diodes (LEDs) and laser diodes [1,2]. The binary semiconductor compounds with bivalent metal chalcogenides ($M^{2+}X^2$, where typically M = Zn, Cd, Be, Mg, and X = O, S, Se, Te) are the simplest class of WBG chalcogenides and the most common for electronic applications [1]. One of the most typical II VI semiconductors is zinc oxide (ZnO), which has been largely studied for flexible electronics due to good optical transparency, piezoelectricity, direct energy bandgap, excellent electron mobility, and the possibility to synthesize into different nanoarchitectures [2,3]. Another common semiconductor of this class is the CdS, which have been widely studied for optoelectronic applications, due to their low direct energy bandgap, piezoelectricity, and long charge carrier diffusion length [1].

The II VI compounds can crystallize in wurtzite (WZ), zinc blende (ZB), rock salt (RS), or nickeline (NC) structures (Figure 13.1) with typical space groups of $P6_3mc$, $F\bar{4}3m$, $Fm\bar{3}m$, and $P6_3/mmc$, respectively [1]. The WZ and NC will have a hexagonal close-packed structure, while the cubic closed packing is observed in ZB and RS. These structures will also have different cation coordination, which is tetrahedral in WZ and ZB, and octahedral in RS and NC. Most II VI compounds are either WZ or ZB, and the structures are associated with attractive piezoelectric properties due to central asymmetry [2,3].

Although commonly an sp^3 covalent bonding is observed in structures with tetrahedral coordination, these WBG semiconductors have substantial ionic character [3]. The p valence energies tend to increase going down group VI (O – 2p, S – 3p, Se – 4p, Te – 5p), while the ionicity tends to decrease. From the molecular orbital theory, when the orbitals have similar energies they are more likely to hybridize. Additionally, the tetrahedral coordination observed for most II VI compounds allows the hybridization of the orbitals p and d [5]. Therefore, going down group VI, there is a greater p-d orbital overlap and the hybridization becomes stronger, increasing the covalency of the M-X bond and the delocalization of valence bands [1]. As a consequence of the p-d hybridization, there is the reduction of the direct bandgap (see below Section 13.3 – Table 13.1) turning these materials strong candidates to optoelectronic devices [5].

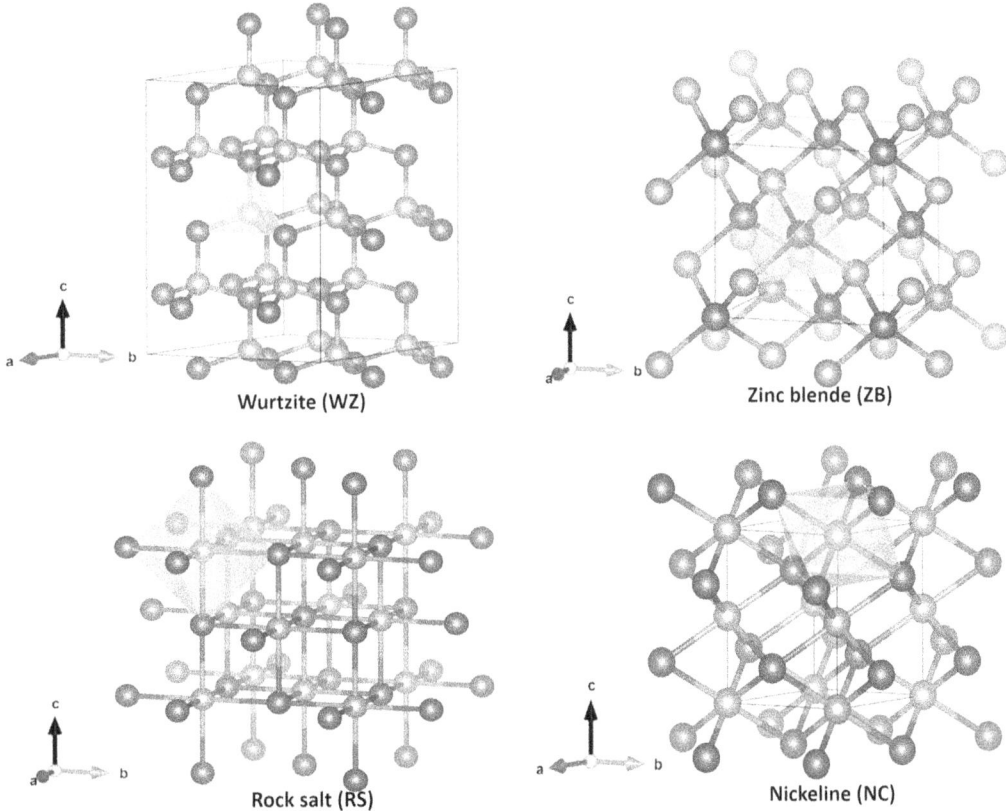

FIGURE 13.1
Crystal structures found in common WBG materials. Structures drawn using VESTA software [4].

TABLE 13.1

Typical Properties of Common WBG Semiconductors from Each Family [1,2,6–12]

	II–VI family		III-nitride family			SiC family		
	ZnO	CdS	AlN	GaN	InN	3C-SiC	4H-SiC	6H-SiC
Bandgap (eV)	3.37	2.50	6.20	3.40	0.70	2.36	3.26	3.02
Melting point (°C)	1,975	1,750 (100 atm)	3,000	2,500	1,100	2,830	2,830	2,830
Breakdown electric field (MV/cm)	4.0	1.0–2.5	1.8	5.0	–	1.2	2.0	2.4
Electron mobility ($cm^2\ V^{-1}\ s^{-1}$)	210	210	300	1,000	3,200	1,000	1,000	450
Thermal conductivity ($W\ cm^{-1} K^{-1}$)	0.6–1.16	0.2	2.5	2.27	1.2	4.5	4.5	4.5

13.2.2 III–Nitride

The group III-nitride compounds belong to group III–V compound semiconductors, and the more common materials include AlN, GaN, InN, and their alloys. The high structural quality, flexibility, spontaneous and piezoelectric polarization, direct bandgap, and good biocompatibility of III-nitride compounds increased the interest for applications in wearable UV detectors and biosensing. Additionally, the III-nitride compounds exhibit considerable bond energies of 2.28 eV for AlN, 2.2 eV for GaN, 1.93 eV for InN [13], resulting in a high melting point, greater chemical stability, and good mechanical strength.

The III-nitride semiconductors can crystallize in the thermodynamically stable WZ, and the ZB structure is metastable [13]. For all the three compounds, although the WZ phase is energetically favorable, the calculated energy difference between the WZ and ZB is small [14]. At high pressures, the crystal RS structure can be formed from the WZ phase, and in this process, the covalent bond character changes to ionic [14].

The polarizations present in a structure will have direct effects on the optical and electrical properties of the materials. In the III-nitrides, besides their piezoelectric properties (where a strain is required), the central asymmetry and the significant ionicity of III-N bonds result in spontaneous polarization (polarization at zero strain) along the c-axis ([0001] – the axis that is perpendicular to the hexagonal layers) [14]. Additionally, the crystal structure of these materials also exhibits crystallographic polarity, and the choice of the correct plane polarity is essential depending on the desired property of the material. A [0001] plane when terminated by group III atoms is denominated by c-plane, while a [000$\bar{1}$] plane terminated by nitrogen atoms is denominated by N-polar, and both of them are polar planes. The c-plane structure results in high electron mobility (see Section 13.3 – Table 13.1), and it is commonly applied in electronic devices, such as heterojunction field-effect transistors (HFETs) [2]. Although the c-plane in WZ of nitrides is more common, the literature showed greater optical efficiency in structures with nonpolar or semipolar planes, enabling LED applications [15]. The *m*-plane (or [10$\bar{1}$0] plane) and *a*-plane (or [11$\bar{2}$0] plane) are nonpolar, while the other planes are semipolar (Figure 13.2), and in these cases, the internal electric field under the planes is induced by the reduction of the polarization.

13.2.3 Silicon Carbide – SiC

Formed by earth-abundant elements, silicon carbide compounds are a very well-known class of wide-band-gap semiconductors due to their unique physical and chemical

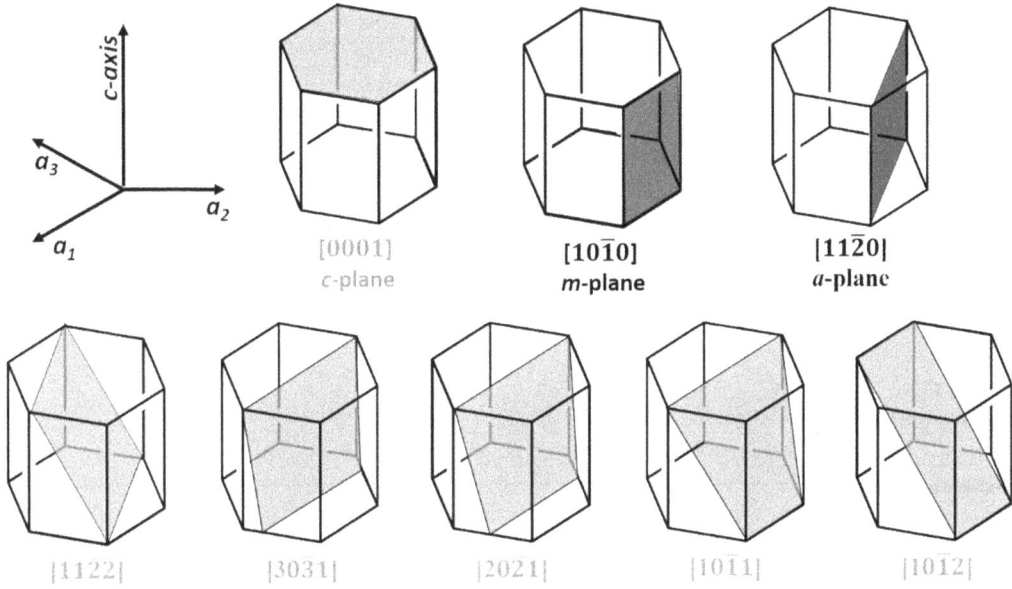

FIGURE 13.2
The different polar, nonpolar , and semipolar plane orientations.

properties, which overcomes silicon materials for applications in high-power and high-temperature electronics [16]. Compared to silicon, SiC has three times the thermal conductivity, ten times the critical electric field strength, and three times the bandgap [16]. Additionally, SiC exhibits a short bond length of 1.89 Å for Si-C bond, which is 88% covalent and 12% ionic [6]. These strong bonds give the SiC materials high chemical inertness, hardness, thermal conductivity, and critical electric field strength, enabling applications in extreme environments (see main properties at Section 13.3 – Table 13.1). The stability and oxidation tolerance of SiC allows it to work at an elevated temperature up to 600°C, being useful for applications in piezoresistive and thermoresistive sensors and long-term implantation.

Silicon carbide has over 250 polytypes of crystalline structures that will change depending on the stacking sequence of the tetrahedrally bonded Si-C bilayers [2]. Each Si-C bilayer is composed of two coupled planar sheets, one of the silicon atoms and another of carbon atoms, and this bilayer is the basal plane in direction of the c-axis. The SiC bilayer planes can be stacked to form either a ZB (cubic) or WZ (hexagonal) crystal structures, and they will have two polar planes referred to as Si-plane and C-plane. A common polytype with cubic structure is the 3C-SiC, also known as β-SiC, and it will have a stacking of three bilayer periodicities (Figure 13.3) [17]. The family of polytypes with WZ (hexagonal) crystal structure is referred to as α-SiC, and it includes polytypes with purely hexagonal structure or mixtures of cubic and hexagonal structures. The pure wurtzite polytype is the 2H-SiC with a stacking periodicity of two bilayers [17]. The common compounds 4H-SiC and 6H-SiC (Figure 13.3) have in their structure a portion of cubic elements; however, the overall is hexagonal crystal symmetry. The 4H-SiC is composed of an equal proportion of cubic and hexagonal bonds, while 6H-SiC for two-thirds of cubic bonds, and each compound will have four and six bilayers stacking periodicity, respectively [17]. Additionally, the silicon carbide can also form rhombohedral structures, the 15R- and 21R-SiC.

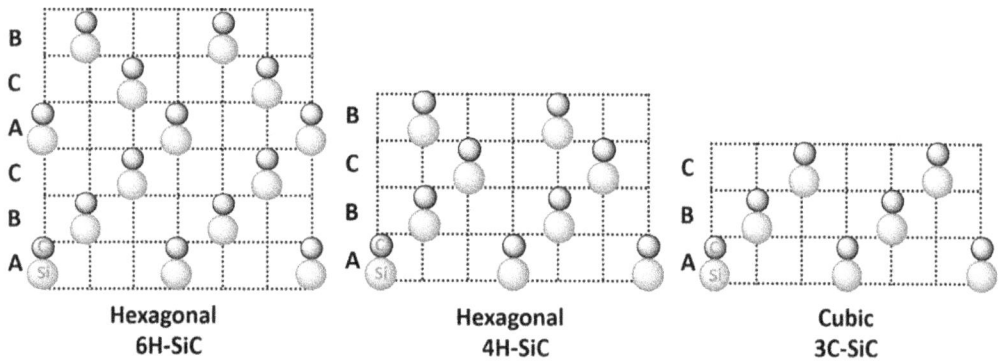

FIGURE 13.3
Bilayers stacking sequence of 6H-Sic, 4H-SiC and 3C-SiC.

13.3 Fundamental Concepts and Properties of Wide Bandgap Semiconductors

Each family of WBG semiconductors has a notable chemical, electrical, and optical characteristics, and therefore the materials should be chosen according to the properties that are required for each application in implantable and wearable devices. Table 13.1 exhibits the typical properties of common WBG materials. These properties could be changed and improved with the formation of tertiary and quaternary alloys, or with the addition of dopants, allowing to form of p-type or n-type materials. Knowing the basics of the main properties of the semiconductors is fundamental for later understanding how these properties will make them efficient for bioelectronics applications. Thus, in this section, basic concepts of the main properties of WBG materials will be present.

13.3.1 Piezoelectric Effect, Piezoelectric Polarization, and Piezoresistive Effect

Discovered by Jacques and Pierre Curie in 1880, the piezoelectric effect is the ability of a material to generate an electric field (or electric displacement) as a response to mechanical stress (or strain). G. Lippmann in 1881 predicted that the piezoelectric effect is a reversible process, and later in 1882, the Curies confirmed it experimentally. Therefore, a reverse piezoelectric effect is the generation of a mechanical strain in response to an electrical charge application.

The linear electromechanical interaction can only be observed in a crystalline compound with no inversion symmetry, thus it is an anisotropic material such as the wide bandgap compounds with WZ and ZB crystal structures. When the pressure is applied to these crystals, the molecules will re-align, generating a voltage across the crystal along the c-axis. Thus, the WBG materials with piezoelectric properties are pressure-sensitive for application in mechanical sensing in the context of bioelectronics. Additionally, the low dielectric losses and high breakdown field of AlN and ZnO (Table 13.1) make these piezoelectric semiconductors of high interest to researchers for applications in high temperatures [7].

The III-nitrides WBG semiconductors show excellent piezoelectric properties, especially AlN [18]. Besides it, the III-nitride compounds also show spontaneous polarization. The spontaneous polarization occurs in two types of materials, the ferroelectric and pyroelectric. In the ferroelectric materials, with the application of an electrostatic field, the polarization can be inverted, while in the pyroelectrics not, where the polarization is parallel to the low symmetry axis of the crystal [19]. Thus, III-nitrides are pyroelectric materials with spontaneous polarization. This property is naturally intrinsic and it corresponds to the bonding nature, where the geometric center of the negative and positive charges of the crystal are not coincident. In other words, the bonding between the atoms in these compounds should be asymmetric, and usually, in the hexagonal crystals, the bond along the c-axis shows to be longer and with different ionicity compared to other ones. On the other hand, the cubic crystal structure with tetrahedral coordination shows four equivalent bonds due to the sp^3 hybridization, explaining why most of the binary III–V and II–VI semiconductors do not have spontaneous polarization, only a piezoelectric effect.

When a mechanical strain induces a change in the electrical resistivity of a material this phenomenon is denoted by the piezoresistive effect, and the SiC compounds are the most favorable choice among the WBG materials. The piezoresistance also has a strong dependence on the crystal orientation, and it is quantified by the parameter gauge factor (GF). This change of resistance in response to applied stress is a function of geometry and resistivity changes.

In other words, the GF is the ratio of the per unit change in the resistance to the per unit change in length. The gauge factor for SiC compounds is considerable, where 3C-SiC showed to be ca. 30 for both p-type and n-type, increasing the importance of this class of WBG semiconductors for applications in bioelectronics, such as radiofrequency wireless communication devices [2].

13.3.2 Direct Bandgap and High Optical Transmittance

Semiconductors can have direct or indirect band gaps. In semiconductors with a direct bandgap, the momentum of the electrons in the highest states of the valence band is practically the same as the momentum of the holes in the lowest states of the conduction band. In this case, the optical transitions occur right after the photon energy exceeds the bandgap energy, and it is observed that the absorption coefficient increase together with the photon energies. On the other hand, in the materials with indirect bandgap, the momentum of the electrons in the valence band does not match the momentum of the holes in the conduction band, requiring an additional emission of a phonon (collective motion of atoms in a crystal) for change the electron momentum, and allowing the recombination.

The II–VI and III-nitride materials are known for their direct band gaps, allowing their application in UV photosensors and optogenetics LED [2]. The possibility of synthesizing different nanostructures of ZnO enables tuning and broadening its emission and absorption wavelength. Further in ZnO nanostructures, combining the direct bandgap and the large optical absorption can result in an efficient and sensitive photodetector over the UV spectral range [2]. Additionally, III-nitrides and their alloys (e.g., InAlN and AlGaN) also exhibit a tunable bandgap that can vary from the visible spectrum to infrared, highlighting the GaN-based materials that show to be an efficient UV photodetector [2].

Materials with a bandgap greater than ca. 3.1 eV usually is considered transparent [1]. Optical transmittance can be defined as the ability for light to be conducted through a material. Therefore, a material with high optical transmittance is essential for applications in optoelectronics, including in optogenetics. However, it is important to keep in mind that transmittance is dependent on the thickness, which can result in different accessible dynamic ranges for measurements of the absorption coefficient [1]. Some WBG materials have shown good transparency, such as ZnO [20]. From the III-nitride family, bulk GaN has been reported to form a material with high transparency, being useful for *in-vitro* studies with observation on-chip of several cells process [2]. SiC compounds are transparent to visible wavelengths and have been used for studies of *in-vitro* electrical stimulation concurrently with an optical observation of SiC electrodes [2].

13.3.3 High Electron Mobility

Electron mobility could be defined as how fast an electron can move through a semiconductor material under an applied electric field. Therefore, the carrier mobility (μ, Equation 13.1) is the average velocity per unit electric field, considering the intrinsic dispersion of the electronic bands (or electronic charge, q), the effective mass (where, m_e^* for electron effective mass in n-type conductivity, and m_h^* hole effective mass in p-type conductivity), and the scattering time (or relaxation time, τ). The relaxation time is defined as the rate of change in electron momentum as it moves through a semiconductor, and this process can occur through different mechanisms, such as phonon scattering and ionized impurity scattering. These scattering mechanisms can be understood through temperature-dependent carrier mobility and concentration experiments. Additionally, the carrier mobility and concentration are proportional to the electron conductivity, showing the importance of high electron mobility for electronic devices.

$$\mu = \frac{q\tau}{m^*} \tag{13.1}$$

Some WBG semiconductors have a more dispersed conduct band than the valence band, and exhibit lower m_e^*, resulting in greater n-type conductivity. In WBG oxides, such as ZnO, the low dispersion of the valence band results in lower electron mobility (Table 13.1). On the other hand, the III-nitride compounds have shown interesting conductive properties, highlighting the GaN-based devices. A device of the two-dimensional electron gas (2-DEG) containing stacking layers of GaN and AlGaN generates space charges due to the piezoelectric effects, and ultrahigh electron mobility [2]. This property enables the application of AlGaN/GaN in high electron mobility transistors (HEMT), and especially field-effect transistors (FET) for highly sensitive biomolecular detection [2]. Further, crystalline SiC can also exhibit excellent electron mobility, and this high conductivity has been studied for electrodes and sensing applications, such as in neural recording electronics using 4H-SiC, and using 3C-SiC in neural interfaces and long-lived cellular monitoring [21].

13.3.4 Biocompatibility and Biodegradability

Biocompatibility and biodegradability are crucial properties of materials to be evaluated for bioelectronics applications. Biocompatibility of materials is the ability of a material to be inserted or in contact with a living system without causing an adverse effect to the surrounding biological environment. Therefore, a biocompatible material must be non-toxic, non-immunogenic, non-allergenic, and non-carcinogenic. Biodegradability of a material is the degradation of the initial compound through biological processes, which can happen inside the living system. Additionally, in biodegradable materials, the resulting products from the degradation also need to be compatible with the biological system. A typical investigation of the biocompatibility of a material is through cell culture assays *in vitro*.

Besides all the unique electronic and optoelectronic properties of WBG materials, some of them also exhibit excellent biocompatibility and biodegradability, enabling them for wearable and implantable applications. Among the WBG semiconductors, the ZnO stands out due to its biodegradability. ZnO can be dissolved not only in water, but also in NaOH solution, ammonia, and blood serum of horses [2]. Besides the ZnO biodegradability in the environmental impact, it is also useful for biomedical devices, which can degrade in the body after serving its purpose [2]. In contrast, due to their chemical inertness, GaN and SiC have been extensively studied for wearable and implantable devices, where they can work properly for several decades *in situ* [2]. Although Al is known for its toxicity, studies showed that in the AlGaN/GaN heterostructures, a low composition of Al does not result in adverse effects on the cell's culture [22]. Further, SiC electronic devices are able to work efficiently in a biofluid without any encapsulation layers [21].

13.4 Which Techniques Have Been Used to Fabricate These Devices?

Even though WBG devices require specific properties already mentioned, a factor as important as their application in bioelectronics is manufacturing. The mechanical capacity of these materials interferes directly with their effectiveness, such as stretchability and flexibility [2]. Therefore, the biggest challenge over the years is to manufacture these devices on flexible substrates [23] since each mechanism has its limitations. Thus, the preparation of WBG semiconductors can be performed by different techniques directly on the flexible substrate or pre-prepared on another material and transferred to the main substrate. Several methods have been developed and improved, and the most common techniques are described (Table 13.2) with their highlights and limitations.

13.4.1 Direct Growth of Nanostructures on Flexible Substrates

Various methods were developed aiming to promote the growth of nanostructures directly on flexible substrates. The main challenge here is the reaction temperature that the nucleation process requires once the soft substrate does not tolerate such high temperatures as those of the direct growth reactions. To overcome this obstacle, techniques were developed and reported involving a combined process.

Examples of low-temperature techniques that are promising are electrochemical deposition (ECD) and chemical solution growth along with atomic layer deposition, for instance. These processes can be combined in three steps of seeding-annealing-growth (SAG). Reddy et al. [24] related the combined SAG method in which seed layers of ZnO were deposited on a nickel-coated flexible substrate using ECD. Then the material was annealed in the air to obtain a pure crystalline ZnO phase, and in the third step, the ZnO nanorods were developed using the chemical deposition process. Pradhan et al. [25] report a successfully direct synthesis of two different structures, nanopillars and nanowalls, of ZnO on a plastic substrate (polyester) by using ECD at low temperature without templates.

Another widely used method is the hydrothermal process (Figure 13.4), which consists of a process where the substrate is coated and dried, and subsequently, it is soaked in a solution with nanoparticles of interest, repeating the deposition process for the concentrated film. The nucleation of these sites occurs, and at a determined ideal temperature, it favors the growth of nanostructures, which depends directly on the main parameters as bath temperature, growth time, and seed coating condition [26].

TABLE 13.2

Main Different Fabrication Methods of WBG Nanostructures and Their Highlights and Limitations

Classification	Technique	Highlights	Limitations
Direct Growth Methods	Electrochemical Deposition	Simple, fast, and low-cost method; The large surface area of treatment	Possible instability of voltage and current;
	Seeding-Annealing-Growth	Low-temperature; Well-controlled morphology	Quality of nanostructures in different reaction parameters
	Hydrothermal or Solvothermal	Scalability; Well-controlled morphology	Usually requires high synthesis time
Bottom-Up Methods	Vapor-Liquid-Solid Mechanism	The growth parameters of nanowires can be manipulated and controlled by varying the conditions of reactions	The formation of defects due to the chosen catalyst
	Chemical Vapor Deposition	Catalyst-free reaction; High-quality crystalline nanowires	High-temperature vacuum-chamber process
	Thermal Evaporation	Simple process; Low-cost method	Morphology control
	Molecular Beam Epitaxy	Suitable for wide materials system	Expensive technique; Low growth rates
	Sol-Gel Technique	Simple process; Highly controlled approach	Expensive raw materials; Time-taking process
Top-Down Methods	Photolithography	Highly aligned nanostructures; Control of the electrical properties	Resolution of nanostructures due to the limitation of optical systems (which can be worked around in a derivative technique)
	Focused Ion Beam	Very precise for nanostructure fabrication; A pre-prepared nanostructure patter is not required	Low yield as it is a serial process
	Electron Beam Lithography	High resolution	Low yield as it is a serial process; Not ideal for large-scale fabrication

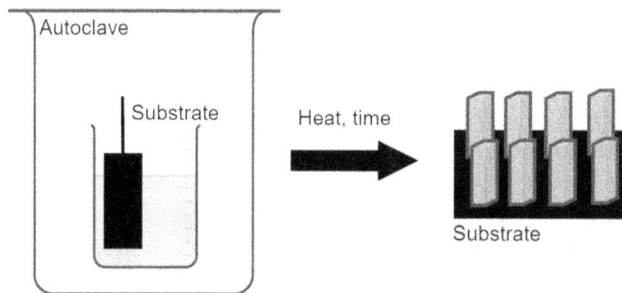

FIGURE 13.4

Schematic mechanism of the preparation of WBG semiconductors through the hydrothermal technique.

Araujo et al. [27] show the use of hydrothermal method assisted by microwave radiation, aiming to reduce the reaction time, where ZnO nanorods are grown on a paper substrate at low temperature and faster than the commonly used typical method. Wang et al. [28] reported a low temperature operated direct growth method as hydrothermal assisted by a ZnO seed layer to fabricate nanorods, which will be used as a flexible micro-supercapacitor.

13.4.2 Fabrication Methods of Nanostructures Followed by Transferring Processes

The materials can be synthesized by different techniques (including those already mentioned) but followed by an additional step of transferring it to a flexible substrate. Fabrication device techniques can be divided mainly into two types that will be described below.

13.4.2.1 Bottom-Up Growth

It consists of physical and/or chemical methods to promote the growth of micro- or nanostructures. The methodology has this name because it starts with small structures such as atoms and molecules, followed by clusters, and sophisticated nanostructures are obtained in the end [29].

The most widely exploited technique is the vapor-liquid-solid (VLS) mechanism [23], which occurs in three stages: alloying, nucleation, and axial growth stage (Figure 13.5). This methodology has a disadvantage in the choice of a specific catalyst. If the catalyst is poorly chosen, it can promote the formation of defects that directly and significantly affect the properties of the manufactured nanomaterial. To avoid this challenge, some catalyst-free methods can be used, such as chemical vapor deposition (CVD) (Figure 13.6), thermal evaporation, molecular beam epitaxy, and others [23,26]. Another technique

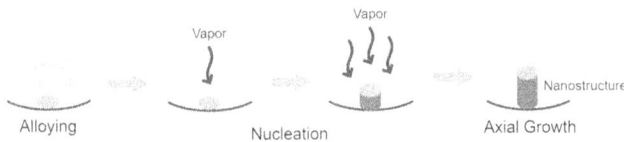

FIGURE 13.5
Schematic mechanism of the preparation of WBG semiconductors through the Vapor-Liquid-Solid (VLS) technique.

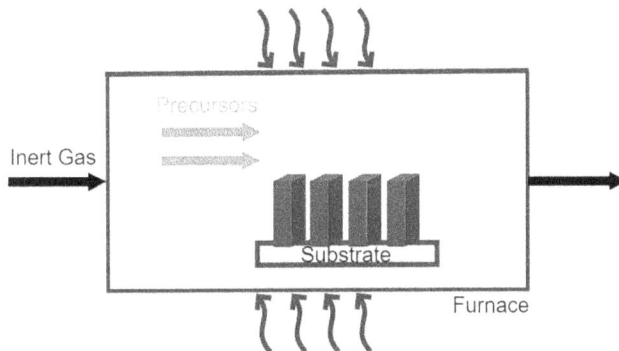

FIGURE 13.6
Schematic mechanism of the preparation of WBG semiconductors through the Chemical Vapor Deposition (CVD) technique.

broadly reported is the sol-gel method, which has several advantages, such as the low-cost, simple, and highly controlled approach [30].

Lin et al. [31] used the sol-gel technique to develop a ZnO thin film for organic solar cells on flexible plastics substrates. First, it was prepared as a ZnO sol-gel by dissolving zinc acetate dihydrate (ZAD) and ethanolamine (MEA) in ethylene glycol monomethyl ether (EGME). It was investigated the molar ratio of ZAD to MEA, and the characteristics of the resulting ZnO thin films. Feng et al. [32] demonstrate for the first time the fabrication of SiC nanowires with precise growth control by tailoring the cooling rates based on the VLS process, aiming to provide a new strategy for the growth of one-dimension nanowires with well-controlled morphology. Low et al. [33] synthesized GaN nanowires on Ni-coated sapphire substrate using the CVD method at different growth temperatures, which studied its influence on the morphological, structural, and optical characteristics of the nanowires.

13.4.2.2 Top-Down Growth

Top-down growth consists basically of a subtractive process through mostly physical methods, such as lithography and derivatives, focused ion beam (FIB), electron beam lithography (EBL), gas-phase condensation, and others, combined with another process [2]. In the same way as the previous technique, this one has this name because it starts from larger structures, converts into smaller ones (e.g., powder), and then into nanostructures with control of some parameters, such as shape and size [29].

Conventional lithography creates patterns on the surface through some processes like coating, irradiation (and because of this, it is commonly named photolithography), and etching [34]. The FIB lithography technique is one of the most advanced and efficient processes for surface modifications and fabrication of semiconductor nanomaterials. It consists of an application of highly focused ion beams (Figure 13.7a) aiming to modify the surface of the target via the sputtering method [23]. Another similar technique widely reported is the EBL, in which the patterns are formed by scanning a focused beam of electrons on a treated surface (Figure 13.7b).

Since the presented mechanisms in this chapter have great advantages and some drawbacks, all these methods can be combined into a hybrid fabrication technique, which offers an improved alternative to prepare WBG semiconductors for bioelectronics. Phan et al. [35] reported the fabrication of silicon nanowires for microelectromechanical systems applications through the FIB process followed by wet etching and thermal annealing. The manufactured materials in this study had an electrical conductivity magnitude enhanced

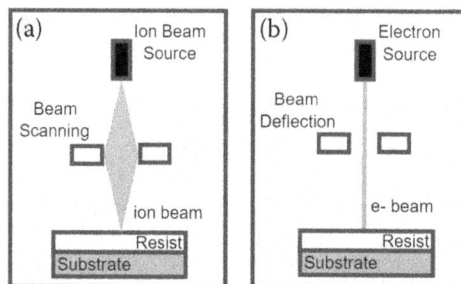

FIGURE 13.7
Schematic mechanism of a (a) focused ion beam and (b) electron beam lithography techniques.

significatively and a largely achieved piezoresistance. Later, the same author published a study developing SiC nanowires using a photolithography process and FIB. Before the nanowire fabrication, it was growth of a thin film of SiC on a substrate by low-pressure CVD, showing that the techniques can be successfully combined, and then, the micro-patterns were etched, followed by the subsequent processes [36].

13.4.2.3 Transferring Processes

The process of transferring nanostructures to flexible substrates can be realized mainly in two ways: through a dry or wet transfer method. The dry transfer method can be carried out through a process of segregation a nanowire because of the adhesion force between them and the substrate, and an alignment process due to the directional shear force (named as contact printing method). The technique can be extended to different processes, including a roll printing method towards larger areas.

The wet transfer method is an alternative to transferring the nanostructures to flexible substrates. In this way, a nanowire-based solution can form a film into a pre-patterned substrate based on the drop-casting process. Nevertheless, there are some disadvantages, such as the low device yield and poor contact with electrodes. To overcome these barriers, alternatives have been studied, such as the Langmuir-Blodgett technique [29].

13.5 Applications – Where They Can Be Used in Bioelectronics?

Due to the diverse properties and advances in the development of these materials, WBG semiconductors are being used in several areas, such as in ultraviolet devices [37–39] and sensors [40–42]. In addition, the possibility of transferring WBG thin films/nanowires onto substrates that are preferentially flexible and biocompatible, has further expanded the applications of these materials, especially in bioelectronics devices. In this section, the advancement of the most widely used bioelectronics applications of WBG compounds will be described (Figure 13.8).

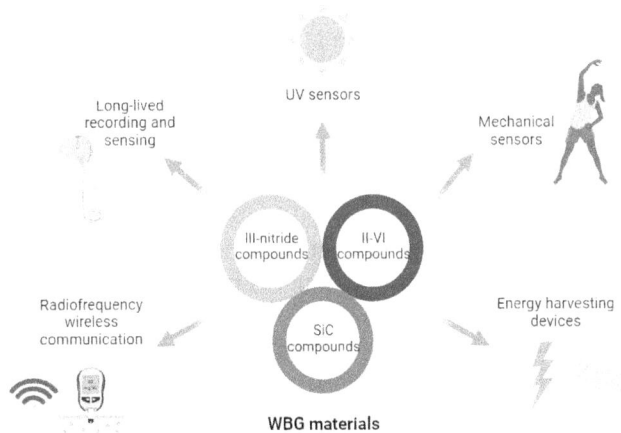

FIGURE 13.8
Main applications of wide bandgap (WBG) compounds.

Starting with SiC compounds, one of the applications in which they have been most used is the development of devices that present long-lived recording and sensing. These devices should have a lifetime of decades *in situ*, in addition to capability to an integrated stimulant function, being interesting, for example, to the measurement of cardiac activities, deep brain stimulators, and pacemakers [21,43,44]. Silicon nanomembranes-on-polymer (Si) [45] and silicon dioxide (SiO_2) [46] are being explored for this type of application. However, Si undergoes a hydrolysis reaction, with the gradual degradation of Si-nanomembranes, and SiO_2 has a limited function, making its application in detection and stimulation devices difficult [2]. To optimize these long-lived implants, recent research shows that SiC exhibits superior properties to Si and SiO_2, being promising for this application. For example, Liu et al. [43] prepared SiC films in memristor medium, for use in neuromorphic systems and artificial nociceptors, important receptors to recognize harmful stimuli, such as extreme temperatures and mechanical stress. Phan et al. [21] were the first to develop flexible SiC nanomembrane platforms. The crystalline cubic SiC nanomembranes were grown on a Si wafer and then physically transferred to a polyimide substrate. The interesting system showed water impermeability and mechanical flexibility, in addition to not undergoing the hydrolysis process, making it an important attraction for application as long-lived flexible implants. Also, in this work, the authors observed that the sensor based on SiC-polyimide can measure small mechanical strains, due to the significant piezoresistive effect of SiC. With this ability to convert mechanical strain into an electrical signal, it is possible to observe the potential of SiC as flexible mechano-physiological sensors to monitor processes such as pulmonary respiration and cardiac contractions.

SiC compounds have also been studied as radiofrequency wireless communication applications. The interesting thing about these devices is that besides detecting/monitoring any signal, they are capable of wireless communication. Afroz et al. [47] developed a continuous glucose sensor that uses radio frequency (RF) signals using SiC. Sensor detection is based on a change in resonance frequency due to changes in glucose levels, causing modifications in blood permittivity and conductivity. For *in-vitro* sensor performance tests, measurements were performed using synthetic body fluid (blood plasma equivalent) and pig blood. The sensor demonstrated that its response is dose-dependent at a glucose concentration between 120 to 530 mg/dl, with a shift of 40 and 26 MHz for simulated blood and pig blood, respectively. This corresponds to a shift of 97 and 67 kHz per 1 mg/dl change in blood glucose.

Still in this application, another type of wide bandgap compound widely used is GaN, belonging to the group III-nitride. As GaN has high electron mobility and a high breakdown field, this material becomes promising for application in RF devices. Chang et al. [48] reported flexible GaN HEMTs (high electron mobility transistors) with high thermal dissipation (0.5 W) operating up to 115 GHz without device degradation. This heat dissipation is an interesting property for RF devices since they need high power for their operation. Glavin et al. [49] demonstrated a stretchable GaN HEMT device that can be stretched uniaxially to 0.85% without damage. High cutoff frequencies and maximum oscillation frequencies greater than 42 and 74 GHz, respectively, at up to 0.43% strain were achieved, demonstrating a breakthrough in the development of flexible RF devices.

GaN compounds have a high piezoelectric polarization and flexibility, being investigated for the fabrication of flexible piezotronic strain sensors. Chen et al. [50] developed a flexible pulse sensor using single-crystalline III-nitride film. The arterial pulse sensor proved to be more sensitive than traditional sensors when tested *in vivo*. In another work, Cheng et al. [51] used GaN p-n junction microwires for a sensitive strain sensor attachable to the elbow joint to detect the biomechanics of human arms. In this sensor, the authors observed a greater piezoelectric output with the increase of the bending angle of the arms, leading to sensor deformation.

Another functional application in GaN is in UV sensors. Heo et al. [52] presented UV light (sun exposure) and blue light (phototherapy in neonatal intensive care units) sensors based on AlGaN and wireless modules on a flexible substrate. Although the microdevice is composed of a chip for near-field communication, a radiofrequency antenna, photo-diodes, supercapacitors, and a transducer, it is still compact, being easily used in sunglasses and earrings, for example.

As WBG materials have optoelectronic properties within the UV wavelength range, other compounds can be used, such as ZnO, belonging to the II-VI compounds. Li et al. [53] developed flexible UV photodetectors based on a metal-semiconductor-metal sandwich structure. Vertically aligned ZnO nanowires were grown in silver nanowire networks, with the deposition of another layer of silver nanowires on top of the ZnO one. With this structure, the authors achieved a transparent and flexible material, with a transparency of 75%, and good mechanical stability. The photodetector could operate at a low voltage of 0.5 V and exhibited a high photocurrent to a dark current ratio of 9756, and fast photo-response time (1.83 s rise time and 1.75 s decay time). Song et al. [54] also developed flexible photodetectors using ZnO nanowires grown on polyester fabric. This controlled cultivation can be carried out using a low-temperature hydrothermal method, and the photodetectors exhibited a stable response with high photocurrent to dark current ratios.

Some of the aforementioned devices may require a power source to operate. However, these battery-powered devices typically have a short operating time, which is a problem for implantable devices as they may require additional surgery to replace this source. An interesting source of energy would be from the movements of the human body, such as muscle movement, which is a form of energy that can be easily converted by piezoelectric materials, such as WBG compounds. ZnO is the most studied compound for this application, and Voiculescu et al. [55] described an elastic device that can be attached to the skin and produces energy through body movements. The system is based on a thin film of ZnO deposited on a polymeric substrate coated with an elastic gold electrode. At 8% voltage, the device output voltage was 2 V, with a power of 160 µW and power density of 1.27 mW/cm^2, demonstrating the potential of ZnO for manufacturing flexible energy-harvesting devices. In contrast, Qin et al. [56] reported the use of ZnO nanowire to obtain piezoelectric energy harvester. The device had an open-circuit voltage and short-circuit current of 1–3 mV and 5 pA, respectively. Despite the great potential of the use of ZnO for this application, its chemical instability in aqueous media can make it difficult to use these devices *in vivo* [2]. Therefore, there is a need for further studies to overcome this problem and allow the use of storage devices based on ZnO for practical applications.

References

1. R. Woods-Robinson *et al.*, "Wide band gap chalcogenide Semiconductors", *Chem. Rev.*, vol. 120, no 9, pp. 4007–4055, 2020, doi: 10.1021/acs.chemrev.9b00600
2. N.K. Nguyen *et al.*, "Wide-band-gap semiconductors for Biointegrated electronics: Recent advances and future directions", *ACS Appl. Electron. Mater.*, vol. 3, pp. 1959–1981, 2021, doi: 10.1021/acsaelm.0c01122

3. Ü. Özgür *et al.*, "A comprehensive review of ZnO materials and devices", *J. Appl. Phys.*, vol. 98, pp. 041301/1–041301/103, 2005, doi: 10.1063/1.1992666

4. K. Momma, F. Izumi, "VESTA 3 for three-dimensional visualization of crystal, volumetric and morphology data", *Journal of Applied Crystallography*, vol. 44. pp. 1272–1276, 2011.

5. S.-H. Wei, A. Zunger, "Role of metal d states in II-VI semiconductors", *Phys. Rev. B*, vol. 37, no 15, p. 8958, 1988.

6. J. Jian, J. Sun, "A review of recent Progress on silicon carbide for photoelectrochemical water splitting", *Sol. RRL*, vol. 4, pp. 2000111/1–2000111/10, 2020, doi: 10.1002/solr.202000111

7. M.A. Fraga, H. Furlan, R.S. Pessoa, M. Massi, "Wide bandgap semiconductor thin films for piezoelectric and piezoresistive MEMS sensors applied at high temperatures: An overview", *Microsyst. Technol.*, vol. 20, no 1, pp. 9–21, 2014, doi: 10.1007/s00542-013-2029-z

8. Q. Hua, B. Ma, W. Hu, "Aluminum, gallium, and indium Nitrides", in *Encyclopedia of Materials: Technical Ceramics and Glasses*, M. Pomeroy, Org. Elsevier, 2020, pp. 1–10.

9. M. Isshiki, J. Wang, "Wide-bandgap II-VI semiconductors: Growth and properties", in *Springer Handbook of Electronic and Photonic Materials*, S. Kasap, P. Capper, 2017, pp. 365–383.

10. M.N. Yoder, "Wide bandgap semiconductor materials and devices", *IEEE Trans. Electron Devices*, vol. 43, no 10, pp. 1633–1636, 1996, doi: 10.1109/16.536807

11. R. Williams, "High electric fields in CdS", *J. Phys. Chem. Solids*, vol. 22, pp. 129–133, 1961.

12. S. Kasap, P. Capper, *Electronic and Photonic Materials*, 2nd Edition. Cham, Switzerland: Springer Nature, 2017.

13. S.N. Mohammad, H. Morkoç, "Progress and prospects of group-III semiconductors", *Prog. Quantum Electron.*, vol. 20, no 5–6, pp. 361–525, 1996.

14. A.R. Acharya, "Group III – nitride semiconductors: Preeminent materials for modern electronic and optoelectronic applications", *Himal. Phys.*, vol. 4, no 4, pp. 22–26, 2013.

15. D. Feezell, S. Nakamura, "Nonpolar and semipolar group III-nitride lasers", in*Semiconductor lasers: Fundamentals and applications*, Woodhead Publishing Limited, 2013, pp. 221–271.

16. B.N. Pushpakaran, A.S. Subburaj, S.B. Bayne, J. Mookken, "Impact of silicon carbide semiconductor technology in photovoltaic energy system", *Renew. Sustain. Energy Rev.*, vol. 55, pp. 971–989, 2016, doi: 10.1016/j.rser.2015.10.161

17. H. Morkoç and I.-V. Z. semiconductor device technologies Strite, SLarge-band-gap SiC, III–V nitride, G.B. Gao, M.E. Lin, B. Sverdlov, M. Burns, "Large-band-gap SiC, III-V nitride, and II–VI ZnSe-based semiconductor device technologies", *J. Appl. Phys.*, vol. 76, pp. 1363–1398, 1994, doi: 10.1063/1.358463

18. V. Cimalla, J. Pezoldt, O. Ambacher, "Group III nitride and SiC based MEMS and NEMS: Materials properties, technology and applications", *J. Phys. D. Appl. Phys.*, vol. 40, no 20, pp. 6386–6434, 2007, doi: 10.1088/0022-3727/40/20/S19

19. F. Bernardini, "Spontaneous and piezoelectric polarization: Basic theory vs. practical recipes", in *Nitride Semiconductor Devices: Principles and Simulation*, Piprek J., 2007, pp. 49–68.

20. J. Miao, B. Liu, "II-VI semiconductor nanowires: ZnO", in *Semiconductor Nanowires*, J. Arbiol, Q. Xiong, no 2, Elsevier, 2015, pp. 3–28.

21. H.P. Phan *et al.*, "Long-lived, transferred crystalline silicon carbide nanomembranes for implantable flexible electronics", *ACS Nano*, vol. 13, no 10, pp. 11572–11581, 2019, doi: 10.1021/acsnano.9b05168

22. X. Li, X. Liu, "Group III nitride nanomaterials for biosensing", *Nanoscale*, vol. 9, pp. 7320–7341, 2017, doi: 10.1039/c7nr01577a

23. T.A. Pham *et al.*, "Nanoarchitectonics for wide bandgap semiconductor nanowires: Toward the next generation of nanoelectromechanical systems for environmental monitoring", *Adv. Sci.*, vol. 7, no 21, pp. 1–30, 2020, doi: 10.1002/advs.202001294

24. N. Koteeswara Reddy, M. Devika, C.W. Tu, "Vertically aligned ZnO nanorods on flexible substrates for multifunctional device applications: Easy and cost-effective route", *Mater. Lett.*, vol. 120, pp. 62–64, 2014, doi: 10.1016/j.matlet.2014.01.029

25. D. Pradhan, M. Kumar, Y. Ando, K.T. Leung, "One-dimensional and two-dimensional ZnO nanostructured materials on a plastic substrate and their field emission properties", *J. Phys. Chem. C*, vol. 112, no 18, pp. 7093–7096, 2008, doi: 10.1021/jp800799b

26. K. Yoo *et al.*, "Low-temperature large-area fabrication of ZnO nanowires on flexible plastic substrates by solution-processible metal-seeded hydrothermal growth", *Nano Converg.*, vol. 7, no 1, 2020, doi: 10.1186/s40580-020-00235-6

27. A. Araújo *et al.*, "Direct growth of plasmonic nanorod forests on paper substrates for low-cost flexible 3D SERS platforms", *Flex. Print. Electron.*, vol. 2, no 1, pp. 1–12, 2017, doi: 10.1088/2058-8585/2/1/014001

28. Y. Wang *et al.*, "A low-temperature-operated direct fabrication method for all-solid-state flexible micro-supercapacitors", *J. Power Sources*, vol. 448, no October 2019, 2020, doi: 10.1016/j.jpowsour.2019.227415

29. D. Shakthivel, F. Liu, C.G. Nunez, W. Taube, R. Dahiya, "Nanomaterials processing for flexible electronics", *IEEE Int. Symp. Ind. Electron.*, no October, pp. 2102–2106, 2017, doi: 10.1109/ISIE.2017.8001581

30. P. Rong, S. Ren, Q. Yu, "Fabrications and applications of ZnO nanomaterials in flexible functional devices–A review", *Crit. Rev. Anal. Chem.*, vol. 49, no 4, pp. 336–349, 2019, doi: 10.1080/10408347.2018.1531691

31. C.C. Lin, S.K. Tsai, M.Y. Chang, "Spontaneous growth by sol-gel process of low temperature ZnO as cathode buffer layer in flexible inverted organic solar cells", *Org. Electron.*, vol. 46, pp. 218–225, 2017, doi: 10.1016/j.orgel.2017.04.006

32. W. Feng, J. Ma, W. Yang, "Precise control on the growth of SiC nanowires", *CrystEngComm*, vol. 14, no 4, pp. 1210–1212, 2012, doi: 10.1039/c2ce06569j

33. L.L. Low, F.K. Yam, K.P. Beh, Z. Hassan, "The influence of growth temperatures on the characteristics of GaN nanowires", *Appl. Surf. Sci.*, vol. 258, no 1, pp. 542–546, 2011, doi: 10.1016/j.apsusc.2011.08.071

34. Q.J. Wang, Y.-W. Chung, *Encyclopedia of Tribology*, vol. 150, no 1–2. Springer, 2013.

35. H.P. Phan *et al.*, "Piezoresistive effect of p-type silicon nanowires fabricated by a top-down process using FIB implantation and wet etching", *RSC Adv.*, vol. 5, no 100, pp. 82121–82126, 2015, doi: 10.1039/c5ra13425k

36. H.P. Phan *et al.*, "The piezoresistive effect in top-down Fabricated p-type 3C-SiC nanowires", *IEEE Electron Device Lett.*, vol. 37, no 8, pp. 1029–1032, 2016, doi: 10.1109/LED.2016.2579020

37. M. Shur, R. Gaska, A. Dobrinsky, M. Shatalov, "Deep ultraviolet light emitting diodes: Physics, performance, and applications", *ECS Trans.*, vol. 61, pp. 53–63, 2014, doi: 10.1149/06104.0053ecst

38. M. Shatalov *et al.*, "High power AlGaN ultraviolet light emitters", *Semicond. Sci. Technol.*, vol. 29, p. 084007, 2014, doi: 10.1088/0268-1242/29/8/084007

39. I. Gaska, O. Bilenko, S. Smetona, Y. Bilenko, R. Gaska, M. Shur, "Deep UV LEDs for public health applications", *Int. J. High Speed Electron. Syst.*, vol. 23, pp. 1–10, 2014, doi: 10.1142/S0129156414500189

40. G. Cai, H. Luo, L. Guo, L. Li, S. Zhang, "MoOx-si heterojunction with wide-band-gap MoOx contact layer in the application of low-intensity visible-light sensing", *Mater. Sci. Semicond. Process.*, vol. 131, p. 105879, 2021, doi: 10.1016/j.mssp.2021.105879

41. V. Belwanshi, A. Topkar, "Quantitative analysis of MEMS piezoresistive pressure sensors based on wide band gap materials", *IETE J. Res.*, pp. 1–11, 2019, doi: 10.1080/03772063.2019.1620641

42. H. Kind, H. Yan, B. Messer, M. Law, P. Yang, "Nanowire ultraviolet photodetectors and optical switches", *Adv. Mater.*, vol. 14, pp. 158–160, 2002, doi: 10.1002/chin.200214011

43. L. Liu, J. Zhao, G. Cao, S. Zheng, X. Yan, "A memristor-based silicon carbide for artificial nociceptor and neuromorphic computing", *Adv. Mater. Technol.*, vol. 6, pp. 1–9, 2021, doi: 10.1002/admt.202100373

44. J. Li *et al.*, "Conductively coupled flexible silicon electronic systems for chronic neural electrophysiology", *Proc. Natl. Acad. Sci. U. S. A.*, vol. 115, pp. E9542–E9549, 2018, doi: 10.1073/pnas.1813187115

45. S.W. Hwang *et al.*, "Dissolution chemistry and biocompatibility of single-crystalline silicon nanomembranes and associated materials for transient electronics", *ACS Nano*, vol. 8, pp. 5843–5851, 2014, doi: 10.1021/nn500847g
46. H. Fang *et al.*, "Ultrathin, transferred layers of thermally grown silicon dioxide as biofluid barriers for biointegrated flexible electronic systems", *Proc. Natl. Acad. Sci. U. S. A.*, vol. 113, pp. 11682–11687, 2016, doi: 10.1073/pnas.1605269113
47. S. Afroz, S.W. Thomas, G. Mumcu, S.E. Saddow, "Implantable SiC based RF antenna biosensor for continuous glucose monitoring", in *IEEE Sensors*, 2013, pp. 1 4.
48. T.H. Chang *et al.*, "High power fast flexible electronics: Transparent RF AlGaN/GaN HEMTs on plastic substrates", *2015 IEEE MTT-S Int. Microw. Symp.*, pp. 2–5, 2015, doi: 10.1109/MWSYM.2015.7167085
49. N.R. Glavin *et al.*, "Flexible gallium nitride for high-performance, strainable radio-frequency devices", *Adv. Mater.*, vol. 29, no 47, pp. 1–7, 2017, doi: 10.1002/adma.201701838
50. J. Chen *et al.*, "High durable, biocompatible, and flexible piezoelectric pulse sensor using single-crystalline III-N thin Film", *Adv. Funct. Mater.*, vol. 29, no 37, pp. 1–10, 2019, doi: 10.1002/adfm.201903162
51. S. Cheng, S. Han, Z. Cao, C. Xu, X. Fang, X. Wang, "Wearable and ultrasensitive strain sensor based on high-quality GaN pn junction microwire arrays", *Small*, vol. 16, pp. 1–8, 2020, doi: 10.1002/smll.201907461
52. S.Y. Heo *et al.*, "Wireless, battery-free, flexible, miniaturized dosimeters monitor exposure to solar radiation and to light for phototherapy", *Sci. Transl. Med.*, vol. 10, p. eaau1643, 2018, [Online]. Available at: https://www.researchgate.net/publication/329449204_Wireless_battery-free_flexible_miniaturized_dosimeters_monitor_exposure_to_solar_radiation_and_to_light_for_phototherapy.
53. Y. Li *et al.*, "Full-solution processed all-nanowire flexible and transparent ultraviolet photodetectors", *J. Mater. Chem. C*, vol. 6, pp. 11666–11672, 2018, doi: 10.1039/c8tc04044c
54. W. Song *et al.*, "ZnO ultraviolet photodetector based on flexible polyester fibre substrates by low-temperature hydrothermal approach", *Micro Nano Lett.*, vol. 14, no 2, pp. 215–218, 2019, doi: 10.1049/mnl.2018.5342
55. I. Voiculescu, F. Li, G. Kowach, K.L. Lee, N. Mistou, R. Kastberg, "Stretchable piezoelectric power generators based on ZnO thin films on elastic substrates", *Micromachines*, vol. 10, pp. 1–11, 2019, doi: 10.3390/mi10100661
56. Y. Qin, X. Wang, Z.L. Wang, "Microfibre-nanowire hybrid structure for energy scavenging", *Nature*, vol. 451, pp. 809–813, 2008, doi: 10.1038/nature06601

14

Recent Advancements in MOF-Based Nanogenerators for Bioelectronics

Ajith Mohan Arjun

School of Materials Science and Engineering, National Institute of Technology Calicut, Kerala, India

Kiran Kumar Garlapati

Center for Interdisciplinary Programs, Indian Institute of Technology Hyderabad, Hyderabad, India

Pathath Abdul Rasheed

Department of Biological Sciences and Engineering, Indian Institute of Technology Palakkad, Kerala, India

CONTENTS

14.1 Introduction

Metal-organic frameworks (MOFs) are a class of porous materials that are composed of metal ions or clusters linked by organic ligands. These materials possess ultra-high porosity combined with large internal surface areas of more than 6,000 m^2/g. In addition to this, the large degree of variability in terms of both organic and metal nodes provides huge potential for applications in diverse fields [1]. Fields like adsorption of antibiotics, pollutants, biomolecules, gas adsorption, photo and electrocatalysis, biosensors, fuel cells, supercapacitors, and batteries have all benefited from the application of MOFs. The MOF materials are made using facile synthesis strategies like solvothermal methods, layer-by-layer growth, microwave, electrochemical, mechanochemical, and high throughput methods [2]. The properties of MOFs like porosity, flexibility in materials design, and availability of large surface areas offer immense possibilities for various applications. The conductivity and functionality of these materials can also be engineered using various strategies, which makes these materials ideal candidates for wearable sensing and nanogenerator applications.

This chapter deals with the application of MOFs for bioelectronics applications. Bioelectronics is the branch of science concerned with the use of electronic devices in living systems. Specifically, the application of MOFs for wearable standalone

DOI: 10.1201/9781003263265-14

electrochemical sensors and nanogenerators will be discussed as wearable devices have seen substantial growth in the past few years. Wearable sensors are those devices, which can be worn on the body of the user while performing user-based diagnostics. Wearable sensors monitor levels of physiologically important molecules like glucose, dopamine, adrenaline, sodium, and potassium levels in sweat, biomarkers for various diseases, and foreign substances like ethanol and opioids, etc. [3]. To power such wearable sensors, a compact and flexible power source is needed. Most of the conventional wearable sensors are powered by batteries that limit their sustainability. Nanogenerators harness the mechanical motions of humans to generate electricity, which makes them a sustainable alternative to batteries. Moreover, these nanogenerators can be used for power generation and self-powered sensing. For instance, triboelectric nanogenerators can scavenge the mechanical energy of human pulse to generate electricity, which can be used to monitor human health conditions.

14.2 MOFs as Sensing Materials

The use of MOFs has been reported extensively for electrochemical sensor applications as both in environmental and physiological sensors [4]. On the environmental front, MOFs have been used for the detection of pesticides and antibiotics in water bodies. Li et al. constructed an electrochemical sensor composed of Cu MOF for the simultaneous detection of hydroquinone and catechol in contaminated water. They were able to achieve a detection limit of 590 nM and 3.30 nM [5]. Fang et al. reported a nanocomposite of Zr (IV)–based MOF (NH$_2$-UiO-66) and reduced graphene oxide (rGO) for the detection of ciprofloxacin (Cip) in water [6]. This electrode combined the large surface area of MOF and the high electrical conductivity of graphene. Anodic stripping voltammetry was used for the detection of Cip and the limit of detection (LOD) achieved was 6.67 nM. The Cip was able to form complexes with Cu^{2+} and the anode stripping voltammetry sensed Cip by the deposition of Cu on the NH$_2$-UiO-66/rGO composite. A Fe$_3$O$_4$@MIL-100(Fe) was used for the detection of chlorogenic acid [7]. A LOD of 50 nM was achieved using this material. The existence of unsaturated iron centers and a large number of complex organic chains led this material to possess a large density of redox-active sites, large pore volume, and water stability. Recently, Zhao et al. have reported conductive two-dimensional (2D) MOFs as sensors for the detection of paraquat [8]. This MOF was based on 2,3,7,18,12,13-hexahydroxyl truxene and copper ions. The MOF was synthesized by a liquid-liquid interfacial reaction. The limit of detection achieved was 41 nM.

The use of MOFs has been used for the detection of physiologically important molecules also. Gao et al. have reviewed the use of MOFs for sensing neurotransmitters such as dopamine, acetylcholine, tyrosine, and histamine in detail [9]. Li et al. reported the use of MOF carbon nanotube composites for the sensitive detection of ascorbic acid [10]. The MOF used in this study was Zn-based nitroimidazole MOF. The MOF was used as the redox mediator owing to the presence of oxidizing nitro groups on the frameworks. The LOD achieved was 1.03 µM. A Cu-hemin MOF was reported, which possessed peroxidase-like bioactivity and good electrical conductivity [11]. This MOF was used for the detection of peroxide with LOD of 0.019 µM. The electrical conductivity of the Cu-hemin MOFs was greatly enhanced when it was combined with CS-rGO. Duan et al. reported a molecularly imprinted electrochemical sensor for the ultra-trace detection of bovine serum albumin (BSA) [12]. This sensor was based on AuNPs@NH$_2$-MIL-125 (Ti)-graphene composite in which the MOF was prepared by a rapid ultrasonic method. The 3D porous framework, which was obtained not only provided a highly conducting MOF due to the presence of Au NPs but also provided a large surface area due to the presence of MOFs. The electrode under optimal conditions provided a low detection limit of 4.147 × 10^{19} g/mL. This electrode was used for the detection of BSA in milk samples also. A porphyrin encapsulated HKUST-1 (Cu) was reported by Ling et al. and this composite can catalyze o-phenylenediamine to 2,2'-diamonoazobenzene, which was then conjugated with streptavidin as a recognition element [13]. Upon the addition of target DNA, the stem of the hairpin DNA was unfolded to form a structure with the strepta-vidin. This activated DNA was then able to bind to the recognition element to greatly enhance the activity of peroxidase towards o-phenylenediamine oxidation in the presence of peroxide. This report presented a versatile "signal on" sensor with a detection limit of 0.48 fM. Recently a dopamine sensor was reported by Kang et al. who used hemin doped HKUST-1 rGO composite as a redox mediator for the detection of dopamine with a LOD of 3.27 nM [14]. The presence of rGO combined with the HKUST-1 was reported to enhance the electrocatalytic activity of the material towards dopamine oxidation. Gumilar et al. reported the use of MOFs based on benzene dicarboxylic acid (BDC) with hierarchical 3D morphologies composed of 2D nanosheets and nanoplates [15]. Multiple metal ions were used for constructing the MOF like Cu, Mn, Ni, and Zr. The constructed MOFs were used for electrochemical glucose sensing with a LOD of 6.68 μM. In keeping with the demands of recent times, MOFs have also been used for the detection of viruses [16].

Despite the immense potential of this material, which has been proved through a multitude of papers reporting lab-scale detection, very limited efforts have been successful in achieving the application of these materials for nanogenerators and wearable sensors.

14.3 MOFs for Nanogenerators

The design of wearable sensors necessitates an energy source for the functioning of these devices and these energy sources comprise batteries, solar cells, biofuel cells, super-capacitors, and nanogenerators [17]. A composite of fuel cells and supercapacitors known as super capacitive biofuel cells have also been used for various applications [18]. Although these devices are very attractive options for powering wearable sensors, they do not form a part of the nanogenerator family, which forms the crux of this book chapter. Nanogenerators are energy-harvesting devices that generate electricity from mechanical or thermal energy from our surroundings. Wang et al. demonstrated the working piezoelectric zinc oxide nanogenerator in 2006 for the first time [19]. Later, different nanogenerators were developed based on triboelectricity, thermoelectricity, pyroelectric, etc. While piezoelectric nanogenerators (PENG) and triboelectric nanogen-erators (TENG) function on converting mechanical energy into electricity, the pyroelectric nanogenerators convert thermal energy into electricity. A typical example of the scale of energy availability during human motion was reported by Yang et al. who were able to light 40 LEDs by using a self-powered backpack that integrated these nanogenerators [20]. This shows that highly sustainable and eco-friendly power generation devices could be built if nanogenerators are employed for power generation. These nanogenerators offer ideal power sources for converting ambient energy to a useful form.

TENG and PENG are extensively studied and potential devices to harness abundantly available mechanical energy in the environment. These can power electronics without an external power source under continuous mechanical input in integration with capacitors. Recent advancements in nanotechnology promoted the advancement and miniaturization of nanogenerators. These devices can be integrated into wearable electronics for energy generation and sensing applications (Figure 14.1).

TENG works on the dual principles of triboelectric charging and electric induction. When two dissimilar materials come into contact, static charges will be produced at their interface that makes one material positively charged and the other one negatively charged based on their tendency to gain or lose electrons and generates a potential difference between the materials. When they are separated, electrons flow from negatively charged material to positively charged material through the external circuit producing electricity. Based on the position of material in the triboelectric series, it can be used as either positive material or negative material. Materials that are far away from each other in the series generate stronger charges when they come to contact. The common working modes of TENG are metal-on-dielectric and dielectric-on-dielectric pairs. These can be assembled in various configurations such as (i) contact sliding mode, (ii) linear sliding mode, (iii) single electrode mode, and (iv) free-standing mode, as shown in Figure 14.2(i) [25].

Many materials such as wool, rabbit fur, hair, mustard seeds, poly(vinylidene fluoride) (PVDF), Kapton, lead, etc. show triboelectric effect. Singh et al. developed TENG using mustard seeds as a positive layer and PVDF as a negative layer which delivered an open circuit voltage of 84 V and power density of 334 mW/m^2 at a force of 40 N at 25 Hz frequency [26]. The major advantages of TENG are cost-effectiveness, easy design, large output power, and high conversion efficiency. It was established that the performance and application of TENG greatly depend on the material used for fabrication.

The use of nanomaterials in these nanogenerators has been reported extensively for a wide variety of sensing applications [27]. Recently Hao et al. used a flexible self-rebound

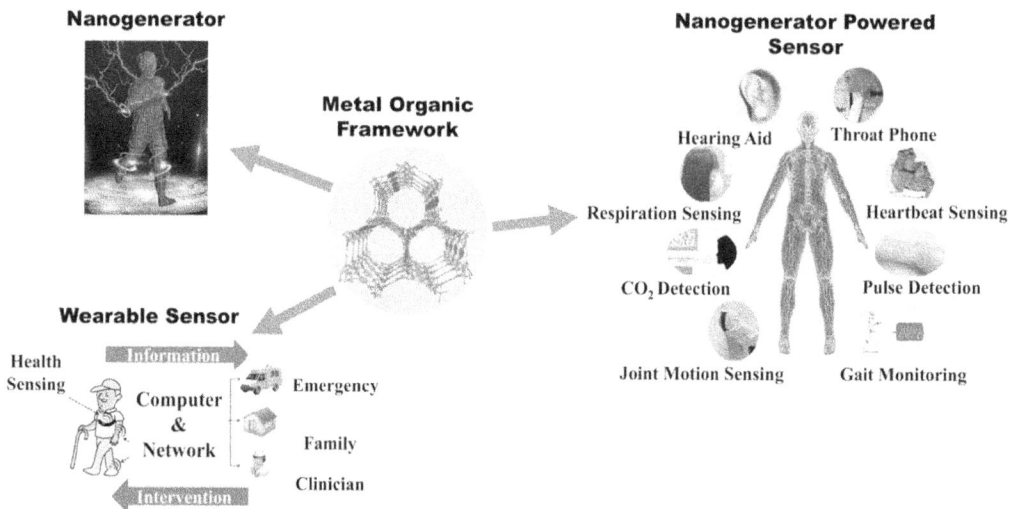

FIGURE 14.1
Metal organic framework ecosystem based on nanogenerators for powering wearable biosensors. Adapted with permission [21], Copyright (2011) Elsevier, [22], Copyright (2012) Springer Nature, [23]. Copyright (2020) Elsevier and [24], Copyright (2019) Elsevier.

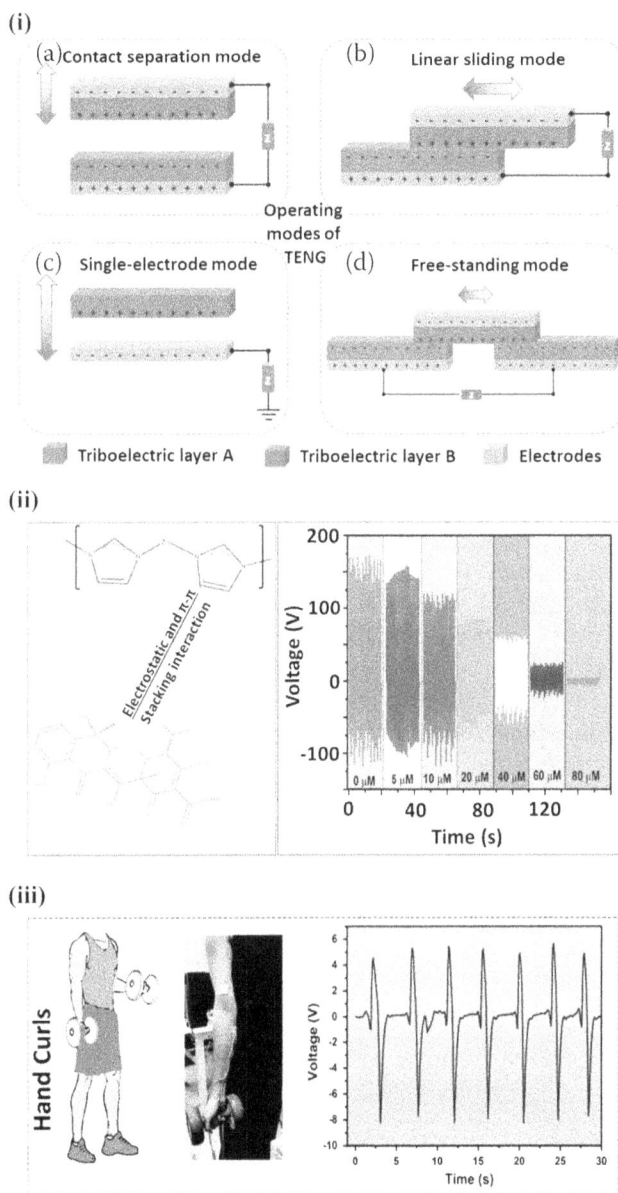

FIGURE 14.2
(i) Schematic image showing the basic operating modes of TENG. Adapted with permission [25], Copyright (2020) The Author(s), some rights reserved exclusive licensee (IntechOpen). Distributed under the terms of the Creative Commons Attribution 3.0 (CCBY). (ii) Schematic showing the π–π interacting mechanism of the benzene ring in tetracycline with imidazole ring of ZIF-8. Reprinted with permission [34], Copyright (2019) John Wiley & Sons, Inc. (iii) Image showing the TENG location during hand curls exercise and its voltage vs time profile. Reprinted with permission [35]. Copyright (2020) Royal Society of Chemistry.

cambered triboelectric nanogenerator for kinematic analysis for equestrian sports applications. A fluorinated ethylene propylene thin film was employed as the triboelectric later with a copper electrode as the contact. The second electrode was an aluminum electrode which served both as the triboelectric layer and as the contact. This device simulated the pressure points when a rider sits on the saddle of the horse and provides data through wireless transmission to know the state of the rider while riding [28]. The power density produced by the device was 1.25 mW/cm^2 under an external load of 60 MΩ. Vijoy et al. used room temperature cured polydimethylsiloxane (PDMS) and Cu electrodes for producing 14 μW power across a load of 20 MΩ. A capacitance model was employed to evaluate the use of this device as an impact detector [29]. Cao et al. developed a self-powered pressure and strain sensor by utilizing MXene film as a single electrode mode TENG. MXene was brushed into a pre-stretched latex substrate followed by releasing of this substrate to obtain crumpled structures. These structures enhanced the surface roughness leading to a higher energy-harvesting property with a power density of 2.89 μW/cm^2, which was higher than the TENG based on a flat MXene film. This system was applied to a wireless motion monitoring system to obtain feedback about the motion state of the human body [30].

The use of MOFs in nanogenerators offers advantages like fine pore-size distribution, ultra-high surface area, and good chemical stability [31]. In addition, there have been multiple reports on the use of MOFs for the improvement of the performance of TENGs [32]. From the analysis of the available reports, it can be concluded that MOFs can help in improving the performance of nanogenerators in addition to helping in the functioning of a wide spectrum of sensors. However, there have been limited reports utilizing MOF for nanogenerator-powered sensors, especially in the wearable domain. This chapter aims to summarize attempts that have been reported for the use of MOFs in wearable sensing and nanogenerator domains so that a clear view of the present scenario can be obtained for ascertaining future directions of research.

The performance, durability, and cost-effectiveness of TENG always depend on the materials used for the fabrication. Dielectric polymers such as PVDF, polyaniline (PANI), polytetrafluoroethylene (PTFE), etc., and some metals are widely studied for TENG applications. Functionalizing polymers is very difficult and this limits the development of multifunctional TENG. MOFs hold a special interest in this field owing to their ease of functionalization by changing their metal centers and organic ligands, and offer high surface area and flexibility. The surface functionalities of MOF-based TENG enable the development of self-powered sensors.

Khandelwal et al. studied the triboelectric performance of zeolite imidazole framework (ZIF) family MOFs as a positive layer and Kapton as a negative layer in vertical contact separation mode [33]. The surface roughness of the ZIF MOF layer was measured using atomic force microscopy (AFM) as it is a crucial factor that affects the performance of TENG. They have synthesized different MOFs (ZIF-7, ZIF-9, ZIF-11, and ZIF-12) by using different reagents with different concentrations. The ZIF-7 showed higher surface roughness than other ZIF MOFs. The ZIF-7/Kapton TENG delivered the highest performance of 1.1 μA and 60 V and it powered a wristwatch and hydro thermometer. In another work by the same group, a ZIF-8/Kapton TENG was developed that showed 164 V and 70 μA [34]. ZIF-8 ligand i.e., 2-methylimidazole is sensitive to tetracycline due to the π–π interactions that take place between them that affect the output voltage of the TENG. With an increase in tetracycline concentration, the output voltage was reduced due to the reduction in electron density at the benzene ring of ZIF-8, as shown in Figure 14.2(ii). This kind of selective MOF enables multifunctional wearable TENG for power generation and sensing applications. In another work, the same group developed ZIF-62 based TENG using benzimidazole and imidazole ligands, further demonstrating its usage as a fitness tracker, as shown in Figure 14.2(iii) [35]. It delivered a performance of 62 V, 14 μA, and 16 nC and by deposition stream of ions using a Zerostat 3 gun, its performance enhanced to 175 V and 10 μA. ZIF-62/Teflon charges a 1 μF capacitor in 150 s and showed endurance for 21 h with good stability till a relative humidity of 60%. ZIF-62/ Teflon TENG was integrated with the human body for energy harvesting based on body motions during exercises and the number of voltage peaks helps as a fitness tracker.

Hajraet al. investigated cyclodextrin (CD) MOF having Na as the metal centers [36]. This is a major development towards bio-compatible MOF TENG as the biocompatibility of ZIF-based MOF is not consistent. They have studied the α, ß, and γ CD MOF as a positive layer and Teflon as a negative layer in multiunit Z-shape vertical separation mode. Kelvin probe force microscopy (KPFM) is used to characterize the surface potentials of α, ß, and γ CD MOFs. They followed the trend α > γ > ß CD MOF. The difference in surface potentials originated due to the structure of ligands as all CD MOFs showed similar surface roughness at higher scan rates. The TENG performances of the devices agree with KPFM analysis showing the high output voltage of 152 V for α CD MOF/ Teflon TENG with 1.3 μA current and 14.3 nC charge. The α CD MOF/Teflon TENG was used to charge a capacitor using a bridge rectifier to convert the AC output of the TENG to DC power. It was attached to the human body and shoes to harness the energy produced during daily activities like walking and jogging.

PENG works on the principle of piezoelectricity i.e., the voltage difference will be generated across the materials under the application of force. The voltage across the material will be generated due to the change in the center of mass of anions and cations in the material. The reverse process is also possible where voltage difference across the material will induce stress in the material named the inverse piezoelectric effect. The applications of PENG are more versatile than TENG. They can be used in smart textiles, ultrasonic transducers, and the transportation sector. The structure of the piezoelectric device is very simple with piezoelectric material sandwiched between two electrodes. Piezoelectric devices can be operated in different modes based on the nature of applied pressure like compression, shear, and expansion. Ceramics that does not have a center of symmetry such as quartz, ZnO, etc.; polymers such as PVDF, PTFE, etc.; and biomaterials such as cellulose, onion skin, etc. show piezoelectric properties. Piezoceramics show higher conversion efficiencies than piezopolymers, but they cannot handle high strains due to their brittle nature. So, composites of both were developed to combine their benefits. Multifunctional PENG sensors are more accurate than TENG-based sensors as they suffer from static electricity, humidity, and temperature changes. MOFs are used as nanofillers in piezopolymers owing to their crystalline nature, porosity, and surface functionalities. MOFs have also been introduced in PENG to improve the properties of PENG for different applications.

Moghadam et al. developed zirconium-based MOF PVDF composite PENG by the electrospinning method for self-powered arterial pulse monitoring [37]. Incorporation of MOF into PVDF increased the piezoelectric constant by 3.4 times with 3% MOF loading and 4.4 times with 5% MOF loading owing to the increased order of crystallinity and polar β phase PVDF content in the composite. PVDF MOF composite nanofibers were sandwiched between copper-coated aluminum foils. The PVDF-MOF composite showed a peak-to-peak voltage of 600 mV under an applied force of 5 N. They used it as a wearable sensor for monitoring the pulse signals of a human, which is discussed in the next section.

Ferroelectric materials are analogous to ferromagnetic materials that produce electric field polarization in absence of an electric field. All ferroelectric materials show a piezoelectric effect due to the absence of center symmetry. In this aspect, Roy et al. developed a self-polarized ferroelectric device for non-invasive health monitoring applications using MOF-PVDF composite [38]. They used CdI_2-INH=CMe_2 MOF as a nanofiller to create pores in the β-phase PVDF matrix to obtain a synergistic effect of nanodiploes (originated from β-phase PVDF) and microdipoles (originated from the porous structure) by solution casting method. PVDF@MOF formed a porous and flexible film while PVDF alone is rarely porous. The PVDF@MOF showed a fourfold increase in its dielectric constant and a fivefold increase in the piezoelectric coefficient than the bare PVDF. The PVDF@MOF film sandwiched between the silver electrodes showed an open circuit voltage of 12 V and a short circuit current of 60 nA under vertical stress of 10 kPa. It shows a quick response time of 8 ms and a sensitivity of 8.52 V/kPa. By utilizing this property, MOF-PVDF ferroelectret film has been used as an ultra-sensitive pressure sensor with mechano-sensitivity of 8.52 V/kPa within 1 kPa pressure range as well as a high-power density of 32 $\mu W/cm^2$. The application of PVDF@MOF PENG as a wearable sensor is explained in the next section.

In another work by the same group, they have developed CdI_2-NAP MOF@PVDF nanofibers by electrospinning [39]. The developed TENG delivered an open circuit voltage of 22 V and a short circuit current of 0.1 μA under periodic stress of 22 kPa with a quick response time of 5 ms. Along with mechanoelectrical conversion, acoustoelectric conversion studies were also done by sandwiching the nanofiber sheet between the ITO-coated PET sheet. A 1 cm diameter hole was made to the device and placed ahead of the speaker. The device produced 6 V at 120 Hz frequency and 110 dB sound pressure level.

14.4 Wearable MOF-Based Sensors

The important requirements of a wearable electronic device are flexibility and lightweight soft material, being able to make direct contact with the skin, the stretchability of the device, and the stability of the material [40]. Considering the properties of MOFs such as ultrahigh porosity, structural flexibility, and large surface areas, MOFs and MOF-derived materials have been utilized for wearable sensor applications with enhanced performance.

A flexible and wearable sensor based on MOFs coupled with multiwalled carbon nanotube (MWCNT) fibers has been developed for the sensitive detection of NO_2 gas [41]. Here, the MOFs were introduced as the precursors of the metal oxides (MO), and well-aligned MWCNT fibers were used as a support for gas-sensing nanocrystals. Both the MOF/MWCNT and as-derived MO/MWCNT hybrid fibers showed a remarkable detection sensitivity for NO_2 down to 0.1 ppm without external heating. In addition, this flexible fiber device can be bent into different angles without loss of sensor performance, and hence it can be further intertwined into smart textiles for NO_2 sensing. Also, the MO/MWCNT hybrid fibers exhibited a high specific capacitance of 110 F/cm^3 which can be utilized in energy storage applications. The dual functions of MO/MWCNT hybrid fibers validate the promising application for integrated wearable devices for safety and healthcare purposes.

In a similar way, Rauf et al. developed a smart textile sensor using a MOF as an active thin-film layer for humidity detection with high selectivity [42]. The deposition of a thin layer of MIL-96 (Al) MOF particles onto interdigitated electrode-based fabrics was done using the Langmuir-Blodgett method for the first time. The developed textile sensor exhibited a sensitivity of 0.6 femtofarad (fF) per % relative humidity with a limit of detection around 0.71% relative humidity. In addition, the sensor exhibited promising stability over several sensing cycles and a very minute change in the sensing response observed after being stored for 3 weeks without loss of sensor properties. The authors proposed the possibility of developing similar other sensors by changing the type of MOF material specific to a particular analyte and this sensing modality can be used to develop smart textiles and safety suits for the personnel working in laboratories and vulnerable industries.

Recently, flexible wearable pressure sensors have received remarkable research interest towards different applications such as wearable electronic skins, disease diagnostics, human-machine interfaces, touchable displays, and artificial intelligence [43]. The sensing mechanisms in wearable pressure sensors include capacitive, piezoresistive, piezoelectric, and triboelectric effects. Among these sensing mechanisms, wearable piezoresistive pressure sensors have attracted researchers owing to their simple device assembly, reliable piezoelectric effect, and relatively low energy consumption [44]. Considering the high specific surface area, mechanical and thermal stability, and permanent porous structure, MOFs have been considered as promising candidates for flexible piezoresistive sensors to deliver excellent sensing performance with the enhanced sensing response time and sensitivity [45].

A wearable, sensitive, and breathable pressure sensor has been made by Wang et al. by sandwiching the interconnected nanocomposites of carbonized metal-organic framework (C-MOF) and polyaniline nanofiber (PANIF) on a polyurethane (PU) sponge between the breathable fabric and the fabric patterned with an interdigitated conductive electrode (Figure 14.3(a–c)) [44]. The developed sensor has been denoted asa C-MOF/PANIF@PU pressure sensor and it exhibited a broad sensing range of up to 60 kPa, high sensitivity of 158.26 kPa ^{1}, a fast response/recovery time of 22 ms/20 ms, and outstanding repeatability over 15,000 cycles. The sensing mechanism is based on tunable changes in the contact resistance between the interdigitated electrode-coated fabric and the C-MOF/PANIF@PU under external pressure, which causes a change in current. The deformation of C-MOF/PANIF@PU provides more conductive paths between the C-MOF/PANIF@PU and the interdigitated electrodes, resulting in increased current. When the pressure is unloaded, both the interdigitated electrodes and the C-MOF/PANIF@PU sponge return to their original shapes, which leads to a reduction in current and sensor response. The compressive deformation of the three-dimensional (3D) C-MOF/PANIF@PU could be obtained under external pressure, resulting in more contact and conductive paths between the C-MOF/PANIF@PU and the interdigitated electrodes. This led to increased current and improved sensing performance. This pressure sensor could be employed to monitor both tiny human activities such as blood pulse and large human motions such as finger bending and finger pressing. The authors have already developed E-skins, which were successfully assembled from the pressure sensor arrays for detecting various tactile signals and to map spatial pressure distribution (Figure 14.3(d–g)). The authors proposed that this pressure sensor can be connected with a wireless transmitter for wireless sensing. Overall, this approach opens the possibility of assembling wearable breathable pressure sensors for potential versatile applications in clinical diagnosis and personal healthcare monitoring with high sensitivity and reproducibility, wireless, and broad-range performance.

For continuous monitoring of analytes from a human body (e.g., glucose level in sweat), it is highly recommended that the materials should have high stretchability and outstanding electrochemical performance. MOFs synthesized by metal nodes and organic ligands, display excellent mechanical flexibility along with ultrahigh specific surface area, and highly accessible active sites, which can be considered as excellent materials for potential application in stretchable wearable sensors. Towards this aspect, a flexible

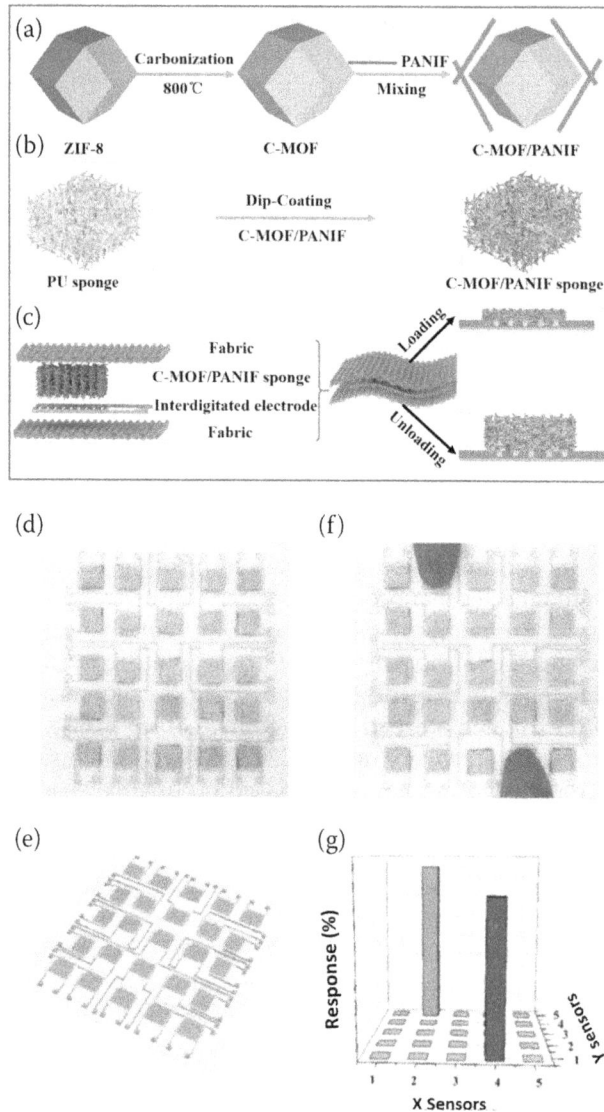

FIGURE 14.3
Schematics showing the fabrication procedure of C-MOF/PANIF@PU based flexible wearable pressure sensors: (a) The synthesis of C-MOF/PANIF, (b) the synthesis of C-MOF/PANIF@PU by dip-coating of C-MOF/PANIF on PU sponge, (c) the assembly of the C-MOF/PANIF@PU based flexible wearable pressure sensors, d) photograph of the E-skin assembled from the C-MOF/PANIF@PU based pressure sensor, (e) schematic illustration of the E-skin assembled from the C-MOF/PANIF@PU based pressure sensor, (f) photograph of two fingers touching the E-skin, and (g) the corresponding pressure distribution mapping from the sensing responses. Reprinted with permission [44]. Copyright (2020) Elsevier.

stretchable electrode has been made by depositing Ni-MOF composite/Au nanoparticles and carbon nanotube (CNT) onto a PDMS film towards real-time monitoring of dopamine [46]. Owing to the superior mechanical flexibility and electrocatalytic activity of the Ni-MOF, the developed stretchable sensor can be utilized for real-time monitoring of dopamine under stretched and unstretched states with a detection limit of 10 nM with a wide linear range of 50 nM to 15 μM. The same research group used an improved wet spinning technology for the production of reduced graphene oxide/polyurethane (rGO/PU) fiber followed by coating conductive Ag glue and as-synthesized Ni-Co MOF nanosheets on the fiber towards developing a stretchable fiber working electrode [47]. The excellent electrocatalytic activity of the developed Ni-Co MOF/Ag/rGO/PU fiber electrode resulted in enhanced electrochemical performance compared to rGO/PU and Ag/rGO/PU fiber electrodes towards glucose detection with a low detection limit of 3.28 μM. In addition, Ni-Co MOF/Ag/rGO/PU fiber electrode showed promising electrochemical performance even under mechanical deformation, which demonstrates its high stretchability. Moreover, they made a wearable nonenzymatic sweat glucose sensor by suturing the Ni-Co MOF/Ag/rGO/PU fiber electrode as a working electrode along with Pt wire as a counter electrode and Ag/AgCl fiber as a reference electrode on an absorbent fabric and fixed on a stretchable PDMS substrate. Overall, the results showed that the Ni-Co MOF/Ag/rGO/PU fiber-based wearable sensor can be used for the accurate and reliable continuous glucose monitoring from sweat.

The major challenge in employing MOFs for the fabrication of electronic devices is their poor conductivity. To overcome this, one option is to use transition metal dichalcogenides (TMDs), which are 2D materials with interesting electronic, chemical, and mechanical properties for developing a composite material. In this method, MoS_2 acts as an active site for electron exchange and transport owing to its excellent electron mobility. Towards this aspect, a MOF-MoS_2 based flexible, low-cost chemiresistive device as a respiration sensor has been developed for sleep apnea monitoring [48]. Here, a highly porous HKUST-1 MOF and a conducting MoS_2 have been combined for the fabrication of an electronic sensor on flexible paper support. MOFs can absorb a greater amount of water molecules exhaled from breath. The HKUST-1 MOF was synthesized by reacting benzene tricarboxlyate with copper nitrate. The developed sensor could detect various kinds of breaths such as normal, deep, fast, slow, and hydrated breath with a fast response time of just ~0.38 s and outstanding stability for a month without any loss in the performance. In addition, they proposed a probable mechanism and fabricated a smartphone-based prototype for real-time applications.

Recently, self-powered wearable piezoelectric sensors have gained much attention in biomedical monitoring applications, in which the mechanical force is converted into electrical energy. A novel wearable piezoelectric sensor has been developed for arterial pulse monitoring based on a poly(vinylidene fluoride) (PVDF) nanofibrous membrane containing microporous zirconium-based MOFs [37]. The PVDF-MOF composite has been attached to the radial artery at normal body conditions and the piezoelectric output of the sensor was evaluated. The results revealed an improved output voltage (568 ± 76 mV) with a sensitivity of 0.118 V/N and this value is highest among flexible energy convertors reported so far. This work explores a new way to develop flexible and lightweight MOF-based piezoelectric nanofibrous sensors for self-powered wearable human pulse monitoring systems.

Recently, flexible and sensitive pressure sensors are also of extensive interest in healthcare monitoring and artificial intelligence. In this context, Roy et al. reported a combination of porous MOF and PVDF to form a ferroelectret film towards the fabrication of mechanical energy harvester [38]. As mentioned in the previous secton, the MOF-PVDF ferroelectret film has been used as an ultra-sensitive pressure sensor with mechano-sensitivity of 8.52 V/kPa within 1 kPa pressure range. This composite ferroelectret film can be used to detect different physiological signals such as coughing, pronunciation, and gulping behavior which plays a significant role in influenza and chronic obstructive pulmonary disease-related symptoms. In addition, it can be used for tracking the subtle pressure change in the wrist pulse by utilizing the effective mechano-sensitivity. They have also tested the wireless transmission of the detected wrist pulse signal using a wireless signal transferring unit and they were able to achieve the displaying of the wrist pulse signal on the screen of a smartphone. Hence, the developed MOF-PVDF ferroelectret can be used in auto-powered electronics, real-time wearable healthcare monitoring devices, and artificial intelligence.

14.5 Future Scope

This chapter has demonstrated that MOFs have great potential in wearable sensing and nanogenerator applications. Owing to the multiple advantages of MOFs, there is scope for translational innovation in standalone wearable sensing. This domain would particularly be attractive in the current healthcare scenario because of the avoidance of complex energy generation devices like batteries and fuel cells. In addition, sensors based on MOFs have been reported to have very low LOD, which makes them very useful in the early-stage detection of diseases like cancer. To realize the potential of MOF for use in biosensors powered by nanogenerators, large-scale processing techniques like 2D and 3D printing, screen printing, and roll-to-roll forming must be introduced. These techniques are widely reported for the large-scale fabrication of devices based on a wide variety of materials [49]. Although these techniques have been reported for the fabrication of MOFs, their applications towards nanogenerators and biosensors need to be studied. Another perspective that needs to be studied is the use of flexible substrates for developing these devices. Since these MOFs will be used for wearable applications, these sensors must adhere to the skin surface. The interaction between MOFs and these flexible substrates needs to be optimized to ensure the proper working of the devices. A large volume of work has been carried out on the optimization of such substrates, and working out the interaction of MOF-based active materials with flexible substrates holds the key to realizing the application of MOFs for use in biosensors powered by nanogenerators [50]. Since the application of 2D materials is being focused on all areas of research, many interesting properties and high-efficiency materials can be obtained if 2D MOFs can be synthesized for applications in wearable biosensors and nanogenerators. Such conducting MOFs and their composites can be used as support materials also thus paving way for highly efficient devices with a small number of constituent layers [51,52]. Due to their high surface area and highly flexible synthesis strategies, MOFs can be used to construct support electronics such as active components of flexible printed circuit boards (PCBs) also. These PCBs hold huge promise during innovation in the device scale as conventional PCBs will be hard to integrate with flexible sensors and nanogenerators [53]. MOFs have already been reported for the construction of diodes, transistors which are very common components of conventional PCBs [54]. If these systems can be integrated into the flexible PCBs, an ecosystem based on MOFs can be constructed. The ability of materials to be used in all components of the ecosystem clearly shows its potential for commercial applications. From all these instances, it can be concluded that the field of MOF-based sensors and nanogenerators is still in its infancy and holds great potential for translational research directed towards battery-free standalone sensors for healthcare applications. Such sensors can form nodes of an IoT (Internet of Things)–based network, which can be used for real-time tracking of the physiological anomalies of the wearer.

References

1. H.-C. Zhou, J.R. Long and O.M. Yaghi 2012 Introduction to metal–organic frameworks *Chemical Reviews* **112** 673–674.
2. Y.-R. Lee, J. Kim and W.-S. Ahn 2013 Synthesis of metal-organic frameworks: A mini review *Korean Journal of Chemical Engineering* **30** 1667–1680.
3. A.J. Bandodkar, I. Jeerapan and J. Wang 2016 Wearable chemical sensors: Present challenges and future prospects *ACS Sensors* **1** 464–482.
4. L. Liu, Y. Zhou, S. Liu and M. Xu 2018 The applications of metal organic frameworks in electrochemical sensors *ChemElectroChem* **5** 6–19.
5. J. Li, J. Xia, F. Zhang, Z. Wang and Q. Liu 2018 An electrochemical sensor based on copper-based metal-organic frameworks-graphene composites for determination of dihydroxybenzene isomers in water *Talanta* **181** 80–86.
6. X. Fang, X. Chen, Y. Liu, Q. Li, Z. Zeng, T. Maiyalagan and S. Mao 2019 Nanocomposites of Zr(IV)-based metal–organic frameworks and reduced graphene oxide for electrochemically sensing ciprofloxacin in water *ACS Applied Nano Materials* **2** 2367–2376.
7. Y. Chen, W. Huang, K. Chen, T. Zhang, Y. Wang and J. Wang 2019 A novel electrochemical sensor based on core-shell-structured metal-organic frameworks: the outstanding analytical performance towards chlorogenic acid *Talanta* **196** 85–91.
8. Q. Zhao, S-H Li, R-L Chai, X. Ren and C. Zhang 2020 Two-dimensional conductive metal–organic frameworks based on truxene *ACS Applied Materials & Interfaces* **12** 7504–7509.
9. L.-L. Gao and E.-Q. Gao 2021 Metal–organic frameworks for electrochemical sensors of neurotransmitters *Coordination Chemistry Reviews* **434** 213784.
10. Y. Li, W. Ye, Y. Cui, B. Li, Y. Yang and G. Qian 2020 A metal-organic frameworks@ carbon nanotubes based electrochemical sensor for highly sensitive and selective determination of ascorbic acid *Journal of Molecular Structure* **1209** 127986.
11. L. Wang, H. Yang, J. He, Y. Zhang, J. Yu and Y. Song 2016 Cu-hemin metal-organic-frameworks/chitosan-reduced graphene oxide nanocomposites with peroxidase-like bioactivity for electrochemical sensing *Electrochimica Acta* **213** 691–697.
12. D. Duan, H. Yang, Y. Ding, D. Ye, L. Li and G. Ma 2018 Three-dimensional molecularly imprinted electrochemical sensor based on Au NPs@ Ti-based metal-organic frameworks for ultra-trace detection of bovine serum albumin *Electrochimica Acta* **261** 160–166.
13. P. Ling, J. Lei, L. Zhang and H. Ju 2015 Porphyrin-encapsulated metal–organic frameworks as mimetic catalysts for electrochemical DNA sensing via allosteric switch of hairpin DNA *Analytical Chemistry* **87** 3957–3963.
14. K. Kang, B. Wang, X. Ji, Y. Liu, W. Zhao, Y. Du, Z. Guo and J. Ren 2021 Hemin-doped metal–organic frameworks based nanozyme electrochemical sensor with high stability and sensitivity for dopamine detection *RSC Advances* **11** 2446–2452.
15. G. Gumilar, Y.V. Kaneti, J. Henzie, S. Chatterjee, J. Na, B. Yuliarto, N. Nugraha, A. Patah, A. Bhaumik and Y. Yamauchi 2020 General synthesis of hierarchical sheet/plate-like M-BDC (M = Cu, Mn, Ni, and Zr) metal–organic frameworks for electrochemical non-enzymatic glucose sensing *Chemical Science* **11** 3644–3655.
16. Y. Wang, Y. Hu, Q. He, J. Yan, H. Xiong, N. Wen, S. Cai, D. Peng, Y. Liu, Z. Liu and Bioelectronics 2020 Metal-organic frameworks for virus detection *Biosensors and Bioelectronics* **169** 112604.
17. G. Rong, Y. Zheng and M. Sawan 2021 Energy solutions for wearable sensors: A review *Sensors (Basel)* **21** 3806.
18. G. Pankratova, P. Bollella, D. Pankratov and L. Gorton 2022 Supercapacitive biofuel cells *Current Opinion in Biotechnology* **73** 179–187.
19. Z.L. Wang and J. Song 2006 Piezoelectric nanogenerators based on zinc oxide nanowire arrays *Science* **312** 242–246.

20. Z. Wu, T. Cheng and Z.L. Wang 2020 Self-powered sensors and systems based on nano-generators *Sensors (Basel)* **20** 2925.
21. T.G. Glover, G.W. Peterson, B.J. Schindler, D. Britt and O. Yaghi 2011 MOF-74 building unit has a direct impact on toxic gas adsorption *Chemical Engineering Science* **66** 163–170.
22. S. Patel, H. Park, P. Bonato, L. Chan, M. Rodgers and Rehabilitation 2012 A review of wearable sensors and systems with application in rehabilitation *Journal of NeuroEngineering and Rehabilitation* **9** 1–17.
23. J. Qi, A.C. Wang, W. Yang, M. Zhang, C. Hou, Q. Zhang, Y. Li and H. Wang 2020 Hydrogel-based hierarchically wrinkled stretchable nanofibrous membrane for high performance wearable triboelectric nanogenerator *Nano Energy* **67** 104206.
24. F. Yi, Z. Zhang, Z. Kang, Q. Liao and Y. Zhang 2019 Recent advances in triboelectric nanogenerator-based health monitoring *Advanced Functional Materials* **29** 1808849.
25. V. Vivekananthan, A. Chandrasekhar, N.R. Alluri, Y. Purusothaman, G. Khandelwal and S.-J. Kim 2020 *Nanogenerators*, ed A C a N R A Sang Jae Kim: IntechOpen.
26. S.K. Singh, P. Kumar, R. Magdum, U. Khandelwal, S. Deswal, Y. More, S. Muduli, R. Boomishankar, S. Pandit and S. Ogale 2019 Seed power: Natural seed and electrospun poly (vinyl difluoride) (PVDF) nanofiber based triboelectric nanogenerators with high output power density *ACS Applied Bio Materials* **2** 3164–3170.
27. V.K. Vashistha, D.K. Das and A. Kumar 2022 Metal–organic frameworks-based nanomaterials for nanogenerators: A mini review *International Nano Letters* 10.1007/s40089-021-003 61-x, In press, 1–7.
28. Y. Hao, J. Wen, X. Gao, D. Nan, J. Pan, Y. Yang, B. Chen and Z.L. Wang 2022 Self-rebound cambered triboelectric nanogenerator array for self-powered sensing in kinematic analytics *ACS nano* **16** 1271–1279.
29. K. Vijoy, H. John and K.J. Saji 2022 Self-powered ultra-sensitive millijoule impact sensor using room temperature cured PDMS based triboelectric nanogenerator *Microelectronic Engineering* **251** 111664.
30. Y. Cao, Y. Guo, Z. Chen, W. Yang, K. Li, X. He and J. Li 2022 Highly sensitive self-powered pressure and strain sensor based on crumpled MXene film for wireless human motion detection *Nano Energy* **92** 106689.
31. M.T. Rahman, S.M.S. Rana, M.A. Zahed, S. Lee, E.-S. Yoon and J.Y. Park 2022 Metal-organic framework-derived nanoporous carbon incorporated nanofibers for high-performance triboelectric nanogenerators and self-powered sensors *Nano Energy* **94** 106921.
32. Y. Guo, Y. Cao, Z. Chen, R. Li, W. Gong, W. Yang, Q. Zhang and H. Wang 2020 Fluorinated metal-organic framework as bifunctional filler toward highly improving output performance of triboelectric nanogenerators *Nano Energy* **70** 104517.
33. G. Khandelwal, N.P. Maria Joseph Raj and S.-J. Kim 2020 Zeolitic imidazole framework: metal–organic framework subfamily members for triboelectric nanogenerators *Advanced Functional Materials* **30** 1910162.
34. G. Khandelwal, A. Chandrasekhar, N.P. Maria Joseph Raj and S.-J. Kim 2019 Metal–organic framework: A novel material for triboelectric nanogenerator–based self-powered sensors and systems *Advanced Energy Materials* **9** 1803581.
35. G. Khandelwal, N.P.M.J. Raj and S.-J. Kim 2020 ZIF-62: A mixed linker metal–organic framework for triboelectric nanogenerators *Journal of Materials Chemistry A* **8** 17817–17825.
36. S. Hajra, M. Sahu, A.M. Padhan, I.S. Lee, D.K. Yi, P. Alagarsamy, S.S. Nanda and H.J. Kim 2021 A green metal–organic framework-cyclodextrin MOF: A novel multifunctional material based triboelectric nanogenerator for highly efficient mechanical energy harvesting *Advanced Functional Materials* **31** 2101829.
37. B.H. Moghadam, M. Hasanzadeh and A. Simchi 2020 Self-powered wearable piezoelectric sensors based on polymer nanofiber–metal–organic framework nanoparticle composites for arterial pulse monitoring *ACS Applied Nano Materials* **3** 8742–8752.

38. K. Roy, S. Jana, S.K. Ghosh, B. Mahanty, Z. Mallick, S. Sarkar, C. Sinha and D. Mandal 2020 Three-dimensional MOF-assisted self-polarized ferroelectret: An effective autopowered remote healthcare monitoring approach *Langmuir* **36** 11477–11489.

39. K. Roy, S. Jana, Z. Mallick, S.K. Ghosh, B. Dutta, S. Sarkar, C. Sinha and D. Mandal 2021 Two-dimensional MOF modulated fiber nanogenerator for effective acoustoelectric conversion and human motion detection *Langmuir* **37** 7107–7117.

40. Y. Gu, T. Zhang, H. Chen, F. Wang, Y. Pu, C. Gao and S. Li 2019 Mini review on flexible and wearable electronics for monitoring human health information *Nanoscale Research Letters* **14** 263.

41. K. Rui, X. Wang, M. Du, Y. Zhang, Q. Wang, Z. Ma, Q. Zhang, D. Li, X. Huang, G. Sun, J. Zhu and W. Huang 2018 Dual-function metal–organic framework-based wearable fibers for gas probing and energy storage *ACS Applied Materials & Interfaces* **10** 2837–2842.

42. S. Rauf, M.T. Vijjapu, M.A. Andrés, I. Gascón, O. Roubeau, M. Eddaoudi and K.N. Salama 2020 Highly selective metal–organic framework textile humidity sensor *ACS Applied Materials & Interfaces* **12** 29999–30006.

43. R. Chellattoan, V. Lube and G. Lubineau 2019 Toward programmable materials for wearable electronics: Electrical welding turns sensors into conductors *Advanced Electronic Materials* **5** 1800273.

44. Y. Wang, M. Chao, P. Wan and L. Zhang 2020 A wearable breathable pressure sensor from metal-organic framework derived nanocomposites for highly sensitive broad-range healthcare monitoring *Nano Energy* **70** 104560.

45. X.-H. Zhao, S.-N. Ma, H. Long, H. Yuan, C.Y. Tang, P.K. Cheng and Y.H. Tsang 2018 Multifunctional sensor based on porous carbon derived from metal–organic frameworks for real time health monitoring *ACS Applied Materials & Interfaces* **10** 3986–3993.

46. Y. Shu, Q. Lu, F. Yuan, Q. Tao, D. Jin, H. Yao, Q. Xu and X. Hu 2020 Stretchable electrochemical biosensing platform based on Ni-MOF composite/Au nanoparticle-coated carbon nanotubes for real-time monitoring of dopamine released from living cells *ACS Applied Materials & Interfaces* **12** 49480–49488.

47. Y. Shu, T. Su, Q. Lu, Z. Shang, Q. Xu and X. Hu 2021 Highly stretchable wearable electrochemical sensor based on Ni-Co MOF nanosheet-decorated Ag/rGO/PU fiber for continuous sweat glucose detection *Analytical Chemistry* **93** 16222–16230.

48. T. Leelasree, V. Selamneni, T. Akshaya, P. Sahatiya and H. Aggarwal 2020 MOF based flexible, low-cost chemiresistive device as a respiration sensor for sleep apnea diagnosis *Journal of Materials Chemistry B* **8** 10182–10189.

49. F. Torrisi and J.N. Coleman 2014 Electrifying inks with 2D materials *Nature Nanotechnology* **9** 738–739.

50. W. Gao, H. Ota, D. Kiriya, K. Takei and A. Javey 2019 Flexible electronics toward wearable sensing *Accounts of Chemical Research* **52** 523–533.

51. R. Dong and X. Feng 2021 Making large single crystals of 2D MOFs *Nature Materials* **20** 122–123.

52. K. Jayaramulu, D.P. Dubal, A. Schneemann, V. Ranc, C. Perez-Reyes, J. Stráská, Š Kment, M. Otyepka, R.A. Fischer and R. Zbořil 2019 Shape-assisted 2D MOF/graphene derived hybrids as exceptional lithium-ion battery electrodes *Advanced Functional Materials* **29** 1902539.

53. B. Meng, W. Tang, X. Zhang, M. Han, W. Liu and H. Zhang 2013 Self-powered flexible printed circuit board with integrated triboelectric generator *Nano Energy* **2** 1101–1106.

54. V. Stavila, A.A. Talin and M.D. Allendorf 2014 MOF-based electronic and opto-electronic devices *Chemical Society Reviews* **43** 5994–6010.

15

MXenes-Based Polymer Composites for Bioelectronics

S.G. Manjushree

Department of Chemistry, Siddaganga Institute of Technology, Karnataka, India

Prashanth S. Adarakatti

Department of Chemistry, SVM Arts, Science and Commerce College (affiliated to Rani Channamma University), Karnataka, India

Abdulraheem S.A. Almalki and A. Alhadhrami

Department of Chemistry, Faculty of Science, Taif University, Al Hawiyah, Saudi Arabia

CONTENTS

DOI: 10.1201/9781003263265-15

15.1 Introduction

The word "bioelectronics" refers to the fusion of biology with electronics and refers to a wide range of bio-related structures utilized within the electrochemical community in broader applications [1]. The term "bioelectronic interface" refers to a variety of bio-integrated electrodes that communicate with biological systems. Bioelectronic interfaces are created on the surface of the human skin, or within the human body. The interfaces can be designed for electro-stimulation [2], as target applications and physiological signal recording [3]. Despite the different modalities and form factors of extant bioelectrodes, some common principles govern the configuration and manufacture of bioelectronic interfaces having high-performance, like minimum interfacial impedance. The fundamental differences between organic tissues and artificial electronics, on the other hand, cannot be overlooked. Human skin is permeable at epidermal interfaces, but electronics normally require tight encapsulation for long life spans. Tissues are ironically conductive, soft, and implanted interfaces, yet traditional electronics are hard, water-exclusive, and electronically conductive. As a result, connecting stiff electrodes with curved, complex, and dynamic tissues of the human body poses substantial obstacles. This field has made significant developments recently, although the extent of that advancement is dependent on material innovation. The appearance of two-dimensional (2D) structured materials has spurred the bioelectronics area of research over the last decade. Following graphene's breakthrough are black phosphorous, transition metal dichalcogenides, graphitic C_3N_4, and metal organic frameworks [1]. MXenes have been applied in different areas, including bioelectronic and biomedical applications, thanks to the attempts made by chemists and materialists. Apart from their two-dimensional layered structure, these new two-dimensional materials have unique physicochemical and electronic properties, large surface areas, two-dimensional tunable architectures, DNA, cells, and they effectively interact covalently with small biomolecules, proteins, and many other small molecules and other biocreatures are just a few of the advantages. As a result of these unique features, 2D materials have a lot of potential in a variety of applications, including drug delivery vehicles, biosensors, bioimaging agents, bioelectronics, and cancer therapy platforms [4].

The recent development of a 2D-layered chemical family known as "MXenes" has piqued the scientific community's interest, owing to special electronic and structural properties, which allow them to be used in a variety of applications. MXenes are the name given to a category of transition metal carbides, nitrides, and carbonatites that are produced by chemical delamination of MAX phases, which are 3D ternary (or quaternary) compounds.

$Ti_3C_2T_x$ (short Ti_3C_2) is the most researched MXene to date, with Tx denoting surface terminations, which are commonly O, OH, and/or F. A novel form of MAX phase, known as i-MAX, was recently identified, resulting in an MXene with in-plane vacancy ordering. The first vacancy MXene, in addition to having a high conductivity, has shown a significant capacity to construct supercapacitors [5]. The use of spontaneous transfers of electrons among MXenes and organic monomers to facilitate the polymerization of the organic monomers to form composite films has proven to be very successful in recent years. These approaches, on the other hand, take a long time and do not produce an ordered composite film in a single step, which must later be achieved through vacuum filtration. MXene, which is normally negatively charged, is extremely similar to electrolyte ions in a colloidal solution [6]. When MXene is added to the electropolymerization process, it can be operated as a counter ion by self-assembling with conductive polymer chains having positively charged to generate a conductive polymer film doped with MXene at the molecular level on the electrode surface in a single step with great efficiency. The MXene-doped conductive polymer has the potential to produce a better electrode architecture for energy storage devices.

The purpose of this work is to present such an overview for Mxenes and MXene/polymer nanocomposites. It gives an overview of the concept, preparation method, and characteristics of MXene; this is followed by MXene/polymer nanocomposites, which elaborates and narrates the preparation technique of the composites, summarizes the properties of the material and details of a variety of applications, including enzyme and non-enzyme sensing, biomedical, and bioelectronics. The last part provides a perspective on the future and challenges for MXenes.

15.2 Synthesis of MXenes

MXenes are produced by the etching method through a wet chemical process that provides fewer defects in the atomic level and higher electronic conductivity according to experiments. The method, however, is only applicable to carbon-based MXenes because from nitride-based MAX phases it does not eliminate the A-layer. The first etching agent employed was hydrofluoric acid (HF), which is toxic to the environment. As a result, the necessity for diverse etchants arose. In 2014, a secured blend of lithium fluoride (LiF) and hydrochloric acid (HCl) was introduced [7]. However, due to HF gas being created in-situ, the problem remained. The problem was solved by the invention of several ways that did not require the usage of HF. These techniques will be explained further.

15.2.1 Chemical Vapor Deposition

Methane was chosen as a source for carbon while Mo foil as a substrate and Cu foil on top of Mo substrate has been devised by Xu et al. by a chemical vapor deposition (CVD) technique to synthesize MXenes in 2015 [8]. They conducted their experiments at a temperature of over 1,085°C or 1,358 K. The breakdown of chemicals on the substrate surface causes the deposition of material layers from the vapor phase during CVD. Due to the high temperature, the Cu foil melted, generating an alloy of molybdenum and copper. Molybdenum atoms dispersed to the surface of the liquid Cu after reacting with the C atoms generated by the breakdown of methane, forming Mo_2C crystals.

Despite its MXene-like structure, the created material was a transition metal based 2D carbide with a greater surface area when compared to the previously synthesized nanosheets. Xu et al. [8] created 2D very thin Mo_2C crystals with lateral diameters more than 100 m and thicknesses of a few nanometers. The thickness has been altered by adjusting the methane content. The resulting MXene material was defect-free, and its superconductivity remained stable after a few months in contact with air [8].

15.2.2 Hydrothermal Synthesis

Li et al. [9] described a method in which from the Ti_3AlC_2 MAX phase, Ti_3C_2Tx MXene, can be obtained with the use of sodium hydroxide (NaOH) [10]. The hydroxide anions react with the layers of Al in this technique, causing the Al to be oxidized. Further, hydroxyl or oxygen radicals were formed with titanium atoms, after dissolving the Al(OH)$_3$ hydroxides in alkali. The procedure, on the other hand, allows the production of new Al hydroxides, which are further confined in the titanium layer and does not react with hydroxyl ion anymore. The ease of reaction has been carried out by using sodium hydroxide and varying the temperature of the hydrothermal in an argon atmosphere. In this method, more hydroxyl and oxygen ions were found in the MXenes than in the HF etching technique, which further enhances the overall activity.

15.2.3 Electrochemical Synthesis

Yang et al. proposed the first electrochemical approach for delamination of Ti$_3$C$_2$ in a binary aqueous electrolyte without the need of F in 2018. They used titanium aluminum carbide as the cathode and anode in a two-electrode setup. Only the anode went through the etching procedure, yielding Ti$_3$C$_2$T$_x$. They utilized a pH-balanced mixture of 1M NH$_4$Cl and 0.2M tetramethylammonium hydroxide (TMAOH) to avoid etching solely on the surface [11] which further helps in the deeper reaching of electrolytes towards the layer of anode [7]. The bulk anode was gradually delaminated using a low voltage of 5 V. To make individual sheets of Ti$_3$C$_2$T$_x$, the sediment and suspended powders of Ti$_3$C$_2$Tx were crushed and put into a 25% weight/weight tetramethylammonium hydroxide solution. The electrical conductivity of the MXenes generated was comparable to that of those synthesized using HF or HCl/LiF [7]. However, in terms of overall etching yield, the electrochemical approach looks to be the most promising, as up to 60% of the bulk material can be converted into Ti$_3$C$_2$T$_x$ [12].

15.2.4 In-situ Polymerization

By using monomers, initiators, and curing agents via a wet approach to the MXene nanosheets, in-situ polymerization can be done and from this MXene can be evenly distributed throughout the polymer hosts. The blending can significantly improve the dispersion of MXene within the polymer matrix. The said protocol is widely used to produce MXene-contained polymer nanocomposites. In the composites, the polymers are thermosetting polymers containing cyclic or heterocyclic units or linear macromolecules, which can be polymerized in mild conditions [13]. Wang et al. reported in-situ blending of Ti$_3$C$_2$Tx/epoxy resin nanocomposites [14]. Polyaniline (PANI), polythiophene (PT), PEDOT and/or its derivatives, polydopamine (PDA), polypyrrole (PPy), and other complex cyclopolymers usually can also be polymerized in-situ for preparing MXene/in-situ polymerization polymer nanocomposites to be applied as electrodes, catalysis, shielding functional materials, and other purposes. Qin et al. [15] have used the pyrrole and MXene component to synthesize the MXene/PPy via the electrodeposition technique. Further, in-situ polymerization techniques have been used by Wang et al. to produce the Ti$_3$C$_2$Tx/ PDA composite [16]; similar protocols have been used by Tong et al. [17] to synthesize the Ti$_3$C$_2$Tx/PPy composite. In-situ polymerization mixing improved MXene dispersion in polymers strengthened the interaction between MXene and the polymer matrix and improved the polymer's thermal, mechanical, and electrical properties.

15.3 Mxenes: Structure and Properties

15.3.1 Structure

MXenes were discovered in 2011. These are transition metal nitrides and carbides [18]. MXenes are related to the process of extracting layers of $M_{n+1}X_n$ (n = 2, 3, 4) from the metal-ceramic $M_{n+1}AX_n$ phase by removing interlayer A atoms (MAX, where M = generally denotes an early transition metals Sc, Ti, Mo, Cr, Zr, Hf, Ta, V, and Nb); A indicates element like Ga, Ti, Pb, S, Ge, Si, P, As, Cd, Sn, In, and Al, X = C, N. $M_{n+1}X_nT_x$ 2D layers named MXenes are formed when the "A" layer is selectively removed by etching. The letters T stand for -O, -OH, and –F. Furthermore, the layered structure possesses hexagonal as well as anisotropic features along with p63/mmc space group [19].

The structure and composition of the MXenes are represented in Figure 15.1. In the MAX phase, the arrangement of atoms has been observed in a hexagonal lattice that includes M and X atoms, where metal atoms are shared by the edges and X atoms located in the center. The $M_{n+1}X_n$ layer can still preserve the hexagonal lattice rather than the cubic structure of MX when the A atom is removed; hence, the $M_{n+1}X_n$ layer can be created by extracting the A atoms. M_2X, M_3X_2, M_4X_3, and M_5X_4 are the models depicted (Figure 15.1). MXenes thin films are often oriented horizontally, as was the case with its predecessor MAX. The majority of MXenes have excellent mechanical qualities, and they are predicted to be employed in nano-devices that require mechanical properties.

15.3.2 Properties

The largest range of Young's modulus, increased electric conductivities, adjustable bandwidth, and higher thermal conductivities are acknowledged as characteristic features of MXene. MXenes are distinguished from other 2D materials, such as graphene, by their hydrophilic nature combined with improved thermal conductivities. Finally, (i) composition (different transition metals "M" and "X" elements), (ii) surface and morphology

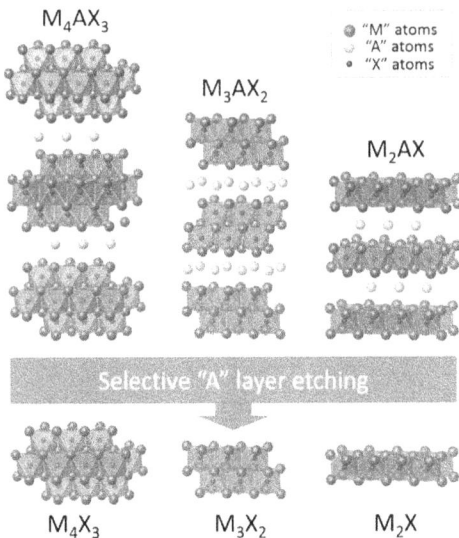

FIGURE 15.1
MXenes: Types and composition.

conversion can be used to tune their properties and applications performances [20]. Furthermore, MXenes exhibits a very high metallic conductivity, which has been measured at 10,000 S/cm in Ti_3C_2Tz spin-cast films. The key properties of the MXenes family are mentioned here.

15.3.2.1 Mechanical Properties

MXene's mechanical properties are of utmost interest because of the greater bonding between metal nitrides and metal carbides. A previous modeling study suggested that parameters related to elasticity be twice as big as MAX systems, including 2D motifs such as cadmium sulfide [21]. These components exhibit elastic character and which is lower than graphene and also which possesses the highest bending feature, indicating that they can be used as composite reinforcing materials. Due to the included capabilities, for composite applications, MXenes have a good contact ability with polymeric matrix than graphene. The hydrophilic characteristic of MXene's titanium-based thin discs intruded with distinct contact angles. Further research found that when the layer number increased, Young's modulus of both MXene nitrides and MXene carbides decreased. Furthermore, as compared to carbide MXenes, nitride-based components have the highest values [22].

Despite the availability of a variety of methodologies for the characterization of bulk materials, evaluating 2D-dimensional materials and their mechanical properties remains difficult. The majority of these experimental results are calculated with the nanoindentation method, which involves applying force to the center point of a 2D material using an AFM tip. The experimental Young's modulus of the $Ti_3C_2T_x$ monolayer was 33,320 GPa, which is slightly higher than the 386 GPa value of $Ti_3C_2O_2$ but lower than graphene oxide and MoS_2. As a result, fresh experimental discoveries should concentrate on the synthesis procedure's development to estimate different functional groups and defects in the pure components. Perhaps, based on theory and experiments, a thorough estimation of mechanical traits as well as significant functional groups has yet to be established.

15.3.2.2 Chemical Properties

Chemical resistivity and toxicity are the most important chemical qualities for bioelectronic applications. Many factors influence the chemical stability of 2D materials, including environment, lattice structure, functional groups, doping, bonding states, and defect density. More crucially, the stability of 2D materials may be controlled by manipulating defect doping, density, and bonding states, because doping elements and defects are frequently used as chemically active sites in which deterioration begins. In addition, by controlling the active spots during synthesis, the chemical stability of the two-dimensional materials could be improved [23]. External circumstances can also be used to regulate chemical stability, such as controlling the environment, using alternative substrates, strain engineering, or changing the relative thickness of constituent components [24]. However, degradation of some unstable two-dimensional materials via an oxidation layer could be prevented, paving the way for further research in this sector [25].

15.3.2.3 Electronic Properties

Functional groups, stoichiometry, and solid solution formation can all be used to adjust two of the most important aspects of MXenes: electrical and electric properties. MXene-pressed discs had electric conductivities that were nearer to multi-layered graphene and greater than carbon nanotubes and reduced graphene oxide materials in experiments [26]. Furthermore, the presence of functional groups and the number of layers were found to enhance resistivity values. As a result, the simulated conductivities are often higher than those measured experimentally.

Due to changes in d-spacing, defect concentration between MXenes flakes, surface functional groups, and their lateral diameters generated by each etching technique, $Ti_3C_2T_x$ observed electrical conductivities ranging from 850 to 9,880 S/cm. In general, MXenes with lower HF concentrations and etching periods have fewer defects and greater lateral diameters, resulting in higher electronic conductivity. Furthermore, humidity in the environment may affect their conductivities, indicating the potential for relative humidity sensing material applications [27].

Modification of surfaces using alkaline and thermal treatments is a good way to improve electrical characteristics. Conductivities increase by two orders of magnitude, according to their findings. The removal of functional groups (particularly –F) and intercalated molecules are responsible for this rise [28].

15.3.2.4 Magnetic Properties

In contrast to MAX phases, investigations of MXenes' magnetic characteristics were broadened due to the potential of magnetization. Magnetic moments are expected in several virgin compounds, including Ti_4C_3, Ti_3N_2, Ti_3CN, Zr_2C, Fe_2C, Cr_2C, Ti_2N, and Zr_3C_2. However, after terminations, each MXene and functionalization group must be examined individually. For example, the functional groups make Ti_3CNT_x and $Ti_4C_3T_x$ non-magnetic, whereas the OH and F groups make Cr_2CT_x and Cr_2NT_x ferromagnetic at ambient temperature, and Mn_2NT_x is ferromagnetic regardless of the surface terminations [29].

15.3.2.5 Optical Property

Photovoltaic, photocatalytic, transparent conductive electrode devices, and optoelectronic all benefit from visible and UV light absorption. Ti_3C_2Tx films absorbed light in the UV–vis range and had a transmittance of up to 91.2% at 5 nm thickness. In addition, depending on the film thicknesses, it may have an intense and wider absorption band at roughly 700–800 nm, which produces a pale greenish film hue and is important for photothermal treatment (PTT) applications. It's worth noting that the transmittance values could be improved by adjusting the thickness and ion intercalation [30].

The optical properties of these two-dimensional materials could be altered by the functional groups, according to first-principles calculations. In reality, unlike oxygen terminations, fluorinated and hydroxyl terminations have identical properties. When compared to virgin MXene, the fluorine and hydroxyl terminations lower absorption and reflectivity in the visible range, while all terminations increase reflectivity in the UV range. Furthermore, the absorbance value could be decreased by reducing the lateral flake size of MXenes [31].

MXenes are intriguing prospects for flexible transparent electrode applications because of their optical transparency in the visible range and metallic conductivity, but their significant reflection in the ultraviolet range signals anti-ultraviolet rays coating materials. Finally, a remarkable 100% light-to-heat conversion efficiency was achieved, which is critical for biomedical and water evaporation applications. To improve MXenes' applications, certain optical qualities such as luminescence efficiency, emission colors, plasmonic, and non-linear optical aspects must be addressed [32].

15.4 Classes of Bioanalytical Sensors Based on MXenes

15.4.1 Bioelectronics

In recent years, two-dimensional MXenes have gained much attention owing to their excellent electrical properties and good mechanical stability and hence they have been utilized in biomedical applications. MXenes exhibit excellent qualities for fabricating bioelectronics devices; however, self-restacking and agglomeration reduce their specific surface area and stability, limiting their use in biomedical applications [33]. The most effective technique to address such challenges is to transform 2D MXenes into 3D MXenes. It has been found that converting accordion-like Ti_3C_2 MXene into urchin-like sodium titanate (M-NTO) via oxidation and alkalization efficiently prevents MXene self-stacking. However, the produced M-NTO tends to impair conductivity due to the wide bandgap of sodium titanate (3.7 eV), and such problems could be efficiently managed by inserting additional conductive materials into M-NTO. Because of their superior electrical conductivity, ease of manufacture, and light weight, CPs are explored extensively among various conductive materials and/or polymers [34]. PEDOT was an obvious candidate for bioelectronics due to its superior stability, biocompatibility, and electrochemical catalytic activity [34]. Incorporating conductive PEDOT with advanced nanomaterials could produce synergistic effects, improve electrochemical sensitivity, and keep the morphologies of the base substrates intact. Because of all of these factors, PEDOT is an excellent option for incorporating M-NTO to enhance electrical conductivity. These materials (M-NTOP-EDOT) generate a huge surface area possessing quick transportation of electrons that could be exploited to make biomedical gadgets [34]. For example, Xu et al. [35] described label-free immunosensors based on gold nanoparticles (AuNPs) and M-NTO-PEDOT to detect prostate-specific antigen (AuNPs/M-NTO-PEDOT) (PSA). The oxidation and alkalization of HFetched Ti_3C_2 MXene nanosheets, followed by in situ oxidation to integrate PEDOT with M-NTO, were used to make macroporous M-NTO in this study. They also added AuNPs to the surface of M-NTO-PEDOT to increase the number of binding sites for PSA antibodies. Hence, AuNPs/MNTO-PEDOT combination, which possesses a huge surface area and good electrical conductivity, allowed the modified electrode to load substantial amounts of PSA antibodies and transmit charge quickly. The immunosensor's advantages included increased electrochemical test sensitivity and signal amplification. PSA was injected into human serum samples and detected within an acceptable range of 96.13% to 107.1% by the immunosensor.

15.4.2 Enzyme Sensors

The creation of electrochemical biosensors requires direct electron transfer of electrons directly among enzymes and electrodes. MXene has a variety of unique features, including a higher specific surface area and excellent electrical conductivity; hence, its addition could be an effective means of facilitating direct electron transfer. It is worth mentioning that, for the first time, Ti_3C_2 has been used in the construction of an electrochemical sensor towards hydrogen peroxide as a MXene [36]. Moreover, encapsulation of enzyme hemoglobin, which directly correlates to the protein to keep it stable and active has been done by using Ti_3C_2. Additionally, for mediator-free enzyme-based sensors, Ti_3C_2 MXenes were suitable candidates for direct electron transfer of hemoglobin. Other enzymes such as tyrosinase and acetylcholinesterase were also immobilized onto the surface of a Ti_3C_2 MXene [37]. According to their findings, Ti_3C_2 MXene, which has good metallic conductivity, huge surface area, and hydrophilic surface, is a viable choice for constructing enzyme-based biosensors. Many studies have followed the technique of mixing a Ti_3C_2 MXene and its functionalized materials, particularly different nanomaterials, to increase the activity of enzyme-based biosensors based on Ti_3C_2 MXene. Wang, F. et al., for example, modified TiO_2 nanoparticles (NPs) on a Ti_3C_2 MXene to increase the active surface area accessible for protein adsorption while maintaining enzymatic stability and activity. When compared to a biosensor without TiO_2 NPs, their constructed Hb-based biosensor had a greater detection capability towards hydrogen peroxide.

Glucose sensing is critical since it is a predictor of diabetes. Because of their hydrophilic nature, huge surface area, and unusual electrical conductivity, MXene nanosheets have been used to make glucose sensors. Gu et al. produced a hybrid of $Ti_3C_2T_x$ with graphene nanocomposite to avoid stacking in 2D graphene [38]. The suggested nanomaterial was deposited on the surface of a glassy carbon electrode for the construction of a glucose sensor, followed by 10 mL glucose oxidase enzyme immobilization. In this method, the proposed sensor has shown a controlled electrochemical process, which can be ascribed by the potential scan rate and electron transfer rate, which is superior to previously reported 2D graphene sheet–based GO_x biosensors [38].

It is well recognized that the use of GO_x is influenced by the environment, which may have an impact on its efficiency. As a result, Li et al. suggested that MXene nanosheets be replaced with nickel-cobalt double-layer hydroxide, which has been useful towards glucose determination because of its huge surface area and greater electrochemical activity. In addition, the two-layer hydroxide produces multiple catalytic sites and an ion diffusion pathway. The suggested sensor featured a three-second glucose response time and good selectivity [39].

The lower detection limit and sensitivity of the sensing platform could be created by oxygen shortage in sweat, as well as the stability of sensors employing all-in-one working electrodes produced using traditional methods, making detecting glucose and lactate in sweat difficult. Using a foldable wearable sensor composed of MXene-Prussian blue hybrid, Lei and colleagues developed a novel method for detecting hyperglycemia and lactate in sweat perspiration. Carbon nanotubes (CNTs) were also used to improve the sensor's mechanical strength [40].

15.4.3 Non-enzymatic Sensors

Non-enzymatic biosensors are electrochemical devices that can be used to determine biological chemicals and can catalyze spontaneous redox behavior of a variety of biological compounds by generating a significant voltage and electrical current. MXenes have been used to construct the biosensor towards many small biomolecules as it favors the electron transfer at the electrode interface in a quick manner, in this direction glucose sensor has been performed by using a MXene/NiCo-LDH composite [39]. Due to the many advantages of glucose oxidase-based sensors, much work has been done until recently, and hydrogen peroxide (H_2O_2) is created during the catalytic activity of GO_x, as well as many other oxidases. Non-enzymatic PB/Ti_3C_2 hybrid nanocomposites may easily evaluate hydrogen peroxide, according to some recent publications in this field [41].

Manufacturing an alternative non-enzymatic sensors using MXene with graphite composite paste to form modified carbon paste electrodes that were responsive to adrenaline and the detection limit was found to be 9.5 nM by chronoamperometry [42]. Differential pulse voltammetry (DPV) allowed for the precise assessment of adrenaline, ascorbic acid, and serotonin, with distinct DPV peaks for them. Acetaminophen and isoniazid pharmaceuticals have been determined together using screen-printed electrodes modified by a $Ti_3C_2T_x$ MXene were used. The use of DPV as a detection method allowed for the separation of acetaminophen and isoniazid and the proposed sensor has shown a wide working linear range and acceptable detection limit for both analytes. The amazing characteristics of MXenes to adsorb gaseous materials were extensively exploited in the development of several MXene-based NH_3 sensors [43]. Furthermore, MXenes' catalytic capabilities can be used to catalyze the determination of a variety of chemical and biological substances.

15.4.4 Electrochemical Immunosensors

In 2019, the first MXene-based immunosensor for the sensing of an antigen such as prostate was created [44]. Then, using a nanocomposite ($CuPtRh/NH_2$- Ti_3C_2) made up of trimetallic hollow CuPtRh cubic nanoboxes (CuPtRh CNBs) and a few stacked ultrathin ammoniated Ti_3C_2 layers. To support this, Dong, H. et al. constructed the immunosensor towards the determination of cardiac troponin I [45]. CuPtRh CNBs embedded in NH_2-Ti_3C_2 served not only as a spacer to prevent the NH_2-Ti_3C_2 layer from irreversibly restacking, but also as a connector to fix more Ab2 via stable Pt-N and Rh-N bonds, and the CuPtRh CNBs embedded in NH_2-Ti_3C_2 served not only as a spacer to prevent the NH_2-Ti_3C_2 layer from irreversibly As an Ab_2 label, CuPtRh CNBs/NH_2-Ti_3C_2 has a strong catalytic activity for lowering H_2O_2, considerably enhancing the electrochemical response. Furthermore, H. Medetalibeyoglu et al. [46]. For procalcitonin detection, a sandwich-type electrochemical immunosensor was designed. To increase the amount of PCT Ab1, they used a delaminated sulfur-doped MXene (d-S-Ti_3C_2 MXene) modified glassy carbon electrode (GCE) with AuNPs as an immunosensor platform and carboxylated graphitic carbon nitride (c-g-C_3N_4) to label PCT Ab_2 as signal amplification.

15.4.5 DNA-Based Biosensors

Biosensors detect nucleic acids and monitor the hybridization process through optical or electrical output as an efficient electrochemical tool towards the measurement of bioanalysis assay and in many other applications. The studies revealed that the MXenes could be utilized as an electrochemical interface towards the greater improvements in the detection sensitivity and monitoring of hybridization. Zheng et al. used a DNA/Pd/Pt nanocomposite to electrochemically detect dopamine (DA) [47]. Typical DA levels can indicate schizophrenia, Parkinson's disease, and Alzheimer's disease, to name a few neurological disorders and acute and chronic diseases. By in situ process, palladium and platinum nanoparticles were synthesized in presence of DNA/MXene nanocomposite. The inclusion of DNA prevents Ti_3C_2 nanosheets from restacking and enhances the even growth of PdNPs and Pd/Pt NPs, according to the findings. The electrocatalytic activity of the nanocomposites towards DA was also improved by depositing Pd/Pt NPs onto Ti_3C_2 nanosheets [48].

15.4.6 Application of MXene Modified Surfaces for Urea, Uric Acid, and Creatinine

On-site and real-time analysis of biomarkers is paramount important to analyze the target analytes and which is much essential in the clinical field. On-site applications are limited by the poor signal response, battery life limits, electrode leaching, low biocompatible longevity, and poor repeatability. In this direction, Liu et al. [49] recently published an MXene-based microfluidic biosensor for continuous multicomponent whole blood analysis. The fabrication approach combines $Ti_3C_2T_x$–MXene/SPE with a low-cost microfluidic device. The MXene/SPE electrode measured creatinine, while the urease/MB–MXene/SPE electrode recognized urea and uric acid. Three important biomarkers are used to detect serious kidney impairment and the requirement for hemodialysis: urea, UA, and Cre. The developed electrochemical biosensor enabled excellent sensitivity and selectivity simultaneous multi-component measurement of urea, UA, and Cre in whole blood. $Ti_3C_2T_x$–MXene was created utilizing a wet etching technique with HF etchant. The EIS of SPE revealed a well-defined semicircle with an interfacial resistance of 372.71, which nearly vanished after SPE was changed with MXene, indicating that the $Ti_3C_2T_x$ had a high electron transfer capacity. When MB was immobilized on the MXene/SPE, the charge transfer resistance was unaltered. After immobilizing urease on it, the resistance increased to 963.41, revealing that the enzyme that restricts the transfer of electron pathway was successfully immobilized.

15.5 Conclusions and Future Perspectives

MXene is a versatile 2D nanomaterial that can significantly improve the mechanical, electrical, and thermal properties of polymers. A MXene has very significant hydrophilic properties, which makes it very suitable for the preparation of nanocomposites. However, owing to the macromolecular structure of the polymer, the mixing effect of MXene in the polymer matrix still needs to be improved. As a result, in situ polymerization mixing can be used to make MXene/polymer nanocomposites. This solution is ideal for thermosetting and linear polymers that can be polymerized at low temperatures and blended with MXene.

MXenes are opening up a new route for the production of conducting composites with metallic conductivity, which could improve the sensing capabilities of amperometric enzymatic biosensors, thanks to direct charge transfers between MXenes and heme-based redox proteins. This finding offers up new possibilities for MXene-based biosensors and biofuel cells that use additional redox enzymes that can transmit direct charge. Furthermore, MXenes' ability to adsorb redox enzymes in 2D planes should be advantageous in biofuel cell applications since enzyme orientation would be less important in such a system, resulting in significantly greater electrochemically active surface areas of biofuel cell electrodes. MXenes have the drawback of being only available in very small sheets (up to 1 m in length and breadth).

References

1. S. Li, L. Ma, M. Zhou, Y. Li, Y. Xia, X. Fan, C. Cheng, H. Luo, New opportunities for emerging 2D materials in bioelectronics and biosensors, *Current Opinion in Biomedical Engineering*, 13 (2020) 32–41.
2. A. Chortos, J. Liu, Z. Bao, Pursuing prosthetic electronic skin, *Nature Materials*, 15 (2016) 937–950.

3. T. Someya, M. Amagai, Toward a new generation of smart skins, *Nature Biotechnology*, 37 (2019) 382–388.

4. C. Anichini, W. Czepa, D. Pakulski, A. Aliprandi, A. Ciesielski, P. Samorì, Chemical sensing with 2D materials, *Chemical Society Reviews*, 47 (2018) 4860–4908.

5. Q. Tao, M. Dahlqvist, J. Lu, S. Kota, R. Meshkian, J. Halim, J. Palisaitis, L. Hultman, M.W. Barsoum, P.O.Å. Persson, J. Rosen, Two-dimensional Mo1.33C MXene with divacancy ordering prepared from parent 3D laminate with in-plane chemical ordering, *Nature Communications*, 8 (2017) 14949.

6. M. Zhu, Y. Huang, Q. Deng, J. Zhou, Z. Pei, Q. Xue, Y. Huang, Z. Wang, H. Li, Q. Huang, C. Zhi, Highly flexible, freestanding supercapacitor electrode with enhanced performance obtained by hybridizing polypyrrole chains with MXene, *Advanced Energy Materials*, 6 (2016) 1600969.

7. M. Ghidiu, M.R. Lukatskaya, M.Q. Zhao, Y. Gogotsi, M.W. Barsoum, Conductive two-dimensional titanium carbide 'clay' with high volumetric capacitance, *Nature*, 516 (2014) 78–81.

8. C. Xu, L. Wang, Z. Liu, L. Chen, J. Guo, N. Kang, X.L. Ma, H.M. Cheng, W. Ren, Large-area high-quality 2D ultrathin Mo2C superconducting crystals, *Nat Mater*, 14 (2015) 1135–1141.

9. T. Li, L. Yao, Q. Liu, J. Gu, R.-C. Luo, J. Li, Y. Xudong, W. Wang, P. Liu, B. Chen, W. Zhang, W. Abbas, R. Naz, D. Zhang, Fluorine-free synthesis of high purity $Ti_3C_2T_x$ (T = -OH, -O) via alkali treatment, *Angewandte Chemie*, 130 (2018).

10. T. Li, L. Yao, Fluorine-free synthesis of high-purity Ti(3) C(2) T(x) (T = OH, O) via alkali treatment, *Angewandte Chemie International Edition*, 57 (2018) 6115–6119.

11. W. Sun, S.A. Shah, Y. Chen, Z. Tan, H. Gao, T. Habib, M. Radovic, M.J. Green, Electrochemical etching of Ti2AlC to Ti2CTx (MXene) in low-concentration hydrochloric acid solution, *Journal of Materials Chemistry A*, 5 (2017) 21663–21668.

12. J. Peng, X. Chen, W.-J. Ong, X. Zhao, N. Li, Surface and heterointerface engineering of 2D MXenes and their nanocomposites: Insights into electro- and photocatalysis, *Chem*, 5 (2019) 18–50.

13. L. Qin, Q. Tao, A. El Ghazaly, J. Fernandez-Rodriguez, P.O.Å. Persson, J. Rosen, F. Zhang, High-performance ultrathin flexible solid-state supercapacitors based on solution processable Mo1.33C MXene and PEDOT:PSS, *Advanced Functional Materials*, 28 (2018) 1703808.

14. L. Wang, L. Chen, P. Song, C. Liang, Y. Lu, H. Qiu, Y. Zhang, J. Kong, J. Gu, Fabrication on the annealed Ti3C2Tx MXene/epoxy nanocomposites for electromagnetic interference shielding application, *Composites Part B: Engineering*, 171 (2019) 111–118.

15. L. Qin, Q. Tao, X. Liu, M. Fahlman, J. Halim, P.O.Å. Persson, J. Rosen, F. Zhang, Polymer-MXene composite films formed by MXene-facilitated electrochemical polymerization for flexible solid-state microsupercapacitors, *Nano Energy*, 60 (2019) 734–742.

16. H. Wang, L. Li, C. Zhu, S. Lin, J. Wen, Q. Jin, X. Zhang, In situ polymerized Ti3C2Tx/PDA electrode with superior areal capacitance for supercapacitors, *Journal of Alloys and Compounds*, 778 (2019) 858–865.

17. Y. Tong, M. He, Y. Zhou, X. Zhong, L. Fan, T. Huang, Q. Liao, Y. Wang, Hybridizing polypyrrole chains with laminated and two-dimensional Ti3C2Tx toward high-performance electromagnetic wave absorption, *Applied Surface Science*, 434 (2018) 283–293.

18. M. Naguib, M. Kurtoglu, V. Presser, J. Lu, J. Niu, M. Heon, L. Hultman, Y. Gogotsi, M.W. Barsoum, Two-dimensional nanocrystals produced by exfoliation of Ti3AlC2, *Advanced Materials*, 23 (2011) 4248–4253.

19. M.W. Barsoum, The MN+1AXN phases: A new class of solids: Thermodynamically stable nanolaminates, *Progress in Solid State Chemistry*, 28 (2000) 201–281.

20. J. Halim, J. Palisaitis, J. Lu, J. Thörnberg, E.J. Moon, M. Precner, P. Eklund, P.O.Å. Persson, M.W. Barsoum, J. Rosen, Synthesis of two-dimensional Nb1.33C (MXene) with randomly distributed vacancies by etching of the quaternary solid solution (Nb2/3Sc1/3)2AlC MAX Phase, *ACS Applied Nano Materials*, 1 (2018) 2455–2460.

21. R.M. Ronchi, J.T. Arantes, S.F. Santos, Synthesis, structure, properties and applications of MXenes: Current status and perspectives, *Ceramics International*, 45 (2019) 18167–18188.

22. E. Pargoletti, V. Pifferi, L. Falciola, G. Facchinetti, A. Depaolini, E. Davoli, M. Marelli, G. Cappelletti, A detailed investigation of MnO_2 nanorods to be grown onto activated carbon. High efficiency towards aqueous methyl orange adsorption/degradation, *Applied Surface Science*, 472 (2018).

23. H. Lin, Q. Zhu, D. Shu, D. Lin, J. Xu, X. Huang, W. Shi, X. Xi, J. Wang, L. Gao, Growth of environmentally stable transition metal selenide films, *Nature Materials*, 18 (2019) 602–607.

24. Z. Dai, L. Liu, Z. Zhang, Strain engineering of 2D materials: Issues and opportunities at the interface, *Advanced Materials*, 31 (2019). DOI: 10.1002/adma.201805417

25. H. Lin, Q. Zhu, D. Shu, D. Lin, J. Xu, X. Huang, W. Shi, X. Xi, J. Wang, L. Gao, Growth of environmentally stable transition metal selenide films, *Nature Materials*, 18 (2019) 602–607.

26. R. Li, L. Zhang, L. Shi, P. Wang, MXene Ti_3C_2: An effective 2D light-to-heat conversion material, *ACS Nano*, 11 (2017) 3752–3759.

27. M. Lu, H. Li, W. Han, J. Chen, S. Wen, J. Wang, X.-M. Meng, J. Qi, H. Li, B. Zhang, W. Zhang, W. Zheng, 2D titanium carbide (MXene) electrodes with lower-F surface for high-performance lithium-ion batteries, *Journal of Energy Chemistry*, 31 (2018) 148–153.

28. J. Halim, S. Kota, M.R. Lukatskaya, M. Naguib, M.-Q. Zhao, E.J. Moon, J. Pitock, J. Nanda, S.J. May, Y. Gogotsi, M.W. Barsoum, Synthesis and characterization of 2D molybdenum carbide (MXene), *Advanced Functional Materials*, 26 (2016) 3118–3127.

29. H. Kumar, N.C. Frey, L. Dong, B. Anasori, Y. Gogotsi, V.B. Shenoy, Tunable magnetism and transport properties in nitride MXenes, *ACS Nano*, 11 (2017) 7648–7655.

30. K. Hantanasirisakul, M.-Q. Zhao, P. Urbankowski, J. Halim, B. Anasori, S. Kota, C.E. Ren, M.W. Barsoum, Y. Gogotsi, Fabrication of Ti3C2Tx MXene transparent thin films with tunable optoelectronic properties, *Advanced Electronic Materials*, 2 (2016) 1600050.

31. K. Maleski, C.E. Ren, M.-Q. Zhao, B. Anasori, Y. Gogotsi, Size-dependent physical and electrochemical properties of two-dimensional MXene Flakes, *ACS Applied Materials & Interfaces*, 10 (2018) 24491–24498.

32. K. Huang, Z. Li, J. Lin, G. Han, P. Huang, Two-dimensional transition metal carbides and nitrides (MXenes) for biomedical applications, *Chemical Society Reviews*, 47 (2018) 5109–5124.

33. P. Yu, G. Cao, S. Yi, X. Zhang, C. Li, X. Sun, K. Wang, Y. Ma, Binder-free 2D titanium carbide (MXene)/carbon nanotube composites for high-performance lithium-ion capacitors, *Nanoscale*, 10 (2018) 5906–5913.

34. A. Fethi, Novel materials for electrochemical sensing platforms, *Sensors International*, 1 (2020) 100035.

35. Q. Xu, J. Xu, H. Jia, Q. Tian, P. Liu, S. Chen, Y. Cai, X. Lu, X. Duan, L. Lu, Hierarchical Ti3C2 MXene-derived sodium titanate nanoribbons/PEDOT for signal amplified electrochemical immunoassay of prostate specific antigen, *Journal of Electroanalytical Chemistry*, 860 (2020) 113869.

36. F. Wang, C. Yang, C. Duan, D. Xiao, Y. Tang, J. Zhu, An organ-like titanium carbide material (MXene) with multilayer structure encapsulating hemoglobin for a mediator-free biosensor, *Journal of The Electrochemical Society*, 162 (2014) B16–B21.

37. L. Wu, X. Lu, Dhanjai, Z.S. Wu, Y. Dong, X. Wang, S. Zheng, J. Chen, 2D transition metal carbide MXene as a robust biosensing platform for enzyme immobilization and ultrasensitive detection of phenol, *Biosensors & Bioelectronics*, 107 (2018) 69–75.

38. H. Gu, Y. Xing, P. Xiong, H. Tang, C. Li, S. Chen, R. Zeng, K. Han, G. Shi, Three-dimensional porous Ti3C2Tx MXene–Graphene hybrid films for glucose biosensing, *ACS Applied Nano Materials*, 2 (2019) 6537–6545.

39. M. Li, L. Fang, H. Zhou, F. Wu, Y. Lu, H. Luo, Y. Zhang, B. Hu, Three-dimensional porous MXene/NiCo-LDH composite for high performance non-enzymatic glucose sensor, *Applied Surface Science*, 495 (2019) 143554.

40. Y. Lei, W. Zhao, Y. Zhang, Q. Jiang, J.-H. He, A.J. Baeumner, O.S. Wolfbeis, Z.L. Wang, K.N. Salama, H.N. Alshareef, A. MXene-based wearable biosensor system for high-performance in vitro perspiration analysis, *Small*, 15 (2019) 1901190.

41. Y. Dang, X. Guan, Y. Zhou, C. Hao, Y. Zhang, S. Chen, Y. Ma, Y. Bai, Y. Gong, Y. Gao, Biocompatible PB/Ti3C2 hybrid nanocomposites for the non-enzymatic electrochemical detection of H₂O₂ released from living cells, *Sensors and Actuators B: Chemical*, 319 (2020) 128259.

42. S.S. Shankar, R.M. Shereema, R.B. Rakhi, Electrochemical determination of adrenaline using MXene/graphite composite paste electrodes, *ACS Applied Materials & Interfaces*, 10 (2018) 43343–43351.

43. B. Xiao, Y.-c. Li, X.-f. Yu, J.-b. Cheng, MXenes: Reusable materials for NH₃ sensor or capturer by controlling the charge injection, *Sensors and Actuators B: Chemical*, 235 (2016) 103–109.

44. P. Liu, H. Meng, G. Zhang, L. Song, Q. Han, C. Wang, Y. Fu, Ultrasensitive dual-quenching electrochemiluminescence immunosensor for prostate specific antigen detection based on graphitic carbon nitride quantum dots as an emitter, *Microchimica Acta*, 188 (2021) 350.

45. H. Dong, L. Cao, Z. Tan, Q. Liu, J. Zhou, P. Zhao, P. Wang, Y. Li, W. Ma, Y. Dong, A signal amplification strategy of CuPtRh CNB-embedded ammoniated Ti3C2 MXene for detecting cardiac troponin I by a sandwich-type electrochemical immunosensor, *ACS Applied Bio Materials*, 3 (2020) 377–384.

46. H. Medetalibeyoglu, M. Beytur, O. Akyildirim, N. Atar, M. Yola, Validated electrochemical immunosensor for ultra-sensitive procalcitonin detection: Carbon electrode modified with gold nanoparticles functionalized sulfur doped MXene as sensor platform and carboxylated graphitic carbon nitride as signal amplification, *Sensors and Actuators B: Chemical*, 319 (2020) 128195.

47. Y. Liang, M. Khazaei, A. Ranjbar, M. Arai, S. Yunoki, Y. Kawazoe, H. Weng, Z. Fang, Theoretical prediction of two-dimensional functionalized MXene nitrides as topological insulators, *Physical Review B*, 96 (2017) 195414.

48. J. Zheng, B. Wang, A. Ding, B. Weng, J. Chen, Synthesis of MXene/DNA/Pd/Pt nanocomposite for sensitive detection of dopamine, *Journal of Electroanalytical Chemistry*, 816 (2018) 189–194.

49. J. Liu, X. Jiang, R. Zhang, Y. Zhang, L. Wu, W. Lu, J. Li, Y. Li, H. Zhang, MXene-enabled electrochemical microfluidic biosensor: Applications toward multicomponent continuous monitoring in whole blood, *Advanced Functional Materials*, 29 (2019) 1807326.

16

Bioelectronics with Graphene Nanostructures

Sobhi Daniel

Postgraduate and Research Department of Chemistry, T.M. Jacob Memorial Govt. College, Manimalakunnu, Ernakulam, India

Praveena Malliyil Gopi and Mohammed Essac Mohamed

Postgraduate and Research Department of Physics, Maharaja's College, Ernakulam, India

CONTENTS

16.1 Introduction

Bioelectronics is an emerging field of materials science, which integrates novel and smart materials with the biological world and will act as a bridge between the electronic and biological domains. With the progress in the development of intelligent bioelectronic devices, the field of bioelectronics has revolutionized the 21st century and has been emerged as an exhilarating field. [1–3]. The technology behind bioelectronics encompasses the synergy of biological materials and biological architecture for information processing and device fabrication. The significant perception of bioelectronics is the transduction of the biological signals to electrical signals at the sensing interface and the functionality of these devices is controlled by the chattels of the interface between the bioelectronic materials and biological systems [4,5].

Bioelectronic applications have gained excessive interest in recent years owing to their mesmerizing characteristics such as flexibility, low cost, nontoxicity, large-volume electronic components, sustainability, biocompatibility, biodegradability, and bioresorbable nature [6]. The miniaturization of nanomaterials such as semiconductors together with biological moieties has opened new horizons in biomedical research, health care, and commercial medical applications. The adaptability of bioelectronics applications in the arena of organic field-effect transistors and biosensors, promises a bright future. Nanoscale bioelectronics has led to the development of molecular-based personalized medicines. Also, nanoscale electrical measurements were found to be enormously important in genomics and proteomics for recognizing the function of proteins and their reaction pathways inside cells, as well as on cell membranes. The biosensor electronic systems can also be integrated with sensors, actuators, and computers with the progress in novel technological interventions. Highly integrated systems also brand conceivable developments in the creation of implantable devices having stimuli-responsive sensing devices and targeted drug delivery devices. Enormous applications will arise from the sustained integration of electronics with biology, which will create innovative biomedical expansions. Besides, the advance of nanoscale metrologies for the semiconductor industry may well find diverse applications in biological and biomedical research areas [7–10].

Carbon-based nanomaterials have the competence to bridge the gap between the biological and the electronic environment together with the fabrication of bioelectronic devices such as bio-actuators, biofuel cells, and biosensors, providing new horizons and prospects towards the future of bioelectronics [11,12]. The carbon-based materials have the potential to perform as a suitable interface by coordinating the biological entities to the electronic system. The interface will serve as a shuttle between biological and electrical entities and enhance the electron transfer rate in bioelectronic devices. Carbon-based materials have emerged as a well-suited candidate in the fabrication of bioelectronic interfaces, as they significantly exhibit a prime role in exploring the basics of material estates. The incredible properties of carbon-based nanomaterials such as their larger surface area, morphological and structural characteristics, chemical interaction, physical properties, thermodynamics, and electron transfer rate enhanced the integration of these materials in bioelectronic devices [13–15].

Among carbon-based nanomaterials, graphene has seized significant consideration in the fabrication of numerous bioelectronic devices owing to its rapid electron transfer characteristics, outstanding chemical and thermal stability, high surface-to-volume ratio, and superior mechanical properties like softness, flexibility, and mechanically robustness [16–18]. The unique structure allows graphene to have many scarce and striking properties such as quantum Hall effect (QHE), large surface area, superior intrinsic electron mobility, and excellent thermal conductivity. The promising applications of graphene-based nanomaterials include bioimaging, drug delivery, antibacterial coating, tissue engineering, 3D scaffolds for tissues, DNA-sequencing, etc. [19,20]. Also, recently graphene and reduced graphene oxide have emerged as brilliant nanomaterials in the development of epidermal and implantable bioelectronic devices. The inherent biocompatibility of graphene is also a fascinating attribute towards the fabrication of bioelectronic devices as it benefits to reduce inflammatory responses and facilitates stable and long-term skin-mounting or implantation. The biocompatibility of graphene can be efficiently tuned via surface chemical functionalization to expand the interaction of graphene with biological tissue [21]. This chapter will give an overview of the allotropic form of carbon-based graphene materials, their synthesis, mesmerizing properties, and diverse applications in bioelectronic devices.

16.2 What are Graphenes?

Graphene is the thinnest two-dimensional wonder carbonaceous nanomaterial with a unique chemical structure, brilliant physical properties, and excellent thermal properties [22].

Graphene, the allotropic form of carbon comprised of sp^2-bonded carbon atoms in a sheet-like hexagonal lattice arrangement in a two-dimensional plane. Three atomic orbitals, from carbon atoms viz. 2s, 2p$_x$, and 2p$_y$ orbitals are hybridized to form sp^2-hybridized orbitals, which form covalent bonds with the neighboring carbon atoms. These arrangements of hybridized orbitals lead to a hexagonal honeycomb lattice planar structure in graphene. The 2p$_z$ orbital is oriented perpendicular to the planar structure and form π bond and these π bonds are hybridized together to form the π-band which contributes to the astonishing electrical conductivity of graphene. Thus, graphene is composed of a closely packed single layer of carbon atoms, creating a 2D honeycomb lattice plane. In single-layer graphene, carbon atoms bond with adjacent carbon atoms with sp^2 hybridization forming a benzene ring in which each atom donates an unpaired electron. Graphene is theoretically a non-metal, but is frequently described as a quasi-metal due to its properties being like that of a semi-conducting metal.

The graphene carbon atoms are bonded to only three other carbon atoms, although they can bond to a fourth carbon atom. This ability with high tensile strength and high surface area to volume ratio brands graphene as one of the promising materials in the fabrication of composites. The inimitable physical properties such as appallingly high carrier mobility, mechanical strength, flexibility, and thermal conductivity positioned graphene as a supreme material [23]. This wonderful material has promising application in the field of bioelectronics owing to its superb electromechanical properties.

The oxidized form of graphene is known as graphene oxide (GO) and the surface of GO is decorated with oxygen-bearing functional groups such as hydroxyl (-OH) and epoxy ($\triangle$) groups on sp^3 hybridized carbon, on the basal carbon plane and carbonyl(-C=O) and carboxyl(C-OOH) groups were attached at the edge's sheets of sp^2 hybridization carbon. The presence of these functional groups enhances the hydrophilicity of graphene and widens their applications in biological fields such as sensing, drug delivery, and implantable devices [24]. The structures of graphene-based materials are shown in Figure 16.1.

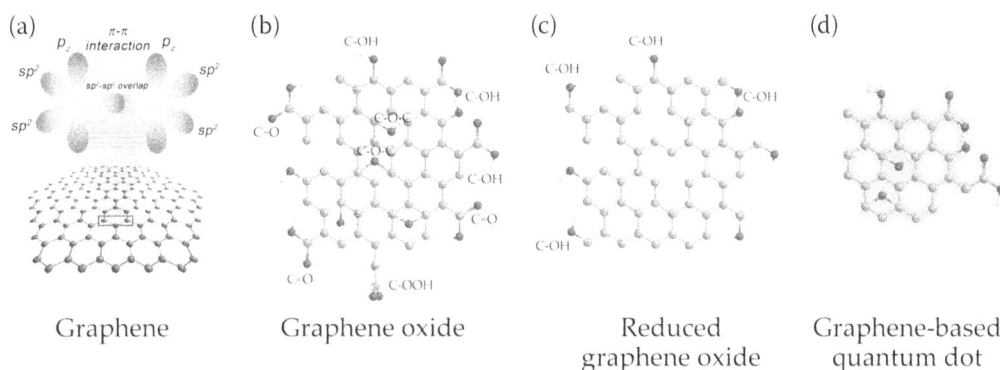

(a)	(b)	(c)	(d)
Graphene	Graphene oxide	Reduced graphene oxide	Graphene-based quantum dot

FIGURE 16.1

Structures of graphene-based materials: (a) the pristine graphene (pure-arranged carbon atoms) with sp^2-hybridized carbon atoms, and the chemically modified graphene, including (b) graphene oxide (GO); (c) reduced graphene oxide (RGO); and (d) graphene quantum dot (GQD).

Source: (Reproduced from Sensors 2017, 17, 2161; doi:10.3390/s17102161: licensed under creative commons attribution (CCBY) (http://creativecommons.org/licenses/by/4.0/).

16.3 Synthesis of Graphene

Analogous to all other nanomaterial synthesis procedures, graphene can also be synthesized by top-down and bottom-up approaches. The synthetic approaches adopted for the synthesis of graphene are schematically represented in Figure 16.2. The top-down synthetic strategy involves breaking down the starting materials into graphene layers and is a destructive technique.

The major top-down approaches adopted for the synthesis of graphene include exfoliation of graphite and graphite derivatives creating nano-sized graphene sheets [4]. Other top-down approaches adopted for the synthesis of graphene are mechanical exfoliation, liquid-phase exfoliation, arc discharge, oxidative exfoliation, reduction, and unhooking of carbon nanotubes (CNTs) [25–27]. Top-down approaches were adopted for the synthesis of graphene isolates and split the graphite layers into single, bi-, tri-, and multilayers of graphene. The major disadvantages encountered in the top-down synthetic strategy are its poor yields and uneven properties, which are related to the quality of the precursors adopted during the synthesis.

Another synthetic method is known as the bottom-up technique, which customs atomic-sized carbon precursor rather than graphite to nurture graphene and its derivatives and is regarded as the construction technique of graphene synthesis. In the bottom-up method, the assembly of graphene was produced from minor carbonaceous materials. Graphene can be generally synthesized utilizing numerous bottom-up methods, namely, chemical vapor deposition (CVD) substrate-free gas-phase synthesis (SFGP), epitaxial growth, template route, and total organic synthesis [28]. The advantages of the bottom-up technique over the top-down approach include the production of uniform and perfect graphene layers possessing a high surface area. Bottom-up synthetic methods were relatively expensive compared to the top-down approach.

Diverse materials can be employed as precursors towards the synthesis of graphene, with variable gradations of success. Solid forms are the widely studied and conventional precursors used for the synthesis of graphene, but liquid and gas precursors were also found to be effective. The ideal precursors suitable for the synthesis of graphene were found to be renewable resources but these materials should be systematically estimated, and the environmental impacts connected with the renewable resource should be thoroughly investigated. The precursors chosen can be of various types, ranging from conventional precursors to advanced starting materials such as carbon nanotubes. Figure 16.3 describes the potential precursors adopted for the synthesis of graphene.

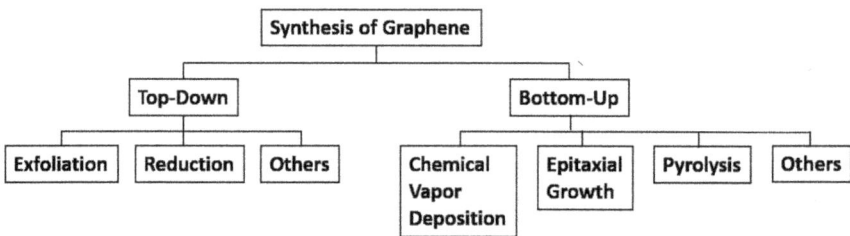

FIGURE 16.2

Schematic representation of the synthetic approaches adopted for graphene.

Source: (Reproduced from Nanotechnology Reviews 2020; 9: 1284–1314: licensed under creative commons attribution 4.0).

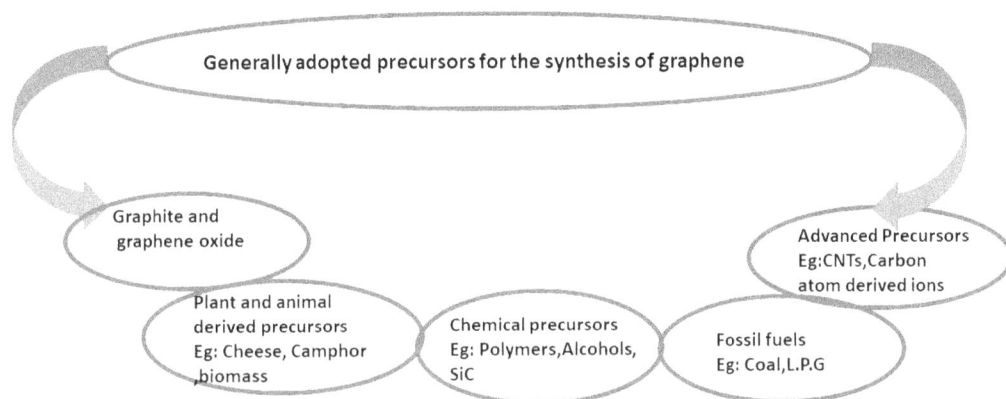

FIGURE 16.3
Potential precursors adopted for the synthesis of graphene.

16.4 Characterization Techniques of Graphene-Based Nanostructures

Characterization of graphene is crucial to investigate the number of layers and defects and to tailor its properties regarding the intended applications. Characterization encompasses both microscopic as well as spectroscopic measurements. The most convincing approaches embrace Raman spectroscopy, X-ray photoelectron spectroscopy (XPS), Fourier transforms infrared spectroscopy (FTIR), X-ray diffraction (XRD), X-ray absorption near edge structure (XANES), X-ray absorption fine structure (XAFS), atomic force microscopy (AFM), scanning electron microscopy (SEM), transmission electron microscopy (TEM), high-resolution transmission electron microscopy (HRTEM), ultraviolet-visible spectroscopy (UV-vis), X-ray fluorescence (XRF), inductively coupled plasma mass spectrometry (ICP), thermogravimetric analysis (TGA), Brunauer–Emmett–Teller (BET), and scanning tunneling microscopy (STM) [29–31]. Microscopic characterizations techniques include optical microscopy, scanning electron microscopy (SEM), TEM, and AFM sheen light on the morphology, flake size, and the number of layers. Figure 16.4 shows the schematic representation of various characterization techniques adopted for graphene-based nanomaterials.

The crystal structure of graphene can be investigated through an optical method known as Raman spectroscopy. This method delivers an idea about the hybridization of the carbonaceous structure as well as the level of disorder and number of layers present in graphene. Raman spectroscopy is a simple, fast, and non-invasive technique, which is highly sensitive to minute changes in the structure and by this technique, vibrant information on the number of layers, defects, and functionalization of graphene can be achieved. Two characteristic bands namely the D and G bands were observed in the Raman spectrum. The D peak ($\sim$1,335 cm^{-1}) was attributed to the defects and disorder while the G band ($\sim$1,593 cm^{-1}) was ascribed to the first-order scattering of the E2g phonon of sp2 carbons atoms and the intensity ratio of both peaks (ID/IG), usually used to qualitatively compare the density of structural defects present in graphene.

Fourier transform infrared spectroscopy (FTIR) is another most accessible and fastest technique, which is complementary to Raman spectroscopy to identify the type of oxygen functionalities and bonding configuration existing in graphene, GO, and its derivatives.

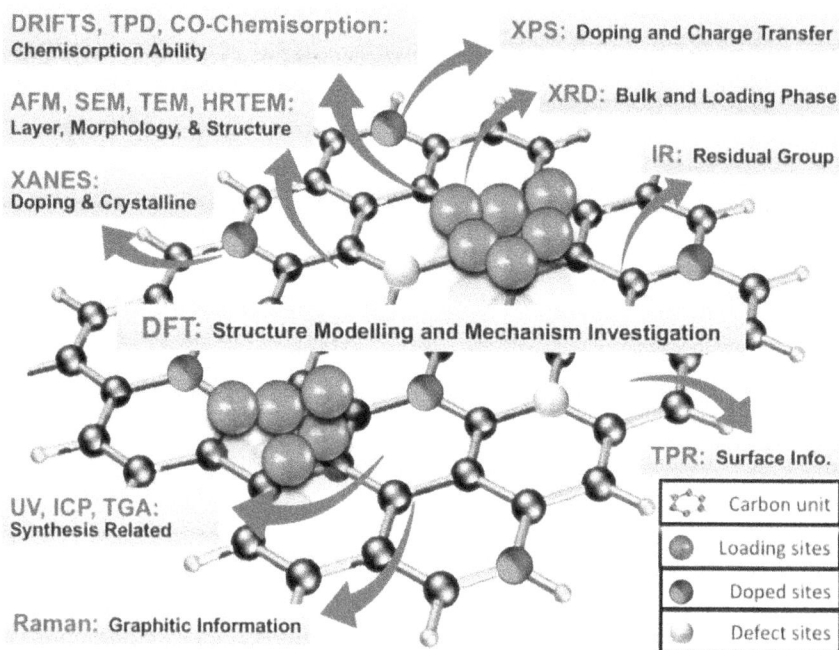

FIGURE 16.4
Schematic diagram of characterization techniques for graphene-based materials.

Source: (Reproduced from AIMS Materials Science, 4(3): 755–788. DOI: 10.3934/matersci.2017.3.755: licensed under creative commons attribution license (http://creativecommons.org/licenses/by/4.0).

From the FTIR spectral analysis, the typical peaks corresponding to functional groups present in GO comprised of O–H stretching (3,400 cm^{-1}), C–H stretching (2,910 cm^{-1}), C=O stretching (1,687, 1,710 cm^{-1}), C=C stretching (1,542, 1,568 cm^{-1}), C–O stretching (1,208 cm^{-1}), C–OH stretching (1,113 cm^{-1}), C–O–H bending (1,409 cm^{-1}), and C–H system stretching (2,875 cm^{-1}).

Ultraviolet-visible spectroscopy (UV-vis) is the most appropriate method to confirm the effective synthesis of graphene and GO. The graphitic structure generally exhibits an absorption peak at ~262 nm while a monolayer of GO exhibits absorption at ~230 nm in the UV-vis spectrum, which is accredited to the $\pi-\pi^*$ transitions of aromatic C–C bond.

X-ray photoelectron spectroscopy (XPS) is a surface-sensitive and prevailing quantitative spectroscopic technique and can be used to characterize the chemical state, elemental composition, and electronic state of the elements present on the surface of graphene. XPS is regarded as a precise technique to determine the quantity of carbon and oxygen compared to elemental analysis. It has become the standard method to prove the successful doping of heteroatoms on the surface of graphene. X-ray diffraction (XRD) and X-ray absorption near-edge spectroscopy (XANES) measurements are enlightening tools to investigate the structure, oxidation state, and local symmetry. From the X-ray absorption fine structure (XAFS) and extended X-ray absorption fine structure (EXAFS) spectroscopy, the accurate percentage of specific bonds present in graphene can be determined.

The morphological characteristics, structural excellence, and crystallinity of graphene and its derivatives can be investigated from the microscopic analysis. The frequently used microscopic methods are scanning electron microscopy (SEM), transmission electron microscopy (TEM) including high-resolution transmission electron microscopy (HRTEM), atomic force microscopy (AFM), and scanning tunnelling microscopy (STM). Scanning electron microscopy (SEM), transmission electron microscopy (TEM), and high-resolution transmission electron microscopy (HRTEM) are typically explored to envisage the morphology and structure of graphene-based materials. In addition to the morphological geographies of the nanostructures, the SEM scanned images additionally help to find the possible mechanisms responsible for the formation of specific structural characteristics, which are correlated to the end property of the material. Energy dispersive spectrometry (EDS) provided with FE-SEM is frequently used for the elemental composition of graphene-based nanostructures. The topographical and structural features exposed by the STM help in perusing the presence of defects, folds, and periodicity in addition to the number of graphene layers and recognizing the lattice disparity and effect of interface between the substrate and graphene.

HRTEM is also an operative technique to perceive surface defects of graphene-based materials. Furthermore, HRTEM elemental mapping is a powerful tool to distinguish the elemental distribution of graphene-based materials. AFM is broadly used to acquire the three-dimensional images, lateral dimensions, thickness, and the number of layers present in graphene films. AFM is also used to characterize the surface roughness, which will provide some evidence of surface area and the active area available in graphene-based materials.

X-ray fluorescence (XRF, non-destructive) and inductively coupled plasma mass spectrometry (ICP, destructive) are two exceedingly suggested techniques to investigate the residual metal concentration present in graphene-based materials. One superficial and practical technique adopted to analyze the mass loss of the functional groups present in graphene can be quantitatively estimated from the is thermogravimetric analysis (TGA). Also, by combining TGA with FTIR or mass spectra (MS), accurate informative data regarding the structural characteristics of graphene-related materials can be obtained.

Brunauer–Emmett–Teller (BET) surface achieved from nitrogen adsorption-desorption experiments at 77 K can quantify the surface area of the graphene-related materials proficiently and reliably, which can provide indirect support for the layer number identification qualitatively. The determination of layer number can be partially used to epitomize the surface area condition and vice versa. The theoretical calculations indicate that the highest surface area of monolayer graphene is 2,630 m^2/g.

The reaction mechanisms of graphene-based materials can be gathered by studying the mechanism by experimental techniques based on the bulk and surface structure analysis and chemisorption ability determination, theoretical computations with density functional theory (DFT), and from the combination of both experimental and theoretical investigations.

16.5 Properties of Graphene

Graphene holds several outstanding properties in terms of optical transparency, electric conductivity, mechanical strength, and thermal conductivity. The graphene revolution has commenced with the development of outstanding electrical and electronics properties. The properties of graphene materials are extremely contingent on the number of layers used to create graphene sheets. Graphene is a semi-metal or zero-gap semiconductor [32,33]. Electronic properties separate graphene from other condensed matter systems.

One of the most promising properties of graphene is that it is a zero-overlap semimetal (with both holes and electrons as charge carriers) with very high electrical conductivity. Graphene is exceedingly appropriate for transistors applications due to the electron-hole effect. Graphene is a semiconductor with zero bandgaps for the π/π^* bands crossing at the Fermi level. Another fascinating property of graphene is electron mobility. Graphene is the utmost conductive material so far at room temperature, with a conductivity of 106 S/m and a sheet resistance of 31 Ω/sq. This is credited to its ultrahigh mobility of graphene which is almost 140 times the mobility in silicon.

According to the refraction and interference of light, graphene with several layers would display different colours and contrasts which can be used to distinguish the layers of graphene. Graphene is a transparent material as it can absorb a 2.3% fraction of light. Graphene and its associated materials spectacle brilliant mechanical properties. Graphene is the strongest material, because of its superior mechanical properties of graphene. It is imperative to note that mechanical properties were dependent on the purity of graphene sheets. Thermal conductivity of graphene is contingent on the diffusive and ballistic conditions at higher and lower temperature ranges respectively. Better thermal conductivity of graphene materials is highly dependent on the quality of graphene sheets.

From a chemical reaction point of view, the pristine form of graphene is mostly not reactive. The chemical properties of graphene are disparagingly influenced by the surface characteristics and thickness of graphene layers. Single-layer graphene materials are highly chemically reactive than multi-layer graphene materials. Researchers unexpectedly found that graphene-based nanomaterials hold exceptional antibacterial properties. Graphene oxide, graphene oxide, and reduced graphene oxide can efficiently inhibit bacterial growth [34]. Graphene has a tremendously high specific surface area and high porosity, making them ideal for the adsorption of different gases such as hydrogen (H_2). Graphene has the capacity of fluorescence quenching. This characteristic of graphene can be exploited for the selective recognition of biomolecules. Graphene can be cast off as a novel effective SERS active substrate with exceptional biocompatibility and chemical inertness. Pristine graphene is insoluble in liquids such as water, polymer resins, and other common solvents. Therefore, it is essential to attach certain functional groups on graphene either physically or chemically to disperse in various common solvents without suggestively altering its required properties. Functionalization of graphene can be conducted with the help of suitable functional groups and by innovative synthetic approaches. Graphene exhibits the property of molecular self-assembly at the liquid-liquid interface. Self-assembly of two-dimensional graphene sheets is an imperative approach for creating macroscopic 3D graphene architectures for practical applications, such as thin films and layered paper-like materials.

16.6 Graphene-Based Bioelectronics

Graphene-based electronics offer an optimistic substitute to conventional bioelectronic device materials to meet the challenging device requirements in biomedical applications. Sustained progress in graphene nanostructure synthesis and micro-fabrication techniques permit innovative device architectures with tuneable physiochemical properties. The monolithic combination of graphene permits nanoscopic field-effect detection of chemical and biological signals with mechanically flexible and robust interfaces with biological systems. Switchable and flexible bioelectronics based on graphene nanostructures broadens the natural biochemical interface and mimic the biochemical reactions along with electron transfer phenomenon under the influence of external stimuli. Recent research works focused on graphene-based materials unlocked significant progress in bioelectronics with large-scale, low-cost, high-quality methods for the identification, detection, and quantification of biomolecules. Biochemical sensors based on graphene nanostructures have lately made substantial progress in this regard, exhibiting specific recognition in complicated biological fluids, remarkable temporal and spatial resolution, and adaptation to *in-vivo* platforms. This section explores contemporary research that incorporates graphene nanostructures in biochemical sensing systems and flexible bioelectronic interfaces to improve diagnostics and expand clinical applications.

Among the graphene-based nanostructures, the most widely explored materials in the production of graphene-based electrochemical biosensors are graphene oxide and reduced graphene oxide. Graphene oxide has a lot of oxygen-containing groups; thus, it's biocompatible and has a lot of active sites for immobilizing enzymes and other compounds. These oxygen-containing groups, however, would reduce their conductivity, necessitating the use of other conductive particles or polymers in the systems used to build electrochemical biosensors. Because of its bigger conjugated structures and fewer oxygen-containing functional groups, reduced graphene oxide has a greater conductivity than graphene oxide. It has been claimed that reduced graphene oxide can be utilized to directly change glassy carbon electrodes, which has proved to have more effects than other carbon nanomaterials like carbon nanotubes.

T. Zhang et al. [35] used the ultrasonication technique to yield a Pd NPs/rGO composite, which can be used as a sensitive tool to detect H_2O_2 and as a label-free immunosensor to identify alpha-fetoprotein selectively. Xiao et al. [36] originally transformed the graphene paper with electrodeposited MnO_2 nanowires and the as-built electrode was effectively used to detect H_2O_2 from living cells with an amperometry response variation of less than 5%. Gan et al. [37] explored the self-assembly of poly(3,4-ethylenedioxythiophene) on the polydopamine-reduced and sulfonated graphene oxide template for preparing a water-soluble, conductive, and redox-active nanosheets. This polydopamine-reduced and sulfonated graphene oxide greatly improve the conductivity and hydrophilic property of nanosheets. This material exhibited the highest conductivity of 108 S/m and was found to be stable for long-term storage under 4°C. The presence of numerous catechol groups makes the nanosheets redox-active and they can be employed as versatile nanofillers in the development of conductive and sticky hydrogels. Inside the hydrogel networks, the nanosheets produce a mussel-inspired redox environment, endowing the hydrogel with long-term and reproducible adhesiveness. This biocompatible hydrogel can be placed in the body for *in-vivo* biosignal detection. The adhesiveness and conducting nature of a prepared hydrogel makes it a suitable adhesive electronic skin for sensing electromyogram, electrocardiogram, and electroencephalogram signals.

The sensitive, speedy, and less expensive biomolecule analysis is critical in clinical diagnosis and therapy. For this, carbon nanostructures including carbon nanotubes, carbon nanodots, and carbon nanofibers have been employed. Lu et al. [38] recently reported that graphene and single-stranded DNA assemblies can be employed to detect biomolecules homogeneously. The electrochemical detection of four free bases viz adenine, thiamine, guanine, and cytosine has been addressed in the discussions of DNA sensors. With the rapid progress in the field of biosensors, graphene nanostructures have been easily integrated into ordinary 3D-printing procedures. Marzo et al. [39]. employed fused deposition modeling to create 3D-printed graphene with polylactic acid (PLA) electrodes for the sensing of H_2O_2. When introduced to 1:4 diluted human serum and five days after the exposure, the developed sensors could retain 98% and 84% of its observed sensitivity to H_2O_2 in buffer solution.

The advances in GO-based colorimetric biosensors have a larger surface area as well as intrinsic peroxidase-like activity. GO was also modified with a probe to create a target-specific colorimetric biosensor. Based on target separation and superior catalytic activity of GO/PtAu nanoparticles, Jungho Kim, et al. [40] prepared a sensitive and selective colorimetric biosensor for ATP detection and is shown in Figure 16.5. Both aptamer-modified GO/PtAuNP and aptamer-connected magnetic beads bind to ATP. The complex is formed from GO/PtA nanoparticles and magnetic beads by the binding of ATP. The complex reacts with H_2O_2 and TMB after the magnetic separation which results in a blue color supernatant. The low-density detection value of this colorimetric sensor is 0.2 nM, which is the lowest value among other ATP colorimetric sensors. Furthermore, at the 50 nM level, the color change could be distinguished with naked eyes.

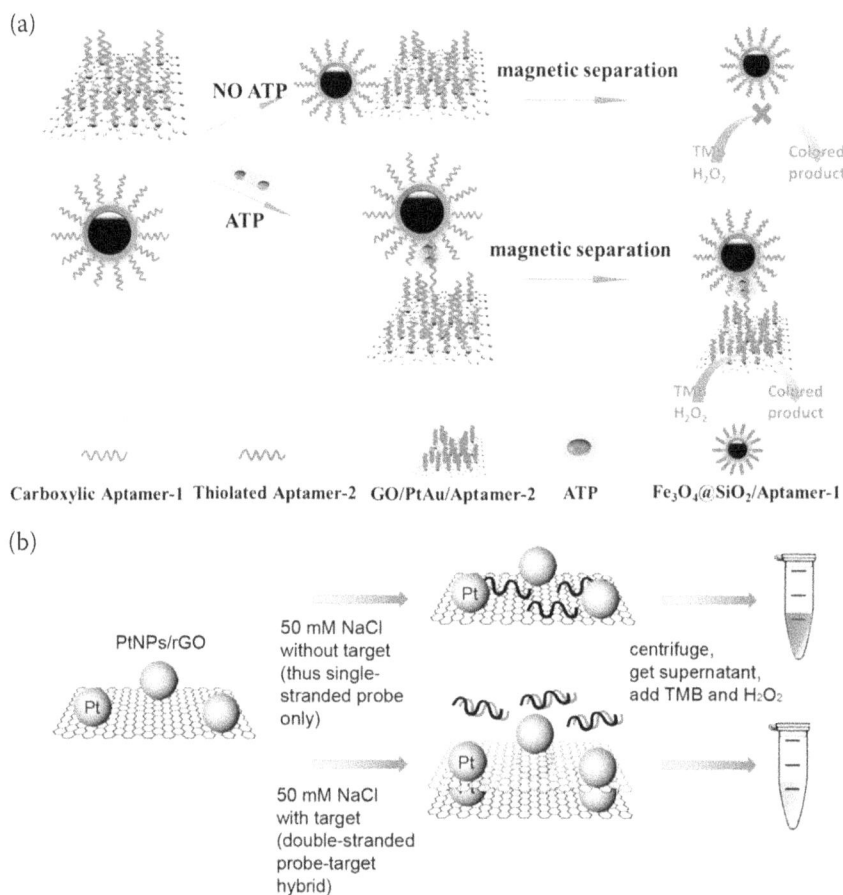

FIGURE 16.5

Colorimetric biosensors based on surface modification with target probe: (a) Scheme for colorimetric detection of ATP and (b) scheme for sequence-specific DNA colorimetric sensor by noncovalent modification of DNA on PtNPs/rGO.

Source: (Reproduced from Analytical Chemistry, 2017:89, 232–48, https://doi.org/10.1021/acs.analchem. 6b04248).

Kahlouche et al. [41] showed that electrophoretic deposition of reduced graphene oxide and polyethyleneimine can be used to selectively modify a gold (Au) microelectrode in a microsystem with a Pt counter and an Ag/AgCl reference electrode. With a detection limit of 50 nM, the functionalized microsystem was effectively used to detect dopamine. The microsystem was employed to detect dopamine levels in meat (beef and chicken) samples. Akkaya et al. [42] proposed a biosensor based on direct electrochemistry of glucose oxidase on a tannic acid–reduced graphene oxide nanocomposite modified glassy carbon electrode coated with Pt nanoparticles. Tannic acid was used to provide a switchable surface with changes in both pH and temperature. It also helps for green reduction of Pt^{4+} and graphene oxide and then altering the reduced GO for GOx immobilization. The redox peaks were found at a formal potential of 0.462 V with a peak separation (Ep) of 56 mV which indicates that there is a quick electron transport. The glucose oxidation response was linear and was in the range of 210 mM with a sensitivity of 27.51 A $mM^{-1}cm^2$, and the detection limit was 1.21 mM. The development of the shrunken and compact globule poly(N-isopropyl acrylamide) structure and variable surface charge resulted in the fabrication of an on-off biosensor with zipperlike interfacial properties after the deposition of poly(N-isopropyl acrylamide) onto the created biosensor via hydrogen bonding. The cyclic voltammetric response of the developed biosensor is shown in Figure 16.6.

Due to the signal transduction mechanism and unique working principles of functionalized graphene field-effect transistors (gFETs), functionalized graphene field-effect transistors (gFETs) have recently exhibited astonishingly low detection limits for trace biomarkers using crumpled graphene channels, which greatly increase gFET device performance for sensitive nucleic acid detection. The authors create wrinkled gFET channels using both substrate deformation and no substrate distortion. DNA is immobilized on the graphene channel via a pyrenebutanoic acid succinimidyl ester linker, and the target DNA is hybridized with a probe strand of DNA to allow for selective detection. Wu et al. [43], for example, developed dual-aptamer modified gFET biosensors for label-free detection of HCC-derived microvesicles in clinical blood samples. For the collection and measurement of these microvesicles, 62 gold nanoparticles containing both HCC-derived microvesicles cell-specific TLS11a aptamer and epithelial cell adhesion molecule aptamer (AptEpCAM) were attached to the gFET channel. Using their gFET biosensing platforms, the scientists discovered substantial differences in microvesicles' amounts between healthy control groups and HCC patients, indicating a promising potential for early HCC detection.

Lian et al. [44] developed a novel piezoelectric sensor for quick and selective detection of *Staphylococcus aureus* with an aptamer/graphene interdigitated gold electrode. 4-mercaptobenzene-diazonium tetrafluoroborate salt was used for molecular crosslinking to bind graphene with the gold electrodes which is coupled to piezoelectric quartz crystal electrodes. When *Staphylococcus aureus* was put onto the surface of graphene, the detection signal was recorded in the oscillator frequency of the quartz crystal (piezoelectric) electrodes. The good electronic conductivity provided by graphene resulted in a variation in the electric properties of the prepared electrode. The graphene-based nanostructures have been used for the recording of electrical activity both *in vivo* and *in vitro*. The greatest branded two-dimensional graphene electrode assemblies comprised of graphene as a passive electrode, such as electrode material in multi-electrode arrays or used as an active electrode, such as a semiconducting channel in field-effect transistors. Furthermore, the mechanical properties of graphene enable the development of bioelectronics on both rigid and flexible surfaces. The high transparency of this

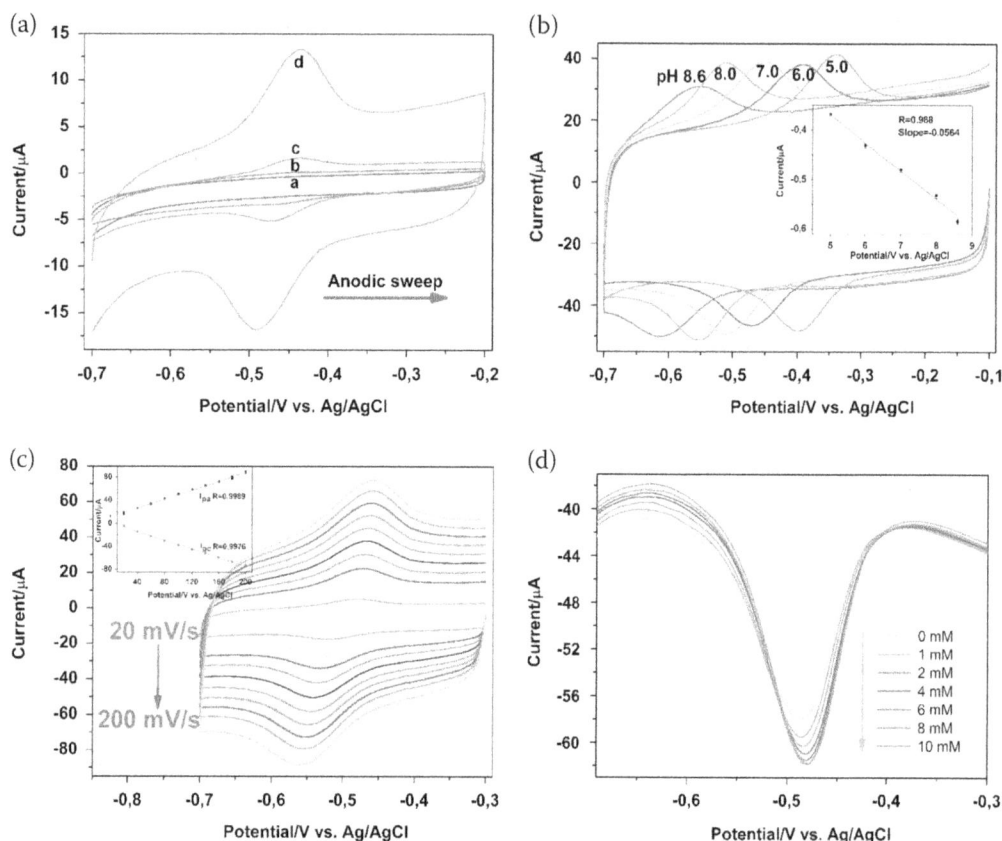

FIGURE 16.6
(A) CV curves of GOx/GCE: (a), GO-GOx/GCE; (b), rGO-GOx/GCE; (c), and rGO-Pt NPs-GOx/GCE; (d) in deoxygenated 0.1 M PBS (pH 7.4). (B) pH effect of the solution. (C) Scan rate effect of the experiment. (D) Glucose measurement.

Source: (Reproduced from ACS Sustainable Chemistry and Engineering 2018, 6, 3805–14, https://doi.org/10. 1021/acssuschemeng.7b04164).

low-dimensional graphene allows for the optical and electrophysiological recordings from electrodes, such as monitoring Ca^{2+} signaling with fluorescent dyes. The various dimensionality provided by graphene nanostructures has a significant impact on the electrical, optical, and mechanical properties of the materials. Two-dimensional graphene nanostructures are chosen for simultaneous electrophysiological, electrical, and optical recordings. Three-dimensional graphene nanostructures, on the other hand, are favored for a smaller sensor footprint and higher limit of detection because they provide effective electrical interactions and low electrode impedance [6].

To illustrate the notion of frequency-division multiplexing of brain impulses, Garcia-Cortadella et al. [45] combined graphene transistors with custom-built front-end amplifiers. It was accomplished by using graphene transistors to perform on-site amplitude modulation of the recorded brain signals. The Long Evans rat's cortex was interfaced with a 4 × 8 array of graphene solution-gated FETs to capture the spatial patterns map of cortical spread depression events. The proposed approach removes the need for switches, minimizing the limits imposed by slow switching speeds and reducing the platform's

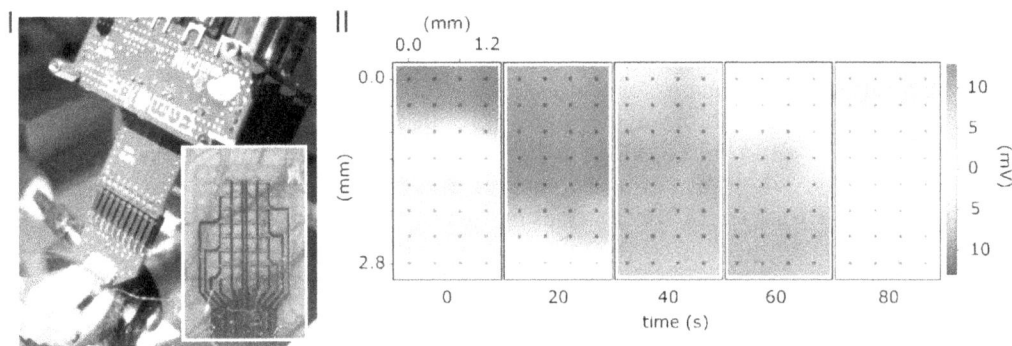

FIGURE 16.7
(I) The graphene solution-gated FETs array connects the brain to the front-end amplifier; (II) color maps showing the signal amplitude during the propagation of the cortical spreading depression.

Source: (Reproduced from reference *Nano Letters* 20, no. 5 (2020): 3528–37, https://doi.org/10.1021/acs. nanolett.0c00467.)

overall complexity. Figure 16.7 depicts the two-dimensional graphene solution-gated field-effect transistors array connects the brain to the front-end amplifier, which was custom-built, and signal amplitude on the array at various stages during the propagation of the cortical spreading depression event.

The reduction of impedance in ultra-micro electrodes (UMEs) is a tedious task and many methods including the deposition of surface coatings such as Pt black and conductive polymers have been adopted in different studies. The long-term stability of graphene bioelectronic interfaces is harmed by the delamination of surface coatings. By extending the topography of two-dimensional graphene to three dimensions, the material's effective surface area can be greatly expanded. Rastogi et al. [46] developed nanowire templated three-dimensional fuzzy graphene-based ultra-micro electrodes (UMEs) as a unique platform for recording extracellular field potentials from human embryonic stem cells-derived cardiomyocytes. The increase in the effective surface area of the electrodes caused by the three-dimensional out-of-plane arrangement of graphene flakes helps to reduce the impedance of the electrodes with a geometric footprint of $50 \times 50\ \mu m^2$ to a value of $9.4 \pm 2.7\ k\Omega$, which is very low compared to Au-based electrodes with the same geometric footprint.

The capacity to manipulate the electrophysiology of cells and tissues aids in the development of a better knowledge of the functional processes that occur in both healthy and diseased organisms. Clinical trials have shown that electrical stimulation of the central and peripheral nervous systems can improve tremors and motor rigidity in people with neurological illnesses. Capacitive charge injection from the surface of the electrode to the target is accomplished by charging and discharging the electrode-electrolyte double layer. To better understand the mechanism behind the charge transfer from graphene electrodes to target tissues and develop therapeutic tools, many graphene-based platforms have been developed for electrical stimulation of *in-vitro* and *in-vivo* systems.

At a negative polarisation potential of 0.6 V, Park et al. [47] calculated the charge injection capacity for manufactured graphene electrodes to be $57.13\ C/cm^2$. The exceptional optical transparency provided by the two-dimensional graphene allows simultaneous spatial and temporal imaging of brain responses to better understand the working of electrical stimulation. The change in fluorescence intensity increased as the amplitude of the stimulation pulse was increased, as seen by temporal mapping of cellular activity using fluorescent markers. This points to a direct link between brain activation and the charge injected.

Another important application of graphene bioelectronics is in the field of fabrication of interfaces inflexible and conformal graphene-graphite integrated devices. Sung Woo Nam et al. [6] developed ultra-thin monolithic graphene-graphite structures, which permitted the transfer of the whole device onto various non-planar substrates. Also, they have demonstrated the transfer of the monolithic device on a human eye model, which is having a potential application in the fabrication of artificial retina where the softness of the electronic material lends itself for conformal interface with the corresponding mechanical properties of biological systems.

Sung Woo et al. [2] also reported the synthesis of three-dimensional (3D) graphene-based biosensors fabricated via 3D transfer of monolithic graphene-graphite structures. They found that the developed materials were mechanically flexible; all-carbon structures were a potential candidate for intimate 3D interfacing with biological systems. The arena of switchable bioelectronics on graphene interface is at the phase of graphene-stimuli-responsive polymer hybrids proficient enough to regulate and control the enzyme-based biomolecular reaction under the effect of temperature, pH, light, etc. Recently, Meenakshi Choudhary et al. [7] reviewed the progress of switchable graphene-based bioelectronics interfaces.

Vinod Kumar et al. [13] highlights the existing advances in graphene and graphene hybrid-based bioelectronics and their properties (in terms of stretchability and conductivity), encounters, and future perspectives. In the arena of graphene-based flexible and stretchable bioelectronics in health care systems. Danker et al. [48] provided some perception on fundamental aspects of graphene solution-gated field-effect transistors and explored them as transducers for the recording of the electrical activity of living cells. The brilliant chemical, electrical, and mechanical properties, of graphene brand it as a supreme material towards the fabrication of bioelectronic devices based on field-effect transistors. Taemin Kim et al. [17] examined several types of flexible and/or stretchable substrates that are integrated with CNTs and graphene for the building of high-quality active electrode arrays and sensors. Young-Tae Kwon et al. [18] recently illustrated the first demonstration of all printed, nanomembrane electronics employing multiple nanomaterials to construct high-performance, wearable sensors, and wireless circuits. Three-dimensional, flexible graphene bioelectronics were fabricated on planar substrates by a wet-transfer method by using a thin Au film as a transfer layer to achieve the 3D graphene structure by Sung Gyu Chun et al. [49]. Dace Gao et al. [1] summarized the emerging soft conductors for bioelectronic interfaces including CNTs and graphene, which are customized to interface with skin and other tissues. Graphene nanostructures for input-output bioelectronics were recently reviewed by Garg et al. [50].

16.7 Conclusion and Outlook

The synergy of graphene-based materials and biology guarantees scalability and cooperativity in diverse fields of bioelectronics. The promising estates of graphene-based materials together with the simplicity of integration and functionalization brand them as suitable candidates in the fabrication of bioelectronic devices. With the advancement in the field of novel technological devices, graphene-based materials have exposed brilliant commercial applications in the field of bioelectronics within a short period. Thus, in recent years, graphene and its derivatives aroused as a rich source for the construction and use of bioelectronics and bioelectrochemical sensors. In sensing applications, graphene-based materials offered excellent conductivity, large specific surface area, and easily functionalizable surfaces. These materials deliver precise, quick, selective, sensitive, and even single-molecular-sensing abilities compared to traditional biosensing platforms. Sensors based on bioelectronics can accomplish a picomolar detection limit extendable up to a low femtomolar concentration range. Even though developments in graphene-based materials have shown remarkable electrical and electrochemical biosensor features, different challenges are still to be overcome to enhance sensitivity and sensitivity. Another challenging area is the performance of graphene-based materials in real biological samples where the presence of high salt concentrations and proteins may interfere with the sensing process. Also, the non-specific interactions present in proteins and the reproducibility of the fabrication of graphene-based biosensor interfaces are the restraining factor for the commercialization process. Thus, the progress in graphene-based bioelectronics is still in its infancy. Graphene-based materials essential for bioelectronic applications should be preferably defect-free and monodispersed concerning lateral dimensions and the number of layers. Also, the bulk scale production of graphene must focus on more environmentally friendly and green synthetic approaches. Toxicity and biocompatibility issues of graphene-based materials and interfaces are also to be addressed prudently to dodge the secondary health effects in clinical diagnosis and device fabrication. With the emergence of novel technologies and integration techniques, the fabrication of portable analytical quantification, wireless sensing devices in real personalized diagnosis, and wearable devices will revolutionize bioelectronics applications in the near future.

References

1. D. Gao, K. Parida and P.S. Lee, Emerging soft conductors for bioelectronic interfaces, *Adv. Funct. Mater.* 2019, 30, 1907184.
2. S. Nam, S. Chun and J. Choi, All-carbon graphene bioelectronics, 35th Annu. Int. Conf. IEEE Eng. Med. Biol. Soc., Osaka, Japan, 2013, pp. 5654–5657.
3. P. Suvarnaphaet and S. Pechprasarn, Graphene-based materials for biosensors: A review, *Sensors* 2017, 17, 2161. doi: 10.3390/s17102161
4. S. Trivedi, K. Lobo and H.S.S.R. Matte, Synthesis, properties, and applications of graphene, M. Hywel, C.S. Rout and D.J. Late (Eds.), *Fundamentals and sensing applications of 2D materials* 2019.
5. G. Liao, J. Hu, Z. Chen, R. Zhang et al., Preparation, properties, and applications of graphene-based hydrogels, *Front. Chem.* 2018, 6, 450. doi: 10.3389/fchem.2018.00450
6. D.S. Roman, R. Garg and T. Cohen-Karni, Bioelectronics with graphene nanostructures, *APL Mater.* 2020, 8, 100906. doi: 10.1063/5.0020455
7. M. Choudhary, S.K. Shukla, J. Narang, et al., Switchable graphene-based bioelectronics interfaces, *Chemosensors* 2020, 8, 45. doi: 10.3390/chemosensors8020045
8. K.A. Madurani, S. Suprapto, N.I. Machrita, et al., Progress in graphene synthesis and its application: History, challenge and the future outlook for research and industry, *ECS Journal of Solid-State Science and Technology* 2020, 9, 093013.
9. N. Patelis, D. Moris, S. Matheiken, et al., The potential role of graphene in developing the next generation of endomaterials, *Hindawi Publishing Corporation BioMed Research International* 2016, Article ID 3180954, 7 pages. doi: 10.1155/2016/3180954

10. A.R. Cardoso, A.C. Marques, L. Santos, et al., Molecularly imprinted chloramphenicol sensor with laser-induced graphene electrodes, *Biosens. Bioelectron.* 2019, 124–125, 167–175.
11. F.A. Pennacchio, L.D. Garma, L. Matino, et al., Bioelectronics goes 3D: New trends in cell–chip interface engineering, *J. Mater. Chem. B* 2018, 6, 7096–7101.
12. C.N.R. Rao, K.S. Subrahmanyam, H.S.S.R. Matte, A. Govindaraj, Graphene: Synthesis, functionalization and properties, *Modern Physics Letters B* 2011, 25, No. 7, 427–451.
13. V. Kumar and G. Khandelwal, Graphene-based flexible and stretchable bioelectronics in health care systems, *J. Anal Pharm Res.* 2016, 3, 12–14.
14. S. Szunerits and R. Boukherroub. Graphene-based bioelectrochemistry and bioelectronics: A concept for the future? *Current opinion in electrochemistry* 2018, 12, 141–147.
15. H. Hess, M. Seifert and J.A. Garrido, Graphene transistors for bioelectronics, in *Proceedings of the IEEE*, 2013, 101, 1780–1792. doi: 10.1109/JPROC.2013.2261031
16. J. Peña-Bahamonde, H.N. Nguyen, S.K. Fanourakis et al., Recent advances in graphene-based biosensor technology with applications in life sciences, *Nanobiotechnol* 2018, 16, 75.
17. T. Kim, M. Cho and K.J. Yu, Flexible and stretchable bio-integrated electronics based on carbon nanotube and graphene, *Materials* 2018, 11, 1163. doi: 10.3390/ma11071163
18. Y.T. Kwon, Y.S. Kim, S. Kwon et al., All-printed nanomembrane wireless bioelectronics using a biocompatible solderable graphene for multimodal human-machine interfaces, *Nature communications* 2020, 11, 3450. doi: 10.1038/s41467-020-17288-0
19. S. Nosheena, M. Irfanb, F. Habibc, et al., Graphene: The material of today and tomorrow, *International Journal of Sciences: Basic and Applied Research (IJSBAR)* 2021, 58, 44–53.
20. C. Zhao, X. Song, Y. Liu et al., Synthesis of graphene quantum dots and their applications in drug delivery, *J Nanobiotechnol* 2020, 18, 142.
21. G. Yang, L. Li, W.B. Lee et al., Structure of graphene and its disorders: A review, *Science and Technology of Advanced Materials* 2018, 19, 613–648. doi: 10.1080/14686996.2018.1494493
22. D. Sahu, H. Sutar, P. Senapati, R. Murmu and D. Roy, Graphene, graphene-derivatives and composites: Fundamentals, synthesis approaches to applications, *J. Compos. Sci.* 2021, 5, 181. doi: 10.3390/jcs5070181
23. X. Huang, Z. Yin, S. Wu, et al., Graphene-based materials: Synthesis, characterization properties, and applications, *Small* 2011, 7, 1876–1902.
24. Y. Yan, F.Z. Nashath, S. Chen, et al., Synthesis of graphene: Potential carbon precursors and approaches, *Nanotechnology Reviews* 2020, 9, 1284–1314.
25. S. Trivedi, K. Lobo and H.S.S.R. Matte, Synthesis, properties, and applications of graphene, chapter 3, *Fundamentals and Sensing Applications of 2D Materials* 2019, Elsevier. doi: 10. 1016/B978-0-08-102577-2.00003-8
26. M. Hu, Z. Yao, and X. Wang, Characterization techniques for graphene-based materials in catalysis, *AIMS Materials Science*, 2017, 4, 755–788. doi: 10.3934/matersci.2017.3.755
27. B. Huang, Q. Wang, Y. Li, M. Zhang et al., Preparation and characterisation of graphene, *Materials Research Innovations* 2015, 19, SUPPL 9. S9-344–S9-350.
28. T.M. Radadiya, A properties of graphene, *European Journal of Material Sciences* 2015, 2, 6–18.
29. M. Kaur and P.K. Tripathi, The basic properties of graphene and its applications, 2018. www. ijrar.org (E-ISSN 2348-1269, P- ISSN 2349–5138).
30. U.K. Sur, Graphene: A rising star on the horizon of materials science, *International Journal of Electrochemistry* 2012, Article ID 237689, 12 pages. doi: 10.1155/2012/237689
31. S. Niyogi, E. Bekyarova, M.E. Itkis, et al., Solution properties of graphite and graphene, *Journal of the American Chemical Society* 2006, 128, 7720–7721.
32. S.K. Tiwari, S. Sahoo, N. Wang et al., Graphene research and their outputs: Status and prospect, *Journal of Science: Advanced Materials and Devices* 2020, 5, 10e29.
33. A.K. Geim, Science, graphene: Status and prospects, *Science* 2009, 324, 1530–1534. doi: 10.1126/science.1158877
34. P. Kumar, P. Huo, R. Zhang et al., Antibacterial properties of graphene-based nanomaterials, *Nanomaterials (Basel)* 2019, 9, 737.

35. T. Zhang, J. Liu, C. Wang, et al., Synthesis of graphene and related two-dimensional materials for bioelectronics devices, *Biosensors and Bioelectronics*2017 89, 28–42. doi: 10.1016/j.bios.2016.06.072
36. F. Xiao, Y. Li, X. Zan, et al., Growth of metal-metal oxide nanostructures on Freestanding graphene paper for flexible biosensors, *Advanced Functional Materials* 2012, 22, no. 12, 2487–2494. doi: 10.1002/adfm.201200191
37. G. Donglin, H. Ziqiang, W. Xiao et al., Graphene oxide-templated conductive and redox-active nanosheets incorporated hydrogels for adhesive bioelectronics, *AdvancedFunctionalMaterials* 2020, 30, 110. doi: 10.1002/adfm.201907678
38. C. Lu, H.H. Yang, C.L. Zhu et al., A graphene platform for sensing biomolecules, *Angewandte Chemie - International Edition* 2009, 48, 4785–4787. doi: 10.1002/anie.200901479
39. A.M. López Marzo, C.C. Mayorga-Martinez and M. Pumera, 3D-printed graphene direct electron transfer enzyme biosensors, *Biosensors and Bioelectronics* 2020, 151. doi: 10.1016/j.bios.2019.111980
40. J. Kim, S.J. Park and D.H. Min, Emerging approaches for graphene oxide biosensor, *Analytical Chemistry* 2017, 89, 232–248. doi: 10.1021/acs.analchem.6b04248
41. K. Kahlouche, R. Jijie, I. Hosu, et al., Controlled modification of electrochemical microsystems with polyethylenimine/reduced graphene oxide using electrophoretic deposition: Sensing of dopamine levels in meat samples, *Talanta* 2018, 178, 432–440. doi: 10.1016/j.talanta.2017.09.065
42. B. Akkaya, B. Çakiroğlu and M. Özacar, Tannic acid-reduced graphene oxide Deposited with Pt nanoparticles for switchable bioelectronics and biosensors based on direct electrochemistry, *ACS Sustainable Chemistry and Engineering* 2018, 6, 3805–3814. doi: 10.1021/acssuschemeng.7b04164
43. D. Wu, Y. Yu, D. Jin et al., Dual-aptamer modified graphene field-effect transistor nanosensor for label-free and specific detection of hepatocellular carcinoma-derived microvesicles, *Anal Chem.* 2020, 3, 4006–4015. doi: 10.1021/acs.analchem.9b05531
44. Y. Lian, F. He, H. Wang et al., A new aptamer/graphene interdigitated gold electrode piezoelectricSensor for rapid and specific detection of staphylococcus aureus, *Biosensors and Bioelectronics* 2015, 65, 314–319. doi: 10.1016/j.bios.2014.10.017
45. R. Garcia-Cortadella, N. Schäfer, J. Cisneros-Fernandez et al., Switchless multiplexing of graphene active sensor arrays for brain mapping, *Nano Letters* 2020, 20, 3528–3537. doi: 10.1021/acs.nanolett.0c00467
46. S.K. Rastogi, J. Bliley, L. Matino, et al., Three-dimensional fuzzy graphene ultra-microelectrodes for subcellular electrical recordings, *Nano Res.* 2020. 13, 1444–1452. doi: 10.1007/s12274-020-2695-y
47. D.W. Park, J.P. Ness, S.K. Brodnick et al., Electrical neural stimulation and simultaneous in vivo monitoring with transparent graphene electrode arrays Implanted in GCaMP6f mice, *ACS Nano.* 2018, 23,148–157. doi: 10.1021/acsnano.7b04321
48. M. Danker, M.V. Hauf, A. Lippert et al., Graphene solution-gated field-effect transistor array for sensing applications, *Advanced functional functional Materials* 2010, 20, 3117–3124.
49. S.G. Chun, J. Choi, A. Ashraf, et al., IEEE, three-dimensional, flexible graphene bioelectronics, *Annu Int Conf IEEE Eng Med Biol Soc.* 2014, 5268–5271. doi: 10.1109/EMBC.2014.6944814. PMID: 25571182.
50. R. Garg, D.S. Roman, Y. Wang, et al., Graphene nanostructures for input–output bioelectronics, *Biophysics Rev.* 2021, 2, 041304. doi: 10.1063/5.0073870

17

Nanomaterial-Assisted Bioelectronic Devices towards Biocomputer

Jinho Yoon and Joungpyo Lim

Department of Chemical & Biomolecular Engineering, Sogang University, Mapo-Gu, Seoul, Republic of Korea

Jinmyeong Kim

Department of Chemical Engineering, Kwangwoon University, Nowon-Gu, Seoul, Republic of Korea

Minkyu Shin

Department of Chemical & Biomolecular Engineering, Sogang University, Mapo-Gu, Seoul, Republic of Korea

Taek Lee

Department of Chemical Engineering, Kwangwoon University, Nowon-Gu, Seoul, Republic of Korea

Jeong-Woo Choi

Department of Chemical & Biomolecular Engineering, Sogang University, Mapo-Gu, Seoul, Republic of Korea

CONTENTS

DOI: 10.1201/9781003263265-17

17.1 Introduction

Since its first discovery, nanomaterials have been broadly used in scientific fields with huge attention. For example, nanomaterials are utilized as the template for efficient drug delivery, an electrode component of the battery, and enhanced stem cell differentiation [1]. Particularly, at the nanometer scale, nanomaterials sometimes have properties that were not present in the bulk state; thus, nanomaterials are being used in fields where the properties generated in the nanoscale are advantageous. For instance, the metal enhanced fluorescence (MEF), in which the strong fluorescent emission can be achieved by control of the distance between the fluorescent-emitting molecule and metal surface at the nanometer scale, is normally utilized in the development of fluorescent biosensors, and the nanoparticle (NP) with a maximized surface area created, adding a nanoporous structure, is used for effective drug delivery. In recent years, as research to develop nanomaterials with superior properties continues, several 2D nanomaterials, such as transition metal dichalcogenide (TMD) and MXene, have been reported with excellent and unique properties beyond metal or carbon nanomaterials [2].

Among the myriad of fields in which nanomaterials can be utilized, the field of bioelectronics is particularly expected to benefit from the introduction of nanomaterials. Bioelectronics is the convergent research field of biology and electronics that studies the demonstration and implementation of electronic functions on the biochip using biomaterials [3]. Since nanometer-sized biomaterials such as enzymes and nucleic acids are directly used for the demonstration of electronic functions by themselves without a combination of lots of electronic components, bioelectronics may overcome the current issues of conventional silicon-based electronic devices that will hit limits in terms of physics (e.g., production process problems in high-density integration of electronic circuits or the limitation of the thickness of the current electronic circuits). Accordingly, several types of bioelectronic devices have been developed using biomaterials like biomemory, biologic gates, bioprocessors, and biotransistors corresponding to core electronic devices (Figure 17.1). However, due to the usage of biomaterials, bioelectronic devices face problems derived from biomaterials including the poor electric or electrochemical signal-to-noise ratio, instability in harsh conditions, or limitation of bioelectronic functional expansion [4]. These limitations may hinder the development of novel functional bioelectronic devices that can be used for developing the biocomputer, which could conduct the overall computing functions through the combination of properties of various biomaterials. To address these issues, nanomaterials have recently been introduced in bioelectronics. Nanomaterials offer advantages that can solve the limitations of biomaterials. For example, nanomaterials can provide the stable template for the immobilization of biomaterials, highly conductive electrodes, and diversification of electronic functions implemented through the expansion of signals derived from biomaterials. Therefore, it is expected that nanomaterial-assisted bioelectronic devices may contribute to the development of the biocomputer.

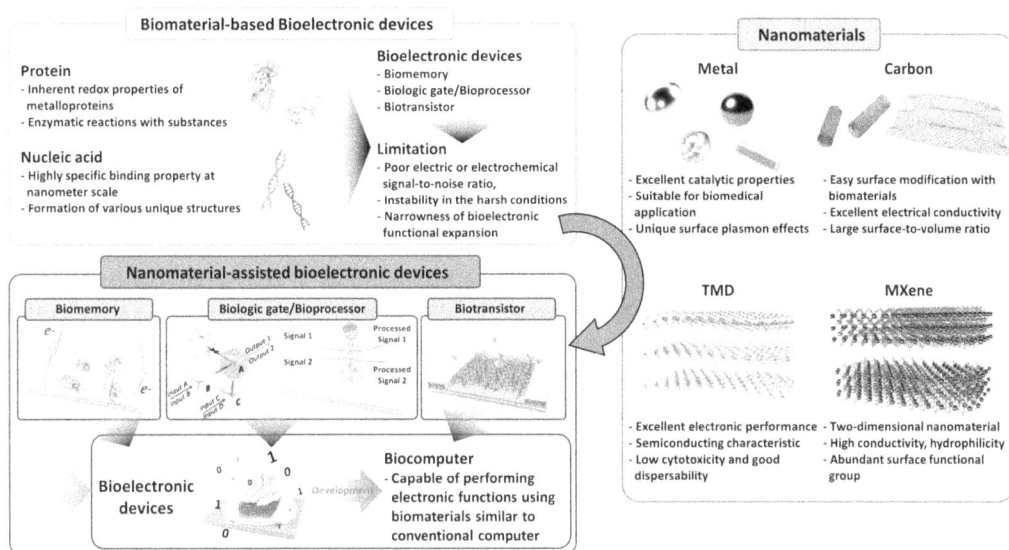

FIGURE 17.1
Nanomaterial-assisted bioelectronic devices towards bioelectronics.

In this chapter, nanomaterial-assisted bioelectronic devices are discussed, focusing on the application to the biocomputer. Specifically, bioelectronic devices developed using only biomaterials, particularly using the representative biomaterials including protein and nucleic acids, are discussed first. Next, several nanomaterials, utilized largely for developing bioelectronic devices, are provided with the classified sections composed of metal, carbon, and 2D nanomaterials (TMD and MXene). Then, nanomaterial-assisted protein-based bioelectronic devices are described based on the classification divided by widely studied types of bioelectronic devices such as biomemory, biologic gate/bioprocessors, and biotransistors. Next, nanomaterial-assisted nucleic acid–based bioelectronic devices are described according to the previous division. Finally, future perspectives are provided, such as the current limitations of nanomaterial-assisted bioelectronic devices and technologies that are considered suitable to combine with bioelectronic devices for future bioelectronics towards the biocomputer.

17.2 Biomaterial-Based Bioelectronic Devices

17.2.1 Protein-Based Bioelectronic Devices

The main purpose of bioelectronics is to implement the electronic functions of conventional silicon-based electronic devices such as memory and logic gate functions on the biochip using biomaterials. Among various biomaterials, proteins have several inherent properties suitable for realizing this concept. For example, metalloproteins have metal ions in their structures, and those metal ions have a huge potential for being applied in biological fields from biosensing to bioelectronics [5]. Due to the metal ions, the metalloprotein has its essential redox property through the switch of its metal ion states by external stimulation. Using this switch of the metal ion, metalloproteins can exist with two different states, which can be distinguished and defined as "0" and "1." This demonstrates the binary-based memory functions in conventional electronic devices [6]. Moreover, since some metalloproteins have different types of metal ions, a higher-order multibit biomemory can be developed through the simultaneous introduction of different metalloproteins. In one study, Choi's group developed the multilevel biomemory device by using two metalloproteins composed of a recombinant azurin and cytochrome c [7]. Using the cysteine residue of a recombinant azurin and electrostatic interaction between azurin and cytochrome c, the heterolayer of metalloproteins was prepared on the gold (Au) substrate, and the redox states of two metalloproteins were regulated by electrochemical stimulation to implement the multilevel memory functions (Figure 17.2a). In addition, metalloproteins have been used to develop other types of bioelectronic devices such as a biotransistor using their inherent redox properties with excellent reproducibility (Figure 17.2b) [8].

Another important protein that can be used for bioelectronic devices is an enzyme. An enzyme acts as a biological catalyst in the metabolic processes of living organisms. Various enzymes conduct lots of enzymatic reactions to maintain living things. These numerous enzymatic reactions between enzymes and substances can be used to implement the logic gate functions on the biochip. The logic gate is one of the core components

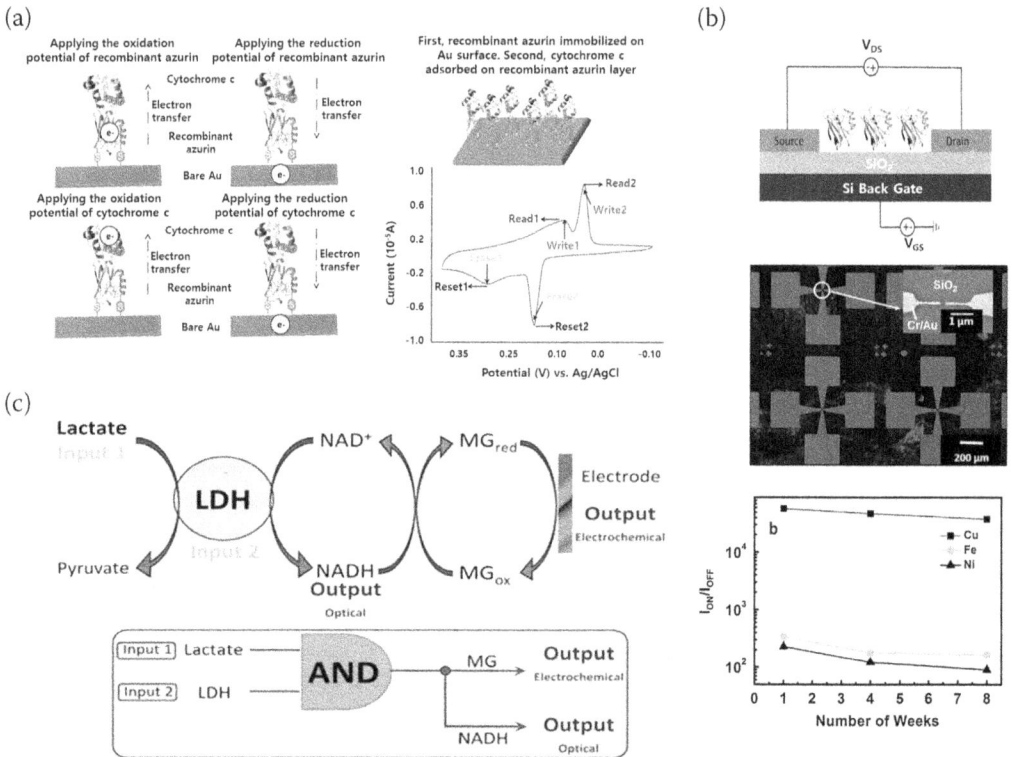

FIGURE 17.2
(a) A multilevel biomemory device. Adapted with permission [7]. Copyright (2010) John Wiley and Sons. (b) An azurin-based field-effect biotransistor and transistor properties. Adapted with permission [8]. Copyright (2017) Elsevier. (c) A biologic gate based on enzymatic reactions. Adapted with permission [9]. Copyright (2010) American Chemical Society.

of the computer that conducts logical operations including AND, NOR, and OR logic functions through the conversion of input signals to the one binary output signals. These logical operations can be demonstrated by using enzymatic reactions for implementing Boolean functions on biochips to develop a biologic gate. For instance, by combining various enzymes (e.g., lactate dehydrogenase, LDH) and their reactions, output signals from logic operations were determined by added input substances (e.g., lactate) to demonstrate certain logic gates such as AND or NAND gates (Figure 17.2c) [9]. However, as discussed previously, bioelectronic devices implemented using only proteins have limitations such as weak signals or difficulties in implementing into more complex electronic devices and the inherent instability of biomaterials. Recently, a lot of research on the fusion of protein-based electronic devices and nanomaterials has been conducted, which will be the focus of later sections.

17.2.2 Nucleic Acid–Based Bioelectronic Devices

A transistor is one of the most essential electronic devices that can amplify or switch current to operate a computing system. The increase of transistor density is an important issue because Si-based electronic devices typically face physical limitations at sizes below 100 nm. Therefore, the demand for materials that can replace Si is increasing, and nucleic acids are one of the most attractive candidates for replacing Si due to their unique properties such as charge transfer and molecular rectification [10].

Gottarelli's group developed the field-effect transistors (FETs) using guanosine (Figure 17.3a) [11]. Guanosine has the lowest oxidation potential among the nucleobases and a unique sequence of hydrogen bonding sites. The low oxidation potential of guanosine is suitable for charge carrier transport and forms long ribbon-shaped supramolecular assemblies via hydrogen bonding. In addition, a strong dipole moment can be formed along the ribbon axis, which induces a commutation of the current for enhancing the transistor density. Stefanović's group developed an array of three ribozyme-based biologic gates to realize an artificial decision-making network in a biocompatible and autonomous manner (Figure 17.3b) [12]. A Boolean algebra was performed with a total of three fluorescence dye–modified ribozymes by applying two ribozymes for the XOR gate construction and another ribozyme for the AND gate construction to generate different outputs. Two oligonucleotides were used as random two inputs, which allosterically activate the ribozyme. The output was also an oligonucleotide, and two different colorimetric fluorescence detection systems had applied to distinguish these two output values. In addition, Lee's group fabricated a global positioning system (GPS) using a DNA bioprocessor that designated two physical locations, the current location of the processor and the final destination, and specified the optimal or shortest route based on the six routes stored in the database (Figure 17.3c) [13]. For simplicity, the map was simplified into six main pieces of information. An indication that connected the physical location with the connection route was made by utilizing the length of single-stranded DNA, which represents the length of the linkage pathway.

In addition, Suyama's group has developed a biomemory using DNA hybridization [15]. The memory strand was composed of DNA with a hairpin structure. The data strand consisted of "address" and "content," where the address was a linear DNA sequence that can complementarily be hybridized with the memory strand, and the content was a DNA or RNA sequence (state 1). "Writing" and "erasing" of the DNA-based biomemory were performed by temperature control. The data strand was hybridized with the memory strand as the hairpin structure of the memory strand changed by writing temperature (T_W)

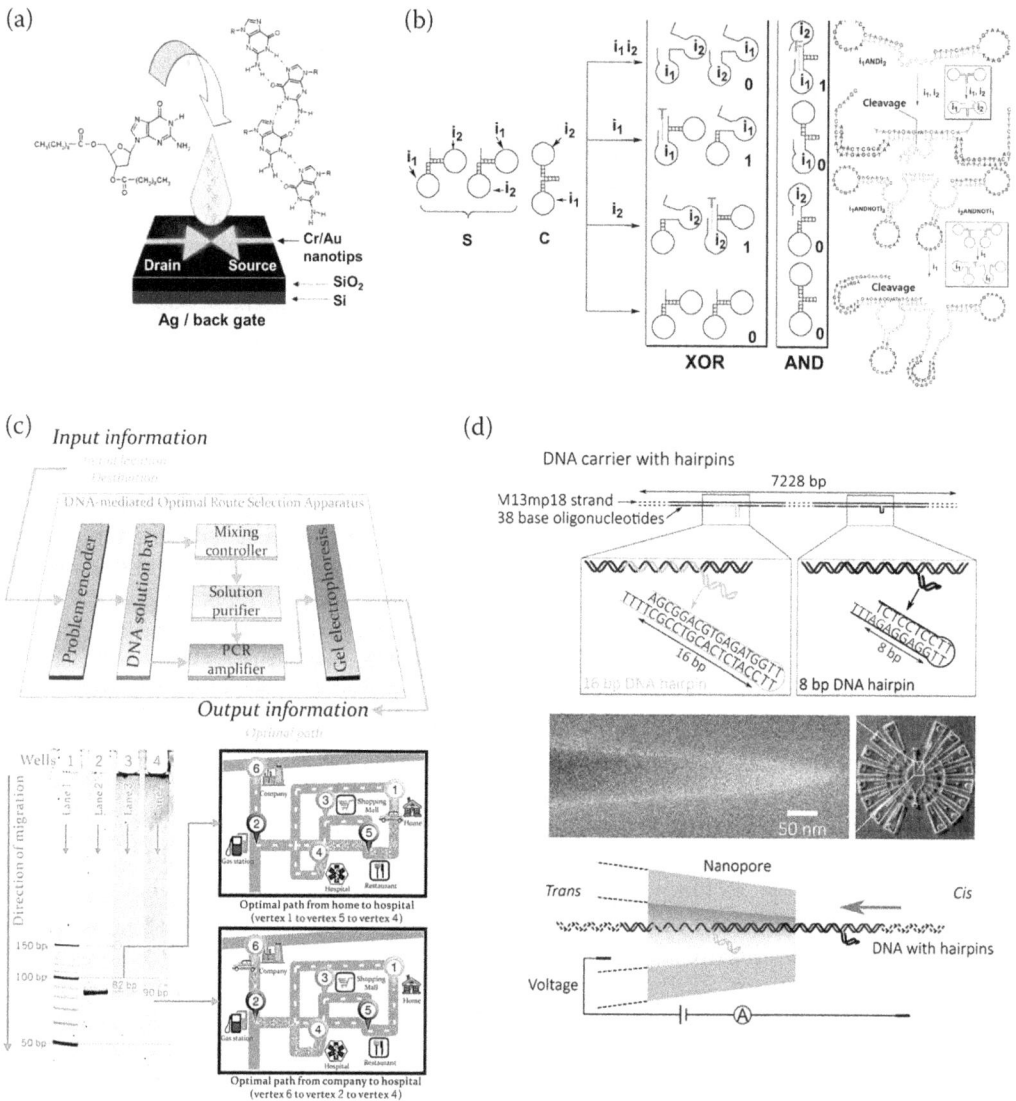

(a)

Drain   Source
— Cr/Au
  nanotips
← SiO₂
← Si
Ag / back gate

(b)

i₁i₂   i₂   i₁   0   1
i₂   i₁   1
S   C
i₂   i₂   1   0
0   0
XOR   **AND**

(c)

Input information

DNA-mediated Optimal Route Selection Apparatus

Problem encoder | DNA solution bay → Mixing controller
Solution purifier
PCR amplifier → Gel electrophoresis

Output information

Wells 1 2 3 4

Optimal path from home to hospital
(vertex 1 to vertex 5 to vertex 4)

Optimal path from company to hospital
(vertex 6 to vertex 2 to vertex 4)

(d)

DNA carrier with hairpins
7228 bp
M13mp18 strand →
38 base oligonucleotides

AGCGGACGTGAGATGGTT
TTTCGCCTGCACTCTACCTT
16 bp DNA hairpin

TCTCCTCCTT
TTTAGAGGAGGTT
8 bp

16 bp DNA hairpin   8 bp DNA hairpin

50 nm

Nanopore
Trans   *Cis*
DNA with hairpins
Voltage   —A—

FIGURE 17.3
(a) A guanosine-based FET. Adapted with permission [11]. Copyright (2003) American Chemical Society. (b) A ribozyme-based biologic gate Adapted with permission [12]. Copyright (2003) American Chemical Society. (c) A DNA bioprocessor. Adapted with permission [13]. Copyright (2015) American Chemical Society. (d) A DNA carrier-based biomemory device. Adapted with permission [14]. Copyright (2018) American Chemical Society.

(state 2). When erasing temperature (T_E) was applied, it was split into two strands and formed a hairpin structure again as temperature decreased (state 3). Keyser's group reported a different approach to DNA-based biomemory (Figure 17.3d) [14]. A short hairpin DNA of eight base pairs (DATA) was attached along a double-stranded DNA called a DNA carrier (Figure 17.3d). Then the DNA carrier carrying the DATA passed through a nanopore acting as an electrode. The electrochemical signal read from the nanopores was different depending on the structure of the DATA, so it was possible to know which DATA was presented in the DNA carrier. As shown here, nucleic acids are an attractive material for

TABLE 17.1

Representative Biomaterials and Their Characteristics Used for Developing Bioelectronic Devices

Types	Property	Type of bioelectronic devices	Reference
Protein	• Redox properties from metal ions inside metalloproteins • Biological catalysts in metabolic processes • Enzymatic reactions with certain substances	• Biomemory • Biologic gate • Biotransistor	[7–9]
Nucleic acid	• High stability • Programmable sequences • Various functionalities (ribozyme, aptamer, etc.)	• Biomemory • Biologic gate • Biotransistor • Bioprocessor	[11–13], [14]

manufacturing bioelectronic devices as it is easy to modify and form various structures with high stability. However, nucleic acid–based bioelectronic devices have some functional limitations, such as low signal and electrical properties. Therefore, numerous novel nanomaterials have been introduced to compensate for these limitations. Table 17.1 shows representative biomaterials and their characteristics used for developing bioelectronic devices.

17.3 Nanomaterials for Bioelectronic Devices

17.3.1 Metal Nanomaterials

Metal nanomaterials have received scientific attention for bioelectronic applications due to their unique physical, optical, and electrical properties. The small size of the metal nanomaterials (under 100 nm) provides excellent properties compared with bulk-scale materials and has potential in many biological fields [16]. For example, metal NPs such as Au, silver (Ag), and platinum (Pt) NPs have been studied due to their optical properties called surface plasmon resonance (SPR) or localized SPR (LSPR). SPR is one of the unique phenomena occurring at the nanoscale of noble metal NPs that emits the light combined with the electron at the surface of the metal NPs to generate strong electron oscillations. As shown in Figure 17.4a, Bintinger's group developed a dual monitoring platform by combining the SPR and electrolyte gate FET (EG-FET) [17]. For this, a 50 nm thin Au layer was fabricated and was used for a gate electrode and the SPR active interface. Furthermore, various types of metal nanomaterials have been studied for biosensors based on the merits of metal nanomaterials such as the excellent catalytic properties, large surface-to-volume ratio, and easy surface modification, which are also equally useful for bioelectronics. Jiang's group reported an easy fabrication strategy of porous noble metal NPs for biosensing [18]. To fabricate the porous noble metal NPs, laser ablation toward water (LATW) with dealloying was performed. The fabricated porous noble metal NPs had 45 times higher local electric field intensity compared with pure noble metal NPs. In addition, metal nanomaterials in the form of nanorods (NRs) have been hugely studied [19]. The metal NRs have several exceptional properties such as the efficient surface plasmon effect that depends on the aspect ratio of the NRs. Besides, numerous metal

(a)

(b)

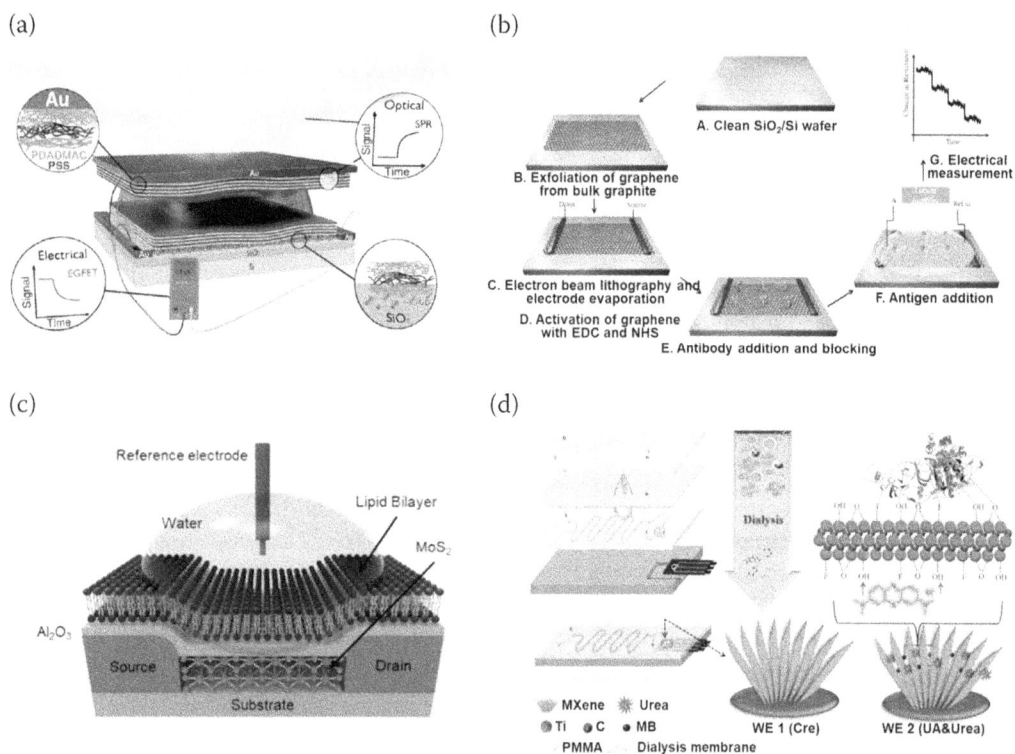

(c)

(d)

FIGURE 17.4
(a) The Au-based SPR and EG-FET gate. Adapted with permission [17]. Copyright (2020) American Chemical Society. (b) A GraFET biosensor. Adapted with permission [20]. Copyright (2020) Springer Nature. (c) The MoS$_2$ FET device. Adapted with permission [21]. Copyright (2020) Elsevier. (d) The MXene nanosheet-based biosensor. Adapted with permission [22]. Copyright (2020) John Wiley and Sons.

nanomaterials with unique compositions or structures are being reported as useful for improving the functions of bioelectronic devices.

17.3.2 Carbon Nanomaterials

Carbon nanomaterials have several attractive properties such as the well-defined electronic property, compatibility with biological molecules, and catalytic effects [23]. Among them, the carbon nanotube (CNT) and graphene are being largely applied to bioelectronic devices due to their unique electrochemical properties. Graphene, a 2D hexagonal lattice structural single layer made of sp^2 hybridized carbon atoms, has a large surface-to-volume ratio and exists in a simple chemical and atomic bonding composition that is suitable for easy surface modification and conjugating with biomaterials. Based on these, graphene exposes a large number of carbon atoms to the environment and exhibits different electrical properties even with small changes to its surface or structure that are suitable for the demonstration of bioelectronic functions. For example, Gandhi's group developed a graphene-based FET (GraFET) for the detection of Japanese encephalitis virus (JEV) and avian influenza virus (AIV) [20]. The surface of the graphene was functionalized with JEV and AIV antibodies by covalent bonding. Due to the large surface-to-volume ratio, a large quantity of antibodies can absorb on the surface to achieve the highly sensitive target detection (Figure 17.4b). The carbon nanodot (CND) is another example of the carbon-based nanomaterials applicable in biological fields. The CND is a spherical NP less than 10 nm in size, usually in the form of nanocrystals with sp^2/sp^3 carbon clusters. The CND has merits for the fabrication of bioelectronic devices such as electrical conductivity, high solubility in various solvents, and large active areas. By using the CND, Ramadan's group fabricated a CND-based FET biosensor for ultrasensitive detection of exosomes [24]. In this research, the CND was introduced to promote the capturing efficiency of exosomes and increase the sensitivity of the FET biosensor. In addition, various types of carbon-based nanomaterials such as the multi-well carbon nanotubes (MWCNTs), crumpled graphene, and graphene quantum dots (GQDs) have been reported to be used in biological fields [25], particularly in the development of bioelectronic devices.

17.3.3 TMD Nanomaterials

Recently, TMD nanomaterials including molybdenum disulfide (MoS_2), tungsten diselenide (WSe_2), molybdenum diselenide ($MoSe_2$), and tungsten disulfide (WS_2) have received intensive attention due to the fascinating physicochemical and electrochemical properties resulting from quantum size effects in ultrathin-layered structures [26]. The TMD nanomaterials are classified into 2H phase and 1T phase, according to the crystal structure, and each has unique properties. The 2H phase of TMD nanomaterials shows excellent catalytic, electronic performance, and semiconducting characteristics for energy-related applications including super-capacitor and battery. The 1T phase of TMD nanomaterials generally has metallic properties such as enhancement of charge transfer efficiency and electrochemical performance. Also, the TMD nanomaterials have a direct bandgap that enables them to overcome the bandgap problem of graphene. Accordingly, TMD nanomaterials are used to develop bioelectronic devices such as FET, biomemory, and biosensors. As shown in Figure 17.4c, Kim's group reported a bioelectronic platform using the MoS_2 nanosheets for FET based ion channel activity monitoring [21]. For this, the liquid-gated MoS_2 FET array was fabricated, and the developed device detected the changes in electrolytes through changes in the electrical properties of MoS_2 nanosheets. The electrical properties of MoS_2 nanosheets were affected by proton transport through the lipid bilayer on the surface of the MoS_2 nanosheets. In another study, Kim's group developed a soft bioelectronic device using high-density MoS_2-graphene heterostructure [27]. Here, an atomically thin MoS_2-graphene heterostructure was developed as a phototransistor, which had two to three times higher photosensitivity compared to a silicon photodiode of the same thickness, due to the efficient photo-absorption of MoS_2. As briefly discussed here, MoS_2 nanosheets are studied the most, but WSe_2, WS_2, and other structures of MoS_2 (quantum dot (QD), NR) are also being gradually studied to combine with biomaterials for developing bioelectronic devices [28].

17.3.4 Mxene Nanomaterials

Since the discovery of graphene, 2D nanomaterials have received a lot of attention for applications in various fields due to their high anisotropy and chemical function. In particular, 2D transition metal carbides (or nitrides) named MXene have been studied [29]. The MXene consists of $M_{n+1}X_nT_x$, and in that composition, M is a transition metal (e.g., Ti, V), X is carbon and nitrogen, and T_x is a functional group (e.g., -F, -OH). The MXene exhibits high dispersibility in an aqueous solution because it has a layered structure and a

TABLE 17.2

Representative Nanomaterials Used for Developing Bioelectronic Devices

Types	Materials	Structure	Property	Reference
Metal nanomaterials	Au, Ag, Pt	NPs	• Excellent catalytic properties	[16,17]
			• Suitable for biomedical applications	
		NRs	• Polarized and directional emission	[19]
			• Unique surface plasmon effects	
Carbon nanomaterials	Carbon	Nanosheet	• 2D nanomaterial	[20]
			• Easy surface modification	
			• Large surface-to-volume ratio	
		Nanodots	• One-dimensional nanomaterial	[24]
			• Excellent electrical conductivity	
			• High solubility in various solvents	
TMD nanomaterials	MoS_2, WS_2, $MoSe_2$, WSe_2	Nanosheet	• Excellent electronic performance	[21,26,27]
			• Semiconducting characteristic	
		QD	• Excellent quantum confinement effects	[28]
			• Low cytotoxicity and good dispensability	
MXene nanomaterials	$M_{n+1}X_nT_x$	Nanosheet	• 2D nanomaterial	[22,31]
			• High conductivity, hydrophilicity	

hydrophilic surface, which is suitable for applications in various fields including energy storage and biosensing. However, despite the excellent hydrophilicity and high conductivity of MXene, there are some limitations in the application to bioelectronics due to MXene's high aggregation tendency [30]. Zhang's group developed an MXene nanosheet-based biosensor for monitoring uric acid, urea, and creatinine in whole blood [22]. Here, MXene nanosheets were simply synthesized through a wet etching technique, and multiple enzymes were immobilized on the MXene for the detection of biological targets (Figure 17.4d). Due to the multi-architecture structure like an accordion, the loading rate of the enzyme was improved and immobilization efficiency was also facilitated by abundant reactive groups on the MXene surface. Hao's group developed an MXene sheet-based biosensor for the detection of phosmet, a type of organophosphorus pesticide [31]. Notably, an MXene nanosheet was synthesized by a facile strategy of electrochemical etching (E-etching) exfoliation instead of the introduction of HF solution. MXene nanosheets synthesized by this method had high biocompatibility as well as excellent capacity for enzyme loading. In brief, due to its conductance, abundant active regions, and short ion diffusion distances, MXene has a high potential for the development of bioelectronic devices. Table 17.2 shows representative nanomaterials used for developing bioelectronic devices.

17.4 Nanomaterial-Assisted Protein-Based Bioelectronic Devices

17.4.1 Biomemory

Various structures and types of nanomaterials have been introduced to the development of bioelectronic devices. Accordingly, by combining with proteins, nanomaterials enhance the electronic properties derived from proteins through high electron transfer efficiency and distinctive energy bandgap characteristics, particularly in the development of protein-based biomemory. Güzel's group developed the photo-induced biomemory device. [32]. Ferritin-based Fe and Mn containing bionanocages (FeMnFBNC) immobilized on the graphene surface by electrostatic bonding were fabricated using photosensitive cross-linkers. The ferritin in the FeMnFBNC acted as an electron bridge, enabling electron transfer between graphene and the FeMnFBNC. Besides, Fe and Mn were able to capture the moving electrons for a long time through redox reaction properties. Using a developed biomemory device, multi-state biomemory behavior was demonstrated through regulation of the oxidation potential (write state), open-circuit potential (read state), and reduction potential (erase state) by UV light irradiation.

Zhang's group developed a biomemristor (a word blending of memory and resistor) device composed of Ag-doped silk fibroin [33] (Figure 17.5a). Conventional silk fibroin-based biomemristors need a high operating current because silk fibroin forms a random

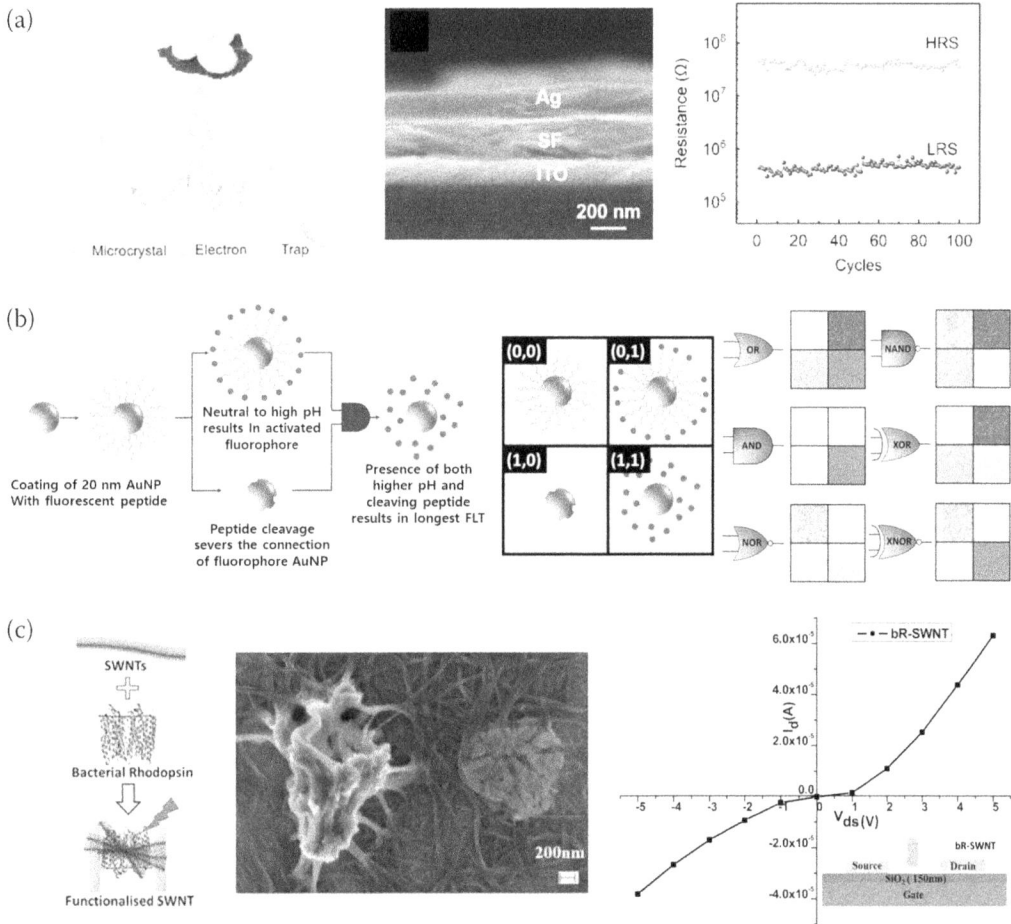

FIGURE 17.5
(a) The Ag-doped silk fibroin-based biomemristor. Adapted with permission [33]. Copyright (2021) American Chemical Society. (b) The AuNP-based biologic gate. Adapted with permission [35]. Copyright (2019) American Chemical Society. (c) A SWCNT-based FET. Adapted with permission [36]. Copyright (2020) American Chemical Society.

structure inside an active layer. To address this issue, here, the doping of Ag on the silk fibroin was done for the formation of the crystal structure of the silk fibroin to promote the carrier transmission along the direction of the formed silk fibroin. This resulted in improved function of the biomemristor device with low operating current, low power, and tunable performance. There was also research on the development of protein-based biomemory utilizing multiple chain reactions between metal NPs and biomaterials. For example, Kwon's group reported a biological bimodal memory device that mimics the cooperative and multimodal activation process of biological memory using a tyrosine-rich peptide assembled film with Ag ions [34]. In this device, multiple redox reactions and movement of Ag ions were facilitated by high proton conductivity and redox capability of tyrosine-rich peptides. As a result, when a positive voltage was applied, Ag ions at the top electrode were formed and migrated to the bottom electrode, showing resistive switching characteristics similar to that of other resistive switching devices.

Wang's group developed a resistance-switching device using graphene oxide (GO) and egg albumen [37]. In this study, GO was used due to its unique properties such as ion migration, redox reactions induced by electrical fields, and carrier trapping/de-trapping characteristics. Egg albumen was used because it can form an active or dielectric layer that is appropriate for the fabrication of resistive switching devices or transistors. Utilizing these properties of each material, the endurance and uniformity of the device were improved, and the resistance switching mechanism was demonstrated. As such, nanomaterials have been applied to the development of protein-based biomemory due to their outstanding properties, overcoming the defects of biomaterials, and improving the function of the biomemory devices.

17.4.2 Biologic Gate/Bioprocessor

The combination of nanomaterials and proteins is frequently utilized to implement the biologic gate functions. Fixler's group developed a biologic gate based on AuNPs and fluorescent molecules linked by peptides (Figure 17.5b) [35]. In this biologic gate, the fluorescence signal generated by the fluorescence molecule (Oregon Green 488) was quenched by the connected AuNPs. However, this signal was recovered by an increase in the surrounding pH or when the proteinase (trypsin) decomposed the peptide. Therefore, by combining the inputs (pH and proteinase), biologic functions (OR, AND, NOR, NAND, XOR, and XNOR) were demonstrated through the change of emitted fluorescent signal.

In another study, Nie's group developed a peptide-mediated NP assembly platform composed of AuNP and a multi-functional peptide for developing a biologic gate [38]. The multifunctional peptide was composed of two functional motifs, the Zn ion-chelating part, and the protease substrate part. When only multifunctional peptides and AuNPs were present in the solution, the multifunctional peptides were attached to the AuNPs to electrically neutralize the AuNPs, which were originally negatively charged, leading to aggregation of AuNPs. However, when Zn ions or chymotrypsin were added as inputs, the structure of the multifunctional peptides was changed so that they cannot be attached to the AuNPs, and the AuNPs maintained a negative charge. As a result, the AuNPs were dispersed well, inducing the change of color. By using this phenomenon, biological operations such as AND, OR, INHIBIT, NAND, and IMPLICATION were performed.

Similarly, Yang's group developed an INHIBIT biologic gate [39]. The melamine and human serum albumin were used as inputs for aggregation and dispersion of AuNPs, respectively. Therefore, the INHIBIT biologic gate was demonstrated by adding only melamine or adding both melamine and human serum albumin, resulting in a change of color of AuNPs based on the degree of aggregation. Tan's group used an organic material to fabricate a copper-organic framework (Cu-MOF) [40]. Due to the strong affinity between Cu NP and pyrophosphate (PPi), PPi inhibited the catalytic activity of Cu-MOF. However, with the addition of alkaline phosphatase (ALP) that hydrolyzes PPi, the catalytic activity of Cu-MOF was recovered. Then, the 2,2'-azinobis(3-ethylbenzothiazoline)-6-sulfonic acid (ABTS) was added to Cu-MOF for investigation of catalytic activity of Cu-MOF. The colorless ABTS turned green when it was oxidized by the catalytic active Cu-MOF. The intensity corresponded to the degree of activity of Cu-MOF. Based on this, an IMPLICATION biologic gate was developed by using PPi and ALP as inputs and the change of the color of ABTS as an output. Taken together, with the unique properties of nanomaterials, high specificity, and the electron transfer efficiency of proteins, research on the multifunctional biologic gate presents the huge potential for further development in the field of bioelectronic devices.

17.4.3 Biotransistor

The transistor plays an important role in operating computing systems through amplifying or switching electronic signals. It is essential to develop a biotransistor for the construction of a biocomputer [41]. To solve the limitations of biomaterials for developing biotransistors, research on the combination of nanomaterials and proteins has been conducted. Das's group fabricated a back-gate biotransistor with a 300 nm-long channel using the Azurin-TiO_2 hybrid nanostructure [42]. Azurin has been widely used in bioelectronic devices because of its intrinsic redox property. TiO_2 is suitable for UV detection due to its wide bandgap and high photocatalytic rate but has some limitations such as low reactivity and weak photocurrent. By combining Azurin and TiO_2, the developed biotransistor exhibited a wide bandgap, high photocatalytic efficiency, fast spectral response, and high photocurrent.

In another study, Chaturvedi's group developed a FET using a hybrid film composed of bacteriorhodopsin and single-walled carbon nanotubes (SWCNTs) (Figure 17.5c) [36]. The 2D structure of the bacteriorhodopsin formed a photo-active center, and SWCNT acted as the highly conductive electronic scaffolds. The developed FET did not exhibit gate control function until the SWCNT/bacteriorhodopsin was immobilized. However, an electrode immobilized with the SWCNT/bacteriorhodopsin had the properties of gate control similar to semiconductors. This phenomenon was manifested by electron transport of SWCNT and further enhanced by bacteriorhodopsin used as an optically active proton pump. The developed FET exhibited the n-type semiconducting characteristics in dark conditions, but in bright conditions, it had p-type semiconducting characteristics because of a proton charge transfer from the bacteriorhodopsin to the SWCNT. Furthermore, the fabricated FET showed an "On" state for positive gate voltages under dark conditions and negative gate voltages under bright conditions.

Protein-based biotransistors have been also applied to biosensing to broaden their applicability. The immunoFET, which uses an antibody fixed on the surface of the oxide between the source and drain electrodes for target molecule sensing, has been reported as achieving label-free target detection. Kim's group developed a biosensor for detection of the SARS-CoC-2 spike protein using an antibody against the SARS-CoV-2 spike protein immobilized on a graphene-based biotransistor [43]. As such, many studies are being conducted to improve the stability and performance of biotransistors through combining nanomaterials and proteins.

17.5 Nanomaterial-Assisted Nucleic Acid–Based Bioelectronic Devices

17.5.1 Biomemory

Nucleic acids are widely used in the development of biomemory due to their unique binding ability and ease of incorporation into nanomaterials. Choi's group developed a resistive switching random access memory device using Cu^{2+}-doped salmon DNA (Cu^{2+}-DNA) as a switching medium [44]. The chelated Cu^{2+} ions were intercalated between DNA base pairs by electrostatically binding to the phosphate backbones of the DNA during the doping process. By applying suitable electrical voltages, the resistance value of the device was changed due to the migration of Cu^{2+} ions as "On state" and "Off state" for demonstration of resistive switching functions. Additionally, DNA, which has high biocompatibility and biodegradable characteristics, had the advantage of being easy to interact with Cu^{2+} ions.

Chen's group introduced two types of metal nanomaterials simultaneously to DNA for the development of the resistive switching memory device [45]. In this research, the CuO and AlNPs were assembled via DNA strands bridge, forming CuO-DNA-Al nanocomposites. Resistive switching characteristics were demonstrated via Al NPs that generated Al ions under an electric field ($Al \rightarrow Al^{3+} + 3e^-$), and Al ions moved, following the direction of the applied electric field. In this device, DNA served as a channel for the movement of Al ions, and the CuO stabilized the movement of Al ions. The developed CuO-DNA-Al nanocomposites-based biomemory device presented the improved resistive switching characteristics through the introduction of both CuO and Al. In addition, Wu's group developed a layered graphene-DNA-based biomemristor device [46]. The graphene had different electronic conductivities depending on the vertical and horizontal directions of the basal plane, and these special physical properties enabled the demonstration of multistate resistive switching behaviors. Moreover, uniformly layered DNA provided the stability and reliability of these behaviors. The developed biomemristor device showed multistate resistive switching behaviors as well as multibit parallel logic operations.

In another study, Choi's group developed a resistive switching device based on a heterolayer composed of carboxyl modified MoS_2 and DNA (Figure 17.6a) [47]. The excellent semiconducting behavior of MoS_2 NPs enabled the realization of the resistive switching function. An insulating layer composed of DNA showed high stability and insulating properties, compared to RNA or protein, for the formation of conducting-insulating-semiconducting layers to demonstrate the resistive property. The developed device showed an electrical bi-stable state with a wide voltage range (4.0 V to 4.0 V) and nonvolatile stability. As such, the nucleic acid can serve as a template for fabricating nanostructures by molecular self-assembly with high stability, and it is easy to combine nucleic acids with various types of nanomaterials to develop the nanomaterial-assisted biomemory.

17.5.2 Biologic Gate/Bioprocessor

The synergistic effects from the combination of nucleic acids and nanomaterials are also used in the development of a biologic gate and bioprocessor. Yi's group developed a biologic gate using AuNP conjugated with cyanine3-tagged aptamer (Cy3-Apt) which can specifically react with chloramphenicol (CAP) [50]. Due to the fluorescence quenching by AuNP, Cy3-Apt could not emit the fluorescence signal. However, in the presence of CAP,

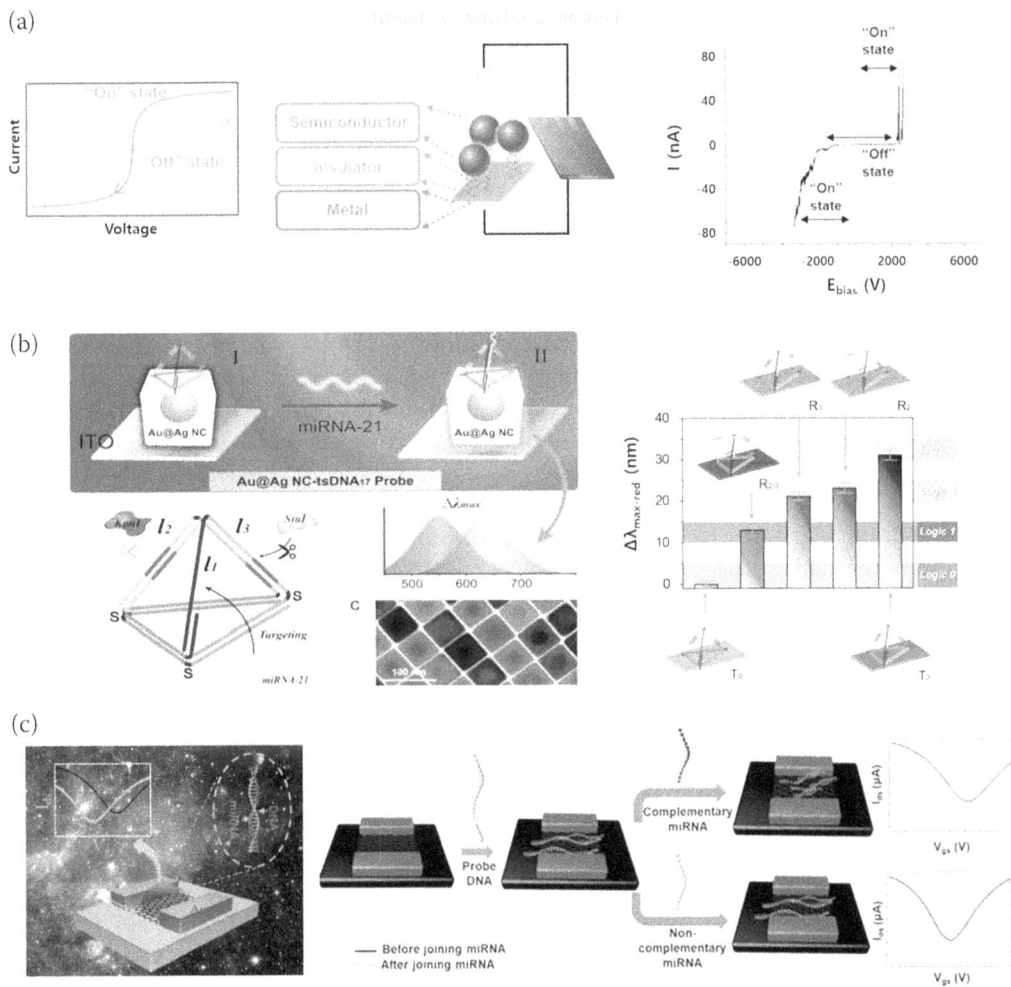

FIGURE 17.6
(a) MoS$_2$ NPs and DNA-based resistive switching device. Adapted with permission [47]. Copyright (2019) Elsevier. (b) Au@Ag core-shell nanocube-based biologic gate. Adapted with permission [48]. Copyright (2018) American Chemical Society. (c) Graphene-based FET. Adapted with permission [49]. Copyright (2020) American Chemical Society.

Cy3-Apt emitted a strong fluorescence signal due to the change of the structural conformation of the Apt by a reaction between Cy3-Apt and CAP. In addition, when heavy metals such as Hg, Ag, and Pb were added together, Apt formed a coordinate bond with them, which induced a fluorescence switching phenomenon, resulting in the regulation of fluorescence intensity. Through these processes, multiple biological functions (YES, PASS 0, INH, NOT, PASS 1, and NAND) were demonstrated successfully.

Wang's group introduced Au@Ag core-shell nanocube to a tetrahedron-structured DNA (tsDNA) for the development of a biologic gate (Figure 17.6b) [48]. Here, a single tsDNA-modified Au@Ag core-shell nanocube was used as a plasmonic probe to react with multiple targets (microRNA (miRNA), endonucleases of *KpnI* and *StuI*). When the target miRNA was hybridized with tsDNA, the plasmonic wavelength value generated in the Au@Ag core-shell nanocube was shifted due to the structural change by double-stranded structure formation. Endonucleases of *KpnI* and *StuI* resulted in changes in plasmonic wavelength values because of the cleavage of certain sequences in tsDNA. Through this, the developed biologic gate performed an OR and XOR logic operation.

Willner's group developed a biologic gate using GO and two types of DNA modified with two different fluorescent materials, respectively [51]. The "AND" biologic gate was initiated by hybridizing these two types of fluorescent modified DNA with complementary DNA (cDNA) and forming a loop structure. Due to the formation of the loop structure, fluorescent modified DNA generated a strong fluorescence signal because of detachment from the GO, which is capable of quenching the fluorescent signal. However, in the presence of target DNA, which had a stronger binding affinity for the cDNA than the fluorescent modified DNA, the fluorescent modified DNA was adsorbed on the GO surface and the fluorescence signal was re-quenched. Using this reaction mechanism, a biological operation was processed using different binding affinities between each single-stranded DNA. Bi's group developed a biologic gate composed of AuNP modified with single-stranded DNA, dumbbell probe (DP), and duplex-specific nuclease (DSN) through the conformational change of DP using different binding affinities between nucleic acids and degradation by DSN [52]. In summary, the unique properties of nucleic acids including complimentary bonds between nucleic acids and differences in binding affinity are suitable for implementing biologic functions and processing of complex functions on the device by combining with functional nanomaterials.

17.5.3 Biotransistor

The performance of the computing system is closely related to transistor density. To improve the integration level of the transistor, it is necessary to manufacture ultracompact transistors. To develop these transistors using biomaterials with nanomaterials, Yin's group manufactured a precise CNT transistor array using DNA as a template [53]. Here, the parallel CNT arrays with a uniform nanometer-sized spacing were constructed by using DNA brick-based nanotrenches to align DNA-wrapped CNTs. For this, the supramolecular assembly method was used to generate a scaffold composed of compacted DNA. In the fabricated scaffold, some part of the DNA was located on the surface to hybridize with other DNA that was immobilized on the surface of the CNT. By placing the CNT on the scaffold, the directionality of individual CNT was precisely controlled. Moreover, by programming the DNA template differently, CNT was arrayed with uniform spacing of 16.8, 12.6, and 10.4 nm using the electrostatic repulsion between DNA and negatively charged CNT with high stability. In addition, this method enabled the fabrication of millions of parallel CNT arrays at the same time, which demonstrated the functionality of the biotransistor.

In addition, Kim's group patterned the chemically modified graphene and bottom-up self-assembly of DNA origami to develop a few nanometer-level DNA-based biotransistors [54]. It was confirmed that a rectangular DNA origami structure with a size of 2 nm × 70 nm × 90 nm was deposited on patterned nitrogen-doped reduced GO (NrGO) without folding or overlapping structures. The nucleic acid-based biotransistors have the potential for developing biosensors by using the property of nucleic acids to hybridize with aptamers or complementary sequences that selectively bind to target molecules [55]. For example, Han's group developed a graphene-based FET for miRNA detection (Figure 17.6c) [49]. In this study, the complementary sequence of the target miRNA was located at the 3' end of the probe DNA, and 10 adenine bases were designed at the 5' end for attachment to the graphene channel via π-π interactions. By investigating the shift of the Dirac point which occurred when target miRNA was hybridized with probe DNA, target miRNAs were detected with high sensitivity within 20 minutes without labeling. Moreover, this FET biosensor was manufactured on a flexible polyimide substrate, and it maintained its properties even after bending it several times which showed the possibility of the development of flexible or wearable FET biosensor by using biomaterials and nanomaterials. As seen so far, the conjugation of nanomaterials and nucleic acids complements each material, leading to the development of functional bioelectronic devices that will be the base to develop a biocomputer.

17.6 Conclusion and Future Perspectives

Bioelectronics is being studied to demonstrate various delicate electronic functions using biomaterials to address issues of current silicon-based electronics and to develop a bio-computer capable of performing various electronic processes similar to a commercialized computer. However, since biomaterials have intrinsic disadvantages such as instability and narrowness of functionalization by themselves, it is hard to implement the sophisticated electronic functions using only biomaterials on the biochip with reproducibility, which is essential for the development of the biocomputer. Nanomaterials suggest a promising approach to address these issues by combining with biomaterials and using their exceptional properties such as the large surface area and high conductivity. Through the introduction of nanomaterials into bioelectronics, it can enhance the electronic signals from biomaterials, improve the biomolecular stability, and expand the electronic functions of biomaterials to demonstrate various bioelectronic functions on the biochip. In recent years, nanomaterial-assisted bioelectronic devices are being studied as a key element in developing various types of functional bioelectronic devices required to develop a biocomputer.

In this chapter, nanomaterial-assisted bioelectronic devices were discussed by the categorized sections. First, we discussed the bioelectronic devices developed using only biomaterials, especially using widely studied biomaterials including protein and nucleic acids. After that, several novel nanomaterials hugely studied in the development of bioelectronic devices were provided, including metal, carbon, TMD, and MXene nanomaterials, with their unique properties suitable for the development of bioelectronic devices. Next, based on the classification divided by widely studied types of bioelectronic devices including the biomemory, biologic gate/bioprocessor, and biotransistor, nanomaterial-assisted protein-based bioelectronic devices and nanomaterial-assisted nucleic acid-based bioelectronic devices were discussed with recently reported studies.

Still, there are obstacles to be addressed for the practical application of nanomaterial-assisted bioelectronic devices. For example, the mass production issue of discussed novel nanomaterials should be addressed to achieve the cost-effective development of bioelectronic devices. Going beyond the implementation of electronic functions at the protein or nucleic acid level, the development of novel nanohybrid material and relevant techniques, such as efficient conjugation methods, is required to demonstrate various delicate electronic functions at a cellular level and for the sophisticated regulation of cell networks and 3D neural cell models for the development of biocomputer. Also, in line with recent research on the development of flexible/wearable electronics, research on the development of excellent flexible electrodes that will serve as suitable and biocompatible supports for biomaterials and nanomaterials in bioelectronic devices is also necessary [56]. Through these efforts, it is expected that a commercially available biocomputer composed of multifunctional bioelectronic components capable of being worn on the body will be developed in the future. In conclusion, this chapter provides the interdisciplinary knowledge of bioelectronics, nanomaterials, and their potential in the development of functional bioelectronic devices, leading to the generation of a biocomputer.

Acknowledgments

This work was supported by the National Research Foundation of Korea (NRF) grant funded by the Korea government (MSIT) (No. 2019R1A2C3002300), and by the National R&D Program through the National Research Foundation of Korea (NRF) funded by the Ministry of Science and ICT(NRF- NRF-2022M3H4A1A01005271).

References

1. A.A. Yaqoob, H. Ahmad, T. Parveen, A. Ahmad, M. Oves, I.M.I. Ismail, H.A. Qari, K. Umar, M.N. Mohamad Ibrahim, Recent Advances in Metal Decorated Nanomaterials and Their Various Biological Applications: A Review. *Front. Chem.* 8, (2020) 341.
2. J. Zhang, L. Liu, Y. Yang, Q. Huang, D. Li, D. Zeng, A Review on Two-Dimensional Materials for Chemiresistive- and FET-Type Gas Sensors. *Phys. Chem. Chem. Phys.* 23, (2021) 15420–15439.
3. M. Rolandi, A. Noy, S. Inal, J. Rivnay, Advances in Bioelectronics: Materials, Devices, and Translational Applications. *APL Mater.* 9, (2021) 070402.
4. J. Zhuang, A.P. Young, C.K. Tsung, Integration of Biomolecules with Metal–Organic Frameworks. *Small* 13, (2017) 1700880.
5. S.E. Lyshevski, *Nano and Molecular Electronics Handbook.* (2007) Florida, USA, CRC Press.
6. J.-W. Choi, B.K. Oh, Y.J. Kim, J. Min, Protein-Based Biomemory Device Consisting of the Cysteine-Modified Azurin. *Appl. Phys. Lett.* 91, (2007) 263902.
7. T. Lee, S.U. Kim, J. Min, J.-W. Choi, Multilevel Biomemory Device Consisting of Recombinant Azurin/Cytochrome c. *Adv. Mater.* 22, (2010) 510–514.
8. N. Kalyani, A. Moudgil, S. Das, P. Mishra, Metalloprotein Based Scalable Field Effect Transistor with Enhanced Switching Behaviour. *Sens. Actuators B Chem.* 246, (2017) 363–369.
9. D. Melnikov, G. Strack, J. Zhou, J.R. Windmiller, J. Halámek, V. Bocharova, M.C. Chuang, P. Santhosh, V. Privman, J. Wang, E. Katz, Enzymatic AND Logic Gates Operated under Conditions Characteristic of Biomedical Applications. *J. Phys. Chem.* 114, (2010) 12166–12174.
10. J. Yin, J. Wang, R. Niu, S. Ren, D. Wang, J. Chao, DNA Nanotechnology-Based Biocomputing. *Chem. Res. Chin. Univ.* 36, (2020) 219–226.
11. G. Maruccio, P. Visconti, V. Arima, S. D'Amico, A. Biasco, E. D'Amone, R. Cingolani, R. Rinaldi, S. Masiero, T. Giorgi, G. Gottarelli, Field Effect Transistor Based on a Modified DNA Base. *Nano Lett.* 3, (2003) 479–483.
12. M.N. Stojanović, D. Stefanović, Deoxyribozyme-Based Half-Adder. *J. Am. Chem. Soc.* 125, (2003) 6673–6676.
13. J.J. Shu, Q.W. Wang, K.Y. Yong, F. Shao, K.J. Lee, Programmable DNA-Mediated Multitasking Processor. *J. Phys. Chem.* 119, (2015) 5639–5644.
14. K. Chen, J. Kong, J. Zhu, N. Ermann, P. Predki, U.F. Keyser, Digital Data Storage Using DNA Nanostructures and Solid-State Nanopores. *Nano Lett.* 19, (2019) 1210–1215.

15. M. Takinoue, A. Suyama, Hairpin-DNA Memory Using Molecular Addressing. *Small* 2, (2006) 1244–1247.
16. A.M. Ealias, M.P. Saravanakumar, A Review on the Classification, Characterisation, Synthesis of Nanoparticles and Their Application. *IOP Conf. Ser.: Mater Sci. Eng.* 263, (2017) 032019.
17. P. Aspermair, U. Ramach, C. Reiner-Rozman, S. Fossati, B. Lechner, S.E. Moya, O. Azzaroni, J. Dostalek, S. Szunerits, W. Knoll, J. Bintinger, Dual Monitoring of Surface Reactions in Real Time by Combined Surface-Plasmon Resonance and Field-Effect Transistor Interrogation. *J. Am. Chem. Soc.* 142, (2020) 11709–11716.
18. Z. Yang, Z. Lin, J. Yang, J. Wang, J. Yue, B. Liu, L. Jiang, Fabrication of Porous Noble Metal Nanoparticles Based on Laser Ablation toward Water and Dealloying for Biosensing. *Appl. Surf. Sci.* 579, (2022) 152130.
19. Y. Lin, M. Zhao, Y. Guo, X. Ma, F. Luo, L. Guo, B. Qiu, G. Chen, Z. Lin, Multicolor Colormetric Biosensor for the Determination of Glucose Based on the Etching of Gold Nanorods. *Sci. Rep.* 6, (2016) 1–7.
20. A. Roberts, N. Chauhan, S. Islam, S. Mahari, B. Ghawri, R.K. Gandham, S.S. Majumdar, A. Ghosh, S. Gandhi, Graphene Functionalized Field-Effect Transistors for Ultrasensitive Detection of Japanese Encephalitis and Avian Influenza Virus. *Sci. Rep.* 10, (2020) 14546.
21. Y. Park, B. Kang, C.H. Ahn, H.K. Cho, H. Kwon, S. Park, J. Kwon, M. Choi, C. Lee, K. Kim, Bionanoelectronic Platform with a Lipid Bilayer/CVD-Grown MoS_2 Hybrid. *Biosens. Bioelectron.* 142, (2019) 11512.
22. J. Liu, X. Jiang, R. Zhang, Y. Zhang, L. Wu, W. Lu, J. Li, Y. Li, H. Zhang, MXene-Enabled Electrochemical Microfluidic Biosensor: Applications toward Multicomponent Continuous Monitoring in Whole Blood. *Adv. Funct. Mater.* 29, (2019) 1807326.
23. S. Liu, X. Guo, Carbon Nanomaterials Field-Effect-Transistor-Based Biosensors. *NPG Asia Mater.* 4, (2012) e23.
24. S. Ramadan, R. Lobo, Y. Zhang, L. Xu, O. Shaforost, D.K.H. Tsang, J. Feng, T. Yin, M. Qiao, A. Rajeshirke, L.R. Jiao, P.K. Petrov, I.E. Dunlop, M.-M. Titirici, N. Klein, Carbon-Dot-Enhanced Graphene Field-Effect Transistors for Ultrasensitive Detection of Exosomes. *ACS Appl. Mater. Interfaces* 13, (2021) 7854–7864.
25. L.H. Nonaka, T.S.D. Almeida, C.B. Aquino, S.H. Domingues, R.V. Salvatierra, V.H.R. Souza, Crumpled Graphene Decorated with Manganese Ferrite Nanoparticles for Hydrogen Peroxide Sensing and Electrochemical Supercapacitors. *ACS Appl. Nano Mater.* 3, (2020) 4859–4869.
26. H.H. Huang, X. Fan, D.J. Singh, W.T. Zheng, Recent Progress of TMD Nanomaterials: Phase Transitions and Applications. *Nanoscale*, 12, (2020) 1247–1268.
27. C. Choi, M.K. Choi, S. Liu, M.S. Kim, O.K. Park, C. Im, J. Kim, X. Qin, G.J. Lee, K.W. Cho, D.H. Kim, Human Eye-Inspired Soft Optoelectronic Device Using High-Density MoS_2-Graphene Curved Image Sensor Array. *Nat. Commun.* 8, (2017) 1–11.
28. C.H. Chu, H.C. Lin, C.H. Yeh, Z.Y. Liang, M.Y. Chou, P.W. Chiu, End-Bonded Metal Contacts on WSe_2 Field-Effect Transistors. *ACS Nano* 13, (2019) 8146–8154.
29. W. Huang, L. Hu, Y. Tang, Z. Xie, H. Zhang, Recent Advances in Functional 2D MXene-Based Nanostructures for Next-Generation Devices. *Adv. Funct. Mater.* 30, (2020) 2005223.
30. Q. Wang, X. Pan, C. Lin, H. Gao, S. Cao, Y. Ni, X. Ma, Modified $Ti_3C_2T_X$ (MXene) Nanosheet-Catalyzed Self-Assembled, Anti-Aggregated, Ultra-Stretchable, Conductive Hydrogels for Wearable Bioelectronics. *Chem. Eng. Sci.* 401, (2020) 126129.
31. M. Song, S.Y. Pang, F. Guo, M.C. Wong, J. Hao, Fluoride-Free 2D Niobium Carbide MXenes as Stable AndBiocompatible Nanoplatforms for Electrochemical Biosensors with Ultrahigh Sensitivity. *Adv. Sci.* 7, (2020) 2001546.
32. R. Güzel, Y.S. Ocak, Ş.N. Karuk, A. Ersöz, R. Say, Light Harvesting and Photo-Induced Electrochemical Devices Based on Bionanocage Proteins. *J. Power Sources* 440, (2019) 227119.
33. Y. Zhang, F. Han, S. Fan, Y. Zhang, Low-Power and Tunable-Performance Biomemristor Based on Silk Fibroin. *ACS Biomater. Sci. Eng.* 7, (2021) 3459–3468.

34. L. Wang, J. Wang, D. Wen, Devices with Tuneable Resistance Switching Characteristics Based on a Multilayer Structure of Graphene Oxide and EGG Albumen. *Nanomaterials* 10, (2020) 1491.

35. E.A. Barnoy, M. Motiei, C. Tzror, S. Rahimipour, R. Popovtzer, D. Fixler, Biological Logic Gate Using Gold Nanoparticles and Fluorescence Lifetime Imaging Microscopy. *ACS Appl. Nano Mater.* 2, (2019) 6527–6536.

36. V. Bakaraju, E.S. Prasad, B. Meena, H. Chaturvedi, An Electronic and Optically Controlled Bifunctional Transistor Based on a Bio-Nano Hybrid Complex. *ACS Omega* 5, (2020) 9702–9706.

37. M.K. Song, S.D. Namgung, D. Choi, H. Kim, H. Seo, M. Ju, Y.H. Lee, T. Sung, Y.S. Lee, K.T. Nam, J.Y. Kwon, Proton-Enabled Activation of Peptide Materials for Biological Bimodal Memory. *Nat. Commun.* 11, (2020) 1–8.

38. Y. Li, W. Li, K.Y. He, P. Li, Y. Huang, Z. Nie, S.Z. Yao, A Biomimetic Colorimetric Logic Gate System Based on Multi-Functional Peptide-Mediated Gold Nanoparticle Assembly. *Nanoscale.* 8, (2016) 8591–8599.

39. Z. Huang, H. Wang, W. Yang, Gold Nanoparticle-Based Facile Detection of Human Serum Albumin and Its Application as an INHIBIT Logic Gate. *ACS Appl. Mater. Interfaces.* 7, (2015) 8990–8998.

40. C. Wang, J. Gao, Y. Cao, H. Tan, Colorimetric Logic Gate for Alkaline Phosphatase Based on Copper (II)-Based Metal-Organic Frameworks with Peroxidase-like Activity. *Anal. Chim. Acta.* 1004, (2018) 74–81.

41. L. Chen, L. Wang, Y. Peng, X. Feng, S. Sarkar, S. Li, B. Li, L. Liu, K. Han, X. Gong, K.W. Ang, A van Der Waals Synaptic Transistor Based on Ferroelectric $Hf_{0.5}Zr_{0.5}O_2$ and 2D Tungsten Disulfide. *Adv. Electro. Mater.* 6, (2020) 2000057.

42. A. Moudgil, N. Kalyani, P. Mishra, S. Das, Azurin-TiO_2 Hybrid Nanostructure Field Effect Transistor for Efficient Ultraviolet Detection. *Nanotechnology* 30, (2019) 495205.

43. G. Seo, G. Lee, M.J. Kim, S.H. Baek, M. Choi, K.B. Ku, C.S. Lee, S. Jun, D. Park, H.G. Kim, S.I. Kim, Rapid Detection of COVID-19 Causative Virus (SARS-CoV-2) in Human Nasopharyngeal Swab Specimens Using Field-Effect Transistor-Based Biosensor. *ACS nano*, 14, (2020) 5135–5142.

44. Y. Abbas, S.R. Dugasani, M.T. Raza, Y.R. Jeon, S.H. Park, C. Choi, The Observation of Resistive Switching Characteristics Using Transparent and Biocompatible Cu^{2+}-Doped Salmon DNA Composite Thin Film. *Nanotechnology.* 30, (2019) 335203.

45. B. Sun, L. Wei, H. Li, X. Jia, J. Wu, P. Chen, The DNA Strand Assisted Conductive Filament Mechanism for Improved Resistive Switching Memory. *J. Mater. Chem. C.* 3, (2015) 12149–12155.

46. B. Sun, S. Ranjan, G. Zhou, T. Guo, Y. Xia, L. Wei, Y.N. Zhou, Y.A. Wu, Multistate Resistive Switching Behaviors for Neuromorphic Computing in Memristor. *Mater. Today Adv.* 9, (2021) 100125.

47. J. Yoon, M. Mohammadniaei, H.K. Choi, M. Shin, G.B. Bapurao, T. Lee, J.-W. Choi, Resistive Switching Biodevice Composed of MoS_2-DNA Heterolayer on the Gold Electrode. *Appl. Surf. Sci.* 478, (2019) 134–141.

48. Y. Zhang, Z. Shuai, H. Zhou, Z. Luo, B. Liu, Y. Zhang, L. Zhang, S. Chen, J. Chao, L. Weng, Q. Fan, C. Fan, W. Huang, L. Wang, Single-Molecule Analysis of MicroRNA and Logic Operations Using a Smart Plasmonic Nanobiosensor. *J. Am. Chem. Soc.* 140, (2018) 3988–3993.

49. J. Gao, Y. Gao, Y. Han, J. Pang, C. Wang, Y. Wang, H. Liu, Y. Zhang, L. Han, Ultrasensitive Label-Free MiRNA Sensing Based on a Flexible Graphene Field-Effect Transistor without Functionalization. *ACS Appl. Electron. Mater.* 2, (2020) 1090–1098.

50. Y. Zhang, C.W. Li, L. Zhou, Z. Chen, C. Yi, "Plug and Play" Logic Gate Construction Based on Chemically Triggered Fluorescence Switching of Gold Nanoparticles Conjugated with Cy3-Tagged Aptamer. *Microchim. Acta.* 187, (2020) 1–11.

51. X. Liu, R. Aizen, R. Freeman, O. Yehezkeli, I. Willner, Multiplexed Aptasensors and Amplified Dna Sensors Using Functionalized Graphene Oxide: Application for Logic Gate Operations. *ACS Nano.* 6, (2012) 3553–3563.

52. S. Yu, Y. Wang, L.P. Jiang, S. Bi, J.J. Zhu, Cascade Amplification-Mediated in Situ Hot-Spot Assembly for MicroRNA Detection and Molecular Logic Gate Operations. *Analytical Chemistry* 90, (2018) 4544–4551.
53. W. Sun, J. Shen, Z. Zhao, N. Arellano, C. Rettner, J. Tang, T. Cao, Z. Zhou, T. Ta, J.K. Streit, J.A. Fagen, T. Schaus, M. Zheng, S.-J. Han, W.M. Shih, H.T. Maune, P. Yin, Precise Pitch-Scaling of Carbon Nanotube Arrays within Three-Dimensional DNA Nanotrenches. *Science* 368, (2020) 874–877.
54. J.M. Yun, K.N. Kim, J.Y. Kim, D.O. Shin, W.J. Lee, S.H. Lee, M. Lieberman, S.O. Kim, DNA Origami Nanopatterning on Chemically Modified Graphene. *Angew. Chem. Inter. Ed.* 51, (2012) 912–915.
55. D. Sung, J. Koo, A Review of BioFET's Basic Principles and Materials for Biomedical Applications. *Biomed. Eng. Lett.* 11, (2021) 1–12.
56. J. Kim, I. Jeerapan, J.R. Sempionatto, A. Barfidokht, R.K. Mishra, A.S. Campbell, L.J. Hubble, J. Wang, Wearable Bioelectronics: Enzyme-Based Body-Worn Electronic Devices. *Acc. Chem. Res.* 51, (2018) 2820–2828.

18

Conductive Hydrogels for Bioelectronics

Meenakshi Singh, Manjeet Harijan, Ritu Singh, and Akriti Srivastava
Department of Chemistry, Mahila Mahavidyalaya, Banaras Hindu University, Varanasi, India

CONTENTS

18.1 Introduction

Bioelectronics is a fast-growing interdisciplinary research field that acts as a bridge between biological systems and electronic devices to get more deep knowledge about biological processes. Bioelectronics came into existence when Galvani in the 1780s showed that connecting electrodes with frog legs can produce contraction of muscles [1]. This early experiment attracted huge attention among the scientific community consequently several bioelectronics materials have been developed to monitor and control biological processes such as glucose sensors for diabetic patients, cardiac pacemakers, brain implants to manage/treat epilepsy, chronic pain, arrhythmia, Parkinson's disease, etc. These bioelectronics devices have tremendous potential for revolutionary diagnostic and therapeutic capabilities. Bioelectronics is a burgeonic field encompassing various disciplines, *viz*. chemistry, physics, material science, biology, data sciences, etc. serving the healthcare industry and society in general. Looking at the scenario today, especially at the brink of a pandemic, billions of people are suffering across the globe, it is a challenge to scientists from across the disciplines to come up united with cost-effective biocompatible devices. Biomedical devices are being explored at a fast pace in the last decades and respectable progress has been made. This progress can be visualized by the

DOI: 10.1201/9781003263265-18

review articles in recent years. Readers are advised to go through these review articles for in-depth details. Here in this chapter, we would limit ourselves to the inclusion of conductive hydrogel materials for bioelectronics.

Reasonable signal transduction traversing the biotic/abiotic interface is vital for current bioelectronics design and operation. Conducting hydrogels are promising materials that can remove the disparity between the biotic and abiotic phases. They can offer effective and reliable signal transduction between bioelectronic devices and tissue. Electronic devices are rigid and dry while biological tissues are soft and wet causing an increase in interfacial impedance due to scar tissue formation. Furthermore reduction in stimulation/recording efficacy is observed due to an increase in tissue–electrode distance. Due to the structural similarity of hydrogels with natural tissue, it can function as an excellent interface between electrode-electrolyte as well as biological soft and synthetic hard materials. Owing to ionic as well electronic conductivity of conducting hydrogel, they find applications in neural electrodes, artificial skin, and electronic tongue as well as in various implants. Furthermore, properties of conducting hydrogels such as toughness, stretchability, and biocompatibility can be easily modulated and additional properties required for bioelectronic applications such as self-healing and shape-memory may also be incorporated. Additionally, their high water holding characteristic facilitates the exchange of biological molecules and markers across interfaces. Earlier inorganic materials such as metal electrodes and silicone were widely used for bioelectronic but they differ intrinsically in terms of chemical and mechanical properties as compared to body tissue. This critical difference causes serious problems such as nonconforming contact between the devices and the skin or tissue, unstable signal collection, as well as causing inflammatory responses in the body. Currently, most bioelectronic devices are used in the form of electrodes that interact with biological systems and collect/deliver various bioelectronic signals in different parts of the body such as skin, brain, spinal cord, and heart.

18.2 Conducting Polymers

Conducting polymers (CPs) facilitate electronic pathways within the polymer backbone. Examples of commercially used CPs are poly(p-phenylene), polyaniline (PANI), polypyrrole (PPy), polythiophene (PTh), poly(3,4-ethylene dioxythiophene) polystyrene sulfonate (PEDOT: PSS), polyphenazine (PPz), polycarbazole (PCz), and their derivatives. CPs show high stable electronic conductivity and thus have gained quite a popularity in the field of bioelectronics. CPs have been widely applied in biosensors, bio-electrodes, enzyme immobilization, and biomedical devices. Among others, PANI, PPy, and PEDOT are the most commonly employed conducting polymers in bioelectronics applications due to their high conductivity, biocompatibility, good water dispersibility, and high stretchability. The PEDOT usually doped with polystyrene sulfonate (PSS) is most popular because of its highly stable electrochemical conductivity combined with a narrow bandgap making it a suitable candidate for several electroanalytical biosensing applications as well as for the fabrication of platforms for tissue engineering applications. Thiophene-based polymers have also gained popularity due to their stability and high conductivity which can be varied with dopants. CPs have been integrated with biosensors for the determination of several chemical species of biological importance including antigens, neurotransmitters, enzyme substrates, DNA fragments, and drug metabolites. These polymeric biosensors can be examined by electrochemical, optical, or piezo-gravimetric detectors with very high sensitivities, and low detection limits.

18.2.1 Conducting Polymer–Based Hydrogels

Conducting hydrogels are often synthesized by mixing insulating polymer matrices (providing structural support and water holding properties) with conducting polymer or filler material (providing electrical conductivity). Metallic nanoparticles, carbon nano-tubes, graphene, and their derivatives have been extensively employed to prepare con-ducting hydrogel due to their electrical and mechanical properties. However, the rigid and fragile nature of conducting polymers hampers the long-time stability of hydrogels and restrains the wider applications in emerging flexible electronic devices. Synthesis of conducting hydrogel along with excellent biocompatibility is highly required for the development of bioelectronics and energy devices.

Several electrically conductive polymers including PPy, PANI, PEDOT, and PTH-based hydrogels with their synthetic flexibility have gained widespread interest in bioelec-tronics applications. Conducting polymer-based hydrogels has the additional benefit of electrical conductivity over conventional hydrogels. Conducting polymers such as PPy have also been widely employed along with dopants for conductive hydrogels designing as they provide conductive pathways for bio-electrocatalysis of enzymes. The first con-ducting hydrogel was synthesized by Gilmore and group by direct electropolymerization of PPy on pre-prepared polyacrylamide hydrogel in the cylindrical gel cell [2], while the Wallace group has prepared a range of conducting polymer-based electroactive hydrogel composites bearing excellent rehydration levels up to 80–95% [3]. The composites based on the growth of conducting film of PPy or PANI throughout hydrogel were investigated. Excellent water-retaining capacity and the stimuli-responsive electrochemical release of larger incorporated counterions provide an open porous structure of the resultant hy-drogel materials. The hydrogel composites, with retained properties of hydrogel, present newer electrochemical applications of these materials. An enzyme-based biosensor was fabricated by an electrosynthetic approach of conducting PPy with alginate as co-dopant of laccase (an oxydoreductase enzyme) and 2,2'-and-bis(3-ethyl benzothiazoline-6-sulfonic acid) (a redox mediator) [4]. The catalytic effect of PPy film as a function of several cycles at various ratios of alginate doped laccase was examined. The catalytic effect was found to enhance the number of cycles from 0 to 10, and further decreased as the number of cycles increased.

PEDOT is a widely used conducting polymer in the field of bioelectronics and has en-abled improvements in the electrical conductivity of metallic electrodes and provided functional versatility of biomolecules. Doping of PEDOT with several counterions was reported. A biocompatible polyurethane hybrid composite (PUHC) hydrogel formed by dispersion of polyurethane with PEDOT:PSS and liquid crystalline graphene oxide shows high conductivity, stretchability, and good mechanical performance. Certain organogels of PEDOT:PSS with polyacrylamide (PAAm) allowed electronic transport within organogel. Conducting polymers incorporated hybrid hydrogels are promising materials for bioactive electrode coatings. A blending of conducting polymers into hydrogels helped in improving the electrical, mechanical, and biological properties of inherent hydrogels, e.g., flexible conducting polymer PEDOT-based sodium alginate hydrogel coated neural electrodes. PEDOT: PSS was added to CS/PVA scaffolds causing a significant enhancement in the mechanical and electrical properties for cardiovascular engineering. Chitosan (CS), a biopolymer, lacked the electrical properties needed for cardiovascular engineering, with the addition of PEDOT:PSS as conductive scaffolds to the CS/PVA, significant electrical conductivity was achieved for heart tissue engineering.

Polydopamine (PDA) and PPy integrated polyacrylamide (PAM) (PDA PPy PAM) hydrogel marked yet another high-performance soft electronic device. They exhibited high intrinsic conductivity (12 S/m), high optical transparency (70% after 3 days), and good UV-shielding performance and may prove beneficial for potential applications in wound dressings, transparent electronic skins, and bioelectrodes.

A conducting hydrogel immobilized enzyme-based amperometric biosensor for glucose determination onto a Pt electrode as a biotransducer was fabricated [5]. An enzyme-loaded electroconductive polymeric hydrogel composite on Pt electrode was chemically modified and functionalized with 3-aminopropyl-trimethoxysilane (APTMS), acryloyl (polyethyleneglycol)-N-hydroxysuccinamide (AC-PEG-NHS), and polyHEMA cross-linked hydrogel scaffold followed by electropolymerization of pyrrole in the presence of glucose oxidase. The polymeric hydrogel composite–based bio-transducer rendered higher catalytic bioactivity.

An injectable self-healing conductive hydrogel as a cell delivery vehicle for cardiac cell therapy for the treatment of myocardial infarction was introduced [6]. CS grafted aniline tetramer (CS-AT) and di-benzaldehyde terminated polyethylene glycol (PEG-DA)–based conductive hydrogel was fabricated for cell treatment. Hydrogels exhibited conductivity similar to that of the myocardium, suitable for cardiac repairing applications by regulating the electrical signals as well as showing self-healing, tissue adhesive, cell proliferation, antibacterial activity, cell delivery ability in chosen H9c2 and C2C12 myoblasts for cardiac repair.

Motivated by the challenges faced during the formation of elastic conducting polymer hydrogel, Lu *et al.* developed conductive PPy hydrogels with extraordinary elasticity of about 70% of compress strain [7] and this added several characteristics to the conducting polymeric hydrogels such as shape memory, facile functionalization, fast removal of dyes from wastewater, etc. They can also be conveniently transformed into pure organic, electronically conductive, and elastic sponges by supercritical fluid drying technique with magnificent stress-sensing performance. Such remarkable characteristics of PPy hydrogels render them an intelligent engineering material.

18.2.2 Conductive Hydrogels

Conductive hydrogel (CH) composites were popular, owing to their electronic functionality and hydrophilic network. As the name implies, a conducting hydrogel is the cross-linked hybrid network of hydrogels incorporated with conducting materials to provide electrical conductivity. CHs have found potential applications in bioelectronics such as implantable and electronic devices at cell/tissue interfaces. They are an ideal candidate for implantable and ingestible devices, as cheap, elastic, and biocompatible, biodegradable materials that are compliant with biological systems. Edible electronics are another feather in the cap for physicians and researchers as a high-performing tool in medical science. Edible devices are digestible within the body, suitable for treating the gastrointestinal (GI) tract without any risk of retention. Various electronic devices based on conducting hydrogels have been explored and employed successfully in biomedical applications for targeted drug delivery, wound dressing, and disease monitoring due to their good electronic properties and tunable mechanical flexibility.

18.2.3 Hydrogels Based on Zwitterionic Polymers

Zwitterionic polymers can mimic cell membranes and can be an ideal candidate to engineer biomaterials able to avert hostile interactions with biological cells. Sulfobetaine/carbobetaine/phosphobetaine polyelectrolytes are highly biocompatible, encompassing some natural analogs such as taurine, glycine betaine, etc. prospects in biomedical devices and other such applications are being explored. Zwitterionic polymer is a special kind of polymer that consists of both cationic and anionic groups on each monomer throughout the polymeric backbone. Due to the presence of an equal number of anionic and cationic groups in the polymeric backbone, they are highly hydrophilic and antifouling. They interact with water via strong ion-dipole interaction and form a stable and dense hydration shell. Polyzwitterions can interact with water molecules *via* electrostatic interactions and the hydration layers around them can "distance" any other biomolecules including protein. They are an ideal replacement for PEG. Their application as a drug delivery vehicle has been recently reviewed [8].

Gels with a polyzwitterionic backbone were extensively reported. The potential use of zwitterionic hydrogels is constrained by their poor mechanical strength. Mechanical properties of non-fouling zwitterionic hydrogels were improved by substituting the methacrylate backbone of sulfobetaine methacrylate (SBMA) by a vinyl imidazole backbone (SBVI)]; the non-fouling characteristics of the zwitterionic sulfobetaine group were retained while aiding on mechanical properties diffusion behavior of fluorescence-labeled model proteins in PEG, polySBMA and mixed PEG-sulfobetaine methacrylate hydrogels (SBMA:PEG 4:1, SBMA:PEG 1:4) was studied [9]. Four hydrogels showed varied diffusion characteristics for either a negatively charged protein or positively charged protein depending on protein-polymer interaction and the labile water content available in the hydrogel matrix.

Protein loading efficiency may increase as stronger interaction between protein-PEG is observed than protein-polySBMA and controlled release is expected by changing the ratio of PEG to SBMA in a hydrogel [10]. A narrowly dispersed zwitterionic poly(amido amine) (PAA) nanogels tethered with N,Ndimethylethylenediamine having a positive surface charge were developed for drug delivery and imaging. They showed excellent stability in serum and minimal cytotoxicity. Stretchable tissue adhesive and antibacterial hydrogels with zwitterionic monomers (strong dipole dipole interaction, electrostatic interaction, and hydrogen bonding with the skin surface) seem promising for wound dressings and implantable devices. A polymer with phosphorylcholine (PC) and poly (propylene glycol) (PPG) showed a steady release of insulin. On injecting the polymer aqueous solution subcutaneously, a hydrogel was formed in the injection site and very mild tissue responses around the injection site were observed. Overall, zwitterionic polymer-based hydrogels possess remarkable characteristics such as being thermo-responsive, good cytocompatibility, anti-biofouling nature, controlled protein adsorption, cell adhesiveness, implantable nature, and many more.

18.2.4 Ion Conductive Hydrogels

Hydrogels consist of free ions from ionic electrolytes usually exhibit higher conductivity and found good application in bioelectronics applications. Ionic salts like NaCl, LiCl, $CaSO_4$, Na_2SO_4, etc. are generally added to hydrogels to make them ionically conductive. The resulting ionic hydrogels exhibit greater ionic conductivity, higher stretchability, and tissue softness. Due to greater electronic conductivity, ionically conductive hydrogels found wide applicability in bioelectronic applications. Ionic electrolytes have been introduced within a hydrogel as a promising material to improve the conductivity of edible electrodes [11]. They fabricated highly swollen, robust, and conductive hydrogel materials made from food material for the enhancement in the edible device. This hydrogel electrode was developed by soaking the alginate-gelatin hydrogels in the electrolytic solution i.e., saturated $CaCl_2$ and NaCl solution. The conductivity of hydrogel was highly enhanced with the addition of ionic species. The conductivity for alginate-gelatin hydrogels from edible supermarket foods was 190 ± 20 mS/cm while that of gelatin/gellan gum soaked in a solution of NaCl or CsCl as ionic species was found to be 200 ± 20 mS/cm and 380 ± 20 mS/cm, respectively. Ionically conductive, robust hydrogel was fabricated by crosslinking polyacrylamide (PAAm) and alginate with calcium sulfate. The PAAm-alginate hydrogel *via* UV irradiation was bonded with Ecoflex elastomer by gelation process which looks to be a valuable candidate for electronic devices under large deformation using soft, flexible, and stretchable conductive material [12] (Figure 18.1).

The electrical conduction within the electronically conducting polymers infused with ionic electrolytes is also monitored using electrical impedance spectroscopy (EIS). Conductance of alginate-based hydrogels as a function of different ionic species using EIS indicated that the lower concentration of electrolyte showed minimal frequency dependence, whereas the higher concentration of electrolyte displays a larger conduction charge between the lower stimulation frequency to higher stimulation frequency [13]. Ionically conductive hydrogel-based circuits using salt-soaked poly (ethylene glycol) diacrylate were designed to generate programmed ionic circuits [14]. High conductivity salt solutions were incubated within a PEG hydrogel to give rise to patterned ionic current to enable localized *in-vivo* muscle electrical stimulation. This strategy offered integrated electronic platforms to distribute ionic electrical signals between tailored and biological systems. The ability of the ionic hydrogel system is displayed for light-emitting diode (LED) activation, localized *in-vitro* cultured cells electrical stimulation, and *in-vivo* skin-mounted skeletal muscle tissue stimulation. A biocompatible, elastic rubber-like ionic conductive hydrogel consisting of polyvinyl alcohol (PVA) and hydroxypropyl cellulose (HPC) biopolymer fibers enhanced the ionic conductivity up to 3.4 S/m, at 1 MHz frequency on ions migration within the hydrogel. It can behave as an artificial nerve in a 3D-printed robotic hand allowing tunable electrical signals.

18.2.5 Conductive Filler–Based Hydrogels

Conductive fillers including graphene, carbon nanotubes, and metal nanoparticles within the hydrogel network are used to augment the conductivity, toughness, and stretchability of hydrogels. These include metallic nanoparticles, graphene-based materials, nanofibers, nanotubes, or conducting polymers. Metallic nanoparticles have been added to attain the desired electrical conductivity of hydrogels. Gold nanoparticles (AuNPs) embedded in thiol 2-hydroxyethyl methacrylate nanocomposite-based conductive hydrogel were designed with tunable electrical and mechanical properties. The neonatal rat cardiomyocytes were grown the conductive scaffold enhanced the expression of connexin-43 with or without any electrical stimulation. Silver nanoparticles (AgNPs) incorporated polyacrylic acid-based hydrogel using methylol

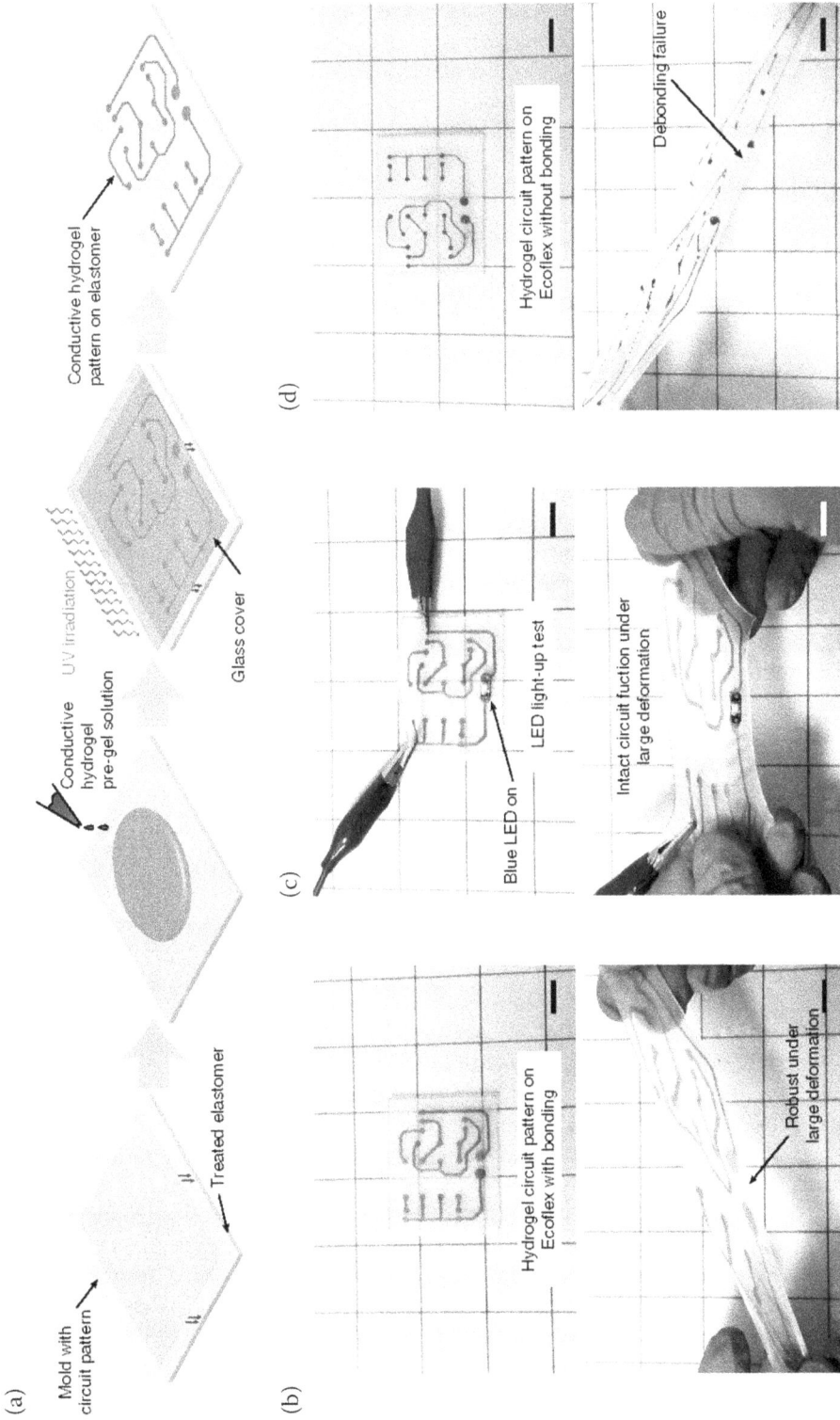

(a)

Mold with circuit pattern

Treated elastomer

Conductive hydrogel pre-gel solution

UV irradiation

Glass cover

Conductive hydrogel pattern on elastomer

(b)

Hydrogel circuit pattern on Ecoflex with bonding

Robust under large deformation

(c)

Blue LED on

LED light-up test

Intact circuit fuction under large deformation

(d)

Hydrogel circuit pattern on Ecoflex without bonding

Debonding failure

FIGURE 18.1

Schematic representation of ion conductive stretchable hydrogel circuit board pattern on the elastomer. Adapted with permission [12], Copyright (2016), Springer Nature.

urea as cross-linker by *in situ* free-radical polymerization [15]. The hydrogel showed excellent improvement in electrical conductivity up to 0.572 S cm^{-1} that can be considered a promising material for nanoelectronic devices.

Platinum nanoparticles (PtNPs)–doped conductive PANI hydrogel enabled the transduction of signals for electrochemical sensing of glucose [16]. An electronically conductive channel allowed efficient charge transfer for sensitive determination of analyte with fast response time. Graphene- and CNT-based materials were engaged as reinforcing filler during the preparation of hydrogel composites for enhancing the electrical conductivity and mechanical properties. A conducting biocompatible chitosan-lactic acid hydrogel composite using graphene as filler material improved the mechanical strength and conductivity of hydrogels [17]. Reduced graphene nanosheets containing biocompatible UV cross-linked methacrylated chitosan (rGO /ChiMA) hydrogels produced conducting 3D-printable scaffolds with good cell adhesion and biodegradable and cytocompatible properties, which can be beneficial. A polyacrylamide (PAM)–based conductive hydrogel with partially reduced graphene oxide/fully reduced graphene oxide (pGO/rGO) using polydopamine (PDA) solution was prepared by controlling the reaction time. The pGO introduced PDA–pGO–PAM hydrogel exhibited the overall highest extension ratio, good toughness (4280 J/m^2), and conductivity (0.08 S/cm) with respect to the unreduced GO and rGO incorporated. The unreduced GO filler forms strong non-covalent interactions with PDA and PAM and also exhibited extremely low conductivity. On the other hand, rGO incorporated PDA–rGO–PAM exhibits good conductivity (0.1 S/cm) but low extension ratio ($\lambda = 20$). Thus the conductive PDA–pGO– PAM hydrogels with high stretchability, self-healablility, and self-adhesiveness potential pave a way as a cell stimulator and implantable bioelectronics for human body (Figure 18.2) [18]. While rGO-containing polyacrylamide, r(GO/PAAm) hydrogel was developed by using mild chemical reduction of GO/PAAm hydrogel in aqueous L-ascorbic acid solution. The r(GO/PAAm) hydrogel exhibited high relative stiffness with a Young's modulus of about 50 kPa. The conductive rGO within the hydrogel network significantly enhanced the electrical and mechanical properties of the hydrogel. The electrical stimulation of C2C12 myoblasts with r(GO/PAAm) hydrogels for seven days greatly enhanced the proliferation and differentiation of myoblasts compared to unreduced hydrogels (GO/PAAm) [19]. As a result, soft and conductive r(GO/PAAm) hydrogels will be useful material for skeletal muscle tissue engineering scaffolds. PEDOT-CNT encapsulated fibrin hydrogel-coated electrodes were designed to record somatosensory induced potentials into a rat cortex through the deflection of multi-whisker [20]. The nanocoating significantly enhanced the electrical conductivity of microelectrode with two orders of magnitude and proved significant for neural recordings. Further, poly(2-hydroxyethyl methacrylate) (pHEMA)-encapsulated PEDOT-PSS-CNT microspheres for neural stimulation and high-quality signal recording in the rat cortex were used [21]. Fractal carbon nanotube (CNT) network tailored gelatin methacrylate (GelMA) hydrogels were found apt for seeding neonatal rat cardiomyocytes onto the conductive CNTs-GelMA hydrogels as functional cardiac patches. CNT–GelMA hydrogels greatly enhanced the electrical signal propagation and synchronous cellular excitability of cardiomyocytes cultured on it. The incorporation of small amounts of CNTs into gelatin-chitosan-based hydrogel supports cardiomyocyte function and helps to attain the electrical conductivity of beating rate of the hearts [22]. Tissue-engineered scaffolds with the combined fascinating properties of CNTs improved the cardiovascular defect repairs.

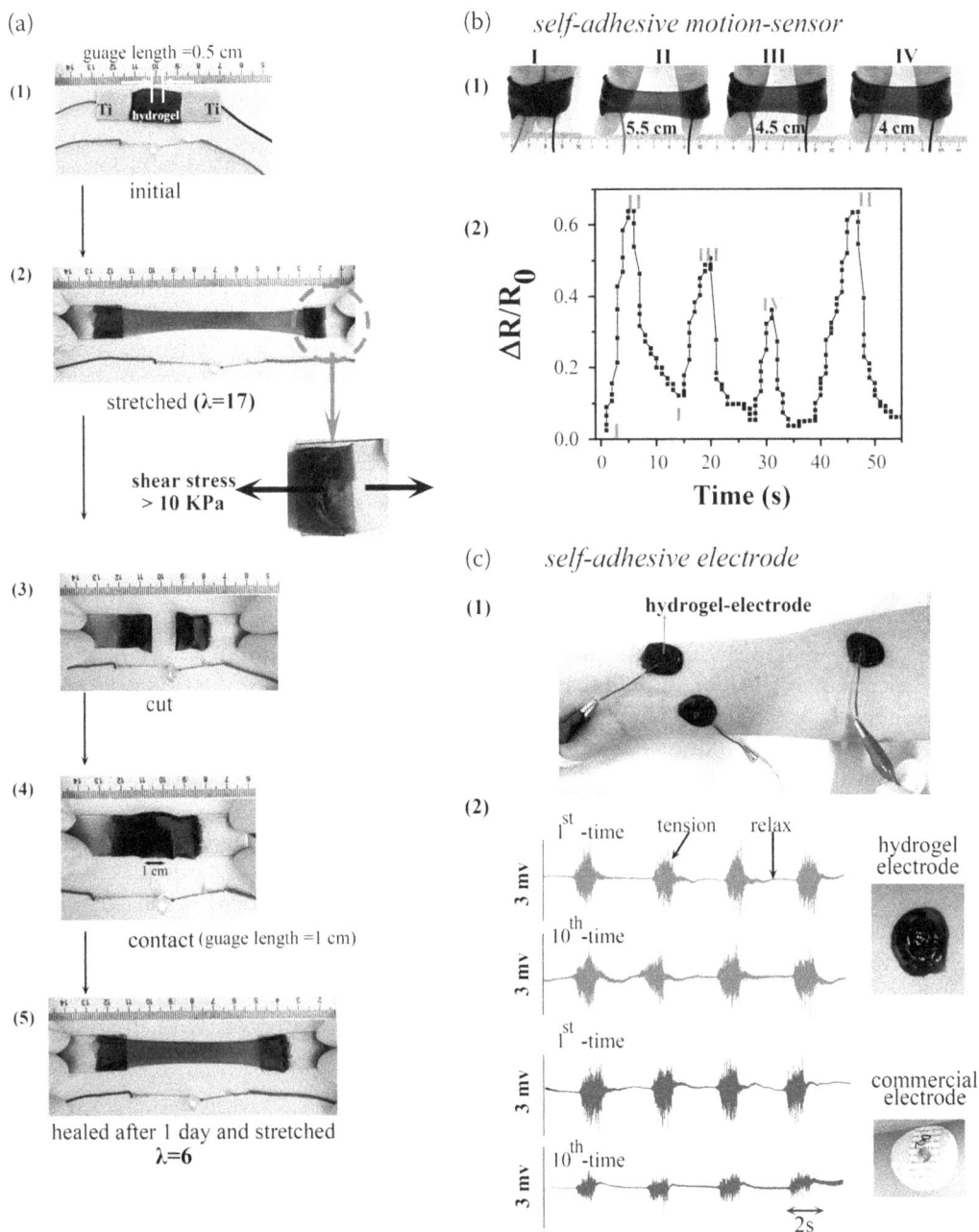

FIGURE 18.2
Demonstration of the PDA–pGO–PAM hydrogel showing (a) integrated high stretchability and self-heal ability, (b) self-adhesive motion sensor and the real-time electrical resistance with the distance between the two fingers, (c) self-adhesion of the electrode to skin and recorded electromyography (EMG) signals. Adapted with permission [18], Copyright (2017) Wiley-VCH.

18.3 Applications of Hydrogels in Bioelectronics

18.3.1 Coating of Hydrogel on the Neural Electrode

Neuron acts as an interface for the communication between the central nervous system and bioelectronics devices. But chemical and the mechanical disparity between neuron and bioelectronics devices cause aggravated inflammation response, an unreliable signal collection due to nonconforming contact between the devices and the surface of skin or tissue. The coating of a hydrogel on neural electrodes improves the functionality of bioelectronics devices by providing intimate cellular integration and mechanical buffer between hard electrodes and soft tissues. But as the thickness of a hydrogel coated on neural electrodes increases, it may hamper the optimal performance of neural electrodes due to lack of neurons near the electrode. The possible solution is to coat a conducting polymer on the electrode to restore loss of functionality by an increase of the thickness of the hydrogel on the electrode. To visualize the effect of hydrogel thickness on the recording quality of neural electrodes, ionically cross-linked alginate hydrogel (AH) having different thicknesses were prepared on the neural electrode by dip coating. It was observed that as the AH thickness increased, the number of clearly detectable units gradually decreased, which could be due to a lack of neurons immediately around the electrode sites. Furthermore, the conducting polymer PEDOT was also deposited on the neural electrode along with AH. This improved the recording functionality of the AH-coated electrodes. The biocompatible hydrogel was also applied for the differentiation of human neural stem cells to enhance neuritogenesis via the electrical stimulation process. Flexible PEDOT-based sodium alginate hydrogel-coated neural electrodes for the sensitive neural recordings in guinea pig auditory were reported. PEDOT-CNT encapsulated fibrin hydrogel-coated electrodes were designed to record somatosensory induced potentials into a rat cortex through the deflection of multi-whisker. While agarose hydrogels doped with surface-modified cellulose nanocrystals were fabricated to produce a diode [23]. A bionic ear via 3D printing of a cell-seeded hydrogel matrix in the geometry of a human ear, with an intertwined conducting polymer embedded with silver nanoparticles, was fabricated [24]. *In-vitro* culturing of cartilage tissue around an inductive coil antenna in the ear was performed, which enabled the readout of inductively coupled signals from cochlea-shaped electrodes. Table 18.1 presents an overview of conductive hydrogels with their specific features and applications.

18.3.2 Artificial Skin

The physiological environment has a huge impact on the performance of hydrogel bioelectronic devices. Some hydrogel bioelectronic devices become unstable and fragile on exposure to aqueous solutions or harsh physiological environments, significantly impeding their desired applications. Biostable hydrogel bioelectronic devices that can maintain their super mechanical and conductive properties, even when exposed to biofluids are highly desirable. By utilizing biocompatible cellulose and conducting reduced graphene oxide (rGO), a biostable conducting hydrogel was prepared. A 2D planar cellulose crystal structure using the polydopamine-reduced graphene oxide was prepared. This 2D planar cellulose crystal after physical and chemical cross-linking self-assembled into a conducting hydrogel. This hydrogel showed high biostability and could withstand long-term immersion in aqueous environments and implantation for over 30 days [45].

TABLE 18.1

Conducting Hydrogel Used in Bioelectronics

S. no.	Conducting hydrogel	Features	Application	Reference
1.	(PEDOT:PSS)/gelatine	Electrical Conductivity Self-Adherent, Biocompatible	ECG Measurement	[25]
2.	CNT/PVA	Electrical Conductivity, Stretchability (Fracture Stain Up To 500%), Room-Temperature Repairable	Wearable Sensor	[26]
3.	PAA	Ion-Conductivity	Artificial Tongue	[27]
4.	PEDOT-based microelectrode	Electrical Conductivity, Stretchability (>200% Strain)	Implantable Bioelectronics	[28]
5.	(Ch-CMC-PDA)	Ion-Conductivity ($0.01\text{–}3.4 \times 10^{-3}$ S/cm) Self-Healing, Adhesive, Injectable Hydrogel	ECG Measurement Triboelectric Nanogenerator	[29]
6.	PANI/PAM	Electrical Conductivity, Light-Stimuli-Responsive Stretchable	Nerve Injury Implants	[30]
7.	P(AA-co-DMAPS)/Al^{3+}	Ion-Conductivity, Thermosensitive	ECG Signal-Monitoring, Temperature Sensor	[31]
8.	PPy-PDA/gelatin-Fe^{3+}	Electrical Conductivity (6.51×10^{4} S/cm)	Cardiac Patches	[32]
9.	PPy rGO PPy/gelatin	Electrical Conductivity, Skin Like Mechanical Compliance Mechanical and Thermal Sensitive	Human Body Movements	[33]
10.	PVA/catechol-Fe^{3+}	Ion-Conductivity, Shape Memory	Intelligent Actuators	[34]
11.	PVA/STB/PEDOT:PSS	Electrical Conductivity, Self-Healing, Stretchable, Highly Adhesive	Epidermal Patch Electrodes	
12.	Gel-UPy/dsCD	Electrical Conductive, Self-Healing, Adhesive	Cancer Detection	[35]
13.	rGO/poly(AMPS-co-AAm)	Ionic and Electronic Conductivity	Strain And Temperature Sensors	[36]
14.	PDMAAp/PEDOT	Electrical Conductivity	Coating Neural Electrode	[37]
15.	PVA/P(AM-co-SBMA), PPS	Electrical Conductivity, Adhesive, Stretchable, Antibacterial	Human Motion Detection	[38]
16.	TiO$_2$@MXene/PAA	Electrical Conductivity, Ultra-Stretchable	ECG And Heart Rate Monitoring	[39]
17.	PDA–pGO-PAM	Electrical Conductivity, Self-Adhesive, Self-Healable	Cell Stimulator	[40]
18.	P(AA-co-DMAPS)/Al^{3+}	Ionic Conductivity, Temperature Responsive	ECG Measurement	[31]
19.	PEDOT:PSS/PAAm	Electrical Conductivity,Ultrasoft, Mass-Permeable	Wearable Bioelectronics	[41]
20.	PANI/PSS 20UPy	Electrical Conductivity, Self-Healable	Strain Sensors	[42]
21.	GO/PAAm	Electrically Conductivity, Hydrogels	Electrical Stimulation Of Cell	[43]
22.	PEDOT:PSS/PHEA/LN	Electrically Conductivity, Tough	Human Motion Sensor	[44]

Another *in-vivo* skin-mounted skeletal muscle tissue stimulation was shown by ionic hydrogel system localized *in-vitro* cultured cells electrical stimulation. Yuk *et al.* reported ionically conductive tough hydrogel for constructing electronic devices under large deformation using soft, flexible, and stretchable conductive material [12]. For the sake of brevity, details of such applications are presented in Table 18.1.

18.3.3 Flexible and Implantable Bioelectronics

Regular and continued monitoring of vital signs of the body such as body temperature, blood pressure, and estimation of analytes in body fluids is necessary for maintaining a healthy life. Currently, electrocardiography (ECG), electroencephalography (EEG), and electromyography (EMG) are used to monitor these vital signs of the body. The acquisition of their signals is typically achieved by metal electrodes which can cause skin damage/irritation. Moreover, these electrodes are rigid and cannot withstand stretching and bending. Therefore, soft and flexible epidermal patches are highly desirable. Conductive hydrogels are tissue-friendly and their tunable electrical properties, flexibility, and biocompatibility make them useful for epidermal patches. A conducting hydrogel was prepared by mixing polyvinyl alcohol (PVA), borax, and PEDOT:PSS screen-printing paste to use in epidermal patches. Prepared hydrogels exhibited high skin adhesion, high plastic stretchability, moderate conductivity, and self-healing properties. The hydrogel was applied for the recording of ECG and EMG signals, which showed high-quality recording. An ion-conducting (Ch-CMC-PDA) hydrogel using chitosan (Ch), cellulose (CMC), and dopamine (DA) [29]. Ch-CMC-PDA the hydrogel was applied for ECG signal detection; the result showed that the ECG pattern obtained using Ch-CMC-PDA was identical to commercial gel Cardijelly.

PEDOT:PSS-PAAm organogels possess a better transport of electrical signals and was highly stretchable. PEDOT:PSS added to CS/PVA scaffolds was introduced for the sake of better mechanical and electrical properties for cardiovascular engineering. The conductive PDA–pGO–PAM hydrogels with high stretchability, self-healing ability, and self-adhesiveness potential pave the way as cell stimulators and implantable bioelectronics for the human body (Figure 18.2) [18]. Soft and conductive r(GO/PAAm) hydrogels were also found to be useful material for skeletal muscle tissue engineering scaffolds [19]. The incorporation of small amounts of CNTs into gelatin-chitosan-based hydrogel supports cardiomyocyte function and helped to attain the electrical conductivity of the beating rate of the hearts [22]. Tissue-engineered scaffolds with the combined properties of CNTs improved the cardiovascular defect repairs. The conductive biopolymer-based hydrogel can behave as an artificial nerve in a 3D-printed robotic hand. This may allow tunable electrical signals to pass and full recovery with robotic hand movements. This natural highly elastic (up to 900 kPa) ionic conductive hydrogel is visualized to contribute to artificial flexible electronics. The conducting 3D-printable scaffolds showed good cell adhesion, are biodegradable, and have cytocompatible properties to be used in tissue engineering. C2C12 myoblasts grown on the hybrid GelMA-vertically aligned CNT hydrogels yielded functional myofibers [46], after applying electrical stimulation in the direction of the aligned CNTs, than cells that were cultured on the GelMA hydrogels with randomly distributed and horizontally aligned CNTs.

The development and application of printed MEA arrays on soft substrates including PDMS and hydrogels were conducted [47]. To this end, a straightforward printing process was introduced that exploits controlled wetting properties of carbon and polyimide inks on PDMS, curtailing major problems that are often faced in printing structures. The soft MEAs were applied for localized recordings of action potentials from HL-1 cells, testifying to the suitability of the printed devices for electrophysiological measurements. This work represents a far-reaching step toward the design of soft hydrogel–based bioelectronic devices using inkjet printing.

An ultra stretchable hydrogel device with custom-designed microchannel patterns perfused with ionic liquids was formed. The hydrophobic ionic liquids were sufficiently conductive and remain stably separated with aqueous surroundings in the air as well as underwater. A hydrogel matrix was prepared using highly water-soluble elastin peptide cryogel to achieve ultra-flexible scaffold, and further reinforced with gelatine, yielding an excellent and biocompatible gelation material [48]. This conductive hydrogel with a fixed shape showed excellent flexibility and injectable property, suggesting its potential application as a syringe-injectable biosensor or bioelectronics. A biocompatible ionic hydrogel made of polyvinyl alcohol, silk fibroin, and borax was prepared, which showed ultrahigh stretchability, water retention, self-healing, tunable conductivity, and adhesion. This hydrogel could be used as a sensing platform to monitor surrounding body motion for applications in healthcare monitoring, soft robotics, and human-machine interfaces. A gelatin/ferric-ion-cross-linked polyacrylic acid (GEL/PAA) dual dynamic supramolecular network was formed, which, on soaking into a NaCl glycerol/water solution to further toughen the gelatin network via solvent displacement, yielded a high toughness and high ionic conductivity [49]. Highly stretchable and multifunctional ionic microdevices are then fabricated based on the organohydrogel electrolytes by simple transfer printing of carbon-based microelectrodes onto the prestretched gel surface. Proof-of-concept microdevices including resistive strain sensors and micro-supercapacitors are demonstrated, which displayed outstanding stretchability to 300% strain, resistance to dehydration for >6 months, autonomous self-healing, and rapid room-temperature degradation within hours.

Smart and robust nanofibrillar poly(vinyl alcohol) (PVA) organohydrogels were fabricated via one-step physical cross-linking. The nanofibrillar network cross-linked by numerous PVA nanocrystallites enables the formation of organohydrogels with high transparency, drying resistance, high toughness, and good tensile strength. For strain sensor application, the PVA ionic organohydrogel, after soaking in a NaCl solution, shows excellent linear sensitivity (GF = 1.56, R2 > 0.998) owing to the homogeneous nanofibrillar PVA network. The potential application of the nanofibrillar PVA-based organohydrogel in smart contact lenses and emotion recognition was demonstrated. Such strategy paved an effective way to fabricate strong, tough, biocompatible, and ionically conductive organohydrogels, shedding light on multifunctional sensing applications in next-generation flexible bioelectronics.

A phenylboronic acid-based, hydrogel-interlayer radio-frequency (RF) resonator is demonstrated as a highly responsive, passive, and wireless sensor for glucose monitoring [50]. Constructs are composed of unanchored, capacitively coupled split rings interceded by glucose-responsive hydrogels. These sensors exhibited no signal drift or hysteresis over the period. This non-degradative, long-term nature of both RF read-out and phenylboronic acid-based hydrogels will enable biosensors capable of long-term, remote read-out of glucose. A conducting hydrogel immobilized enzyme-based amperometric biosensor was devised for glucose determination on to platinum electrode as a viable biotransducer. Dong *et al.* designed injectable self-healing conductive hydrogels as cell delivery vehicles for cardiac cell therapy in case of myocardial infarction [6]. The developed CS-AT and PEG-DA hydrogel exhibited excellent self-healing, tissue adhesive, cell proliferation, antibacterial activity, and cell delivery ability in chosen H9c2 and C2C12 myoblasts for cardiac repair.

18.3.4 Electronic Tongue

As per the IUPAC technical report, "The electronic tongue is an analytical instrument comprising an array of nonspecific, low-selective, chemical sensors with high stability and cross-sensitivity to different species in solution and an appropriate method of PARC and/or multivariate calibration for data processing." A MIP-based electronic tongue for certain phenols was fabricated using chemometrics and an artificial neural network (ANN) [51,52]. An electrically conductive hybrid hydrogel was fabricated with a composite of PPy and alginate and for human mesenchymal stem cell (hMSC) culture [51]. The conductive hybrid hydrogels may be used as a smart interface to stimulate stem cells via the effects of electrical and mechanical signals. The increase in Py and oxidant concentration showed a transition in the color of hydrogels from brown to black and a clear solution obtained after PPy polymerization. In cell culture studies, the results figured out that conductive hybrid hydrogel swells interacted with hMSCs as the hMSCs derived into larger and more elongated shapes when other substrates were used. An electrochemical biosensor using hydrogel-based MIPs for protein detection was used [52]. The coupling of pattern recognition techniques via principal component analysis (PCA) resulted in unique protein fingerprints for corresponding protein templates, allowing for MIP-based protein profiling. This PCA-coupled method was efficient for discriminating four proteins (BHb, Mb, BSA, and Cyt C), confirming that glassy carbon (GC) electrodes modified with MIP film could be used as a fast sensor to segregate between different kinds of proteins.

18.4 Conclusions and Perspectives

In conclusion, conductive hydrogels seem to be an integral part of bioelectronic devices. They are the coupling agent between the bionic and abionic constituents, playing the role of a perfect hinge between the two widely different fields, coupling them together almost perfectly. Although efforts have been made to design adaptable gel networks with higher flexibility, better biocompatibility, and simultaneously transducing the signal(s) from bionic system to abionic sectors for the sake of monitoring the biology, understanding at molecular level details are lacking. Such understandings will pave the way for elucidating the molecular biology of diseases threatening society today. The ignorance lying in our complete understanding of nature/biology forbids us to fabricate foolproof devices. Chemistry can tailor the hydrogels and a more synergistic approach will prove to be a boon, facilitating the transfer of these devices to the common man of society. Conductive hydrogels are on the verge of reaching the diagnostics market and contributing to "theranostics" more efficiently, spreading to other untouched sectors also.

References

1. M. Bresadola, Medicine and science in the life of Luigi Galvani (1737–1798). *Brain Research Bulletin* 46 (1998) 367–380.
2. K. Gilmore, A.J. Hodgson, B. Luan, C. Small, G. Wallace, Preparation of hydrogel/conducting polymer composites. *Polym Gels Networks* 2 (1994) 135–143.

3. C.J. Small, C.O. Too, G.G. Wallace, Responsive conducting polymer-hydrogel composites. *Polym Gels Networks* 5 (1997) 251–265.
4. S.Y. Kim, G.T.R. Palmore, Conductive hydrogel for bio-electrocatalytic reduction of di-oxygen. *Electrochem commun* 23 (2012) 90–93.
5. C.N. Kotanen, C. Tlili, A. Guiseppi-Elie, Amperometric glucose biosensor based on elec-troconductive hydrogels. *Talanta* 103 (2013) 228–235.
6. R. Dong, X. Zhao, B. Guo, P.X. Ma, Self-healing conductive injectable hydrogels with anti-bacterial activity as cell delivery carrier for cardiac cell therapy. *ACS Appl Mater Interfaces* 8 (2016) 17138–17150.
7. Y. Lu, W. He, T. Cao, H. Guo, Y. Zhang, Q. Li, Z. Shao, Y. Cui, X. Zhang, Elastic, conductive, polymeric hydrogels and sponges. *Sci Rep* 4 (2014) 5792.
8. M. Harijan, M. Singh, Zwitterionic polymers in drug delivery: A Review. *J Mol Recogn* 35 (2022) e2944.
9. J. Wu, Z. Xiao, C. He, J. Zhu, G. Ma, G. Wang, H. Zhang, J. Xiao, S. Chen, Protein diffusion characteristics in the hydrogels of poly(ethylene glycol) and zwitterionic poly(sulfobetaine methacrylate) (pSBMA), *Acta Biomaterialia* 40 (2016) 172–181.
10. G. Cheng, L. Mi, Z. Cao, H. Xue, Q. Yu, L. Carr, S. Jiang, Functionalizable and ultrastable zwitterionic nanogels, *Langmuir* 26 (2010) 6883–6886.
11. A. Keller, J. Pham, H. Warren, M. Panhuis, Conducting hydrogels for edible electrodes. *J Mater Chem B* 5 (2017) 5318–5328.
12. H. Yuk, T. Zhang, G.A. Parada, X. Liu, X. Zhao, Skin-inspired hydrogel-elastomer hybrids with robust interfaces and functional microstructures. *Nat Commun* 7 (2016) 1–11.
13. G. Kaklamani, D. Kazaryan, J. Bowen, F. Lacovella, S.H. Anastasiadis, G. Deligeorgis, On the electrical conductivity of alginate hydrogels. *Regen Biomater* 5 (2018) 293–301.
14. S. Zhao, P. Tseng, J. Grasman, Y. Wang, W. Li, B. Napier, B. Yavuz, Y. Chen, L. Howell, J. Rincon, F.G. Omenetto, D.L. Kaplan, Programmable hydrogel ionic circuits for biologically matched electronic interfaces. *Adv Mater* 30 (2018) 1–10.
15. S.J. Devaki, R.K. Narayanan, S. Sarojam, Electrically conducting silver nanoparticle-polyacrylic acid hydrogel by in situ reduction and polymerization approach. *Mater Lett* 116 (2014) 135–138.
16. D. Zhai, B. Liu, Y. Shi, L. Pan, Y. Wang, W. Li, R. Zhang, G. Yu, Highly sensitive glucose sensor based on Pt nanoparticle/polyaniline hydrogel heterostructures, *ACS Nano* 7 (2013) 3540–3546.
17. S. Sayyar, E. Murray, B.C. Thompson, J. Chung, D.L. Officer, S. Gambhir, G.M. Spinks, G.G. Wallace, Processable conducting graphene/chitosan hydrogels for tissue engineering. *J Mater Chem B* 3 (2015) 481–490.
18. L. Han, X. Lu, M. Wang, D. Gan, W. Deng, K. Wang, L. Fang, K. Liu, C.W. Chan, Y. Tang, L.T. Weng, H. Yuan, A mussel-inspired conductive, self-adhesive, and self-healable tough hy-drogel as cell stimulators and implantable bioelectronics. *Small* 13 (2017) 1–9.
19. H. Jo, M. Sim, S. Kim, S. Kim, S. Yang, Y. Yoo, J.H. Park, T.H. Yoon, M.G. Kim, J.Y. Lee, Electrically conductive graphene/polyacrylamide hydrogels produced by mild chemical re-duction for enhanced myoblast growth and differentiation. *Acta Biomater* 48 (2017) 100–109.
20. E. Castagnola, A. Ansaldo, E. Maggiolini, G.N. Angotzi, M. Skrap, D. Ricci, L. Fadiga, Biologically compatible neural interface to safely couple nanocoated electrodes to the surface of the brain. *ACS Nano* 7 (2013) 3887–3895.
21. E. Castagnola, E. Maggiolini, L. Ceseracciu, F. Ciarpella, E. Zucchini, S.D. Faveri, L. Fadiga, D. Ricci, pHEMA encapsulated PEDOT-PSS-CNT microsphere microelectrodes for recording single unit activity in the brain. *Front Neurosci* 10 (2016) 1–14.
22. S. Pok, F. Vitale, S.L. Eichmann, Biocompatible carbon nanotube-chitosan scaffold matching the electrical conductivity of the heart. *ACS Nano* 8 (2014) 9822–9832.
23. K. Nyamayaro, P. Keyvani, F. D'Acierno, J. Poisson, Z.M. Hudson, C.A. Michal, J.D.W. Madden, S.G. Hatzikiriakos, P. Mehrkhodavandi, Toward biodegradable electronics: ionic diodes based on acellulose nanocrystal agarose hydrogel. *ACS Appl. Mater. Interfaces* 12 (2020) 52182 52191.

24. M.S. Mannoor, Z. Jiang, T. James, Y.L. Kong, K.A. Malatesta, W.O. Soboyejo, N. Verma, D.H. Gracias, M.C. McAlpine, 3D Printed bionic ears. *Nano Lett.* 13 (2013) 2634 2639.
25. Y. Lee, S.G. Yim, G.W. Lee, S. Kim, H.S. Kim, D.Y. Hwang, B. An, J.H. Lee, S. Seo, S.Y. Yang, Self-adherent biodegradable gelatin-based hydrogel electrodes for electrocardiography monitoring. *Sensors* 20 (2020) 5737.
26. H. Wang, J. Lu, H. Huang, S. Fang, M. Zubair, Z. Peng, A highly elastic, Room-temperature repairable and recyclable conductive hydrogel for stretchable electronics. *J Coll Interf Sc* 588 (2021) 295–304.
27. J. Yeom, A. Choe, S. Lim, Y. Lee, S. Na, H. Ko, Soft and ion-conducting hydrogel artificial tongue for astringency perception. *Sci Adv* 6 (2020) eaba5785.
28. Y. Liu, J. Liu, S. Chen, T. Lei, Y. Kim, S. Niu, H. Wang, X. Wang, A.M. Foudeh, J.B.-H. Tok, Z. Bao, Soft and elastic hydrogel-based microelectronics for localized low-voltage neuro-modulation. *Nat Biomed Eng* 3 (2019) 58–68.
29. V. Panwar, A. Babu, A. Sharma, J. Thomas, V. Chopra, P. Malik, S. Rajput, M. Mittal, R. Guha, N. Chattopadhyay, D. Mandal, D. Ghosh, Tunable, conductive, self-healing, adhesive and injectable hydrogels for bioelectronics and tissue regeneration applications. *J Mater Chem B* 9 (2021) 6260–6270.
30. M. Dong, B. Shi, D. Liu, J.H. Liu, D. Zhao, Z.H. Yu, X.Q. Shen, J.M. Gan, B.L. Shi, Y. Qiu, Conductive hydrogel for a photothermal-responsive stretchable artificial nerve and coalescing with a damaged peripheral nerve. *ACS Nano* 14 (2020) 16565–16575.
31. Y. Tan, Y. Zhang, Y. Zhang, J. Zheng, H. Wu, Y. Chen, S. Xu, J. Yang, C. Liu, Y. Zhang, Dual cross-linked ion-based temperature-responsive conductive hydrogels with multiple sensors and steady electrocardiogram monitoring. *Chem Mater* 32 (2020) 7670–7678.
32. S. Liang, Y. Zhang, H. Wang, Z. Xu, J. Chen, R. Bao, B. Tan, Y. Cui, G. Fan, W. Wang, W. Wang, W. Liu, Paintable and rapidly bondable conductive hydrogels as therapeutic cardi-acpatches. *Adv. Mater* 30 (2018) 1704235.
33. X. Yang, L. Cao, J. Wang, L. Chen, Sandwich-like polypyrrole/reduced graphene oxide nanosheets integrated gelatin hydrogel as mechanically and thermally sensitive skin like bioelectronics. *ACS Sustain Chem Eng* 8 (2020) 10726–10739.
34. Y. Qian, Y. Zhou, M. Lu, X. Guo, D. Yang, H. Lou, X. Qiu, C.F. Guo, Direct construction of catechol lignin for engineering long-acting conductive, adhesive, and uv-blocking hydrogel bioelectronics. *Small Methods* 5 (2021) 2001311.
35. X. Ren, M. Yang, T. Yang, C. Xu, Y. Ye, X. Wu, X. Zheng, B. Wang, Y. Wan, Z. Luo, Highly conductive PPy–PEDOT: PSS hybrid hydrogel with superior biocompatibility for bioelec-tronics application. *ACS Appl. Mater. Interfaces* 13 (2021) 25374 25382.
36. J. Chen, H. Wen, G. Zhang, F. Lei, Q. Feng, Y. Liu, X. Cao, H. Dong, Multifunctional con-ductive hydrogel/thermochromic elastomer hybrid fibers with a core–shell segmental con-figuration for wearable strain and temperature sensors. *ACS Appl Mater Interfaces* 12 (2020) 7565–7574.
37. C. Kleber, K. Lienkamp, J. Rühe, M. Asplund, Wafer-scale fabrication of conducting polymer hydrogels for microelectrodes and flexible bioelectronics. *Advanced Biosystems* 3 (2019) 1900072.
38. Z. Zhou, Z. He, S. Yin, X. Xie, W. Yuan, Adhesive, stretchable and antibacterial hydrogel with external/self-power for flexible sensitive sensor used as human motion detection. *Composites Part B: Engineering* 220 (2021) 108984.
39. Q. Wang, X. Pan, C. Lin, H. Gao, S. Cao, Y. Ni, X. Ma, Modified Ti3C2TX (MXene) nanosheet-catalyzed self-assembled, anti-aggregated, ultra-stretchable, conductive hydrogels for wearable bioelectronics. *Chem Engg J* 401 (2020) 126129.
40. L. Han, X. Lu, M. Wang, D. Gan, W. Deng, K. Wang, L. Fang, K. Liu, C.W. Chan, Y. Tang, A mussel-inspired conductive, self-adhesive, and self-healable tough hydrogel as cell stimu-lators and implantable bioelectronics. *Small* 13 (2016) 1601916.
41. C. Lim, Y.J. Hong, J. Jung, Y. Shin, S.H. Sunwoo, S., Baik, O.K. Park, S.H. Choi, T. Hyeon, J.H. Kim, Tissue-like skin-device interface for wearable bioelectronics by using ultrasoft, mass-permeable, and low-impedance hydrogels. *Science Advances* 7 (2021) eabd3716.

42. J. Chen, Q. Peng, T. Thundat, H. Zeng, Stretchable, injectable, and self-healing conductive hydrogel enabled by multiple hydrogen bonding toward wearable electronics. *Chem Mater* 31 (2019) 4553–4563.
43. H. Jo, M. Sim, S. Kim, S. Yang, Y. Yoo, J.H. Park, T.H. Yoon, M.G. Kim, J.Y. Lee, Electrically conductive graphene/polyacrylamide hydrogels produced by mild chemical reduction for enhanced myoblast growth and differentiation. *Acta Biomaterialia* 48 (2017) 100–109.
44. Y. Li, X. Xiong, X. Yu, X. Sun, J. Yang, L. Zhu, G. Qin, Y. Dai, Q. Chen, Tough and conductive nanocomposite hydrogels for human motion monitoring. *Polymer Testing* 75 (2019) 38–47.
45. L. Yan, T. Zhou, L. Han, M. Zhu, Z. Cheng, D. Li, F. Ren, K.K. Wang, X. Lu, Conductive cellulose bio-nanosheets assembled biostable hydrogel for reliable bioelectronics. *Adv Funct Mater* 31 (2021) 2010465.
46. S. Ahadian, J. Ramoʹn-Azcoʹn, M. Estili, X. Liang, S. Ostrovidov, H. Shik, H. M. Ramalingam, K. Nakajima, Y. Sakka, H. Bae, T. Matsue, A. Khademhosseini, Hybrid hydrogels containing vertically aligned carbon nanotubes with anisotropic electrical conductivity for muscle myofiber fabrication, *Sci Rep* 4 (2014) 4271.
47. N. Adly, S. Weidlich, S. Seyock, F. Brings, A. Yakushenko, A. Offenhausser, B. Wolfrum, Printed microelectrode arrays on soft materials: From PDMS to hydrogels. NPJ Flexible *Electronics* 2 (2018) 15.
48. Y. Liu, K. Xu, Q. Chang, M.A. Darabi, B. Lin, W. Zhong, M. Xing, Highly flexible and resilient elastin hybrid cryogels with shape memory, injectability, conductivity, and magnetic responsive properties, *Adv. Mater* 28 (2016) 7758–7767.
49. L. Fang, J. Zhang, W. Wang, Y. Zhang, F. Chen, J. Zhou, F. Chen, R. Li, X. Zhou, X.Z. Xie, Stretchable, healable, and degradable soft ionic microdevices based on multifunctional soaking-toughened dual-dynamic- network organohydrogel electrolytes. *ACS Appl. Mater. Interfaces* 12 (2020) 56393 56402.
50. X.J. Zha, S.T. Zhang, J.H. Pu, X. Zhao, K. Ke, R.Y. Bao, L. Bai, Z.Y. Liu, M.B. Yang, W. Yang, Nanofibrillar Poly(vinyl alcohol) Ionic organohydrogels for smart contact lens and human-interactive sensing. *ACS Appl. Mater. Interfaces* 12 (2020) 23514 23522.
51. S. Yang, L. Jang, S. Kim, J. Yang, K. Yang, S.W. Cho, J.Y. Lee, Polypyrrole/alginate hybrid hydrogels:electrically conductive and soft biomaterials for human mesen-chymal stem cell culture and potential neural tissue engineering applications, *Macromol. Biosci* 16 (2016) 1653–1661.
52. L. Bueno, H.F.H.F. El-Sharif, M.O. Salles, R.D. Boehm, R.J. Narayan, T.R.L.C. Paixão, S.M. Reddy, MIP-based electrochemical protein profiling. *Sens.Actuators B* 204 (2014). 88–95.

19

Conducting Polymer Composites for Metabolite Sensing

Zondi Nate

Department of Pharmaceutical Chemistry, College of Health Sciences, University of KwaZulu-Natal, Westville Campus, Durban, South Africa

Department of biotechnology & Chemistry, Vaal University of Technology, Vanderbijlpark, South Africa

John Alake, Darko Kwabena Adu, Blessing Wisdom Ike, and Rajshekhar Karpoormath

Department of Pharmaceutical Chemistry, College of Health Sciences, University of KwaZulu-Natal, Westville Campus, Durban, South Africa

CONTENTS

19.1 Introduction

Metabolites are intermediate or end products of metabolic activities. Metabolic processes lead to the breakdown/degradation of complex material in simpler forms (catabolism) or the building of material from a simpler form into a more complex form (anabolism). Some of the metabolites are essential biomolecules critical for the growth and survival of the biological system known as primary metabolites. The most important primary metabolite produced by plants is glucose. In animals, anabolic processes may generate primary metabolites such as peptides, chemical messengers, nucleic acids, and hormones. On the other hand, secondary metabolites are not critical for the growth and survival of the biological system. They may be produced in response to a particular condition. These metabolites may be a by-product of other metabolic activities or storage biomolecules. Secondary metabolites are most abundant in plants.

Over the years, the application of metabolites in diagnostic tools is increasing. Metabolites are used as biomarkers for various diseases that affect humans; thus, their detection and quantification are important. The detection of metabolites is also vital in the food industry, forensic investigation, and drug discovery. Several methods have been reported for detecting metabolites, such as nuclear magnetic resonance spectroscopy, mass spectrometry, and liquid chromatography coupled with mass spectrometry. Methods such as immunohistochemistry, enzyme-linked immunosorbent assays (ELISA), and immunochromatography are applicable for the detection of some biomarkers. This chapter focuses on biosensors using conducting polymers or a composite consisting of conducting polymers as one of the constituents.

Conducting polymers are organic polymers with unique optical and electrical characteristics composed of conjugated carbon chains of alternating single and double bonds. The highly delocalized, polarized, and electron-dense bonds account for the optical and electrical behavior of conducting polymers. The common examples of conducting polymers that have gained lots of interest due to their unique properties include polyaniline (PANi), polypyrrole (PPy), polyacetylene (PA), polythiophene (PTH), poly(3,4-ethylene dioxythiophene), and polyfuran. Conducting polymers are ranked among the most used materials to modify the surface of the working electrodes in electrochemical sensors. This is due to their unique properties, such as high electrocatalytic activity, flexibility, scalability, corrosion resistance, and they can be custom-made for a particular need. They also have improved mechanical strength, biocompatibility, and environmental stability.

19.2 Classification of Conducting Polymers

19.2.1 Intrinsically and Extrinsically Conducting Polymers

Conducting polymers can be classified as intrinsically or extrinsically polymers (Figure 19.1). Intrinsically conducting polymers are polymers that have a backbone made up of a conjugated system; the conjugated system is responsible for the conductance of the polymer. Intrinsically conducting polymers can be further grouped into polymers with π-electron backbone and doped conducting polymer. Conducting polymers with a conjugated π-electron backbone are defined as types of conducting polymers that contain conjugated π-electron backbone, which is responsible for their electrical properties. This is due to the double bonds and lone pair of electrons present. Under the influence of an electrical field, the conjugated π-electrons of the polymer become excited and then transported through the polymer. Moreover, due to the overlapping of conjugated pi-electrons, valance and conduction bands develop throughout the polymer's backbone, contributing to the conductivity of the polymer.

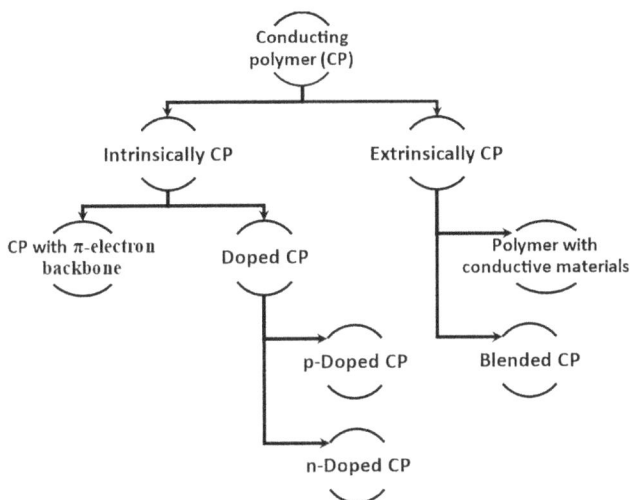

FIGURE 19.1
Classification of conducting polymers (CPs).

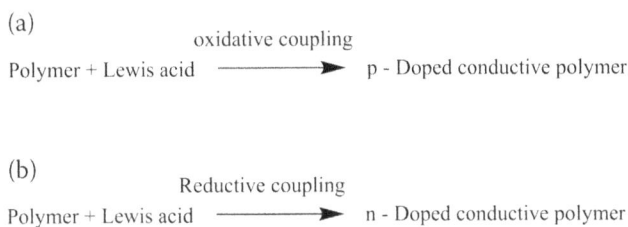

(a)
oxidative coupling
Polymer + Lewis acid ⟶ p - Doped conductive polymer

(b)
Reductive coupling
Polymer + Lewis acid ⟶ n - Doped conductive polymer

FIGURE 19.2
An illustration of the chemical reaction leading to the formation of doped conducting polymers. (a) p-type and (b) n-type conducting polymer.

Doped conducting polymers are grouped into p-doped and n-doped conducting polymers. In p-doped conducting polymers, as shown in Figure 19.2a, when polymers with conjugation in the backbone are treated with electron-deficient species (Lewis acids), oxidation occurs, causing the formation of a positive charge in the polymer. The removal of one electron from the π-backbone of the conjugated polymer results in the formation of a radical cation (polaron). Losing a second electron forms bipolaron. The delocalization of the positive charges is responsible for the electrical conduction. In n-doped conducting polymers, as shown in Figure 19.2b, when the Lewis base is reacted with a conjugated polymer, the reduction of the polymer leads to the formation of a negative charge. By the addition of the first and second electrons, polaron and bipolaron are formed, respectively. The delocalization of the charge causes conductive behavior.

In extrinsically conducting polymers, the conductivity of these polymers is due to the addition of external ingredients. In one type, non-conductive polymers act as binders impregnated with conducting elements like metals to form a single solid polymer filled with the conductive material. The presence of the conductive element confers conductivity on the product. The minimum concentration of the conductive filler added to let the polymer start conducting is called the percolation threshold. In another group, conducting polymers are produced when a nonconducting polymer is blended with a conducting polymer physically or chemically. The conductivity of the resulting product is improved.

19.3 Common Examples of Conducting Polymers

19.3.1 Polyaniline (PANi)

Polyaniline is a conducting polymer that is produced from the oxidative polymerization of aniline. The polymer backbone of polyaniline is composed of both quinoid and benzoid rings in different ratios. The differences in the proportions of quinoid and benzoid ring results in the existence of polyaniline in three different oxidation states. The three different forms of polyaniline are emeraldine, pernigraniline, and leucoemeraldine. Polyaniline in the conductive emeraldine form consist of equal proportions of both quinoid and benzoid rings. In the fully reduced leucoemeraldine form, polyaniline is composed of quinoid rings whereas the fully oxidized pernigraniline form of polyaniline consists of benzoid rings. Emeraldine is the most important form of polyaniline because it is electrically conductive. Emeraldine is produced from the oxidative polymerization of aniline in aqueous acids. This form of polyaniline is also stable as the positive charge units on the aniline are balanced by the negative charges of the chloride ion in the structure. Figure 19.3a-b depicts the structure of polyaniline and its forms.

Several forms of polymerization have been employed in the synthesis of polyaniline. These include electrochemical polymerization, chemical polymerization, plasma polymerization, and interfacial polymerization. Wang et al. [1] used an electrochemical polymerization approach to synthesize polyaniline. They reported that the electrochemical

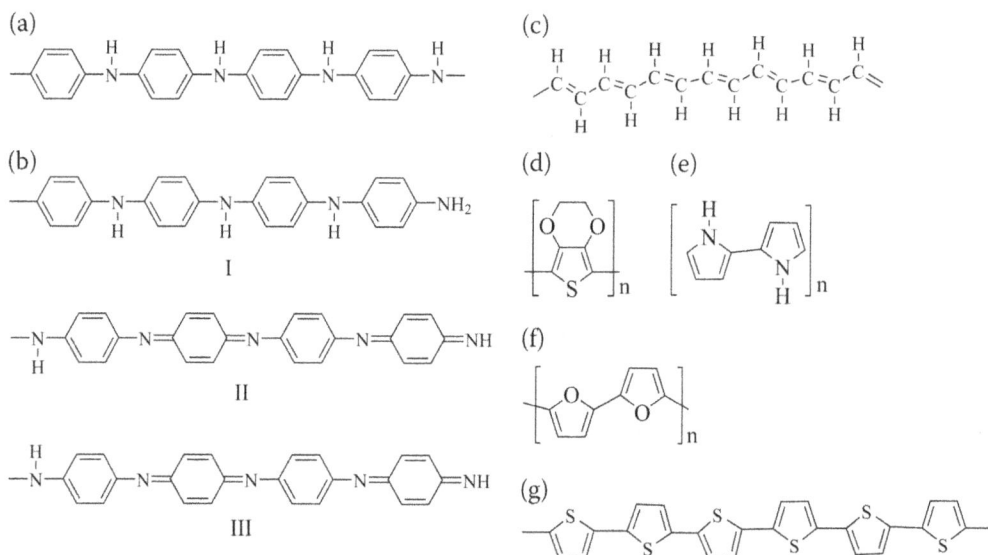

FIGURE 19.3

Chemical structures of conducting polymers. (a) Polyaniline, (b) molecular forms of polyaniline; I. Leucoemeraldine. II. Emeraldine III. Pernigraniline, (c) polyacetylene, (d) poly(3,4-ethylene dioxythiophene), (e) polypyrrol, (f) polyfuran, and (g) polythiophene.

polymerization synthesis of polyaniline occurred directly on the surface of the indium-tin-oxide glass. The chemical polymerization method of synthesis was also employed by Cao et al. [2] to synthesize polyaniline. This study involved the polymerization of aniline, in which different oxidizing agents and protonic acid were used to synthesize polyaniline. The plasma polymerization method was used by Cruz et al. [3] to synthesize polyaniline film. This involved the use of RF glow discharges that has restrictive coupling between the stainless electrodes to fabricate polyaniline film. The report stated that polyaniline was formed at a frequency and pressure range of 13.5 MHz and $(2-8) \times 10^{-2}$ Torr, respectively. Interfacial polymerization, a method in which polymerization occurs at the boundary between the two immiscible phases of the liquid used, was employed by Zang et al. [4] to synthesize polyaniline using aniline in toluene as the upper organic phase and acidic ammonium peroxidisulphate as the lower aqueous phase.

19.3.2 Polyacetylene (PA)

Polyacetylene is a type of conducting polymer which consists of a long molecular chain of repeating C_2H_2 patterns and shows alternating patterns of single and double bonds (Figure 19.3c). Polyacetylene is referred to as a conjugate molecule due to the alternating nature of the single and double bonds in its structure. Two isomeric forms of polyacetylene (trans – polyacetylene and cis – polyacetylene) are available. The conductivity of polyacetylene is enhanced greatly when doped with dopants such as iodine. Despite the high electrical conductivity of this conducting polymer, polyacetylene is unstable and encounters processing challenges in the presence of humidity and other gases. But among the two isomeric forms of polyacetylene, the trans-isomer shows more thermodynamic stability at room temperature than the cis-isomer. The stability of polyacetylene is greatly improved when it is in the form of nanoparticles. Nanoparticles of polyacetylene are fabricated when acetylene is polymerized in a solution saturated with certain polymers [5].

The synthesis of polyacetylene has seen the application of various methods such as catalytic polymerization, non-catalytic polymerization, and precursor-assisted synthesis. The catalytic-polymerization method involves the use of a catalyst such as Ziegler–Natta catalyst or Luttinger catalyst in the synthesis of polyacetylene. Shirakawa [6] used a Ziegler–Natta catalyst solution in the interfacial polymerization method to synthesize polyacetylene from acetylene monomers. Non-catalytic synthesis of polyacetylene encompasses approaches in which catalysts are not used. One such approach is the electrochemical polymerization method. This method was employed by Ma et al. [7] to synthesize poly(o-dihydroxybenzene), a polyacetylene analog. The process involved direct anodic oxidation of o-dihydroxybenzene in boron trifluoride diethyl etherate.

19.3.3 Poly(3,4-Ethylene Dioxythiophene) (PEDOT)

Poly(3,4-ethylene dioxythiophene) is a derivative of polythiophene with a shorter side chain (Figure 19.3d). To improve the stability of polythiophene, the monomer, thiophene is substituted with alkoxyl groups (such as ether). Polymerization of the alkoxyl groups substituted thiophene results in the formation of poly(3,4 ethylene dioxythiophene). Poly(3,4-ethylene dioxythiophene) is more stable than polythiophene. The improved stability of poly(3,4-ethylene dioxythiophene) resulting from the inclusion of alkoxyl group in the thiophene monomer, helps to reduce the oxidizing potential. Owing to the stability and high conductivity of poly(3,4-ethylene dioxythiophene), poly(3,4-ethylene dioxythiophene) is applied in supercapacitors and bioelectronics.

19.3.4 Polypyrrole

Polypyrrole (Figure 19.3e) is a doped polymer that shows good stability in chemical and room temperature, with comparably higher conductivity under physiological conditions and environmental stability. Polypyrrole undergoes polymerization during synthesis, in the presence of n-type dopants, which act as electron donors, or p-type dopants, which act as electron acceptors. Dopants have been reported to confer some good level of conductivity which ranges from 2 to 100 S/cm. Surfactants and nanoparticles are also used to improve the conductivity, catalytic activity as well as crystallinity of the polypyrrole. Methyl orange (MO) is one of the azo dyes used in the preparation of polypyrrole, because of its planar hydrophobic region as well as hydrophilic point group, which interacts by stacking flattened in aqueous solution.

In addition, $FeSO_4$ and $FeCl_3$ are types of oxidants introduced into the reaction environment during synthesis, to counter the electrostatic force repellent between the negatively charged MO aggregates in solution, which results in a complex formation of MO–$FeSO_4$. The outstanding electrical conductivity of polypyrrole has been assigned to the redox interaction of electrostatic cross-linking between the conducting polymer, and the metallic oxidant, as well as the characteristic stacking of the acidic azo dye which enhances the electrical and optical properties of the polypyrrole. Also, the overlapping orbitals of conjugated π-electrons run over the entire backbone of the polypyrrole matrix resulting in the formation of valence bands as well as conduction bands, which runs through the entire polymeric molecules; hence, their presence on the list of first choice conductive and redox-active materials for use in biosensors [8].

19.3.5 Polyfuran

Polyfuran is a type of conducting polymer that consists of furan aromatic rings. Furan is a five-membered heteroaromatic compound whose properties have been studied for application in technology utilization in resins. Polyfuran is a conjugated polymer that is different from non-conjugated resins. Polymerization of furan monomers leads to the formation of polyfuran. Figure 19.3f illustrates the chemical structure of polyfuran. Polyfuran can be synthesized by chemical and electrochemical polymerization.

The electrochemical process of fabricating polyfuran can be done using cyclic voltammetric technique at a constant potential, at constant current density, or by colorimetry. Sherberla et al. [9] used the electrochemical polymerization method to synthesize polyfuran from oligofuran. According to the authors, the use of furan monomers requires a high potential of 1.8 V to achieve oxidation but the use of oligofuran reduces the potential to below 1.0 V required to achieve oxidation. The reduction in oxidation potential by using oligofuran produces a polyfuran of good quality and relevant for their applications. The chemical polymerization method of fabricating polyfuran was used by McConnel et al. [10] to synthesize polyfuran using a mild oxidizing agent, pyridium chlorochromate. The use of nucleophilic agents such as water makes polyfuran less stable. Therefore, the authors of this article reported the use of anhydrous conditions to fabricate a stable polyfuran. The synthesized conducting polymer was characterized using proton nuclear magnetic resonance (^{1}H NMR), infrared (IR) spectroscopy, and electron resonance spectroscopy (ESR). The ^{1}H NMR spectra for polyfuran showed primary aromatic signals at δ 7.40, 7.740, 8.066, and 8.581. The IR spectra showed characteristic bands of the monomers of polyfuran at 1,585 cm^{-1}, 1,535 cm^{-1}, 1,438 cm^{-1}, 1,200 cm^{-1}, 1,160 cm^{-1}, 1,060 cm^{-1}, 940 cm^{-1}, and 730 cm^{-1}. The ESR spectra of polyfuran showed a Gaussian signal ($\Delta H_{PP} = 0.79$ G) with a spin concentration of 8.2×10^{19}. The results obtained from these techniques indicated successful synthesis of polyfuran of good quality and stability.

19.3.6 Polythiophene (PTH)

Polythiophene is produced from oxidative polymerization of thiophene. This type of conducting polymer is an important conjugated polymer whose structure is composed of an aromatic ring with sulphur, a heteroatom present in the aromatic ring. The structure of polythiophene is presented in Figure 19.3g. The sulfur atoms contained in the structure of polythiophene are bonded to sp^2 hybridized carbons, which shows two lone pairs of electrons available for interaction with other molecules. This offers polythiophene, the property to interact and remove pollutants; hence, the application of polythiophene in ridding the environment of pollutants. Polythiophene is a conducting polymer that forms stable materials environmentally and thermally. Owing to this, polythiophene is used in sensors, antistatic coating, solar cells, electrodes, smart windows, artificial noses, and muscles.

Polythiophene synthesis can be carried out by both electrochemical and chemical oxidative-polymerization methods. The chemical oxidative-polymerization method of polythiophene synthesis involves the use of oxidants such as $FeCl_3$ by nickel catalyzed reaction [11]. For example, Karim et al. synthesized polythiophene by gamma radiation-induced chemical oxidative-polymerization method. The synthesis process involved the use of anhydrous $FeCl_3$ as oxidizing agents [12]. The electrochemical oxidative-polymerization of polythiophene synthesis has been employed by Kaneto et al. [13] to synthesize polythiophene films. The report stated that benzonitrile was used as the electrolyte while the polymerization process occurred on an indium-tin-oxide anode. The resultant polythiophene per the report exhibited better electrical conductivity than the one synthesized using the chemical oxidative-polymerization method.

Synthesis methods that have been employed in the synthesis of poly(3,4-ethylene dioxythiophene) include hydrothermal method, interfacial polymerization, and reverse microemulsion polymerization method. For example, Ahmed et al. [14] used the hydrothermal method to synthesize poly(3,4-ethylene dioxythiophene) for application in high-performance supercapacitors. Also, the reverse microemulsion polymerization method has been utilized by Siju et al. [15] to synthesize poly(3,4-ethylene dioxythiophene). The synthesis involved the use of hexane/water reverse microemulsion system, sodium bis(2-ethylhexyl) sulfosuccinate cylindrical micelles as a template, and ferric chloride as an oxidizing agent. Jang et al. [16] applied the surfactant-mediated interfacial polymerization method to fabricate poly(3,4-ethylene dioxythiophene). The morphology of the poly(3,4-ethylene dioxythiophene) fabricated was dependent on the concentration of the surfactant used.

19.4 Application of Conductive Polymers for Metabolite Sensing

Detection of metabolites, is useful for diagnosis, drug analysis, quality and safety control in the food industry, forensic investigation, and drug discovery. Due to their unique properties, conductive polymers have been used in the development of sensors for diverse forms of metabolites. These include glucose, neurotransmitters, hormones, nucleic acid, organic acid, phytochemicals, and food pathogens [17,18]. This section discusses some advances in the use of conducting polymers for the detection of metabolites. The metabolites are discussed in three groups: application of conducting polymers for detection of pharmaceuticals and their metabolites, the use of conducting polymers for intrinsic biogenic molecule and biomarker sensing, and finally the application of conducting polymer-based sensors for food degradation and food spoilage pathogens.

19.4.1 Conducting Polymer-Based Sensors for Pharmaceutical Drug and Their Metabolite

Conducting polymers have attracted tremendous interest in biosensor application. Due to their impressive electrical conductivity, mechanical strength, lightweight, and processability, they have been hugely applied to electrochemical devices and sensors [19]. Over the year, they have become popular in the drug detection field and have been applied in several drug sensors. The conducting poly (3,4-ethylenedioxythiophene) (PEDOT) was used in an amperometric sensor for paracetamol. The MnO_2 nanoflowers doped PEDOT-based sensor was highly sensitive with a low and reproducible detection limit of 31 nM [19]. The veterinary antimicrobial drug sulfamethazine was previously detected using a similar electrode (PEDOT-MnO_2) and techniques, as mentioned. The sensor showed a very wide linear range of 1.0 μM to 500 μM and a detection limit of 0.16 μM with no interference from the commonly known interfering agent [20].

Poly(terthiophene carboxylic acid) (poly-TTCA)) complexed with copper ion was demonstrated as a highly selective electrochemical sensor for acetaminophen by Boopathi et al. [21]. Han et al. fabricated a novel polymer poly(p-aminobenzene sulfonic acid) for electrochemical determination of levofloxacin. The polymer was fabricated through electropolymerization. This polymer-based electrochemical sensor was also sensitive and highly selective [22]. In another antibiotic drug analysis, a tosylate doped poly(3,4-ethylenedioxythiophene) (PEDOT: TsO) was demonstrated as an effective electrode material for an impedimetric ampicillin sensor [23].

There are several other research demonstrating the use of conducting polymers for the detection of drugs such as amoxicillin, dacarbazine, 5-fluorouracil, and alprenolol. Some of these experiments are summarized in Table 19.1.

19.4.2 Conducting Polymer-Based Sensors For Biogenic Molecules and Biomarkers

Sensors for biomolecule such as proteins, hormones, oligonucleotides, neurotransmitters, and organic acids are mostly useful for the diagnosis of various diseases. Conducting polymers have been extensively utilized in this field. For instance, the determination of serum acetylcholine levels is of diagnostic importance for managing, patients suffering from memory loss or Alzheimer's disease. A previous report has shown the detection of the neurotransmitter and acetylcholine using poly(3,4-ethylenedioxythiophene) (PEDOT) based composite [29]. In their research, Chauhan et al. reported exceptional selectivity and sensitivity of an electrode material consisting of ferric oxide, poly(3,4-ethylenedioxythiophene, and reduced graphene oxide. They obtained a limit of detection of 4.0 nM from a linear range of 4.0 nM to 800 μM. In another research, PEDOT is again used in a sensor for dopamine. Xu et al. detected dopamine in the presence of ascorbic acid using a composite of PEDOT and carbon nanotube (PEDOT/CNT). From the differential pulse voltammetry, they obtained a linear range from 0.1 to 20 μM and a detection limit of 20 nM [30]. Another neurotransmitter, histamine was detected by Zeng et al. using the enzyme methylamine dehydrogenase and polypyrrole-based

TABLE 19.1

Some Examples of Conducting Poly-Based Biosensors for Drug Detection

Polymer used	Composite	Analyte	Sensor type	LOD (M)	Ref.
PEDOT	PEDOT-MnO₂	Paracetamol	Electrochemical sensor	3.1×10^{-8}	[19]
PEDOT	PEDOT-MnO₂	Sulfamethazine	Electrochemical sensor	1.6×10^{-7}	[20]
poly(p-ABSA)	poly(p-ABSA)-rGO	Levofloxacin	Electrochemical sensor	1.2×10^{-7}	[22]
poly-TTCA	Cu-poly-TTCA	Acetaminophen	Electrochemical sensor	5.0×10^{-6}	[21]
PEDOT	PEDOT:TsO	Ampicillin	Electrochemical sensor	$<1.145 \times 10^{-8}$	[23]
PANi	PANi/CPE	Amoxicillin	Electrochemical sensor	3.5×10^{-10}	[24]
poly-ATD	poly-ATD/CNPE	Dacarbazine	Electrochemical sensor	3.5×10^{-10}	[25]
poly-TTBA	AuNPs/polyTTBA	Daunomycin	Electrochemical sensor	5.23×10^{-11}	[26]
polythiophene	UCNP@CP	Alprenolol	Optical sensor	2.2×10^{-10}	[27]
PANi	AgNPs@PANINTs	5-fluorouraci	Electrochemical sensor	6.0×10^{-8}	[28]

Notes: **PEDOT**: *poly(3,4-ethylenedioxythiophene),* **poly(p-ABSA)**: *poly(p-aminobenzene sulfonic acid),* **rGo**: *reduced graphene oxide,* **poly-TTCA**: *poly (terthiophene carboxylic acid),* **TsO**: *tosylate,* **PANi**: *polyaniline,* **CPE**: *carbon paste electrode,* **poly-ATD**: *poly(2-amino-1,3,4-thiadiazole),* **CNPE**: *carbon nanotube paste electrode,* **poly-TTBA**: *2,2':5',2"-terthiophene-3'-(p-benzoic acid),* **CP**: *conjugated polythiophene,* **UCNPs**: *upconversion nanoparticles,* **AgNP**: *silver nanoparticles,* **PANINTs**: *polyanilime nanotubes.*

electrochemical sensor [31]. Polyaniline has also been used in an electrochemical sensor for histamine with a low limit of detection of 48.7 μM [32]. There have been several other research works demonstrating the use of conducting polymers such as polyaniline and polypyrrole for the detection of neurotransmitters like epinephrine, dopamine, and serotonin. A detailed review of the works was done by Moon et al. [33].

Conducting polymers have also been utilized in sensors for biomolecules like creatinine and urea, common metabolites from the degradation of muscles and other proteins. In 1995, Yamato et al. reported a creatinine sensor electrode consisting of polypyrrole and three enzymes: creatininase, creatinase, and sarcosine oxidase. They reported that the sensor demonstrated considerable sensitivity towards creatinine under a nitrogen atmosphere [34]. In a relatively more recent study, Kumar et al. reported a PEDOT and β-cyclodextrin-based sensor for creatinine. The sensor showed a low detection limit of 50 μM with a linear range from 0.4 mM to 0.1 M [35]. Urea sensor fabricated from polyaniline and conducting polymer hydrogel has been reported by Das et al. [36]. The highly sensitive sensor showed and detection limit of 60 nM and a wide linear range from 1.5 to 1,000 μM. In another urea sensor experiment, Dervisevic et al. utilized another conducting polymer obtained through electropolymerization of 4-(2,5-Di(thiophen-2-yl)-1H-pyrrol-1-yl)aniline monomers (SNS-Aniline) on a pencil graphite electrode (PGE). The SNS-Aniline/PGE was then modified with di-amino-ferrocene (DAFc). The sensor showed a detection limit of 12 μM [37,38].

Cevik et al. have also demonstrated the usefulness of conducting polymer in sensor development by detecting cholesterol using a conducting polymer. In their work, they used 4-(4H-dithienol [3,2-b:2',3'-d]pyrrol-4)aniline polymer (DTP(aryl)aniline) with cholesterol oxidase enzyme for the detection of cholesterol. The limit of detection was 0.27 μM and a linear range of 2.0 μM–23.7 μM. Conducting polymer-based sensors have been reported for other biogenic molecules such as glucose, uric acid, ascorbic acid, catechol, and oligonucleotides [17]. A summary of some biomolecules and their conducting polymer-based sensors are presented in Table 19.2.

TABLE 19.2

A Summary of Some Conducting Polymer-Based Sensors for Intrinsic Biogenic Molecules

Polymer used	Bioreceptor	Analyte	Sensor type	LOD (M)	Ref.
PEDOT	$Fe_2O_3NPs/rGO/PEDOT$	Acetylcholine	Electrochemical sensor	4.0×10^{-9}	[29]
PEDOT	PEDOT/CNT	Dopamine	Electrochemical sensor	4.0×10^{-9}	[30]
Ppy	MADH-PPy	Histamine	Electrochemical sensor	2.5×10^{-5}	[31]
PANi	CeO_2-PANI/DAO/nafion	Histamine	Electrochemical sensor	4.87×10^{-5}	[32]
PEDOT	PEDOT-βCD	Creatinine	Electrochemical sensor	5.0×10^{-5}	[35]
Poly(SNS-Aniline)	SNS-Aniline/DAFc	Urea	Electrochemical sensor	1.2×10^{-5}	[37]
P(DTP(aryl)aniline)	P(DTP(aryl)aniline)/ChOx	Cholesterol	Electrochemical sensor	2.7×10^{-7}	[39]
Ppy	BOx/GONP@Ppy/FTO	Bilirubin	Electrochemical sensor	1.0×10^{-10}	[40]
PPy-PPa copolymer	PPy-PPa/ G-CNTs	Protein antigen (cTnI)	Electrochemical sensor	1.0 pg/mL^*	[41]

Notes: **Ppy**: *polypyrrole,* **MADH**: *methylamine dehydrogenase,* **DAO**: *diamine oxidase,* **PANI**: *polyaniline,* **βCD**: *β-cyclodextrin,* **SNS-Aniline**: *4-(2,5-Di(thiophen-2-yl)-1H-pyrrol-1-yl)aniline,* **DAFc**: *di-amino-ferrocene,* **P(DTP(aryl)aniline)**: *4-(4H-dithienol[3,2-b: 2',3'- d]pyrrole-4)aniline polymer,* **ChOx**: *cholesterol oxidase,* **BOx**: *bilirubin oxidase,* **FTO**: *fluorine doped tin oxide,* **GONP**: *graphene oxide nanoparticle,* **PPy-PPa**: *poly(pyrrole-co-pyrrolepropylic acid) copolymer,* **G-CNTs**: *graphene-carbon nanotubes.* * *LOD presented in g/mL due to nature of analyte.*

19.4.3 Conducting Polymer-Based Sensors for Foodborne Toxins, Food Spoilage, and Foodborne Pathogens

The presence of pathogens, toxins in food, and food spoilage, in general, are of great concern because they can cause serious health problems. Therefore, there is a continuous effort to develop effective techniques for sensing foodborne toxins and pathogens [18,42]. One of the techniques used in recent times is biosensors. Conducting polymers have been fairly applied in biosensor technologies for toxin and food pathogen detection [43]. Ochratoxin A, a mycotoxin found in food products, meat, and breastmilk, was previously detected by Yu et al. [44]. The research demonstrated for the first time; a chlorine-doped polypyrrole-based surface plasmon resonance sensor for the toxin [44]. Khan et al. also detected ochratoxin A using a composite of polyaniline and chitosan (PANi-CS). They immobilized a rabbit IgG on the composite for the interaction. This impedimetric sensor produced a detection limit of 1 ng/mL [42]. Another research by Khan et al. reported a polyaniline and acacia gum-based ochratoxin sensor [45].

Aflatoxin B1, another mycotoxin, is known to be hepatotoxic and carcinogenic. Determination of the levels of this toxin is very important. Linting et al. proposed graphene and conducting polymer-based immunosensor for aflatoxin B1. The composite was constituted by 2,5-di-(2-thienyl)-1-pyrrole-1-(p-benzoic acid) (DPB) and graphene oxide. The sensitivity of the sensor was very impressive. The detection limit was as low as 1 fM (1×10^{-15}) and a very wide linear range of 3.2 fM to 3.2 Pm [46]. Similarly, PEDOT was used in another immunosensor for aflatoxin B1 [47].

Degradation of food is in principle, accompanied by the release of molecules into their immediate environment. These molecules produced because of degradation are sometimes useful for the detection of food spoilage. Several researchers have demonstrated the prospect of conducting polymers for spoilage sensors. Polyaniline was used in a sensor for the detection of ammonia gas emanating from the spoilage of protein-rich foods [48,49]. Also, there are several commercially available electronic nose sensors such as Cyranose–320™ [50] and Aromascan A32S that make use of conducting polymers. Food spoilage is sometimes caused by microorganisms. The use of conducting polymers for the detection of foodborne microorganisms has been reviewed in detail by Arshak et al. [18]. From their review, they noted that conducting polymers have been used extensively for the detection of foodborne pathogens. Polyaniline and polypyrrole were the most used polymers in this regard.

19.5 Conclusion and Future Prospective

The application of conducting polymers to develop electrochemical sensors for detecting metabolites such as drugs, biomolecules, foodborne toxins, and pathogens is increasing. This is due to their unique properties that include high electrocatalytic activity and good conductivity. However, over the years, it has been discovered that electrochemical sensors made up of pure conducting polymers are affected by some disadvantages such as poor selectivity, low sensitivity, and surface poisoning due to adsorbed intermediates and interface from other species. Also, these polymers are fragile structures with poor adhesion to the electrode. To overcome these drawbacks, nanostructured conducting polymers and nanocomposites consisting of conducting polymers and various nanomaterials are being developed. More studies still need to be done on nanostructured conducting polymers for metabolite sensing.

References

1. X. Wang, W. Liu, C. Li, C. Chu, S. Wang, M. Yan, J. Yu, J. Huang, Synthesis of polyaniline using electrochemical polymerization and application in a sensitive DNA biosensor with [Ru (bpy)3]2+ functionalized nanoporous gold composite as label, *Monatshefte Fur Chemie.* 144 (2013) 1759–1765.
2. M. Zagórska, I. Kulszewicz-Bajer, A. Proń, P. Barta, F. Cacialli, R.H. Friend, Influence of polymerization conditions on the properties of poly(4,4′-dialkyl-2,2′-bithiophenes), *Synth. Met.* 101 (1999) 142.
3. G.J. Cruz, J. Morales, M.M. Castillo-Ortega, R. Olayo, Synthesis of polyaniline films by plasma polymerization, *Synth. Met.* 88 (1997) 213–218.
4. X. Zhang, R. Chan-Yu-King, A. Jose, S.K. Manohar, Nanofibers of polyaniline synthesized by interfacial polymerization, *Synth. Met.* 145 (2004) 23–29.
5. A. Harlin, M. Ferenets, Introduction to conductive materials, in: *Intell. Text. Cloth.*, Mattila, H. R., Elsevier, 2006: pp. 217–238.
6. H. Shirakawa, Synthesis and characterization of highly conducting polyacetylene, *Synth. Met.* 69 (1995) 3–8.
7. M. Ma, H. Liu, J. Xu, Y. Li, Y. Wan, Electrochemical polymerization of o-dihydroxybene and characterization of its polymers as polyacetylene derivatives, *J. Phys. Chem. C.* 111 (2007) 6889–6896.
8. M.E. SantosMiranda, C. Marcolla, C.A. Rodriguez, H.M. Wilhelm, M.R. Sierakowski, T.M. BelleBresolin, R. Alves de Freitas, I. The role of N-carboxymethylation of chitosan in the thermal stability and dynamic, *Polym Int.* 55 (2006) 961–969.
9. A.H. Sherberla, P. Dennis, W. Snehangshu, H. Yair, S. Sharma, Y. Sheynin, A.-E. Haj-Yahia, O. Barak, M.B. Gidron, Chemical Science, *Chem. Sci.* 6 (2015) 360–371.
10. R.M. McConnell, W.E. Godwin, S.E. Baker, K. Powell, M. Baskett, A. Morara, Polyfuran and co-polymers: A chemical synthesis, *Int. J. Polym. Mater. Polym. Biomater.* 53 (2004) 697–708.
11. S. Zuppolini, V. Guarino, A. Borriello, Advanced organic electroactive nanomaterials for bio-medical use, in: *Adv. Nanostructured Mater. Nanopatterning Technol.*, Guarino, V., Focarete, M. L., & Pisignano, D., Elsevier, 2020: pp. 141–165.
12. M.R. Karim, K.T. Lim, C.J. Lee, M.S. Lee, A facile synthesis of polythiophene nanowires, *Synth. Met.* 157 (2007) 1008–1012.
13. K. Kaneto, K. Yoshino, Y. Inuishi, Electrical and optical properties of polythiophene prepared by electrochemical polymerization, *Solid State Commun.* 46 (1983) 389–391.
14. S. Ahmed, M. Parvaz, R. Johari, M. Bilal, S. Ahmad, M. Zaid, S.H., Islamuddin, Z.H. Khan, M. Rafat, Hydrothermal synthesis of poly(3,4-ethylenedioxythiophene) for high-rate performance supercapacitor, *AIP Conference Proceedings*, in: 2018: p. 030072.
15. C.R. Siju, K. Narasimha Rao, R. Ganesan, E.S.R. Gopal, S. Sindhu, Synthesis of poly(3,4 ethylenedioxythiophene) nano structure using reverse microemulsion polymerization, *Phys. Status Solidi.* 8 (2011) 2739–2741.
16. J. Jang, J. Bae, E. Park, Selective Fabrication of Poly(3,4-ethylenedioxythiophene) Nanocapsules and Mesocellular Foams Using Surfactant-Mediated Interfacial Polymerization, *Adv. Mater.* 18 (2006) 354–358.
17. G. Erdoğdu, A.E. Karagözler, Investigation and comparison of the electrochemical behavior of some organic and biological molecules at various conducting polymer electrodes, *Talanta.* 44 (1997) 2011–2018.
18. K. Arshak, V. Velusamy, O. Korostynska, K. Oliwa-Stasiak, C. Adley, Conducting polymers and their applications to biosensors: Emphasizing on foodborne pathogen detection, *IEEE Sens. J.* 9 (2009) 1942–1951.
19. Z. Xu, H. Teng, J. Song, F. Gao, L. Ma, G. Xu, X. Luo, A nanocomposite consisting of MnO2 nanoflowers and the conducting polymer PEDOT for highly sensitive amperometric detection of paracetamol, *Microchim. Acta.* 186 (2019) 2–9.

20. Y.L. Su, S.H. Cheng, A novel electroanalytical assay for sulfamethazine determination in food samples based on conducting polymer nanocomposite-modified electrodes, *Talanta.* 180 (2018) 81–89.
21. M. Boopathi, M.S. Won, Y.B. Shim, A sensor for acetaminophen in a blood medium using a Cu(II)-conducting polymer complex modified electrode, *Anal. Chim. Acta.* 512 (2004) 191–197.
22. L. Han, Y. Zhao, C. Chang, F. Li, A novel electrochemical sensor based on poly(p-aminobenzene sulfonic acid)-reduced graphene oxide composite film for the sensitive and selective detection of levofloxacin in human urine, *J. Electroanal. Chem.* 817 (2018) 141–148.
23. J. Daprà, L.H. Lauridsen, A.T. Nielsen, N. Rozlosnik, Comparative study on aptamers as recognition elements for antibiotics in a label-free all-polymer biosensor, *Biosens. Bioelectron.* 43 (2013) 315–320.
24. P.K. Brahman, R.A. Dar, K.S. Pitre, Conducting polymer film based electrochemical sensor for the determination of amoxicillin in micellar media, Sensors Actuators, B Chem. 176 (2013) 307–314.
25. M. Satyanarayana, K. Yugender Goud, K. Koteshwara Reddy, K. Vengatajalabathy Gobi, Conducting polymer-layered carbon nanotube as sensor interface for electrochemical detection of dacarbazine in-vitro, *Electrocatalysis.* 8 (2017) 214–223.
26. P. Chandra, H.B. Noh, M.S. Won, Y.B. Shim, Detection of daunomycin using phosphatidylserine and aptamer co-immobilized on Au nanoparticles deposited conducting polymer, *Biosens. Bioelectron.* 26 (2011) 4442–4449.
27. S. Ha Lee, S.M. Tawfik, D.T. Thangadurai, Y.I. Lee, Highly sensitive and selective detection of Alprenolol using upconversion nanoparticles functionalized with amphiphilic conjugated polythiophene, *Microchem. J.* 164 (2021) 106010.
28. F.M. Zahed, B. Hatamluyi, F. Lorestani, Z. Es'haghi, Silver nanoparticles decorated polyaniline nanocomposite based electrochemical sensor for the determination of anticancer drug 5-fluorouracil, *J. Pharm. Biomed. Anal.* 161 (2018) 12–19.
29. N. Chauhan, S. Chawla, C.S. Pundir, U. Jain, An electrochemical sensor for detection of neurotransmitter-acetylcholine using metal nanoparticles, 2D material and conducting polymer modified electrode, *Biosens. Bioelectron.* 89 (2017) 377–383.
30. G. Xu, B. Li, X.T. Cui, L. Ling, X. Luo, Electrodeposited conducting polymer PEDOT doped with pure carbon nanotubes for the detection of dopamine in the presence of ascorbic acid, *Sensors Actuators B Chem.* 188 (2013) 405–410.
31. K. Zeng, H. Tachikawa, Z. Zhu, V.L. Davidson, Amperometric detection of histamine with a methylamine dehydrogenase polypyrrole-based sensor, *Anal. Chem.* 72 (2000) 2211–2215.
32. M.B. Gumpu, N. Nesakumar, S. Sethuraman, U.M. Krishnan, J.B.B. Rayappan, Development of electrochemical biosensor with ceria-PANI core-shell nano-interface for the detection of histamine, *Sensors Actuators B Chem.* 199 (2014) 330–338.
33. J.M. Moon, N. Thapliyal, K.K. Hussain, R.N. Goyal, Y.B. Shim, Conducting polymer-based electrochemical biosensors for neurotransmitters: A review, *Biosens. Bioelectron.* 102 (2018) 540–552.
34. H. Yamato, M. Ohwa, W. Wernet, A Polypyrrole/Three-Enzyme Electrode for Creatinine Detection, *Anal. Chem.* 67 (1995) 2776–2780.
35. T. Naresh Kumar, A. Ananthi, J. Mathiyarasu, J. Joseph, K. Lakshminarasimha Phani, V. Yegnaraman, Enzymeless creatinine estimation using poly(3,4-ethylenedioxythiophene)-β-cyclodextrin, *J. Electroanal. Chem.* 661 (2011) 303–308.
36. J. Das, P. Sarkar, Enzymatic electrochemical biosensor for urea with a polyaniline grafted conducting hydrogel composite modified electrode, *RSC Adv.* 6 (2016) 92520–92533.
37. M. Dervisevic, E. Dervisevic, M. Senel, E. Cevik, H.B. Yildiz, P. Camurlu, Construction of ferrocene modified conducting polymer based amperometric urea biosensor, *Enzyme Microb. Technol.* 102 (2017) 53–59.
38. J. Wang, M. Jiang, B. Mukherjee, Flow Detection of Nucleic Acids at a Conducting Polymer-Modified Electrode, *Anal. Chem.,* 71 (1999) 4095–4099.

39. E. Cevik, A. Cerit, N. Gazel, H.B. Yildiz, Construction of an amperometric cholesterol biosensor based on DTP(aryl)aniline conducting polymer bound cholesterol oxidase, *Electroanalysis.* 30 (2018) 2445–2453.

40. N. Chauhan, R. Rawal, V. Hooda, U. Jain, Electrochemical biosensor with graphene oxide nanoparticles and polypyrrole interface for the detection of bilirubin, *RSC Adv.* 6 (2016) 63624–63633.

41. S. Singal, A.K. Srivastava, Rajesh, Electrochemical impedance analysis of biofunctionalized conducting polymer-modified graphene-CNTs nanocomposite for protein detection, *Nano-Micro Lett.* 9 (2017) 1–9.

42. R. Khan, M. Dhayal, Chitosan/polyaniline hybrid conducting biopolymer base impedimetric immunosensor to detect Ochratoxin-A, *Biosens. Bioelectron.* 24 (2009) 1700–1705.

43. C. Apetrei, M.D. Maximino, C.S. Martin, P. Alessio, Sensors based on conducting polymers for the analysis of food products, in: *Polymer for Food Application*, Springer International Publishing, Gutiérrez, T. J., Cham, 2018: pp. 757–792.

44. J.C.C. Yu, E.P.C. Lai, Polypyrrole film on miniaturized surface plasmon resonance sensor for ochratoxin A detection, *Synth. Met.* 143 (2004) 253–258.

45. R. Khan, N.C. Dey, A.K. Hazarika, K.K. Saini, M. Dhayal, Mycotoxin detection on antibody-immobilized conducting polymer-supported electrochemically polymerized acacia gum, *Anal. Biochem.* 410 (2011) 185–190.

46. Z. Linting, L. Ruiyi, L. Zaijun, X. Qianfang, F. Yinjun, L. Junkang, An immunosensor for ultrasensitive detection of aflatoxin B 1 with an enhanced electrochemical performance based on graphene/conducting polymer/gold nanoparticles/the ionic liquid composite film on modified gold electrode with electrodeposition, *Sensors Actuators, B Chem.* 174 (2012) 359–365.

47. A. Sharma, A. Kumar, R. Khan, A highly sensitive amperometric immunosensor probe based on gold nanoparticle functionalized poly (3,4-ethylenedioxythiophene) doped with graphene oxide for efficient detection of aflatoxin B1, *Synth. Met.* 235 (2018) 136–144.

48. S. Matindoust, A. Farzi, M. Baghaei Nejad, M.H. Shahrokh Abadi, Z. Zou, L.R. Zheng, Ammonia gas sensor based on flexible polyaniline films for rapid detection of spoilage in protein-rich foods, *J. Mater. Sci. Mater. Electron.* 28 (2017) 7760–7768.

49. Z. Ma, P. Chen, W. Cheng, K. Yan, L. Pan, Y. Shi, G. Yu, Highly sensitive, printable nanostructured conductive polymer wireless sensor for food spoilage detection, *Nano Lett.* 18 (2018) 4570–4575.

50. S. Balasubramanian, S. Panigrahi, C.M. Logue, M. Marchello, C. Doetkott, H. Gu, J. Sherwood, L. Nolan, Spoilage identification of beef using an electronic nose system, *Trans. ASAE.* 47 (2004) 1625–1633.

20

Self-Powered Devices: A New Paradigm in Biomedical Engineering

Apurba Das

Department of Physics, D. K. College, Mirza, Assam, India

Department of Physics, Indian Institute of Technology Guwahati, Guwahati, Assam, India

Pamu Dobbidi

Department of Physics, D. K. College, Mirza, Assam, India

CONTENTS

20.1 Introduction

State-of-the-art biomedical systems have enormous potential and have driven the miniaturization of several wearables and implantable devices [1]. These miniaturized systems are responsible for the enhanced life span of patients by offering control, diagnostic, and treatment possibilities. The first applications of these biomedical devices were primarily

DOI: 10.1201/9781003263265-20

aimed at controlling malfunction or restoring the lost functions of the body. Common examples of such devices are pacemakers, retinal implants, prosthetic controllers, neuro-stimulators, and cochlear implants. There have been several exciting developments from then on, such as the integration of radio frequency identification (RFID) and near-field communication microchips [2]. These features have been instrumental in monitoring in-situ parameters of organs and transmitting information for rapid diagnostics and treatment of ailments. However, a significant area that has challenged researchers is the power sources in the form of traditional batteries that have poised as a drawback by limiting the lifetime of such devices [1]. The limitations with the conventional batteries have affected the miniaturization as well.

Consequently, when the batteries deplete, the patient needs to undergo revision surgery to replace the current device with a new one, thereby increasing the risk of infections resulting in deaths and, at the same time, the economic burden on the patient [3]. Therefore, there is a growing need for new power sources for biomedical systems' independent and continuous operation. The idea is to implement smaller-sized microelectronic devices that can function with ultra-low power as an alternative to the existing devices. However, the concerns about the power source remain. One option is to harness the energy from the body movements that will power these biomedical devices [4]. This process has altogether given rise to a new area of research that will harvest the energy generated from the various body movements and ultimately complement as the power source for the miniaturized biomedical devices. The devices thus developed will be termed *self-powered biomedical devices* for *in-vivo* and *ex-vivo* applications.

To harness the energy generated from the movements in the body, several processes have been identified, and different supporting mechanisms have been proposed for the same. Fan et al. made a pioneering discovery by designing a piezoelectric nanogenerator (PENG) and subsequently triboelectric nanogenerator (TENG) in 2006 and 2012, paving the way for an alternative source of energy generation other than a conventional battery [5]. After that, the pyroelectric nanogenerators (PyNG) and thermoelectric nanogenerators (TEG) were designed to harvest the waste heat generated from the body. Significant developments in nanogenerators (NGs) have articulated the concept of self-powered devices into reality and, in its current state, have generated widespread interest due to its output performances, cohesiveness in miniaturization, and most importantly, the biocompatibility aspects [6]. This chapter is an attempt at understanding such technologies that demonstrate the potential to power self-powered devices: a milestone of the current state of development.

20.2 Survey of Power Requirements of Biomedical Devices

Portable electronic devices such as implantable radio transmitters, pacemakers, wearable glucose monitors, and pressure sensors require voltages lesser than 100 mV, and the power limits are lesser than 20 µW [4]. In Figure 20.1, we present an illustration that shows a survey of power generated from various human body motions. The Figure shows that harnessing about 1%–5% of the energy associated with the multiple movements would be sufficient for powering the wearable biomedical devices. As shown in Figure 20.1, the energy generated from the arms motion is enough to produce a point of 60 W, which is more than sufficient to power pacemakers [4]. In the current scenario, the

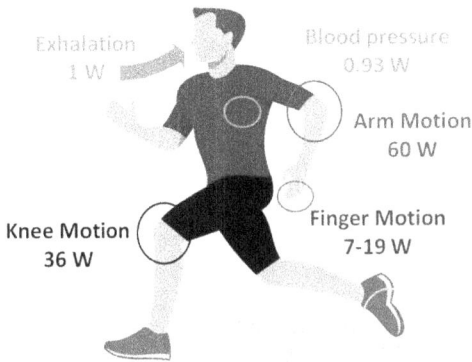

FIGURE 20.1
A schematic of the energy associated with various motions related to the different movements of the body. Adapted with permission [4], Copyright (2021), American Chemical Society.

battery powering such devices occupies almost two-thirds of the volume of the entire device [4]. One of the significant hurdles towards the miniaturization of devices is the battery size, which can be realized in the immediate future with the advent of self-powered devices.

20.3 Emergent Technologies for Self-Powered Generators

In this section, a summary of the various new generation technologies available for powering the self-powered devices is discussed in sufficient detail.

20.3.1 Nanogenerators

Four technologies associated with nanogenerators are identified, and the first two types are the PENGs and TENGs. These devices have the capacity to harvest the mechanical energy generated from the human body. The different mechanical energy sources are the heart beating, internal movement of the organs, breathing, exhalation, and acoustic energy. The other nanogenerator categories focus on converting the power generated from the heat gradient between the body and the environment while performing various functions. These devices are the PyNG and TEG that have the adequate technologies to harvest the energy wasted due to temperature gradients. A broad description of such devices' workings will be presented in the following sections.

20.3.1.1 PENG

The piezoelectric nanogenerators are based on the piezoelectric effect, related to the generation of voltages upon applying mechanical stress to a particular class of crystals [7]. The direct piezoelectric effect and the PENG are based on this principle. Piezoelectric materials have been shown to generate continuous and alternating pulsed electric signals for responding to dynamic mechanical stimuli. This effect has tremendous potential in biomedical applications, from bone regeneration to self-powered devices. However, the primary concern that limits the direct use of these classes of materials is the issues concerning biocompatibility [8]. There have been a lot of advances made in developing

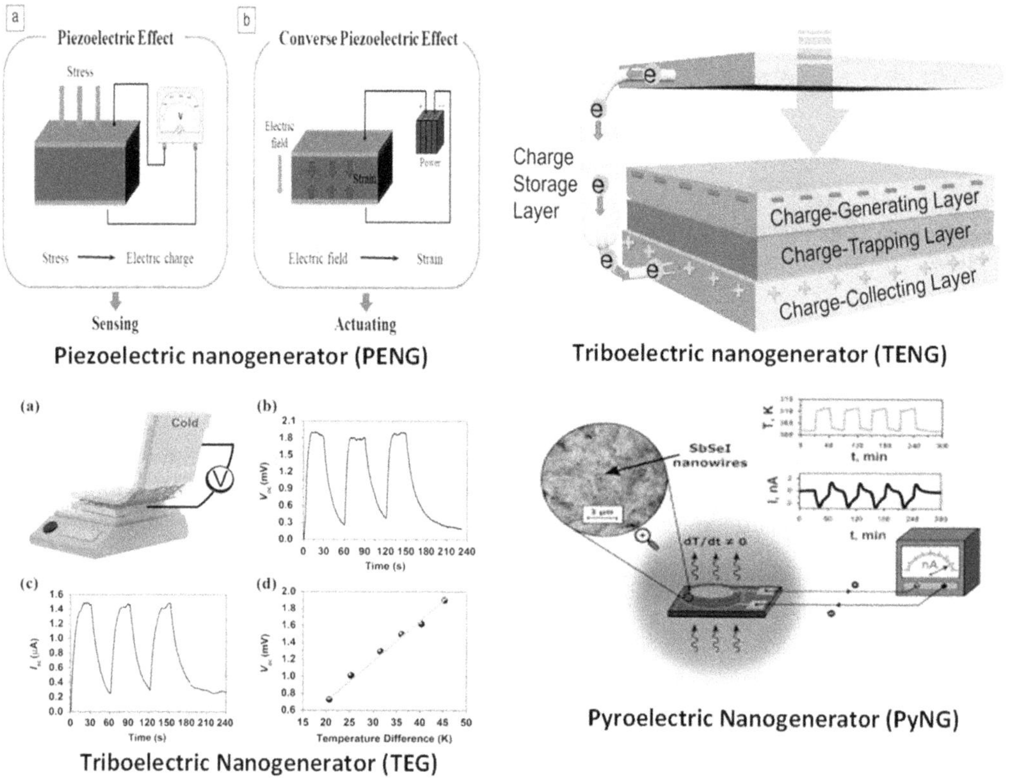

FIGURE 20.2
Illustration of the different sources of energy that can be harvested to power the self-powered devices. Each illustration represents the mechanism by which other physical and biological processes can be utilized to harvest the energy for running the self-powered devices. Adapted with permission [8]. Copyright (2021), The Authors, some rights reserved; exclusive licensee John Wiley & Sons. Distributed under a Creative Commons Attribution License 4.0 (CC BY).

piezoelectric that are biocompatible, and it is not far from now when such biocompatible piezoelectric will be a reality.

For a PENG, as shown in Figure 20.2, the open-circuit voltage (V_{OC}) and the short circuit current (I_{SC}) can be expressed mathematically according to the following equations:

$$V_{OC} = k_1 \times h \times \frac{d_{33}}{\varepsilon_{33}^T} \times \Delta\sigma. \tag{20.1}$$

$$I_{SC} = k_2 \times A \times \frac{\Delta\sigma}{\Delta t} \times d_{33}. \tag{20.2}$$

where k_1 and k_2 are two constants, d_{33} denotes the piezoelectric coefficient (CN^{-1}) , and h is the thickness of the (piezoelectric material used in) PENG. ε_{33}^T Is the permittivity of the material of the PENG when constant stress is applied along the direction of polarization, A denote the area of the opposite faces of the piezoelectric material, and $\Delta\sigma$ indicates the magnitude of the applied mechanical stress. The equations described above are related to the piezoelectric material used in manufacturing the PENG. Wang et al. reported a remarkable discovery on

TABLE 20.1

The Output Characteristics of PENG and TENG Fabricated Using Various Materials

Device	Materials	Matrix	V_{OC} [V]	J_{sc} [μA/cm²]	P_d [μW/cm²]	Ref.
PENG	BaTiO₃/carbon tubes	Polydimethylsiloxane (PDMS)	4.6	1.84 μA	8.8	[9]
	Graphene quantum dot/ Polyvinylidene Fluoride (PVDF)	NA	6	25 nA	NA	[10]
	Polyvinylidene Fluoride trifluoroethylene P(VDF-TrFE)/ZnO	NA	61	2.2 μA	NA	[11]
	BaTiO₃/Bacterial cellulose	NA	14	0.19	0.64	[12]
TENG	PVDF/Polyethylene terephthalate (PET)	NA	1140	9.2	NA	[8]
	Polytetrafluoroethylene (PTFE)/PMMA	NA	233	3.18	NA	[13]
	Fluorinated ethylene propylene (FEP)/Acrylic	NA	1670	13.4	0.016	[13]
	PDMS/PVA	NA	270.2	0.44	NA	[13]
	Kapton/PET	NA	191	NA	8.75	[8]

ZnO to power the nanogenerators, the first PENG [6]. Ever since there have been many developments in the output device performance of PENGs, such as the output power density (P_d) and some of these developments are summarized in Table 20.1.

20.3.1.2 TENG

This class of nanogenerators is based on the triboelectric effect. Certain materials are seen to acquire electric charges after they are separated from a specific material with which it was in contact. When two triboelectric materials are rubbed against each other, the surface connection increases; hence, the magnitude of triboelectricity [8]. The triboelectric charges are seen to move to the surface when there is friction between the materials. When these materials are separated, a potential difference is seen to develop between the surfaces. The external free electrons usually move to screen the effect of this potential difference that results in generating an electrical signal [8]. For a triboelectric nanogenerator, the output parameters are measured by the following parameters [13]:

$$V_{OC} = \frac{Qd}{S\varepsilon_r} \qquad (20.3)$$

$$I_{SC} = \frac{dQ}{dt}, \text{ such that } Q_{SC} = \int I_{SC} dt \qquad (20.4)$$

where Q denotes the charge transferred, d is the displacement on sliding the surfaces, S is the area of the opposite faces, ε_r is the permittivity of the material used in the generation of the TENG, and t is the time required in a complete cycle. To improve the TENGs' performance, various polymers have been developed and used to achieve a high output.

Some common examples of such polymers are polymethyl methacrylate (PMMA), polyamide (PA), and polyvinyl alcohol (PVA). Some performances of the PENGs based on the mentioned polymers are listed in Table 20.1.

20.3.1.3 TEG

TEG nanogenerators are based on the generation of thermoelectricity due to the Seebeck effect. The Seebeck effect usually tells us that a temperature gradient established between two dissimilar electrical conductors or semiconductors leads to a potential difference between the two substances. The potential difference is due to the migration of charge carriers (electrons or holes) from one junction (hot) to the other (cold) [14]. The efficiency of a TEG is determined by the figure of merit (FOM) of a thermoelectric material (which is practically a dimensionless constant), and is mathematically expressed as [14]

$$FOM = \frac{S^2 \sigma T}{k_e + k_{lat}} \qquad (20.5)$$

where k_e and k_{lat} is the thermal conductivity of the electron and lattice, respectively. σ is the electrical conductivity of the materials used in the TEG, is the Seebeck coefficient, and T is the absolute temperature. It is clear from the above equation that to obtain a high conversion rate of thermal to electrical energy, materials with a very high value of S and σ are required [8].

20.3.1.4 PyNG

The pyroelectric nanogenerators are typically based on the pyroelectric effect, which refers to the production of voltages by certain classes of materials when there is a change in temperature [7]. When a temperature gradient is established, the voltages are produced due to the difference in the polarization (in certain materials that naturally possess spontaneous polarization). The temperature change thus leads to a current in the external circuit. From the theory of pyroelectricity, the potential across the electrodes connected to a pyroelectric material is given by [15]

$$U = \frac{\Delta P \times \Delta T}{(\varepsilon_r - 1)\varepsilon_0} \qquad (20.6)$$

where ΔP denote the change in the polarization, ΔT is the change in the temperature, ε_r is the permittivity of the pyroelectric material, and ε_0 is the permittivity of the vacuum. The technology based on PyNG was first demonstrated in 2012 in which a lead zirconium titanate-based PyNG was used for monitoring the temperature changes [16]. However, the toxicity associated with the PZT led to the development of $KbNO_3$ nanowire-based PyNG to harvest the energy from sunlight illumination. These PyNGs were able to generate an output voltage and current of 2.5 mV and 25 pA for a temperature change of 295 to 298 K. It is expected that a higher temperature change shall lead to higher pyroelectric potential, as shown in equation (20.6).

20.3.2 Photovoltaic Energy Harvesting

Light energy is a source of energy that can power portable energy devices. Photovoltaic (PV) cells are sources that can convert light energy into electricity. The photovoltaic effect in this context refers to the transformation of the sunlight to useful voltages or currents that can power any form of the device [17]. In this context, the semi-conducting materials play a crucial role, as they can serve as means that can make the energy conversion possible. Today, most PV cells are fabricated from the monocrystalline or polycrystalline Si in the form of a PN-junction diode. The current research scenario has shown that the PV cells' efficiency based on the Si has reached a level of 18% for polycrystalline Si to 24% for monocrystalline Si. The *I–V* characteristics and the output power generated from the PV cells can be described by the following equations [17]:

$$I(V) = I_{SC} - I_d - \frac{V + I(V)R_s}{R_{sh}} \tag{20.7}$$

$$P_{out} = I_{SC} \cdot V_{OC} \cdot FF \tag{20.8}$$

where R_s is the series resistance of PV cell, R_{sh} is the shunt resistance of the PV cell, I_{SC} is the short-circuit current, is the dark current of the PV cell, V_{OC} is the open-circuit voltage, and *FF* is the fill factor. It must be mentioned here that for implantable device applications, the PV cells are required to be encapsulated in a particular arrangement that will protect the PV cells and, at the same time, save the body from any toxicity [17]. The details of some of the devices that use these PV cells and, in general, all the aforementioned technologies shall be done in the subsequent section.

20.4 Self-Powered Devices Based on the New Technologies

In biomedical applications of the technologies described previously, many factors need special attention. The implantable devices need to be miniaturized and have a long lifetime, both of which are contradictory under the purview of the current technology. This has encouraged researchers to invent technologies that do not require batteries to power devices. We have presented a discussion on the possible technologies that can be used instead of batteries. In the present section, we shall discuss some of the devices based on these technologies that have been used in the biomedical market.

20.4.1 Self-Powered Cardiac and Pulse Sensors

Ma et al. first proposed the first cardiac sensor in 2016 based on the TENG technology used for real-time monitoring of the vital signals [18]. The device was based on nanostructured PTFE and Kapton film that served as the primary friction materials for the triboelectric sensor. The intelligent design of the sensor with flexible packaging enables the sensor to monitor even tiny changes in the signals originating from the vital organs together with incredible biocompatibility and enhanced durability. It has been reported that the device could generate an output voltage of $V_{oc} \sim 10$ V, and $I_{sc} \sim 4$ μA when the sensor is used to monitor the pericardium model of the living porcine model (Figure 20.3). Further, the device could also achieve the added advantage like the monitoring of the blood pressure and the velocity of the blood flow in the subject with fair degree of accuracy [18].

Ouyang et al. in 2017 proposed a wearable ultrasensitive pulse sensor (SUPS) based on a TENG, having a commendable signal-to-noise ratio of 45 dB and long durability of 10^7 cycles (Figure 20.4) [19]. By using Bluetooth, this sensor showed the capability of

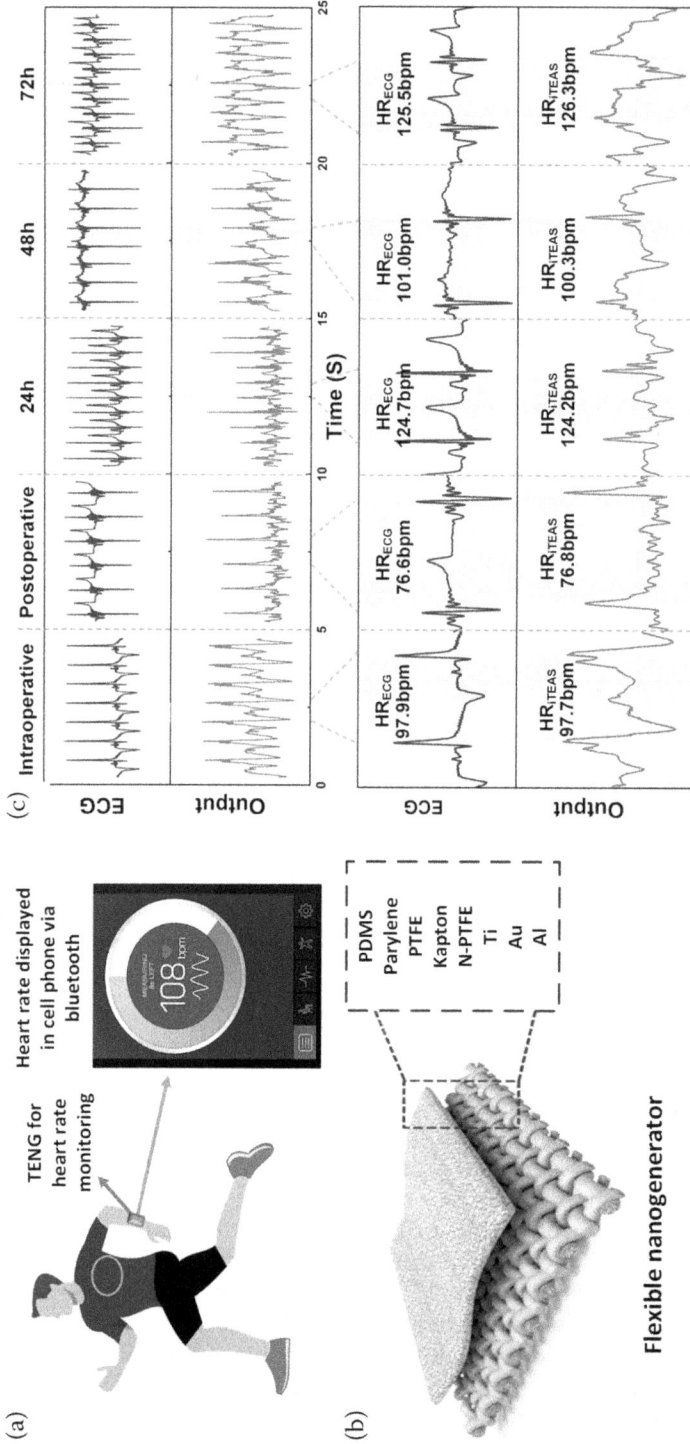

FIGURE 20.3

(a) Illustration of a triboelectric sensor to monitor the real-time conditions of the heart; (b) the schematic diagram of the sensor showing different components of the sensor, which shows its flexibility; and (c) the real-time electro-cardiograph (ECG) reading generated by the pulse sensor during operation and post-operation of the porcine model. Adapted with permission [18], Copyright (2016), American Chemical Society.

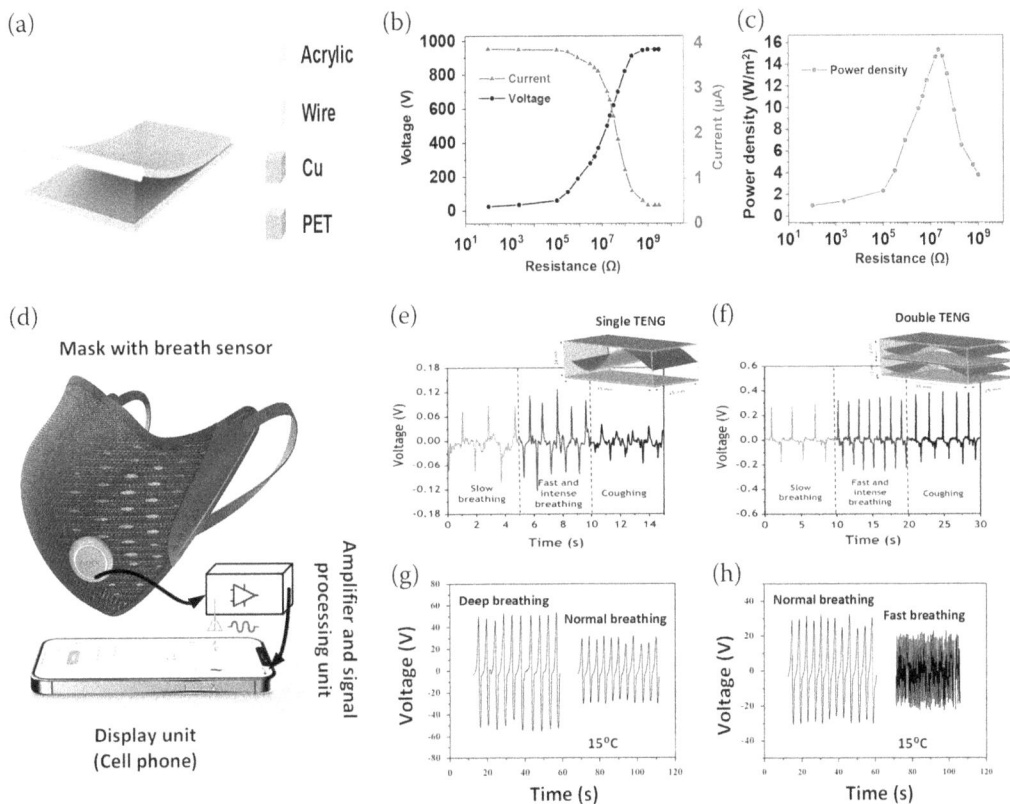

(a)

(b)

(c)

Acrylic

Wire

Cu

PET

(d)

Mask with breath sensor

(e)

(f)

Single TENG

Double TENG

(g)

(h)

Display unit
(Cell phone)

Amplifier and signal
processing unit

FIGURE 20.4
(a) Illustration of a breath sensor fabricated using the TENG technology; (b and c) the output performance of the
TENG in terms of the voltage and power density of the sensor. Adapted with permission from Reference [20],
Copyright (2019), Elsevier; (d) Illustration of biocompatible and disposable smart mask functioning as a breath
sensor and provides additional benefit for human health monitoring; (e and f) the performance of the biocompatible TENG in single and double TENG configuration. Adapted with permission [21], Copyright (2019),
American Chemical Society; (g and h) a breath sensor fabricated using the PyNG and fitted around the region
marked by the curved arrow, along with their performance under normal and fast breathing conditions at 15°C.
Adapted with permission [22], Copyright (2019), Elsevier.

transmitting data over wireless to a smartphone or a PC to monitor the user's real-time
heartbeat. The data received from the SUPS was comparable to the commercial pulse
sensors and included the added advantage of transmitting the information over a
wireless data transmission system to the user's smartphone by a simple homemade
data receiver circuit. The results obtained from the SUPS were highly comparable with
the commercial medical devices and made SUPS a significant candidate.

20.4.2 Self-Powered Breath Sensors

The reparation process is primary for living beings to survive and perform their normal
physiological activities. Thus, monitoring the reparation rhythm is of primary importance
to determine the overall condition of a patient. Over the past years, there have been
several devices, and based on the NGs, these devices have developed into state-of-the-art
devices. The human-machine interface (HMI) plays a critical role in many devices.

However, for the category of patients with disabilities, these interfaces are not suitable due to the problems on the part of the patients to clearly express their intentions either by touching or by language. Zhang et al., in 2019, reported a breath-driven sensor to transmit control commands to the HMI through breathing [20]. This sensor used the TENG-based technology, and the device's total size and weight were measured to be 2.47 g and 0.5 cm × 2 cm × 3.5 cm. The mechanism of the device was that when the airflow is passed through the pipe, the PET film is set to vibrations and cyclical contact with the electrode, thus generating electrical energy. Based on the breathing intensity, the device can produce different electrical signals and identify normal breathing or enhanced breathing. Enhanced breathing has higher electrical signals than normal breathing, with the maximum value of output voltage and current reaching 342 V and 2.3 µA, respectively. The HMI interface can later convert the electrical signals based on human breathing to control electrical applications [20].

Several improvements have been made from the previous designs. In one of the latest designs in 2021, Araz et al. proposed a cellulose nanofibril-based TENG that used diatom biosilica to improve the output characteristics while maintaining the biocompatibility (see Figure 20.4(d–f)) [21]. The biocompatible cellulose nanofibril and PTFE are used as the friction material in the TENG. Compared to cellulose, the nanofibrils used in the TENG provide flexibility, robustness, transparency, and most importantly, unmatched triboelectric performance giving it an edge [21]. Needless to say, the effect of SiO_2 is considered the best triboelectric material in the output performance of this device. The TENG based on this configuration can produce an output voltage (V_{oc}) of 88 V and current (I_{sc}) of 18.6 µA under a constant loading of 8N. Based on the breathing (fast or intense), a maximum voltage of 0.08–0.12 V can be generated using the smart TENG-based devices [21].

Similarly, Xue et al. proposed a wearable PyNG using PVDF thin film that was integrated into the N95 mask to harvest the energy generated during breathing (see Figure 20.4(g–i)) [22]. The PyNG is a three-layered device that includes a PVDF film and two Al film electrodes. The PyNG installed on the mask was able to harness the temperature fluctuation caused by human respiration to generate the voltage of 42 V (V_{oc}) and current (I_{sc}) of 2.5 µA. Thus, the maximum power reached up to 8.31 µW, that however depends upon the intensity of breathing and allows the real-time monitoring of the health patterns of the patient [22].

20.4.3 Implantable Photovoltaic Cells

The PV cells have a long development history and have achieved many milestones since their inception (Figure 20.5). A significant development occurred in 2012, as before this year, PV cells employed CMOS technology that occupied larger areas that limited its application to only a few devices [17]. With time, further developments occurred, and recently the PV cells started to be manufactured from organic compounds with no encapsulation requirements, even for biocompatibility. A significant development in implantable PV cells was achieved in 2004 when Laube et al. tested it in a rabbit [23]. The implantable PV cell was developed in an intraocular microsystem and was encapsulated in a resin. A NIR source powered the device, and it was tested for seven months inside the rabbit, which is still a record for the most extended period any device has been tested inside a subject [23].

Flexible implantable PV cells are a viable option considering the patient's comfort level, and such a system was first designed by Song et al. [24]. This device successfully generated power of 8 mW/cm^2, which was supplied to a commercial pacemaker implanted in a rat [24]. In the field of flexible PV cells, organic photovoltaic (OPV) cells have started

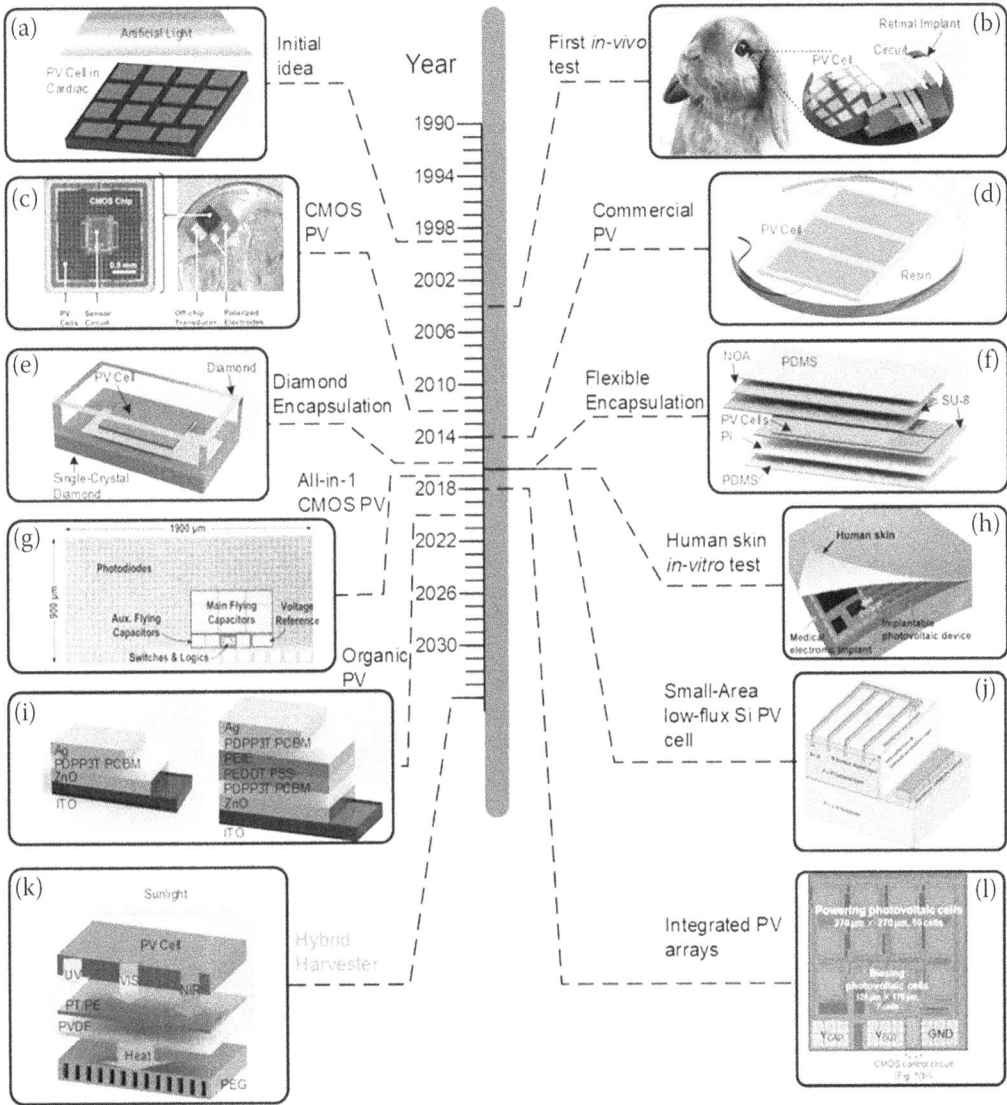

FIGURE 20.5
(a–i) Illustration of the timeline associated with the development of the PV cells from 1990 to 2030. Adapted with permission [17]. Copyright The Authors, some rights reserved; exclusive licensee John Wiley & Sons. Distributed under a Creative Commons Attribution License 4.0 (CC BY).

gaining popularity among researchers due to the versatility of these devices for their sensitivity to NIR light. Single junction and tandem OPV cells based on a bulky hetero-junction were considered, and these cells' voltage and charge storing time were investigated [17]. The efficiency of the tandem cells was reportedly higher than the single junction PV cells (5.6% in comparison to 5.3%). The added advantage of tunability of the tandem OPV cells such as in retinal applications in which the light intensity is limited in the range of 150–600 mW/cm^2. The tandem OPV cells with an active area of 2,500–6,250 μm^2 and electrode diameter of 35 μm can effectively tune the requirements in comparison to the single junction OPV that has an effective diameter of 60 μm of the electrode and limits the implantable resolution [17]. Thus, organic OPV cells are revolutionizing the research of PV cells, and it is not very far from now that we shall see self-powered devices based on these OPV.

20.5 Artificial Sensory Organs and Exquisite Biomedical Devices

Several artificial sensory organs have been developed with significant biomedical applications based on the NG technology described. The new research on the application of self-powered technology has seen a shift in focus from traditional sensors to areas like the stimulation of biological tissues and powering crucial life-saving biomedical devices like pacemakers. A few of these devices have been described in the following section with some detail.

20.5.1 Electronic Skin (e-Skin)

In the field of next-generation wearable electronics, the e-skins are expected to play a prominent role with applications ranging from human-machine interaction to defense equipment and many more. In 2019, Wang et al. considered an e-skin based on PENG technology [25]. The device was designed to be of a single electrode and was fabricated by electrospinning PVDF nanofibers capable of sensing pressure and temperature. During the electrospinning process, it was ensured that the PVDF films were spontaneously polarized. The domains inside the material will be inclined towards the external electric field (Figure 20.6(a–d)). When the sensor is heated or an external force is exerted, the spontaneous polarization within PVDF film changes, resulting in a potential difference [25,26]. To screen this effect, electrons from the external electrodes shall flow, resulting in the generation of electronic signals. The versatility of this device lies in the fact that two different signals due to heat and force can be acquired simultaneously using a single device. The sensitivity of the e-skin lies in the fact that whenever anything touches it, the skin can feel it.

20.5.2 Wound Healing

Severe injuries or traumas are very much troublesome and affect the patient's daily activities. The wounds must heal faster, and the everyday activities are restored quickly. It has been realized that applying an electric field at regular intervals can lead to faster healing of wounds. TENG-based technology can produce low-intensity electrical signals that can be useful for healing skin wounds. Such a TENG was tested on a rat by wrapping it around the chest area such that during the breathing process, an electric current would flow around the dressing electrodes resulting in an electric field (Figure 20.6(e–h)) [27]. Regular monitoring of the rat activity revealed that the produced output voltage reached a maximum level of 2.2 V. Two days of constant monitoring showed that the wound area was completely healed. Thorough studies revealed that the discrete electric field generated by the TENG promoted fibroblast proliferation, migration, and transdifferentiation that led to the faster healing process. Furthermore, the alternating electric field (rather than direct current) produced by the TENG was far more capable and successful in promoting the wound healing process [28].

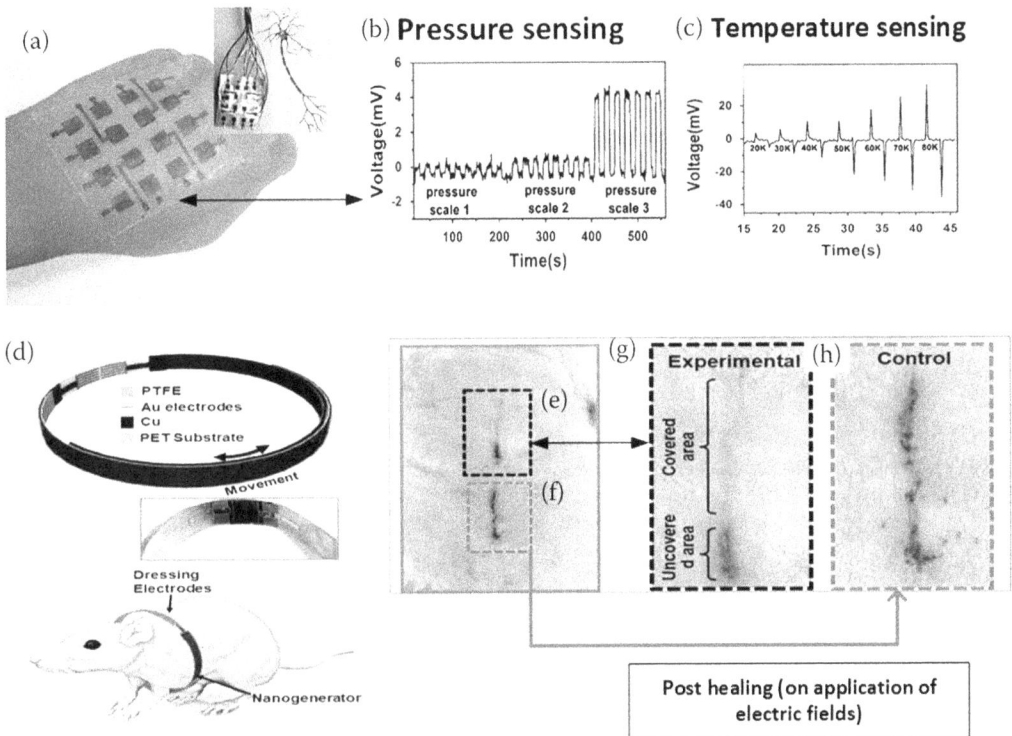

FIGURE 20.6
(a) E-skin and its performance under (b) pressure sensing and (c) temperature sensing. Adapted with permission [26], Copyright (2018), American Chemical Society. (d) The device generated for wound healing using an electric field that is tested on a rat model, (e–h) shows the healing of the wound under application of an electric field in comparison to control. Adapted with permission [27], Copyright (2018), American Chemical Society.

20.5.3 Cardiac Pacemakers

Cardiac pacemakers are considered the essential biomedical device responsible for prolonging the lives of the patient affected by sinus syndrome or heart block by stimulating the cardiac muscle and regulating the heartbeat by using an electric pulse produced by the associated electronic circuit associated with the pacemaker. The main limitations of the present-day pacemakers are the life span of the batteries that can be replaced by using self-powering technology to power the device. Ouyang et al. proposed a TENG-based pacemaker in 2019 that consisted of three parts: TENG, energy management unit, and the pacemaker (Figure 20.7) [29]. The effective functioning of the pacemaker led to decreasing the systolic blood pressure from 100 mm to 60 mm of Hg, thus preventing further decline of the heart condition of the subject. However, studies revealed that compared to TENG, PENG is more effective in converting mechanical energy to electrical energy, especially in very compact spaces (*in-vivo* conditions). The performance of the PENG is independent of the time and location. Recently, Azimi et al. (2021) proposed a pacemaker based on the PENG, which was biocompatible and flexible and was driven by cardiac motions [30]. The PENG was sutured on the pericardium because the left ventricle amplitude is larger than the right ventricle. The PENG reportedly produced a voltage amplitude of approximately 3.9 V and successfully powered a commercial pacemaker.

(a)   (b)   (c)   (d)   (g)

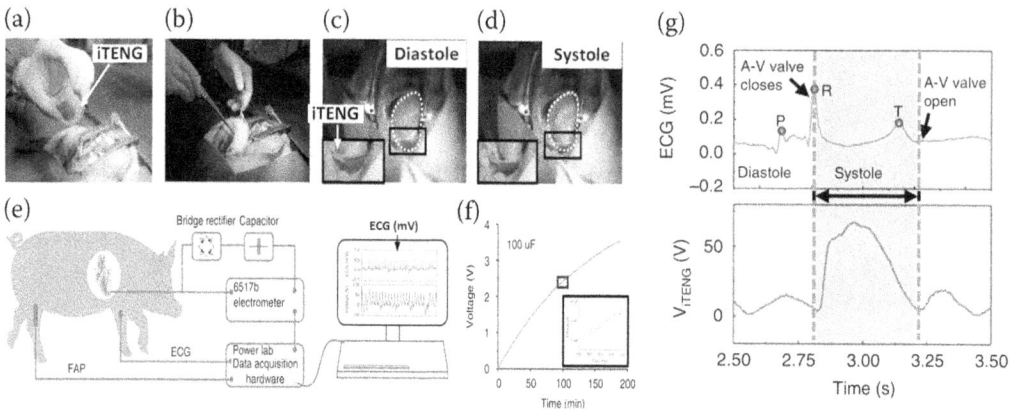

FIGURE 20.7
(a–d) TENG-based cardiac pacemaker implanted in a pig model, (e and f) shows the associated electronics of the TENG model and how it helps in real-time monitoring of the heart rate and (g) shows the ECG and the associated voltage generated from the TENG due to energy harvesting from the heart. Adapted with permission [29]. Copyright, The Authors, some rights reserved; exclusive licensee Nature. Distributed under a Creative Commons Attribution License 4.0 (CC BY).

20.6 Future Developments and Associated Roadblocks

From the discussion conducted so far, it is clear that self-powered technology has tremendous advantages that can potentially revolutionize the entire field of bioelectronics gadgets. A time in the history of the human race where each biomedical device discussed so far runs on such technology is not very far away. However, getting there would require the entire scientific community to identify the challenges that persist at each implementation step. In this section, we compile some of the roadblocks ahead of us and we shall try to provide some of our understanding of how those can be tackled to achieve the goal of advanced medical care for all.

1. The most significant challenge associated with the self-powered biomedical device is that it must meet all the biocompatibility requirements, especially considering that these devices are required to be implanted inside the body. The *in-vivo* conditions are especially harsh considering that the nanogenerators involve certain configurations, which need to be shielded from such environments. Thus, encapsulation is an extreme necessity, and materials providing such tight encapsulation that does not significantly degrade are required. Additionally, the human body has a very complex structure. Therefore, flexible devices that can handle deformations without damaging internal electronics can be a great asset.

2. The nanogenerators shall be primarily based on the piezoelectric/pyroelectric/triboelectric effect to power the devices. Thus, ensuring that the external packaging does not disrupt these devices to tap the mechanical vibrations/temperature fluctuations. Therefore, the encapsulation layers must not be unnecessarily thick, and at the same time, they must be able to maintain the sensitivity of the nanogenerators. Research has suggested that flexible polymers like PDMS and polyimide (PI) films can serve as excellent encapsulation layers. However, the

problem associated with PI is that it has not Food and Drug Administration compliant. However, PI has shown superior biocompatibility for long-term applications. Moreover, the coatings of stable oxide films such as Al_2O_3 over PDMS have been shown to enhance the stability of such encapsulation layers. Hydroxyapatite (HAP) coatings can be an excellent alternative over PDMS or PI polymers as the compound is naturally biocompatible and is highly stable under *in-vivo* conditions.

3. An essential aspect of self-powered technology is the miniaturization of the devices. The miniaturization allows the devices to fit into compact spaces inside the body, along with the added advantage that in the case of sensors, where accurate monitoring of specific vital signs is necessary, the device's bulkiness would lead to measuring uneven stress. This would lead to a wrong interpretation of the results. In addition, in the case of cardiac pacemakers, the maximum allowable size is 16 mm × 16 mm, and its weight should be under 6 g. Thus, it is clear that the quality and the expectancy of a patient's life are significantly affected by the miniaturization of the life-saving devices. Efforts are directed towards developing self-powered devices that are of the size of cells. However, such ambitious projects will require a substantial amount of time.

The discussion clarifies that harvesting the energy from various daily mechanical activities to power devices is an interesting construct and can potentially eliminate an age-old solution relating to batteries. However, there are significant challenges, some of which have been discussed at length in the previous sections. There is always a cost associated with state-of-the-art technologies. To make the technology affordable for each person, significant developments are yet to be made. For instance, in the case of PV cells, the cells are considered rigid and very expensive. Using organic PV has overcome the solution to both issues. The concerns remain about the efficiency of the energy conversion of these cells.

Similarly, in the case of NGs, achieving a cost-effective method to manufacture TENG, PENG, etc., is still a challenge for the researchers. In all these efforts, it has to be ensured that biocompatibility is never compromised; the entire effort shall be rendered useless.

20.7 Conclusions

In this chapter, an effort to discuss emergent technology in the field of self-powered devices has been made. Several technologies like the NGs, and PV cells have addressed the need for alternative sources of power other than the traditional batteries. Some of these technologies are at an advanced stage of development, and some of them have delivered products that have helped clinicians save lives at critical junctions. The development of self-powered technologies also promises to augment some of the already existing technologies with a better lifetime, better functioning, and ease of implantation. Cardiac pacemakers must be mentioned in the context, which is undoubtedly a versatile device. The only limitation that can be thought of this device is its bulky battery, which has a limited lifespan. Self-powered technology holds the potential to eliminate the associated drawbacks. However, despite these developments, there remain areas where the significant thrust is the need of the hour. This chapter introduces the reader to the possibilities of such technologies and identifies some of the core areas where further research can shed light on future developments. A holistic approach to discuss the future devices that can stem from these technologies is made in sufficient detail. Finally, based on our understanding, we propose and identify the areas which would be the hotspot of research in the upcoming years. We also point out some road maps to help young researchers solve specific problems in this domain.

References

1. R. Das, F. Moradi, H. Heidari, Biointegrated and wirelessly powered implantable brain devices: A review, *IEEE Trans. Biomed. Circuits Syst.* 14 (2020) 343–358. 10.1109/TBCAS.2020.2966920
2. B. Shi, Z. Liu, Q. Zheng, J. Meng, H. Ouyang, Y. Zou, D. Jiang, X. Qu, M. Yu, L. Zhao, Y. Fan, Z.L. Wang, Z. Li, Body-integrated self-powered system for wearable and implantable applications, *ACS Nano.* 13 (2019) 6017–6024. 10.1021
3. J. You, L. Dou, K. Yoshimura, T. Kato, K. Ohya, T. Moriarty, K. Emery, C.C. Chen, J. Gao, G. Li, Y. Yang, A polymer tandem solar cell with 10.6% power conversion efficiency, *Nat. Commun.* 4 (2013) 1–10. 10.1038/ncomms2411
4. N. Chodankar, C. Padwal, H.D. Pham, K. (Ken) Ostrikov, S. Jadhav, K. Mahale, P.K.D.V. Yarlagadda, Y.S. Huh, Y.K. Han, D. Dubal, Piezo-supercapacitors: A new paradigm of self-powered wellbeing and biomedical devices, *Nano Energy.* 90 (2021) 106607. 10.1016/J.NANOEN.2021.106607
5. F.R. Fan, Z.Q. Tian, Z. Lin Wang, Flexible triboelectric generator, *Nano Energy.* 1 (2012) 328–334. 10.1016/J.NANOEN.2012.01.004
6. Z.L. Wang, J. Song, Piezoelectric nanogenerators based on zinc oxide nanowire arrays, *Science (80-.).* 312 (2006) 242–246. 10.1126/SCIENCE.1124005
7. A. Das, D. Pamu, A comprehensive review on electrical properties of hydroxyapatite based ceramic composites, *Mater. Sci. Eng. C.* 101 (2019) 539–563. 10.1016/j.msec.2019.03.077
8. Y. Zhang, X. Gao, Y. Wu, J. Gui, S. Guo, H. Zheng, Z.L. Wang, Self-powered technology based on nanogenerators for biomedical applications, *Exploration.* 1 (2021) 90–114. 10.1002/EXP.20210152
9. U. Erturun, A.A. Eisape, S.H. Kang, J.E. West, Energy harvester using piezoelectric nanogenerator and electrostatic generator, *Appl. Phys. Lett.* 118 (2021) 063902. 10.1063/5.0030302
10. M. Venkatesan, W.C. Chen, C.J. Cho, L. Veeramuthu, L.G. Chen, K.Y. Li, M.L. Tsai, Y.C. Lai, W.Y. Lee, W.C. Chen, C.C. Kuo, Enhanced piezoelectric and photocatalytic performance of flexible energy harvester based on CsZn0.75Pb0.25I3/CNC–PVDF composite nanofibers, *Chem. Eng. J.* (2021) 133620. 10.1016/J.CEJ.2021.133620
11. L. Ye, L. Chen, J. Yu, S. Tu, B. Yan, Y. Zhao, X. Bai, Y. Gu, S. Chen, High-performance piezoelectric nanogenerator based on electrospun ZnO nanorods/P(VDF-TrFE) composite membranes for energy harvesting application, *J. Mater. Sci. Mater. Electron.* 2021 324. 32 (2021) 3966–3978. 10.1007/S10854-020-05138-0
12. G. Zhang, Q. Liao, Z. Zhang, Q. Liang, Y. Zhao, X. Zheng, Y. Zhang, G. Zhang, Q. Liao, Z. Zhang, Q. Liang, Y. Zhao, X. Zheng, Y. Zhang, Novel piezoelectric paper-based flexible nanogenerators composed of BaTiO3 nanoparticles and bacterial cellulose, *Adv. Sci.* 3 (2016) 1500257. 10.1002/ADVS.201500257
13. D. Tan, J. Zhou, K. Wang, X. Zhao, Q. Wang, D. Xu, Bow-type bistable triboelectric nanogenerator for harvesting energy from low-frequency vibration, *Nano Energy.* 92 (2022) 106746. 10.1016/J.NANOEN.2021.106746
14. M.N. Hasan, S. Sahlan, K. Osman, M.S. Mohamed Ali, Energy harvesters for wearable electronics and biomedical devices, *Adv. Mater. Technol.* 6 (2021) 2000771. 10.1002/ADMT.202000771
15. C.R. Bowen, J. Taylor, E. Leboulbar, D. Zabek, A. Chauhan, R. Vaish, Pyroelectric materials and devices for energy harvesting applications, *Energy Environ. Sci.* 7 (2014) 3836–3856. 10.1039/C4EE01759E

16. Y. Yang, Y. Zhou, J.M. Wu, Z.L. Wang, Single micro/nanowire pyroelectric nanogenerators as self-powered temperature sensors, *ACS Nano.* 6 (2012) 8456–8461. 10.1021/NN303414U/SUPPL_FILE/NN303414U_SI_001.PDF

17. J. Zhao, R. Ghannam, K.O. Htet, Y. Liu, M.-K. Law, V.A.L. Roy, B. Michel, M.A. Imran, H. Heidari, Self-powered implantable medical devices: Photovoltaic energy harvesting review, *Adv. Healthc. Mater.* 9 (2020) 2000779. 10.1002/ADHM.202000779

18. Y. Ma, Q. Zheng, Y. Liu, B. Shi, X. Xue, W. Ji, Z. Liu, Y. Jin, Y. Zou, Z. An, W. Zhang, X. Wang, W. Jiang, Z. Xu, Z.L. Wang, Z. Li, H. Zhang, Self-powered, one-stop, and multifunctional implantable triboelectric active sensor for real-time biomedical monitoring, *Nano Lett.* 16 (2016) 6042–6051. 10.1021/ACS.NANOLETT.6B01968

19. H. Ouyang, J. Tian, G. Sun, Y. Zou, Z. Liu, H. Li, L. Zhao, B. Shi, Y. Fan, Y. Fan, Z.L. Wang, Z. Li, Self-powered pulse sensor for antidiastole of cardiovascular disease, *Adv. Mater.* 29 (2017) 1703456. 10.1002/ADMA.201703456

20. B. Zhang, Y. Tang, R. Dai, H. Wang, X. Sun, C. Qin, Z. Pan, E. Liang, Y. Mao, Breath-based human–machine interaction system using triboelectric nanogenerator, *Nano Energy.* 64 (2019) 103953. 10.1016/J.NANOEN.2019.103953

21. A. Rajabi-Abhari, J.N. Kim, J. Lee, R. Tabassian, M. Mahato, H.J. Youn, H. Lee, I.K. Oh, Diatom bio-silica and cellulose nanofibril for bio-triboelectric nanogenerators and self-powered breath monitoring masks, *ACS Appl. Mater. Interfaces.* 13 (2021) 219–232. 10.1021/ACSAMI.0C18227

22. H. Xue, Q. Yang, D. Wang, W. Luo, W. Wang, M. Lin, D. Liang, Q. Luo, A wearable pyroelectric nanogenerator and self-powered breathing sensor, *Nano Energy.* 38 (2017) 147–154. 10.1016/J.NANOEN.2017.05.056

23. T. Laube, C. Brockmann, R. Buß, C. Lau, K. Höck, N. Stawski, T. Stieglitz, H.A. Richter, H. Schilling, Optical energy transfer for intraocular microsystems studied in rabbits, *Graefe's Arch. Clin. Exp. Ophthalmol.* 242 (2004) 661–667. 10.1007/S00417-004-0909-8

24. K. Song, J.H. Han, H.C. Yang, K. Il Nam, J. Lee, Generation of electrical power under human skin by subdermal solar cell arrays for implantable bioelectronic devices, *Biosens. Bioelectron.* 92 (2017) 364–371. 10.1016/J.BIOS.2016.10.095

25. X. Wang, Y. Zhang, X. Zhang, Z. Huo, X. Li, M. Que, Z. Peng, H. Wang, C. Pan, A Highly Stretchable transparent self-powered triboelectric tactile sensor with metallized nanofibers for wearable electronics, *Adv. Mater.* 30 (2018) 1706738. 10.1002/ADMA.201706738

26. X. Wang, W.Z. Song, M.H. You, J. Zhang, M. Yu, Z. Fan, S. Ramakrishna, Y.Z. Long, Bionic single-electrode electronic skin unit based on piezoelectric nanogenerator, *ACS Nano.* 12 (2018) 8588–8596. 10.1021/ACSNANO.8B04244

27. Y. Long, H. Wei, J. Li, G. Yao, B. Yu, D. Ni, A.L. Gibson, X. Lan, Y. Jiang, W. Cai, X. Wang, Effective wound healing enabled by discrete alternative electric fields from wearable nanogenerators, *ACS Nano.* 12 (2018) 12533–12540. 10.1021/ACSNANO.8B07038

28. Z. Li, H. Feng, Q. Zheng, H. Li, C. Zhao, H. Ouyang, S. Noreen, M. Yu, F. Su, R. Liu, L. Li, Z.L. Wang, Z. Li, Photothermally tunable biodegradation of implantable triboelectric nanogenerators for tissue repairing, *Nano Energy.* 54 (2018) 390–399. 10.1016/J.NANOEN.2018.10.020

29. H. Ouyang, Z. Liu, N. Li, B. Shi, Y. Zou, F. Xie, Y. Ma, Z. Li, H. Li, Q. Zheng, X. Qu, Y. Fan, Z.L. Wang, H. Zhang, Z. Li, Symbiotic cardiac pacemaker, *Nat. Commun.* 10 (2019) 1–10. 10.1038/s41467-019-09851-1

30. S. Azimi, A. Golabchi, A. Nekookar, S. Rabbani, M.H. Amiri, K. Asadi, M.M. Abolhasani, Self-powered cardiac pacemaker by piezoelectric polymer nanogenerator implant, *Nano Energy.* 83 (2021) 105781. 10.1016/J.NANOEN.2021.105781

21

Implantable Microelectronics

Mario Birkholz

IHP – Leibniz Institut für innovative Mikroelektronik, Frankfurt (Oder), Germany

CONTENTS

21.1 Introduction

A breathtaking development began with the realization of the first integrated circuits [1–3] around 1960, which has reached a level today allowing the integration of billions of transistors on one microchip. In the course of this development, not only were enormous rationalization potentials in industrial processes tapped and an essential basis for the economic prosperity of many people laid, it also opened up new business fields in information and communications technology, such as those associated today above all with the Internet [4]. Microelectronic chips are already being used in various human implants, and it is foreseeable that their use in the human body in the form of sensors and actuators will become increasingly widespread.

The development of intelligent implants is essentially based on advances in microelectronics and its continuous miniaturization. The latter is usually referred to as "Moore's Law" and goes back to the observation, first published by Gordon Moore, that the number of components used in integrated circuits doubles every 1½ to 2 years [5]. For many years, this doubling was possible due to the so-called scaling of CMOS technology (complementary metal-oxide-semiconductor), as first described in 1974 by Dennard et al. for the MOS field-effect transistor MOSFET [6]. This observation gave Moore's law the character of a self-fulfilling prophecy since Moore had stated in his work that there were "no comparable limits to the degree of integration as in thermodynamic processes." It is true that in the leading semiconductor factories, scaling is no longer reflected in the

DOI: 10.1201/9781003263265-21

MOSFET, but in its successor, the so-called FinFET, and its critical dimensions will decrease in the range of a few nanometers in the 2020s. However, the doubling of microelectronic chip performance in a 1.5–2-year cycle continues unabated – and can be seen by all of us regularly when buying new electronic equipment.

Medical implants with microelectronic components have been in use for decades as pacemakers, defibrillators, and cochlear implants for the treatment of heart disease and extreme hearing loss. In addition, so-called wearables, which are worn on the body to continuously track body functions and fitness parameters like heart rate, body temperature, blood pressure, respiration rate, blood oxygen content, deep sleep phases, etc., have become widespread in recent years. Most developments in the use of microelectronics for monitoring bodily functions have been in the field of biosensors. For a large number of analytes, it would be extremely interesting to follow the spatiotemporal distribution patterns in the body directly *in vivo*. This applies in particular to glucose dissolved in the blood, from whose deviations from the normal range (3–5 mMol/L) millions of diabetes patients suffer worldwide. In addition to implantable glucose sensors [7–11], sensors are also being developed for other analytes such as lactate, creatine/creatinine, ethanol [12], O_2, NO_x, etc.

The purpose of these systems is to detect deviation of the analyte from its normal range and to help patients maintain the physiologically beneficial state. In addition, the development of microelectronic implants has already begun not only for diagnosis but also for therapy, of which the insulin pump is a good example [13]. The developments to be presented are always about assistance systems for maintaining the patient's health. The technology drivers here are the high degree of miniaturization, i.e., the extreme reduction in the form factor, and the greater comfort for the patient that microelectronics makes possible.

Various reviews are available on the subject of microelectronic human implants, covering the aspects of biocompatibility [14] or network issues of a body-area network [15]. This work concentrates on Si-based microelectronics, although polymer microelectronics can now also be produced and are becoming increasingly important [16,17]. However, some findings, especially those concerning system architecture, concern bioelectronic implants in general, independent of the material used. The paper does not focus on cardiovascular or cochlear implants, but gives an overview of ongoing research and developments for future systems.

Another fundamental observation relates to the degree of integration of bioelectronic systems into the body. Many of them must be called semi-implants, since for them only the sensor or actuator chip is in contact with the corresponding tissue, and other components are attached extracorporeally. This is the case, for example, with cochlear hearing aids, current glucose sensors, or systems for peripheral nerve stimulation (PNS), in which the transponder or power supply are often not implanted as well. Cardiac pacemakers and derived systems, especially, have reached the level of full implants, where in addition to sensor and actuator functions, transponder and energy supply are also implanted into the body.

First, current examples of sensor and actuator chips are presented, of which functional samples have already been implanted. Also, systems will be considered that are developed for veterinary medicine. Since the application environment in other mammals is very similar to that in humans, some of these are precursor models whose human application is subsequently envisaged. The presentation of the microchips is followed by other modules that are essential for the overall system: the controller and communication chip as well as the power supply and system integration. Figure 21.1 shows an implantable overall system with its components [18]. The paper concludes with a discussion of the societal constraints

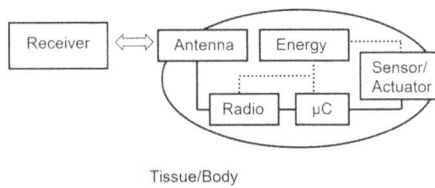

FIGURE 21.1
General scheme for the construction of microelectronic sensor or actuator implants for use in human patients. The interaction between tissue and microelectronic system runs through a window kept as small as possible to protect the other components from corrosion or denaturation; the antenna must also be able to radiate into a permeable medium.

under which bioelectronic systems will find their way into human patients in the future and raises questions about the ethically appropriate approach.

21.2 Sensor and Actuator Designs

Microelectronic implants can be divided into two broad groups of sensor and actuator systems. For example, the sensory function is in the focus of glucose and other metabolite monitors [8,19], but also in systems for physical quantities such as temperature or tensile stress to determine the mechanical load in bone prostheses [20]. Other examples of multisensor systems, such as developments for artificial retina or implantable ECG and EEG systems, can also be counted in this group [21]. The second group of implantable systems, on the other hand, has an actuator component such as stimulators for Parkinson's patients [22] implanted medication dosage devices such as insulin pumps [13] or peripheral nerve stimulators [22], which are used to deliver stimulation pulses to nerve or other tissues. A closer look at actuator systems reveals that most of them have one or more integrated sensors that allow the determination of the time or boundary condition at which they become active.

The dominant semiconductor technology today is CMOS technology, which is used to process about 1 mm thin, single-crystalline silicon wafers. The progress of this technology manifested itself on the one hand in the steady reduction of the processable structures, which have now reached the nm range. The mass production of low-cost microchips initiated with scaling was accompanied by an increase in wafer diameters from 4″ to 300 mm, the transition from μm to nm lithography systems, the decrease in switching times of field-effect transistors (FET) into the ns range, the increase in FET density to more than 10^9 cm $^{-2}$, the introduction of new materials such as Cu instead of Al conductors in the back-end-of-line stack, or the integration of rare earth oxides as high-k dielectrics in the transistor gate, to name just a few of the most important development steps.

Economically, CMOS technology was characterized by a steady increase in the necessary investment costs for a state-of-the-art semiconductor factory (fab) to several 10^9 in the meantime. Due to enormous equipment costs, which can no longer be raised by research institutes, a second development direction has established itself, which follows the claim described as "More than Moore." Frequently, earlier CMOS technology levels run also under this heading, which is characterized by their specific FET gate length. Researchers may develop microelectronic chips for their purposes by designing so-called application-specific integrated circuits (ASIC). Their fabrication can be done in so-called multi-project wafer shuttles (MPW), where the cost is shared among several users by dividing the wafer area. In Europe, the Europractice project provides access to MPW shuttles from various research fabs. The segment of bioelectronic ASICs has grown steadily in recent years.

Sensor systems in the human body can be classified according to whether they need to determine physical quantities such as pressure, temperature and tensile stress, or biological-chemical quantities such as the concentration of certain analytes like glucose [15]. A current example of the first group is provided by the development of blood pressure and heart rate sensor [23], which works by photoplethysmography (PPG), i.e., the back-scattering of monochromatic light by tissue. The technique is commonly used with finger or ear clips, but there are interesting developments for an implantable system, such as that performed by Valero-Sarmiento et al. [23] Several functions could be realized with com-mercially available chips, but two components had to be redesigned as ASICs. Figure 21.2 shows one of the ASICs developed, fabricated using a 0.5 µm CMOS process. It serves as an analog front-end for amplification and readout of the current generated by the photodiode. This made it possible to manufacture a largely miniaturized system that could be integrated into a glass capsule with external dimensions of 25 × 6 mm, making it implantable.

In the development of implantable biosensor chips for monitoring metabolites, hor-mones and biomarkers in general, the additional challenge arises that a biomolecular receptor must be used to specifically recognize the desired molecule and transform it into an electrical signal. In this respect, experience gained in laboratory diagnostics may be used. However, implantable biosensors are subject to different environmental constraints and, when detecting glucose, for example, the enzyme glucose oxidase, which is used under laboratory conditions, cannot be used because it depends on the unhindered access of oxygen. A different enzyme must then be chosen as a bioreceptor, and many activities have therefore focused on the use of the receptor concanavalin A [19,24–26], which re-versibly binds glucose and does not chemically convert the analyte, but only reversibly binds it and releases it again when the concentration decreases.

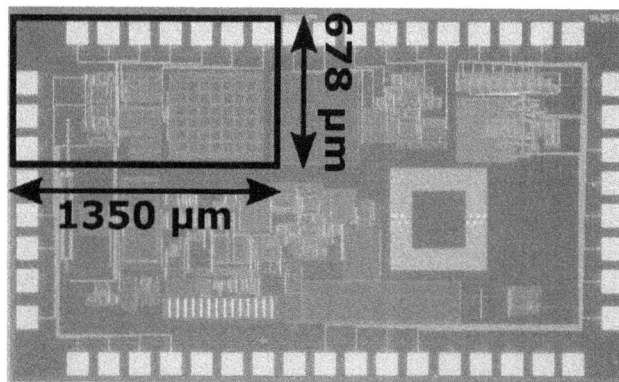

FIGURE 21.2

Micrograph of an ASIC (before being wire bonded to the PCB). The delimited area measures approximately 1.3 × 0.7 mm and represents the transimpedance amplifier, current digital-to-analog converter, and switched integrator [23]. Distributed under a Creative Commons Attribution License 4.0 (CC BY) https://creativecommons.org/licenses/by/4.0/.

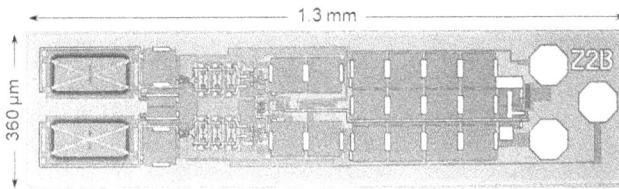

FIGURE 21.3
Glucose sensor chip with X-shaped mechanically bendable beams [9].

The transformation of the analyte to the actual concentration of interest often takes place in two or more steps in biosensors, whereby one part of the transformation can already take place in the implant and another only after data transfer outside the body. In the development of a Berlin-Brandenburg consortium, a microelectronic chip was developed to exploit the transformation of glucose concentration to viscosity [7,9,27]. A microelectromechanical system (MEMS) was developed for this purpose, in which a mechanically deflectable beam made of titanium nitride determines the viscosity of a mixture of ConA, glucose, and dextran [19].

Figure 21.3 shows the top view of the microelectronic chip with lateral dimensions of 1.3 × 0.4 mm, which was produced in a preparation process comprising five metal layers and several hundred individual steps in a 0.25 μm technology [28]. The wafer was ejected from the cleanroom in such a way that, except for the areas of the MEMS cavities to be etched free, the top of the wafer was still covered with a photoresist. Before free etching, however, the wafer was first thinned to 150 μm. The mechanical active structures of TiN were exposed by wet etching of the surrounding SiO_2 sacrificial layers and subsequent critical point drying to avoid stiction (static friction) of the cantilevers. [29]. Subsequently, the bond pads were provided with 50 μm stud bumps of gold to allow later contact of the chip. The separation of the chips had to be done subsequently with a dry process to avoid adhesion of the beam to the base plate, so the laser-based StealthDicing process was used [30].

Examples of actuator systems include implants for peripheral nerve stimulation, for which applications in pain management, cancer, and immunotherapy are envisioned, which are sometimes referred to as electroceuticals [22]. In contrast to brain implants or brain-computer interfaces (BCI), nerve endings on organs or tissues do not have an unmanageable number of billions of nerve cells, but usually only a few 100 or 1,000 nerves. Thus, there is a greater likelihood of arriving at a fundamental understanding of the effect of electrical stimulation patterns and developing effective therapies.

Implants for vagus nerve stimulation (VNS) are already in use today and served as the starting point for development. They have a similar design to cardio implants with a system housing, header, and probe, except that their stimulation impulses are directed at the vagus nerve running in the neck, which connects the brain to many internal organs. Commercially available devices are approved for the treatment of epilepsy and depression. Other applications being studied include migraines, tinnitus, headaches, rheumatoid arthritis, hypertension, and other diseases [22]. A key development step will be to reduce the size of the electrodes, which are currently still in the mm range, but which can be manufactured much more precisely using semiconductor technology and may address selected nerve endings. It is expected that highly integrated CMOS technology will be used in these systems, but the range of materials must be expanded to include materials not yet used in semiconductor fabs, such as gold and flexible plastics like PDMS to be suitable for use in the human body [31]. Other examples of implantable actuator systems are drug dosage devices for hormones such as insulin. The first systems have been used as semi-implants in the form of an insulin pump for the treatment of type I diabetes [13], but fully implantable systems are also under development.

21.3 Biocompatibility

The insertion of microelectronic systems into the body of humans or other mammals is a challenging task because the underlying material systems have emerged from different development processes and are largely incompatible with each other. For example, the tertiary and quaternary structure adopted for the function of proteins is generally destroyed when they come into contact with engineered surfaces [32,33]. On the other hand, the thin-film stacks from which microelectronic chips are constructed tend to corrode and become defunctionalized when they are in contact with electrolyte solutions for extended periods [27,34–36].

In particular, the metallic conductive electrode layers made of Al, Ti, W, and $CoSi_2$ as used in CMOS chips degrade within a short period [34,35]. Figure 21.4 shows the corrosion of a meander-shaped conductor track made of Al:Cu on SiO_2, which was stored for a few days in saline. Of all the materials used in CMOS technologies, only the ceramic, yet electrically highly conductive titanium nitride TiN is sufficiently stable to withstand the harsh environmental conditions in body fluids over extended periods [34–36]. Depth-resolved XPS studies have shown that the effect is associated with a 1–2 nm thin oxidized surface, i.e., the presence of an ultrathin TiO_2 layer [34]. Accordingly, thin TiN films are well suited for coupling voltages into electrolyte solutions. However, currents can only be introduced as dielectric displacement currents and not in the form of charges crossing the interface because the surface TiO_2 coating acts as an insulator. This explanatory model correlates well with other observations such as (i) the very low charge transfers – compared to gold electrodes – observed for TiN layers as working electrodes in an electrochemical cell [34] or (ii) the use of 30 nm thin TiO_2 layers for hermetic encapsulation of implantable needles for voltage measurement in neuronal tissues [37].

However, not only electrically conductive electrode surfaces but also structural materials such as the SiN-based passivation layer are corroded in body fluid. In the backend

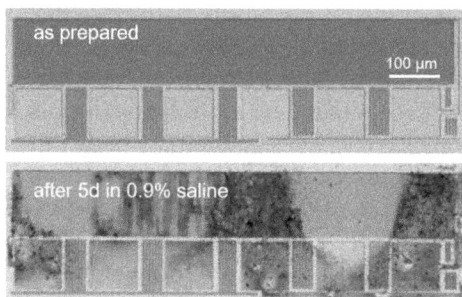

FIGURE 21.4
Optical micrographs of metallic meander structures of TiN/Al:Cu/TiN multilayer stack. Both figures show the same chip section, (top) initial (bottom) after five days in 0.9% saline.

stack of CMOS and BiCMOS chips, the passivation layer forms the top layer to protect the underlying layers from oxidation. However, the protection is only effective against ambient air and not liquid electrolytes. In an *in vivo* test, degradation rates of 50 nm/month were determined for the standard passivation layer fabricated using IHP's SG25V technology [35]. The corrosion rates observed may vary between individual technologies and manufacturers, but measures must always be taken to protect the microchip against corrosion.

For the interaction between sensor and actuator on one side and the biomilieu on the other, a miniaturized window should be provided, while all other components are housed in a hermetically sealed enclosure. The highest durability and diffusion resistance of all materials has so far been shown by housings made of titanium. As miniaturization has progressed, the enclosure issue has become increasingly difficult from a technological point of view. This is because in all cases reliable separation between electrical connections and active surfaces is required, and in many bioelectronic systems, the two areas are separated by only a few dozen or a few 100 µm. And it is this remaining area of space in which safe separation of the liquid biomilieu from the electrical leads must be ensured [19]. It is therefore inevitable to include the modern methods of microsystem integration in implant development projects.

21.4 Intelligence

The central control of measurements or sequence of stimuli, the recording of measurement data, their intermediate storage and forwarding for data transmission as well as the control of the energy supply is carried out in intelligent implants by a microcontroller µC [18]. Depending on the length of the data words exchanged between the components of the µC, 8-, 16- and 32-bit architectures are distinguished. Typically, they are supplied with a working voltage of 3–5 V.

The power consumption of the µC can be reduced by choosing a small clock speed and a simple architecture. This includes small memories (<32kB), few and general instructions, and few interfaces to the outside world (<10) as well as limiting the data bus width to 8- or 16-bit. Interfaces to the outside world include serial ports, analog/digital converters, and input/output pins. Other components are analog to digital converters for digitizing the incoming, usually analog sensor signal, and a timer that sets the clock for processes running on the µC.

Common microcontrollers have different power supply modes. These include the active mode and the sleep mode, which is switched to when no tasks are pending. For optimum system life, the microcontroller should be set to this mode whenever possible. Between both modes, there are usually still various intermediate modes in which only certain components are switched off.

The functional sequence in the µC, i.e. the sequence of measuring-reading-transmitting and all other activities are controlled by the program code, which is stored in the main memory built up from flash cells. Depending on the application of the implant, measurement data are generated. In the case of a continuously operating glucose sensor, for example, one measured value every 1.5 minutes makes sense, which is following the physiological time constants, so that up to 1,440 values must be temporarily stored per day, provided no data retrieval takes place.

Commercially, a large number of different, CMOS-manufactured µCs are available, which can be configured by the user concerning the intended use and measurement sequence [18]. The chip architectures of microcontrollers can also be acquired as software programs in languages commonly used for this purpose, such as VHDL, to tailor them to specific user needs and have them manufactured as ASICs in semiconductor fabs.

21.5 Communication

As is common in wireless data transmission with conventional sensor and actuator systems, solid implants also use a radio module [18] and an antenna [38]. However, special boundary conditions have to be taken into account when radiating out of the body, which is derived from the dielectric properties of muscle and fat tissue. Both have relative dielectric constants of $\varepsilon_r = 58$ and 11.6, which differ significantly from water or air. Important preliminary decisions regarding range and signal level are thus made when the communication frequency is specified.

Various frequency bands have found application in implants such as those at 125 and 134 kHz for RFID tagging of livestock and pets [39] or the MICS band around 403 MHz (Medical Implant Communication Service), which is used for cardio implants and has been approved by regulatory authorities for wireless communication from within the body. RFID modules have a much lower power requirement than MICS radio modules. In return, they show a low data rate and also range. However, this may not be a disadvantage for metabolite monitors with a maximum of a few 1,000 measurement data per day, if the readout device in form of a smartphone is brought close to the subcutaneously positioned implant and data is exchanged at short distances using near-field communication NFC [8].

The antenna is also about four times longer for RFID than for 403 MHz radio modules. This has a decisive influence on the overall size of the implant. The length of the antenna must correspond to a certain fraction of the wavelength of the carrier frequency f, and $\lambda/4$ coils are often used. The miniaturization of the implant benefits from the fact that the antenna length calculated in the air is reduced by $1/\varepsilon_r$ in body tissue. In muscle tissue, a $\lambda/4$ antenna for the MICS band therefore only needs to be 25 mm long. For implants the size of a matchbox, such antennas are acceptable. For smaller implants, the antenna area must be further reduced. Ref. [40] presents an antenna design where the edge lengths of the antenna are 8.1 and 8.2 mm, respectively, which is already well suited for use in small implants.

21.6 Energy Supply

In the case of full implants, the energy supply can be realized in an internal and external variant. In the internal variant, the implant is powered by a battery, which must not be too large but must supply sufficient energy for the intended lifetime. Here, only three possible battery types will be considered. The first is lithium-iodine batteries, which have a high energy density and low self-discharge current. They are available in special versions for implants and provide voltages of about 2.8 V and maximum currents of about 50 µA [41]. Due to the low current, they are rather unsuitable for many biosensor implants.

A second type is zinc-air button cells, which are used in cochlear and other implants. They provide a voltage of 1.4 V, a maximum current of 30 mA, and have capacities in the range of several 100 mAh. Their diameter is 11.6 mm and their height is 5.4 mm. The third option is thin-film batteries. These batteries are characterized by a small thickness (<0.3 mm). The largest thin-film batteries deliver ~5 mA/cm² for 2.7–4.2 V [42]. There have been interesting developments in the field of energy harvesting in recent years. Various concepts have been developed to obtain energy from bodily functions, such as from thermal energy by using Peltier elements, from glucose, or kinetic energy via piezoelectric layers [15]. At present, developments do not appear to have progressed to the point where they are already being used in commercially available implants. However, they could perform important functions in support of battery-powered systems by enabling extended lifetime or further miniaturization.

In the case of the external energy supply, use is made of the impedance coupling of an electromagnetic radiation field, which can be tapped in the implant with a coil. In the case of the development of a subcutaneously placed glucose sensor, this is already being used [8]. The concept has also opened up significant miniaturization potential.

21.7 System Integration

For various applications, the use of semi-implants is currently still considered sufficient, which can be placed easily and without great risk of injury to large blood vessels or organs. For example, metabolites such as glucose can be determined well by measurements in subcutaneous tissue, since their concentration there takes comparable values as in blood with a slight delay. The advantage of semi-implants is that components not directly required for bioelectronic function, such as µC, a radio module, antenna, and power supply, are placed extracorporeally and are easily accessible. [43].

For full implants, RFID systems for animal identification are currently used with the largest numbers, which have the shape of a cylinder with a length of just over 10 and diameters of a few mm. With the small form factor, outpatient implantation with local anesthesia becomes possible as is the case with RFID implants for pets. Migration of the implant can be suppressed by various measures such as rough and hydrophobic surface design that provokes adhesion or anti-migration caps.

The individual components of the implant, i.e., sensor/actuator chip, microcontroller, front end, antenna, and power supply, must be integrated electrically, for which printed circuit boards (PCB) are usually used as platforms. Due to the targeted miniaturization, the packaging is always challenging. In particular, newly developed sensor chips to be integrated into such systems often pose a considerable challenge because all electrically connecting components must be hermetically shielded against access by the surrounding body fluid. Figure 21.5 shows the PCB and integration scheme of a glucose sensor implant.

A decisive aspect related to the topic of biocompatibility concerns of sterilization. According to national and international specifications for medical technology products, a technical system to be implanted must be sterilized. Both a medical device and the test series of implantable biosensors to be used in a clinical study must be demonstrated that all test objects are sterile. Sterilization is also required if the implant or prototype is to be used for functional tests in animal models. Thermal, chemical, and irradiation processes can be considered as sterilization methods. For the latter, irradiation doses on the order of 25 kGy

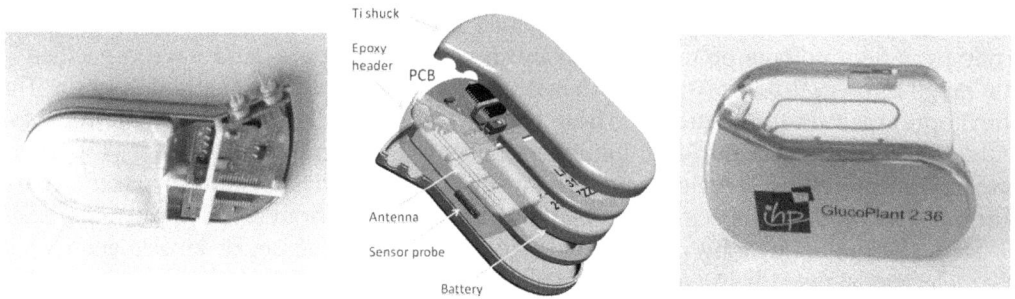

FIGURE 21.5
Biosensor implant in a form mimicking cardio implants: (a) open Ti package with PCB and battery, (b) overall system as exploded view, and (c) photo of the fabricated implant (59 × 45 × 8 mm) with sensor and antenna in the epoxy header [9].

are typically used. This is quite challenging, particularly for biosensor implants as enzymes/proteins used are damaged by ionizing radiation, causing strand breaks and denaturation.

In recent years, the smartphone has become increasingly qualified for the control of the overall system, as it has highly developed interfaces for wireless data transmission via BlueTooth or NFC. The use of apps and the sales realized with them also lead us to expect that most bioelectronic implants will be controlled by smartphone-based apps in the future. Implanted sensors and actuators will then appear to be merely devices in the developing Internet of Things (IoT).

21.8 Ethical Aspects

The development and, in particular, the commercialization of human medical implants require the testing of the system in animal models, i.e., the performance of animal experiments. Animal testing and clinical trials are governed by extensive regulatory requirements and are different for individual states or confederations of states such as the EU or the USA. Approval generally requires a positive vote by an ethics committee, which usually includes physicians and often also members of animal welfare organizations or patient associations. The test series are associated with high costs so many scientific institutes or bioelectronic working groups involved in implant developments do not reach this point. If this is the case, adaptive developments often have to be carried out subsequently, e.g., to improve hermiticity or transponder function. After a successful demonstration in the animal model, clinical studies must be carried out in the course of which the system is implanted in a cohort of patients on a trial basis, who must be continuously monitored.

A number of the problems associated with implants can usually be resolved within the framework of ethics committees. Future developments and applications of human implants, however, are associated with social implications that go far beyond this, cf. the study collection [44]. For example, a large part of the digital world is dominated by Internet corporations with extremely high sales and financial power. The five largest of them generated nearly $1,200 billion in revenue in 2020 and 2021, respectively [45], which exceeds the tax revenues of half of all EU countries [46]. As a result, non-state actors are gaining a high degree of political power, which they also use for their benefit through excessive lobbying. More and more tasks of social services, which until the end of the twentieth century were reserved for local authorities or states, such as telecommunication, information research, news dissemination, food supply, navigation and logistics, and even payment systems and currencies, are being monopolized by some corporations to such an extent that political observers now recognize new feudalism in it [47].

Former employees who have left these companies for ethical reasons point out that sensationalist headlines keep users glued to their devices for as long as possible to play them as much advertising as possible. Reports are presented in an exaggeratedly lurid and emotionally arousing manner, and in many cases, false reports and nonsensical conspiracy theories are put into the world [48]. For example, the rumor has become widespread, which is important in the context discussed here, that microchips are injected with the COVID-19 vaccine to monitor vaccinated persons (which, due to the small inner diameter of vaccination needles in the range of 0.1 mm, would have to be recognized as nonsense from a technical point of view). The sheer flood of this dubious news is eroding the democratic opinion-forming process in many countries so that the influence of populists is increasing and Internet corporations are making profits at the expense of the cohesion of society [49].

In addition, extensive data collections are created of practically all Internet users, ranging from their behavioral patterns to personality profiles. The companies make use of the large volume of communication data (BigData), which provides them with information about the devices used, user name, age, gender, telephone calls, e-mails, geolocation, place of residence, workplace, profession, position, purchases, income, credit card sales, social situation, political preferences, memberships, and other sensitive personality data, as well as their circle of friends and relatives and comparable information from the latter. The data is aggregated through excessive tracking across pages and devices for every user action on the Internet [50], with which the personality profiles become more and more accurate. For the vote on the United Kingdom's exit from the EU (Brexit) and the 2016 presidential election in the United States, there is extensive evidence of how such personality profiles were used to influence the outcome of the election [49,51]. In addition, health or fitness apps also involve medical data, the sensitivity of which is considered particularly high in the European General Data Protection Regulation (Art. 9 (1)). It may be expected that this data will be used to further detail personality profiles, making users/patients predictable and manipulable in their behavior.

For a large area of digital technologies, therefore, an unenthusiastic picture emerges as to whether a patient-friendly use of human implants is possible if implants are designed as microelectronic IoT systems and privacy on the Internet cannot be guaranteed. Given the problems mentioned, the question arises as to whether scientists can still participate in such developments with a clear conscience. To do so, it would have to be ensured that the data of the implant in whose development one is involved remain under the control of the user in any case. As a scientist and developer, one can refer to the UN Sustainable Development Goals, point 16.6, which calls for the development of effective, verifiable, and transparent institutions at all levels.

The ensuing discussion is reminiscent of the one about nuclear armament and the involvement of scientists in the 1980s. At that time, the question of a Hippocratic oath for scientists was discussed, like the one taken by physicians and in which they commit themselves to ethical action [52]. There are corresponding passages in many statutes of scientists' organizations, such as in the case of the German Physical Society, which commits itself "… to be aware of the fact that those working in science are responsible for the shaping of the whole of human life to a particularly high degree."

In 2009, Ellen McGee has already addressed the lack of debate, which in her view does not do justice to the importance of human bioelectronic implants [53]. Particularly in the case of the development of brain implants as computer interfaces, she proposed regulatory intervention and the drafting and conclusion of an international treaty to contain the societal dangers of the technology. While such a treaty has not materialized to date, the approach to regulating research and development, the need to incorporate ethical principles of sustainability into it, is now supported by many researchers. For example, in 2021, the IEEE formulated a new ethical standard for the development of intelligent and autonomous systems. The IEEE 7000 is expected to become the new baseline standard describing the learning processes companies must go through to build values-driven ethical, reliable, risk-aware, and responsible technology. The approach seems to have room for expansion, but it is a start that companies and institutions can use as a guide in the future. As stated by McGee, ethical consideration of societal consequences should accompany any development of human bioelectronic implant to identify the societal context and to allow focusing our efforts on the many positive potential applications.

21.9 Conclusions and Perspectives

Microelectronics is on its way into the human body. In the future, it will not only serve us outside the body as useful technology but will also be integrated into our bodies in the form of intelligent biosensors and other medical implants. Many functions currently associated with wearables and semi-implants will then be performed by implants. Various sensor and actuator systems are currently under development to record and elicit physical and biochemical parameters in body tissues or organs. Actuator systems can be used to readjust substance concentrations that have drifted out of the normal range, or to perform peripheral stimulation of nerve cords for pain relief, etc. Internal and external solutions can be considered for energy supply. If an internal solution is chosen, i.e., the use of a battery to be implanted, it represents the size-determining component of the overall system. A major hurdle for many development projects is the overall system integration, which requires the constructive interaction of various individual disciplines as well as a clever sequence of manufacturing processes that take into account system sterilization. Despite the great benefits that human bioelectronic implants promise for improving patient care, several ethical and societal issues remain unresolved. This is especially true of their connection to the Internet, where patients cannot be guaranteed privacy of their health data under prevailing conditions of use. Also, in the case of implants with functions as brain-computer interfaces, a broad societal debate on the dangers and consequences of such technology is still lacking.

Acknowledgments

This review is partially based on the results of previous BMBF and BMWi funded projects for the development of an implantable blood sugar sensor (contract numbers 0313862 and KF0653901UL8).

References

1. T.H. Lee, *The (Pre-) History of the Integrated Circuit: A Random Walk*, IEEE Solid-State Circuits Newsl **12**, 16 (2007).
2. J.W. Orton, *The Story of Semiconductors* (Oxford University Press, Oxford, 2004).
3. M. Riordan and L. Hoddeson, *Crystal Fire: The Birth of the Information Age*, (Norton, New York, 1997).
4. C. Brown and G. Linden, *Chips and Change: How Crisis Reshapes the Semiconductor Industry* (MIT Press, Cambridge, MA, 2009).
5. G.E. Moore, *Cramming More Components onto Integrated Circuits*, Electronics **38**, 114 (1965).
6. R.H. Dennard, F.H. Gaensslen, H.-N. Yu, V.L. Rideout, E. Bassous, and A. LeBlanc, *Design of Ion-Implanted MOSFETs with Very Small Physical Dimensions*, IEEE J Sol Stat Circ **9**, 256 (1974).
7. M. Birkholz, P. Glogener, T. Basmer, F. Glös, D. Genschow, C. Welsch, R. Ruff, and K.P. Hoffmann, *System Integration of a Silicone-Encapsulated Glucose Monitor Implant*, Biomed EngBiomed Tech **59**(s1), S1089 (2014).
8. M. Mortellaro and A. DeHennis, *Performance Characterization of an Abiotic and Fluorescent-Based Continuous Glucose Monitoring System in Patients with Type 1 Diabetes*, Biosens Bioelectr **61**, 227 (2014).
9. M. Birkholz, P. Glogener, F. Glös, T. Basmer, and L. Theuer, *Continuously Operating Biosensor and Its Integration into a Hermetically Sealed Medical Implant*, Micromachines **7**, 10 (2016).
10. J.K. Nielsen, J.S. Christiansen, J.S. Kristensen, H.O. Toft, L.L. Hansen, S. Aasmul, and K. Gregorius, *Clinical Evaluation of a Transcutaneous Interrogated Fluorescence Lifetime-Based Microsensor for Continuous Glucose Reading*, J Diabetes Sci Technol **3**, 98 (2009).
11. A.J. Müller, M. Knuth, K.S. Nikolaus, R. Krivánek, F. Küster, and C. Hasslacher, *First Clinical Evaluation of a New Percutaneous Optical Fiber Glucose Sensor for Continuous Glucose Monitoring in Diabetes*, J. Diabetes Sci. Technol. **7**, 13 (2013).
12. H. Jiang, X. Zhou, S. Kulkarni, M. Uranian, R. Seenivasan, and D.A. Hall, *A Sub-1 MW Multiparameter Injectable BioMote for Continuous Alcohol Monitoring*, in *2018 IEEE Custom Integrated Circuits Conference (CICC)* (IEEE, San Diego, CA, 2018), p. 1.
13. B. Kovatchev and A. Kovatcheva, *Creating the Artificial Pancreas*, IEEE Spectr. **58**, 38 (2021).
14. M. Frost and M.E. Meyerhoff, *In Vivo Chemical Sensors: Tackling Biocompatibility*, Anal. Chem. **78**, 7370 (2006).
15. H. Dinis and P.M. Mendes, *Recent Advances on Implantable Wireless Sensor Networks*, in *Wireless Sensor Networks – Insights and Innovations*, edited by P. Sallis (InTech, London, 2017).
16. A.-M. Pappa, O. Parlak, G. Scheiblin, P. Mailley, A. Salleo, and R.M. Owens, *Organic Electronics for Point-of-Care Metabolite Monitoring*, Trends Biotechnol **36**, 45 (2018).
17. C. Hassler, T. Boretius, and T. Stieglitz, *Polymers for Neural Implants: Polymers for Neural Implants*, J. Polym. Sci. Part B Polym. Phys **49**, 18 (2011).
18. T. Basmer, P. Kulse, and M. Birkholz, *Systemarchitektur Intelligenter Sensorimplantate*, Biomed Eng/Biomed Tech **55**, P43 (2010).
19. M. Birkholz, K.-E. Ehwald, T. Basmer, C. Reich, P. Kulse, J. Drews, D. Genschow, U. Haak, S. Marschmeyer, E. Matthus, K. Schulz, D. Wolansky, W. Winkler, T. Guschauski, and R. Ehwald, *Sensing Glucose Concentrations at GHz Frequencies with a Fully Embedded BioMEMS*, J. Appl. Phys **113**, 244904 (2013).
20. B. Kienast, B. Kowald, K. Seide, M. Aljudaibi, M. Faschingbauer, C. Juergens, and J. Gille, *An Electronically Instrumented Internal Fixator for the Assessment of Bone Healing*, Bone Jt. Res. **5**, 191 (2016).
21. E. Zrenner, *Fighting Blindness with Microelectronics*, Sci. Transl. Med. **5**, (2013).
22. E. Waltz, *A Spark at the Periphery*, Nat. Biotechnol. **34**, 904 (2016).
23. J.M. Valero-Sarmiento, P. Ahmmed, and A. Bozkurt, *In Vivo Evaluation of a Subcutaneously Injectable Implant with a Low-Power Photoplethysmography ASIC for Animal Monitoring*, Sensors **20**, 7335 (2020).

24. R. Ballerstädt and R. Ehwald, *Suitability of Aqueous Dispersions of Dextran and Concanavalin A for Glucose Sensing in Different Variants of the Affinity Sensor*, Biosens Bioelectr **9**, 557 (1994).

25. H. Xian, L. Siqi, E. Davis, L. Dachao, W. Qian, and L. Qiao, *A MEMS Dielectric Affinity Glucose Biosensor*, Microelectromechanical Syst. J. of **23**, 14 (2014).

26. U. Beyer, D. Schäfer, A. Thomas, H. Aulich, U. Haueter, B. Reihl, and R. Ehwald, *Recording of Subcutaneous Glucose Dynamics by a Viscosimetric Affinity Sensor*, Diabetol **44**, 416 (2001).

27. P. Glogener, M. Krause, J. Katzer, M.A. Schubert, M. Birkholz, O. Bellmann, C. Weber, H. Hammon, C. Metges, C. Welsch, R. Ruff, and K.P. Hoffmann, *Prolonged Corrosion Stability of a Microelectronic Biosensor Implant during in Vivo Exposure*, Biosensors **8**, 13 (2018).

28. D. Knoll, K.-E. Ehwald, B. Heinemann, A. Fox, K. Blum, H. Rücker, F. Fürnhammer, B. Senapati, R. Barth, U. Haak, W. Höppner, J. Drews, R. Kurps, S. Marschmeyer, H.H. Richter, T. Grabolla, B. Kuck, O. Fursenko, P. Schley, R. Scholz, B. Tillack, Y. Yamamoto, K. Köpke, H.E. Wulf, D. Wolansky, and W. Winkler, *A Flexible, Low-Cost, High-Performance SiGe:C BiCMOS Process with One-Mask HBT Module*, in *IEDM Technical Digest* (IEEE, San Francisco, CA, USA, 2002), pp. 783.

29. P. Kulse, M. Birkholz, K.-E. Ehwald, J. Bauer, J. Drews, U. Haak, W. Höppner, J. Katzer, K. Schulz, and D. Wolansky, *Fabrication of MEMS Actuators from the BEOL of a 0.25 Mm BiCMOS Technology Platform*, Microelectr Eng **97**, 276 (2012).

30. M. Birkholz, K.-E. Ehwald, M. Kaynak, T. Semperowitsch, B. Holz, and S. Nordhoff, *Separation of Extremely Miniaturized Medical Sensors by IR Laser Dicing*, J Opt Adv Mat **12**, 479 (2010).

31. A.-H. Lee, J. Lee, F. Laiwalla, V. Leung, J. Huang, A. Nurmikko, and Y.-K. Song, *A Scalable and Low Stress Post-CMOS Processing Technique for Implantable Microsensors*, Micromachines **11**, 925 (2020).

32. M. Birkholz, *Konvergenz in Sicht: Zur Gemeinsamen Perspektive von Mikroelektronik und Biotechnologie*, in *Sensorsysteme 2008.* (LIFIS-online, Lichtenwalde (Sachsen), Deutschland, 2008), pp. 1–11.

33. A. Starzyk and M. Cieplak, *Denaturation of Proteins near Polar Surfaces*, J. Chem. Phys. **135**, 235103 (2011).

34. M. Birkholz, K.-E. Ehwald, D. Wolansky, I. Costina, C. Baristiran-Kaynak, M. Fröhlich, H. Beyer, A. Kapp, and F. Lisdat, *Corrosion-Resistant Metal Layers from a CMOS Process for Bioelectronic Applications*, Surf Coat Technol **204**, 2055 (2010).

35. M. Fröhlich, M. Birkholz, K.-E. Ehwald, P. Kulse, O. Fursenko, and J. Katzer, *Biostability of an Implantable Glucose Sensor Chip*, IOP Conf. Ser. Mater. Sci. Eng. **41**, 012022 (2012).

36. H. Hämmerle, K. Kobuch, K. Kohler, W. Nisch, H. Sachs, and M. Stelzle, *Biostability of Micro-Photodiode Arrays for Subretinal Implantation*, Biomat. **23**, 797 (2002).

37. S. Schroder, C. Cecchetto, S. Keil, M. Mahmud, E. Brose, O. Dogan, G. Bertotti, D. Wolanski, B. Tillack, J. Schneidewind, H. Gargouri, M. Arens, J. Bruns, B. Szyszka, S. Vassanelli, and R. Thewes, *CMOS-Compatible Purely Capacitive Interfaces for High-Density in-Vivo Recording from Neural Tissue*, in *IEEE BioCAS* (IEEE, Atlanta, GA, USA, 2015), p. 1.

38. T. Basmer, N. Todtenberg, F. Popiela, and M. Birkholz, *Antennas For Medical Implant Applications Operating In The MICS Band*, in *Proc. 2013 MTT-S International Microwave Workshop Series on RF and Wireless Technologies for Biomedical and Healthcare Applications (IMWS-Bio 2013)*, (IEEE, online, 2013).

39. A.R. Garcia, D.V. Barros, M.C.M. de Oliveira Junior, W. Barioni Junior, J.A.R. da Silva, J. de B. Lourenço Junior, and J. dos Santos Pessoa, *Innovative Use and Efficiency Test of Subcutaneous Transponders for Electronic Identification of Water Buffaloes*, Trop. Anim. Health Prod **52**, 3725 (2020).

40. J. Abadia, F. Merli, J.-F. Zurcher, J.R. Mosig, and A.K. Skrivervik, *3D-Spiral Small Antenna Design and Realization for Biomedical Telemetry in the MICS Band*, Radioneng **18**, (2009).

41. C.F. Holmes, The Lithium/Iodine-Polyvinylpyridine Battery, in *Handbook of Solid State Batteries and Capacitors* (World Scientific, Singapore, 1995), pp. 157.

42. J. Kawamura, Thin Film Batteries, in *Solid State Ionics for Batteries*, edited by M. Tatsumisago, M. Wakihara, C. Iwakura, S. Kohjiya, and I. Tanaka (Springer, Tokyo, 2005), pp. 64.

43. M. Birkholz, K.-E. Ehwald, M. Fröhlich, P. Kulse, T. Basmer, R. Ehwald, T. Guschauski, U. Stoll, H. Siegel, S. Schmaderer, J. Szeponik, and D. Zahn, *Minimal-Invasiver Blutzuckersensor*, in *Tagungsband 16. GMA/ITG-Fachtagung "Sensoren und Messsysteme"* (GMA ITG VDI/VDE, Nürnberg, Germany, 2012), pp. 177.

44. M.G. Michael and K. Michael editors, *Uberveillance and the Social Implications of Microchip Implants: Emerging Technologies* (IGI Global, Australia, 2014).

45. *Zahlen, Daten, Fakten: GAFAM - Die US-Tech Giganten*, c't Magazin für Comput. Tech. 126 (2021).

46. Central Intelligence Agency, *The World Factbook 2021*, Washington D.C.

47. S. Zuboff, *The Age of Surveillance Capitalism: The Fight for a Human Future at the New Frontier of Power* (Profile books, London, 2019).

48. J. Horwitz, *The Facebook Whistleblower, Frances Haugen, Says She Wants to Fix the Company, Not Harm It*, Wall Str. J. (2021). https://www.wsj.com/articles/facebook-whistleblower-frances-haugen-says-she-wants-to-fix-the-company-not-harm-it-11633304122

49. S. Giusti and E. Piras editors, *Democracy and Fake News: Information Manipulation and Post-Truth Politics* (Routledge, Abingdon, Oxon; New York: Routledge, 2021).

50. T. Libert, *An Automated Approach to Auditing Disclosure of Third-Party Data Collection in Website Privacy Policies*, in *Proceedings of the 2018 World Wide Web Conference –WWW '18* (ACM Press, Lyon, France, 2018), pp. 207.

51. C. Wylie, *MINDF*CK – Inside Cambridge Analytica's Plot to Break the World* (Profile Books, Online, 2019).

52. W. Hirschwald, *Ethical Decisions in Science and Technology –Survey, General Considerations and Consequences*, in *Challenges. Science and Peace in a Rapidly Changing Environment*, Vol. II (BdWi, Berlin, 1992).

53. E.M. McGee, *Bioelectronics and Implanted Devices*, in *Medical Enhancement and Posthumanity*, edited by B. Gordijn and R. Chadwick, Vol. 2 (Springer, Netherlands, Dordrecht, 2009), pp. 207.

22

Printable and Flexible Biosensors

Khairunnisa Amreen and Sanket Goel

Micro-electromechanical systems (MEMS), Microfluidics and Nanoelectronics Lab, Department of Electrical and Electronics Engineering, Birla Institute of Technology and Science Pilani, Jharkhand, India

CONTENTS

22.1 Introduction

Recently, advances and emerging trends in the fabrication of printable and flexible biosensors have gained substantial attention since these can be employed as point-of-care testing (POCT) tools. Significant research for developing methods, materials, and approaches for strategic designing and targeting specific biosensors has taken place [1]. The advent of biosensors started in 1999 when IUPAC regarded these as efficient analytical tools for interference mitigated, both qualitative and quantitative detections [2]. A biosensor is an electro-analytical device comprising of three major components. The first one is a bioreceptor, which is a biological element of choice like an antibody, DNA, enzyme, cell, and aptamer. These act as redox mediators and transfer electrons at electrode/electrolyte junctions. Various matrices like graphene, carbon nanomaterials, nanorods, nanosheets, polymers, metal oxides, composites, etc. are employed to either trap or integrate these bioreceptors in the matrix. The second one is a transducer, whereupon the exposure of biological redox mediators with analytes, electrochemical reaction corresponding to oxidation or reduction takes place. This leads to changes in parameters like pH, temperature, and other chemical changes. The transducer captures these reaction signals and converts them to a measurable electrical response. The third one is the signal processor, which

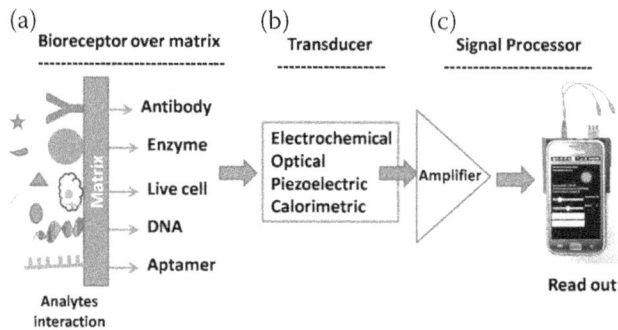

FIGURE 22.1
Schematic representation of biosensor components and working principle.

amplifies the current signals into a readable digital display in the readout device [3]. Figure 22.1 gives a schematic representation of the workings of the biosensor device.

22.1.1 Categories of Biosensors

22.1.1.1 Classification Based on Bioreceptor

As shown in Figure 22.1, mainly five kinds of bioreceptors are used for the fabrication of biosensors. Based on these, there are different types:

1. *Enzyme-based biosensor:* In these, an enzyme is used as a bioreceptor over the matrix. This can detect a specific analyte substrate that can compatibly bind with the enzyme. It has a lock and key model. Enzymes are target analyte-specific. Enzymes that can recognize the analytes are effective biocatalysts. For instance, glucose oxidase for glucose, urease for urea, peroxidases for peroxide, etc. The analyte detection depends upon the attributes like enzyme changing the analyte to a detectable form, pH, temperature, substrate concentration, enzyme concentration, etc. Although enzyme-based biosensors are highly selective and specific, there are certain limitations related to stability and adaptability [4].

2. *Antibody/immunosensor:* These biosensors are used for pathogen and infection analysis. An antibody (Immunoglobin-Ig) is a bioreceptor and is used for the detection of diseases and biomarkers like cancer, cardiovascular diseases, hepatitis, etc. Ig is a target antigen-specific and is immobilized on the matrix. Ig binds with the antigen to form an antigen-antibody complex, which causes electron shuttling [5].

3. *DNA-based biosensor:* Herein, complementary DNA strands, usually single strands, are used as the bioreceptors on the matrix. The target analyte DNA is denatured chemically and mixed with the electrolyte. The matching sequence identifies this strand and forms double-stranded DNA bond causing electron transfer [6].

4. *Cell-based biosensors:* Herein, live microorganisms cells like bacteria and fungi are used as bioreceptors over the matrix. These measures intracellular and extracellular parameters. The major limitation is stability and contamination [7].

5. *Biomimetric biosensor:* Here, synthetic DNA sequences, called aptamers, are used as bioreceptors over the matrix, which mimic the natural DNA sequence. These are used for the detection of proteins, amino acids, etc. These are slightly advantageous as they can be manipulated as needed [8].

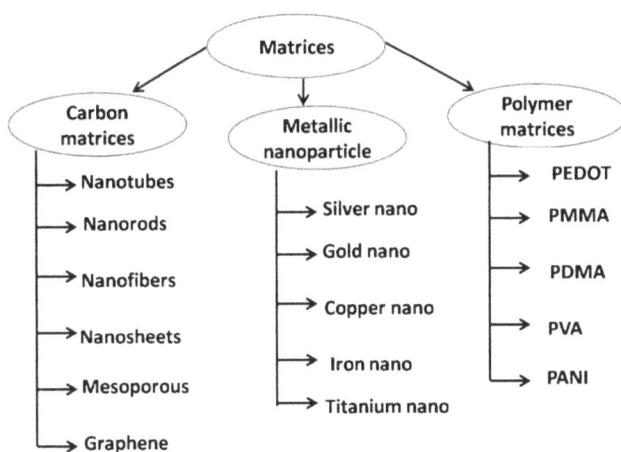

FIGURE 22.2
Schematic representation of different matrices employed for immobilizing bioreceptors.

22.1.1.1.1 *Types of Matrices*

Figure 22.2 gives a schematic presentation of different kinds of matrices employed for immobilizing the bioreceptors. Mostly, carbon nanomaterials are used due to their good electron transferability. The schematic mentions a few commonly used materials. Similarly, metal-based nanoparticles are also useful in immobilizing the bioreceptor. A few common ones are mentioned in Figure 22.2. Likewise, polymer and poly-based nanomaterials composites are also used. A few are mentioned in the schematic.

22.1.1.1.2 *Bioreceptor Immobilization*

The bioreceptor is immobilized over the chosen matrix via chemical or physical approaches. Physical adsorption, entrapment, polymer or sol-gel way, or chemically through covalent binding are some of the methods. The chosen approach depends upon the compatibility of the bioreceptor with the matrix [4]. Figure 22.3 gives the schematic representation of different types of immobilization.
    Following are the methods of immobilization [9]

    i. *Adsorption:* Binding takes place with weak bonds via physical adsorption, a simple and easy approach wherein the matrix can be regenerated. However, limitations in terms of desorption and less efficiency are associated with this type of approach.
    ii. *Covalent bond formation:* Chemical bond is formed between the matrix and a specific functional group of the molecule. It is more stable, has strong linkage, has no diffusion barriers, and gives a rapid response. However, the matrix cannot be regenerated in this case.
    iii. *Cross-linkage:* In this, a bond between the bioreceptor is formed. It is stronger and has more stability. However, these cross-linked bonds between the bioreceptors and matrix will give a loss of activity of the bioreceptor.
    iv. *Entrapment:* In this low-cost and faster approach, a bioreceptor is incorporated in a gel or q polymer matrix. However, limitations in terms of

(a)   (b)   (c)

Matrix   Matrix

Adsorption   Covalent binding   Cross-linking

(d)   (e)

Entrapment   Encapsulation

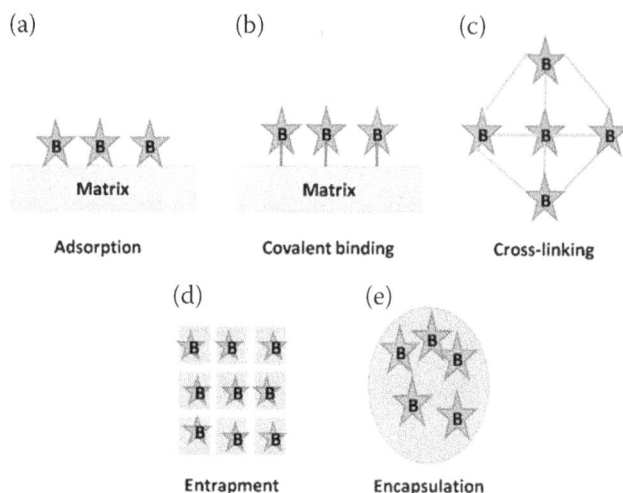

FIGURE 22.3
Schematic representation of various immobilization approaches.

using a high-concentration monomer for polymerization and bioreceptor entrapment, leakage of bioreceptors is observed.

v. *Encapsulation:* In this, a semi-permeable membrane is used, which allows a selective bioreceptor to seep in and form a capsule around it. An inexpensive approach, but limitations in terms of pore size and permeability are observed.

22.1.1.2 Classification Based on Transducer

1. *Electrochemical:* Herein, a systematically modified electrode with various matrices and chemicals or a non-modified electrode is used as a transducer. Potentiostatic techniques like impedance, voltammetry, amperometry, and conductometry are used to measure the signals.

2. *Optical:* In this, optics-dependent sensors act as transducers. Methods like absorption, fluorescence, phosphorescence, photomultiplier tube, etc. are utilized for measuring the signals [10].

3. *Calorimetric:* Heat and temperature-based sensors are used. Changes in these parameters are recorded as signals.

4. *Piezoelectric:* Materials like quartz that resonate at a particular frequency when it comes in contact with the target analyte are used. The bioreceptor is also coated with this piezoelectric substance. Upon reaction, the frequency is altered, which is captured as signals.

22.1.1.3 Classification Based on Electron Transfer

Biosensors are divided into three major categories based upon the electron transfer mechanism:

1. *First-generation:* These are mediator-less sensors. Herein, the analyte concentration or the product of the enzyme-analyte reaction is measured via diffusion to

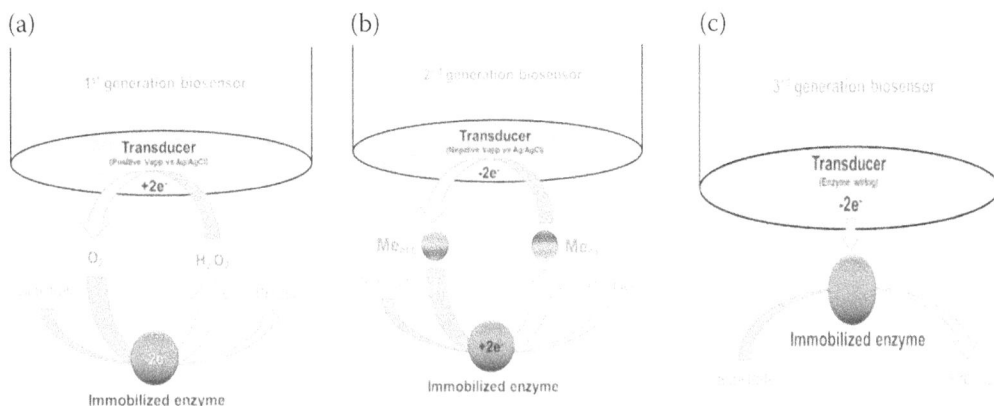

FIGURE 22.4
Schematic representation of (a) 1st-generation, (b) 2nd-generation, (c) 3rd-generation biosensor types. Adapted with permission [11]. Copyright The Authors, some rights reserved; exclusive licensee [MDPI]. Distributed under a Creative Commons Attribution License 4.0@2016.

the transducer surface which in turn gives an electrical response. Figure 22.4a is the schematic representation of this reprinted from [11]. Mostly enzyme-based biosensors are in this category, where an enzyme is immobilized directly over a transducer, and signals of the reaction product are measured.

2. *Second generation:* These are mediator-dependent sensors. Herein, redox mediators like ferricyanide, ferrocene, Prussian blue, thionin, azure, methyl violet, etc. are used to immobilize the bioreceptors or carry out the shuttling of the electron. Redox mediators can be added to electrolytes or can be immobilized on the surface of the electrode depending on the application. Figure 22.4b is the schematic representation of this [11].

3. *Third generation:* Herein, wiring of a bioreceptor on the electrode surface is direct via co-immobilizing the bioreceptor and conductive polymer. This electrodeposition takes place layer by layer. The monomer is mixed with a bioreceptor and electropolymerized. Figure 22.4c is the schematic representation of this reprinted from [11].

22.1.2 Characterization Techniques

Printable, as well as flexible biosensors, have several layers of matrices. Starting with the base electrode usually, carbon or solid metal or flexible polymer, followed by carbon or metallic or polymer matrix. Over this, a bioreceptor and a transducer further interact with the analyte. A synergetic mechanism must exist between these layers. This mechanism plays a key role in electron transfer activity, electro-oxidation/reduction, hence, is the major driving force of sense. The association of each layer can be manipulated based on desired features. Hence, morphological nature has to be examined. To study the morphological and chemical characteristics and features, several techniques mentioned below are employed [12]:

1. *Microscopic:* To study the surface morphology, scanning electron microscopy (SEM) and transmission electron microscopy (TEM) are usually adopted. This shows the basic shape, size of the various matrices used for immobilization.

2. *Spectroscopic:* These give the chemical composition, hybridization, and functional group information. Techniques like Raman, UV-Vis, FT-IR, and NMR are commonly used techniques. These studies also give plausible bond formations amongst the various modified layers.

3. *Morphological/Elemental analysis:* To find out the surface characteristics, dimensions, size, shape, and presence of elements in the biosensors matrices, techniques like XRD, XPS, BET, and EDX are used. The metallic and non-metallic elements have a significant role in enhancing the enzyme activity.

22.1.3 Printable and Flexible Biosensor Fabrication

Printable and flexible biosensor devices are fully integrated, portable, and use low sample and reagent volume for analysis. Hence, these can be employed as a point-of-care testing tool (POCT). Detection of biomarkers, pathogens, and other health parameters can be carried out using these biosensors. These give rapid results with no sample preparation and are hence easy to use. In further, these types of biosensors are robust, highly selective, and cost-effective. Several approaches are being adapted for their fabrication like 3D printing, ink-jet printing, screen printing, lamination, molding, embossing, photolithography, soft lithography, and laser cut. Each approach is described briefly [13,14]:

1. *3D printing (or additive manufacturing)* is an approach in which conductive filaments are deposited layer-by-layer giving a 3D structure. Computer aided design (CAD) software is used for designing the sensor. Filaments like acrylonitrile butadiene styrene (ABS), poly lactic acid (PLA), etc. are used. Various types of 3D printers like fused deposition molding (FDM), extrusion, lamination, stereolithography, and photo-polymerization are used.

2. *Molding:* Liquid polymers are molded and solidified as a sensor. There are two ways for this: (a) injection molding and (b) replica molding. Figure 22.5a shows injection molding schematic. Figure 22.5b gives replica molding. Herein, the liquified polymer is filled in the mold fabricated. This polymer acquires the shape of the mold that has the desired pattern and upon solidification gives a device.

3. *Photolithography:* An optical beam like UV, x-ray, electron beam, or ion beam are used to make the desired electrode patterns over the substrate. A mask with the desired microchannel or electrode pattern is placed over the substrate and the optical beam is exposed. The pattern is drawn over the substrate. Figure 22.5c gives a schematic of this method.

4. *Soft-lithography:* Molten polymers like polydimethylsiloxane (PDMS), poly (methyl methacrylate (PMMA), and polyimide are poured over a master mold of elastomers. These master molds are made up of materials like silicon. The molds have desired shape, pattern, and channel. The molten polymer tends to acquire this. Solidification gives the designed sensor. Figure 22.5d is the schematic representation of this method.

5. *Lamination:* In this, separate cut layers of materials like glass slides, PMMA, PLA, etc. are used, stacked, and bonded together. There are three layers: bottom, intermediate in which microchannels are engraved, and top layer. Adhesives are used for firm bonding and knife plotter or laser are used for designing.

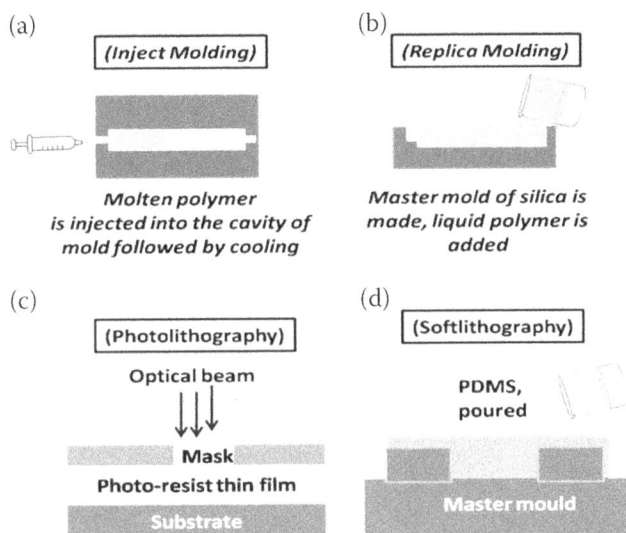

FIGURE 22.5
Schematic representation of (a) injection molding, (b) replica molding, (c) photolithography, and (d) soft lithography.

6. *Screen printing*: In this, flexible substrates like paper, cloth, etc. can be used to draw electrodes. Conductive ink is poured over the designed mask of the electrode. The obtained design on a substrate is dried in an oven. This is the most simplistic approach. Figure 22.6a is the schematic of this approach.

7. *Embossing*: Herein, a mold with cavities for microchannels is made, a thermoplastic polymer sheet is placed over this mold, and a specific temperature and pressure are applied. The sheet melts and occupies the shape of a cavity. Cooling and solidification give a sensor. Figure 22.6b is the schematic of this technique.

8. *Laser-cut*: In this, substrates like paper, glass, carbon, plastic, polymer sheets, etc., are ablated by lasers like CO_2, UV, pulsed, diode, etc., forming laser-induced graphene electrodes and laser-cut microchannel patterns. Figure 22.6c shows the image of a CO_2 laser cutting the polyimide sheet.

9. *Ink-jet printing*: In this, an ink-jet printer is employed and a conductive ink is filled in the nozzle of the printer and sensor electrodes are printed over substrates like paper, glass, etc. Figure 22.6d shows the image of an ink-jet printer.

22.2 Printable and Flexible Biosensors' Applications

22.2.1 Application in Health Management

Several printable and flexible biosensors have been fabricated for monitoring health and diagnosis of ailments. These include the detection of specific disease biomarkers or pathogenic antigens in physiological samples. A few of the recent advances are discussed here. For instance, a screen-printed biosensor was developed by Cao et al. Herein, a paper-based 3D device was reported using a combination of screen printing and

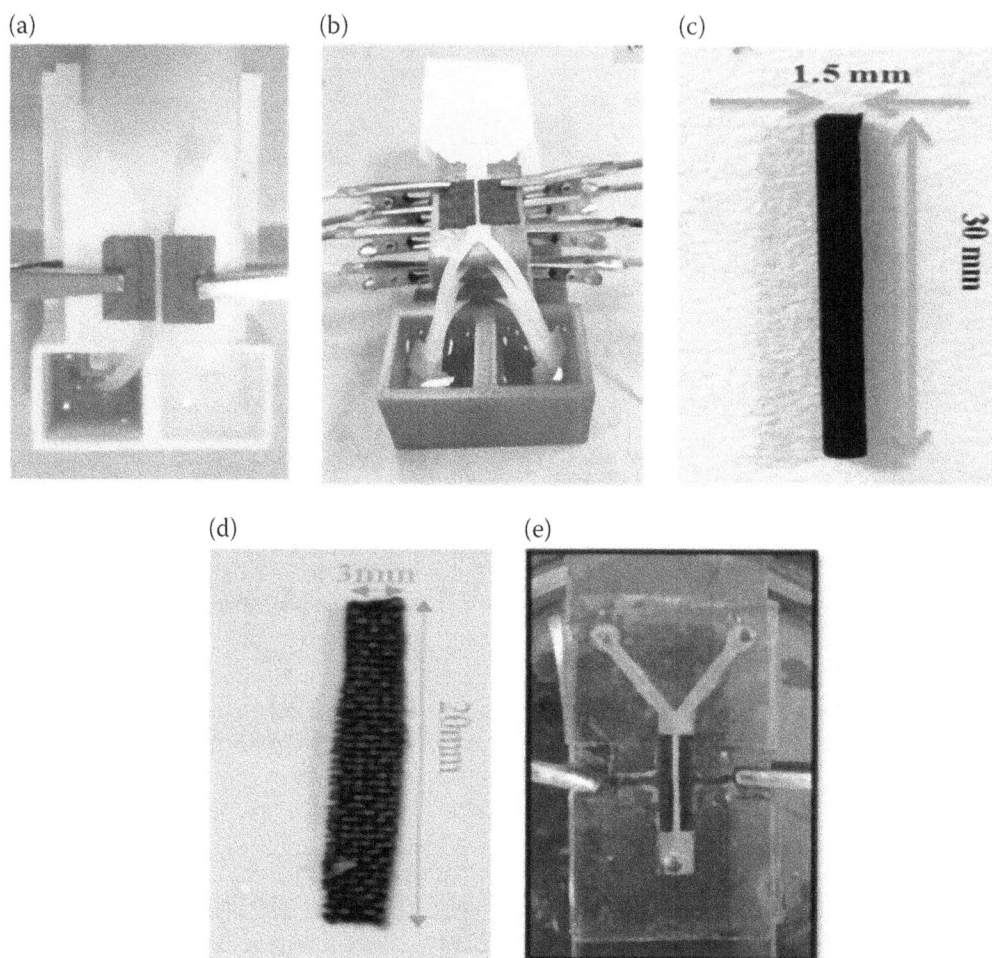

FIGURE 22.6
Reprint of the devices (a) adapted with permission from Reference [15] Copyright (2018), IEEE. (b) Adapted with permission [16], Copyright (2020), ACS. (c) Adapted with permission [17], Copyright (2020), IEEE. (d) Adapted with permission [18], Copyright (2021), IEEE. (e) Adapted with permission [19], Copyright (2021), IEEE.

photolithography technique. The hydrophilic region of the counter and reference electrodes was subjected to aldehyde treatment to functionalize them. A working electrode modified with Prussian blue redox mediator combined with a base of reduced graphene oxide (composite) was used as an electron transfer medium. Glucose oxidase enzyme was immobilized over this matrix and glucose sensing was done. A linear range of 0.1–25 mM and a limit of detection (LoD) was 25 µM. In further, the same electrode was able to sense hydrogen peroxide which was the by-product of the enzyme-substrate reaction. To check the practicality in real time, human blood and urine samples were used for the detection of glucose. To validate, this printable sensor was compared with the market glucose meter and appreciable results were seen [20]. Similarly, a paper-based biosensor with glucose oxidase and horseradish peroxidase composite with copper nanostructure matrix was reported by Zhu et al. A wax printing approach was used here. These copper nanostructures were inorganic, flower-like crystals that improved the co-immobilization of both enzymes. This provided stability to the enzyme activity and enhanced the electron transfer. These were termed μPADS. They exhibited sensitive and selective glucose detection in the linear range of 0.1–10 mM with an LoD of 25 μM. Glucose detection was done in real-time samples of human whole blood and blood serum to check applicability in the clinical analysis [21]. In another work, a biochip was fabricated for the detection of kidney ailment biomarker, creatinine. Herein, PDMS substrate-based microchannels were developed. These were strategically placed over carbon screen-printed electrodes. In further, these electrodes were chemically modified with a matrix of gold nanostructures and multiwalled carbon nanotube composite. This metallic-carbon nanotube composite matrix was used to immobilize the creatinase enzyme. This device gave a linear concentration range of 0.01 mM–1mM with LoD as 0.5 μM. No interference from any other co-existing biochemicals and metabolites was observed. Furthermore, physiological samples were tested for real-time applications [22].

A continuous lactate monitoring wearable biosensor using a screen-printed approach was developed by Shitanda et al. PDMS substrate with MdO-1,2-naphthoqui and lactate oxidize enzyme as a working electrode. A microfluidic, PDMS-based sweat collector was made to collect the sample. The sensor gave a linear range of 0.3–50 mM with an LoD 0.3 Mm [23]. In another interesting work, Zhang et al. developed a microfluidic biosensor for the detection of interleukin-8, a biomarker for cancer. The microchip was connected with two passages via a vertical channel. Antibody against this biomarker was used for capturing which was immobilized in one of the channels and on the other and, the channel was used for cell culture. A linear range of 7.5–120 pg/mL was observed. Real-time tumor cells were used for analysis and the biosensor and the obtained results were compared to the commercial assay results [24]. Likewise, interdigitated printable electrodes chemically modified with gold nanoparticles were designed by Nunna et al. for cancer biomarker detection using impedance analysis [25]. A circuit board-based biosensor was developed for detection of cytokine, a cardiac biomarker by Evans et al. Herein, gold electrodes were employed as working and counter electrodes, Ag/AgCl as a reference electrode [26]. Using a DNA sequence as a capture bioreceptor over nonporous beads matrix, tumor biomarker was detected by Caneira et al. Herein, beads were used for immobilizing the DNA probe. The device gave an excellent LoD of 9.5 pM [27].

In a remarkable work, a microfluidic channel device with multi-walled carbon nanotube-indium-tin-oxide electrodes modified with probe DNA was used over PDMS substrate for detection of leukemia by Ghrera et al. This biochip displayed an appreciable linear range of 1 fm–1μM. A very short response time of about 60 seconds was enough to obtain the results [28]. Pursey et al. designed array electrodes for the detection of a biomarker for bladder cancer using DNA as a bioreceptor. Herein, three different bladder cancer detection DNA biomarkers were detected over a single chip. The device gave a LoD of 250 fM. The microchannel had a facility of integrating 20 sensors simultaneously for detecting different DNA sequences. The response time was about 2 minutes [29]. Apart from ailment biomarkers, biosensors for pathogen detection are also reported in the literature. For example, Funari et al. prepared a chip for the detection of SARS-CoV-2 antibodies. The PDMS-based micro biosensor was prepared which gave a LoD of 0.08 ng/mL [30]. An interdigitated biosensor for detection of Salmonella type B and type D detection was prepared by Liu et al. The fabricated biosensor was subjected to impedance analysis and the signal was recorded as a function of bacteria concentration. The antibody-antigen complex approach was used and the biosensor was selective with zero interference from *E. coli* strains [31]. Same way, PDMS-based micro biosensor was fabricated by Jiang et al. using a dendrimer aptamer for detecting *E. coli*. [32]. Overall, significant printable and flexible biosensors for health monitoring have been reported.

22.2.2 Application in Energy Harvesting

Printable and flexible enzyme-based electrodes platforms have proven to be efficient in energy harvesting; biofuel cell applications. Usually, the glucose oxidase enzyme is used as a bioreceptor on these electrodes for glucose biofuel cells. Off lately, our group has been working extensively to design various paper-based, bioelectrodes for energy harvesting. For instance, Rewatkar et al. developed a microfluidic paper-based Y-shaped microchannel device with bucky paper bioelectrodes modified using glucose oxidase and laccase enzyme as bioreceptors. The device has bioanode and biocathod. Bucky paper electrodes were made with size 15 mm × 8 mm, they were cleaned with isopropyl alcohol. These electrodes were dipped in a linker solution of EDC/NHS. Enzyme solutions were prepared by weighing 5 mg of enzymes separately in 1 mL of 0.1 M PBS. The electrodes were immersed in these enzyme solutions for about 2 hours. Bioanode was dipped in glucose oxidase and laccase on biocathode. These prepared electrodes were then integrated over a paper Y-shaped microchannel. The total size of this μPAD fuel cell device was 50 mm × 25 mm. The device gave a maximum power density of 100 μW/cm^2 (600 μA/cm^2) at 0.505 V for about 50 hours. Figure 22.6 is the reprint of their device [15]. They also developed buck eye composite buckypaper bioelectrodes for developing enzymatic biofuel cells using glucose oxidase and laccase enzyme. This device gave a large current density of 9.79 mA/cm^2 at 0.4 V and 2 mA/cm^2 at 0.3 V using 40-mM of glucose and a scan rate of 10 mV/s [33]. Nath et al. from our group reported paper-based microbial biofuel cells using *Escherichia coli* carbon nanotube-buckypaper electrode. Bucky paper of dimensions 15 mm × 8 mm was cut as bioelctrodes. Further, these were cleaned with isopropyl alcohol and modified with multiwalled carbon nanotubes. A T-shaped microchannel with a single outlet and two outlets was made. One inlet was used for feeding bacterial solution and the other for oxygenated water. The electrodes were placed near the edge of both channels. A 3D printed mini platform was designed to assemble these electrodes. The platform had provisions for electrolytes. The device showed a power density of 20 μA/cm^2 at 0.405 V with 200 μL volume of culture [34].

Jayapriya et al. also demonstrated the fabrication of flexible electrodes using polyimide sheets and CO_2 laser ablation. These give laser-induced graphene which was further used for enzymatic fuel cell application. Polyimide sheet was clenched to the glass slide. A virtual design of microchannel was fed through the software. The CO_2 laser of optimized power and speed was made to ablate the sheet. About 80% of it was burnt. The burnt area was removed to get a channel of 100 μM depth. The same approach was used for fabrication laser-induced graphene (LIG) electrodes, modified with enzymes for studying the energy harvesting application [18]. They also fabricated a 3D-printed, enzymatic microfluidic fuel cell device. Polylactic conductive filament with graphene composite was used as electrodes. A Y-shape device was made of two parts. The device gave a power density of 4.15 μWcm^{-2} and a current density of 13.36 A/cm^2 [35].

Rewatakar et al. also fabricated a shelf-stacked, paper-based, Y-shaped microfluidic device. It had bucky paper and carbon nanotube electrodes immobilized with glucose oxidase and laccase enzymes. This gave a power density of 58 μA/cm^2 at 0.8 V. Figure 22.6B gives the real image of their device reprinted [16]. The same author also developed automated, 3D printed, graphene and polylactic acid filament electrodes modified with glucose oxide and laccase enzyme for biofuel cell study. This gave current density of 1.41 mA/cm^2 at 0.5 V (bioanode) using 40 mM glucose and 0.216 mA/cm^2 at 0.42 V (biocathode). Figure 22.6C is the real image of their electrodes reprinted [17]. Jayapiriya et al. developed a microfluidic enzyme-based biofuel cell using laser-ablated polyimide laser-induced graphene. Further, these were modified with carbon nanotubes and enzymes. This gave a power density of 4.7 µW/cm^2 at 260 mV. Figure 22.6D is the real image of their device reprinted [18]. The same author also developed a carbon cloth electrode-based, enzymatic biofuel cell. This gave a power density of 24.8 µW/cm^2 at 300 mV. Figure 22.6E is the reprint of their real image [19]. Jayapiriya et al. also developed carbon paste electrodes fabricated with a PCB printer. Further, gold nanorods were immobilized on these to form enzymatic glucose biofuel cells. This gave maximum energy of 8.8 µW/cm^2 [36]. Hence, printable and flexible biosensors, especially enzymatic and microbial, have proven to be quite useful in energy-harvesting biofuel cell applications.

22.2.3 Applications in Environmental Monitoring

For spontaneous environmental monitoring, to measure the environmental impact load, real-time, portable detection systems for field applications are crucial. These could reduce the limitations like collection and logistics of a sample, handling, and other such issues. In this context, printable and flexible biosensors have proven to be advantages. Quite a few research groups have worked on developing these types of sensors for monitoring various environmental parameters. McConnell et al. gave a detailed review of aptamer-based biosensors for environmental parameters monitoring. The review covers various biosensors reported for detection of microbial contamination, heavy metal, metal ions, toxins, industrial waste, pesticides, pharmaceutical remains in water and soil [37]. Song et al. also reported a detailed review about array-based biosensors using DNA-, enzyme-, aptamer-, antibody-, and micro-organism-based bioreceptors [38]. Avramescu et al. reviewed graphite screen-printed biosensors for food and environment quality monitoring [39]. Honeychurch presented a view about screen-printed biosensors for metal pollutants detection [40]. Laschi et al. reviewed advances in disposable biosensors for the detection of food and environmental pollutants [41]. In an interesting work, a microfluidic biochip was developed by Brennan et al. Herein, fish cells of rainbow trout gill epithelial cells were used as bioreceptors. These were used for the detection of pesticide toxicity for water quality assessment [42]. Likewise, Lin et al. developed a screen-printed biosensor with a combination of antibody and horseradish peroxide enzyme for selective detection of *E. coli*. Carbon-based electrodes modified with gold nanoparticles were used as a matrix to immobilize these antibodies [43]. In a remarkable work, Rupesh et al. reported a lab on a flexible glove-based, printed biosensor. This had great stretchability and could be used as a point of care wearable sensor. A carbon ink was screen printed over the glove as an electrode. Similarly, Ag/AgCl ink was screen printed and used as a reference electrode. Over the working carbon ink electrode, an enzyme organophosphorus hydrolase (OPH), was coated as a bioreceptor. This enzyme was mixed with Nafion and this solution was coated. This was utilized for the detection of organophosphate, a common pesticide. In further, this biosensor was integrated with electrochemical analysis and wireless transmission of data via smartphone. This could be used in food quality assessment [44].

Similarly, Tirgil et al. prepared an aptamer-based sensor using a single-walled carbon nanotube matrix. This was used for the detection of an antibiotic, oxytetracycline, in water samples. This is used as a medicine for pathogenic infection in livestock. Its portable size, high stability makes it suitable for industry and real-time environmental applications [45]. Huang et al. demonstrated an *E. coli*–detecting biosensor fabricated over graphene matrix. The chemical vapor deposition method was adapted to form a film of graphene. Over this, antibodies were immobilized. The device showed selective and sensitive detection of *E. coli* with a low concentration of 10 cfu/mL. No interference from other strains was obtained. This no-label approach was easy, rapid, and sensitive for real-time bacteria detection in environmental samples [46]. Park et al. reported an immunosensor for the detection of 2,4,6-Trinitrotoluene (TNT). Herein, they used single-walled carbon nanotubes in a conducting channel of device, modified with an antibody against TNT. This could detect TNT in a linear range of 0.5–5,000 ppb. The real water sample analysis was done and they found that it showed great selectivity towards TNT in presence of other nitroaromatic explosives [47]. In another work, Gong et al. prepared a selective and highly sensitive mercury detection biosensor. This was a DNA-based sensor fabricated over single-walled carbon nanotubes based on chemiresistive principle. The device gave a linear range of 100–1,000 nM with LoD as 6.721 nM [48]. García-Aljaro fabricated a chemiresitive immunosensor for the detection of two pathogens, *E. coli* and Bacteriophage T7. Gold electrodes were placed parallelly and bridged with single-walled carbon nanotubes. In further, antibodies corresponding to these pathogens were immobilized. There was a remarkable increase of resistance observed when the device was tested with specified *E. coli* strain. No interference from other strains with LoD of 105 CFU/mL. Whereas, in the case of the virus, LoD of 103 PFU/mL was obtained with no interference [49]. Liu et al. developed a biosensor device using photolithography and PDMS. Graphene oxide sheets were coated over a Si/SiO2 substrate. This graphene oxide was converted to a reduced form via a thermal approach. Rotavirus-specific antibodies were immobilized over this. The sensor was exposed to various rotavirus concentration solutions and has an LoD of 102 PFU/mL [50]. Thus, the literature reveals that printable biosensors have significant importance in environment monitoring and pollutant detections.

22.3 Conclusion and Future Outlook

In recent times, substantial advances for the fabrication of novel analytical platforms with flexible and printable biosensor electrodes have taken place. These have been revolutionizing tools for the estimation of biological and environmental analytes. With the integration of automation, microfluidics to prepare biosensors, point-of-care testing has become feasible. Several advantages, such as instant, selective, and sensitive estimations at the point of sample collection, multiplexed analyte detection, disposability as well as re-usable features, ease of use, cost-effectiveness, smaller sample, and reagent volume, have made them popular. The advances in these types of sensors have made analytical detections laboratory-free. Various matrices and materials are being explored for fabrication. Since, bioreceptor molecules are sensitive and prone to lose activity, the matrices play a significant role in the stability of the biosensors. The tremendous growth in the future, in terms of preparations, materials, and applications is expected. With a special focus on bridging the gap between academia fabrication, application, and industrial production, in the future, printable biosensors can be made commercially viable. The present chapter gives detailed information about the basic working principle of biosensors, types of biosensors based on bioreceptor, generations, and transducers. Brief information on fabrication is also discussed. Recent advances and some remarkable works reported for the application of flexible and printable biosensors in the detection of biomarkers of ailments, pathogens for health monitoring, energy-harvesting fuel cells, and environmental pollutant detections are also discussed. In conclusion, it can be estimated that the onset of wearable biosensors in the near future could be benchmarking game changers in various fields of electro-analytical quality and quantificational analysis.

References

1. P. Panjan, V. Virtanen, A.M. Sesay, Determination of stability characteristics for electro-chemical biosensors via thermally accelerated ageing, *Talanta*. 170 (2017) 331–336. 10.1016/j.talanta.2017.04.011
2. D.R. Thévenot, K. Toth, R.A. Durst, G.S. Wilson, Electrochemical biosensors: Recommended definitions and classification, *Biosens. Bioelectron*. 16 (2001) 121–131. 10.1016/S0956-5663(01)00115-4
3. V. Perumal, U. Hashim, Advances in biosensors: Principle, architecture and applications, *J. Appl. Biomed*. 12 (2014) 1–15. 10.1016/j.jab.2013.02.001
4. D. Grieshaber, R. MacKenzie, J. Vörös, E. Reimhult, Electrochemical biosensors – Sensor principles and architectures, *Sensors*. 8 (2008) 1400–1458. 10.3390/s8031400
5. P.J. Conroy, S. Hearty, P. Leonard, R.J. O'Kennedy, Antibody production, design and use for biosensor-based applications, *Semin. Cell Dev. Biol*. 20 (2009) 10–26. 10.1016/j.semcdb.2009.01.010
6. S. Cagnin, M. Caraballo, C. Guiducci, P. Martini, M. Ross, M. Santaana, D. Danley, T. West, G. Lanfranchi, Overview of electrochemical DNA biosensors: New approaches to detect the expression of life, *Sensors (Switzerland)*. 9 (2009) 3122–3148. 10.3390/s90403122
7. C. Liu, D. Yong, D. Yu, S. Dong, Cell-based biosensor for measurement of phenol and ni-trophenols toxicity, *Talanta*. 84 (2011) 766–770. 10.1016/j.talanta.2011.02.006
8. L. Lu, X. Hu, Z. Zhu, Biomimetic sensors and biosensors for qualitative and quantitative analyses of five basic tastes, *TrAC – Trends Anal. Chem*. 87 (2017) 58–70. 10.1016/j.trac.2016.12.007
9. A. Sassolas, L.J. Blum, B.D. Leca-Bouvier, Immobilization strategies to develop enzymatic biosensors, *Biotechnol. Adv*. 30 (2012) 489–511. 10.1016/j.biotechadv.2011.09.003
10. I. Abdulhalim, M. Zourob, A. Lakhtakia, Overview of Optical Biosensing *Techniques*, (2008). 10.1002/9780470061565.hbb040
11. G. Rocchitta, A. Spanu, S. Babudieri, G. Latte, G. Madeddu, G. Galleri, S. Nuvoli, P. Bagella, M.I. Demartis, V. Fiore, R. Manetti, P.A. Serra, Enzyme biosensors for biomedical applications: Strategies for safeguarding analytical performances in biological fluids, *Sensors (Switzerland)*. 16 (2016). 10.3390/s16060780
12. R. Monošík, M. Streďanský, E. Šturdík, Biosensors – classification, characterization and new trends, *Acta Chim. Slovaca*. 5 (2012) 109–120. 10.2478/v10188-012-0017-z
13. A. Plecis, Y. Chen, Fabrication of microfluidic devices based on glass-PDMS-glass tech-nology, *Microelectron. Eng*. 84 (2007) 1265–1269. 10.1016/j.mee.2007.01.276
14. B.K. Gale, A.R. Jafek, C.J. Lambert, B.L. Goenner, H. Moghimifam, U.C. Nze, S.K. Kamarapu, A review of current methods in microfluidic device fabrication and future commercialization prospects, *Inventions*. 3 (2018). 10.3390/inventions3030060
15. P. Rewatkar, S. Goel, Paper-Based Membraneless Co-Laminar Microfluidic Glucose Biofuel Cell with MWCNT-Fed Bucky Paper Bioelectrodes, *IEEE Trans. Nanobioscience*. 17 (2018) 374–379. 10.1109/TNB.2018.2857406
16. P. Rewatkar, J. U. S. S. Goel, Optimized Shelf-Stacked Paper Origami-Based Glucose Biofuel Cell with Immobilized Enzymes and a Mediator, ACS Sustain. *Chem. Eng*. 8 (2020) 12313–12320. 10.1021/acssuschemeng.0c04752
17. P. Rewatkar, S. Goel, 3D Printed Bioelectrodes for Enzymatic Biofuel Cell: Simple, Rapid, Optimized and Enhanced Approach, *IEEE Trans. Nanobioscience*. 19 (2020) 4–10. 10.1109/TNB.2019.2941196

18. U.S. Jayapiriya, P. Rewatkar, S. Goel, Direct Electron Transfer based Microfluidic Glucose Biofuel cell with CO2 Laser ablated Bioelectrodes and Microchannel, *IEEE Trans. Nanobioscience.* 1241 (2021). 10.1109/TNB.2021.3079238

19. U.S. Jayapiriya, S. Goel, Optimization of carbon cloth bioelectrodes for enzyme-based biofuel cell for wearable bioelectronics, Proc. IEEE Conf. Nanotechnol. 2020–July (2020) 150–154. 10.1109/NANO47656.2020.9183700

20. L. Cao, G.C. Han, H. Xiao, Z. Chen, C. Fang, A novel 3D paper-based microfluidic electrochemical glucose biosensor based on rGO-TEPA/PB sensitive film, *Anal. Chim. Acta.* 1096 (2020) 34–43. 10.1016/j.aca.2019.10.049

21. X. Zhu, J. Huang, J. Liu, H. Zhang, J. Jiang, R. Yu, A dual enzyme-inorganic hybrid nanoflower incorporated microfluidic paper-based analytic device (μPAD) biosensor for sensitive visualized detection of glucose, *Nanoscale.* 9 (2017) 5658–5663. 10.1039/c7nr00958e

22. J. Li, Z. Li, Y. Dou, J. Su, J. Shi, Y. Zhou, L. Wang, S. Song, C. Fan, A nano-integrated microfluidic biochip for enzyme-based point-of-care detection of creatinine, *Chem. Commun.* 57 (2021) 4726–4729. 10.1039/d1cc00825k

23. I. Shitanda, M. Mitsumoto, N. Loew, Y. Yoshihara, H. Watanabe, T. Mikawa, S. Tsujimura, M. Itagaki, M. Motosuke, Continuous sweat lactate monitoring system with integrated screen-printed Mgo-templated carbon-lactate oxidase biosensor and microfluidic sweat collector, *Electrochim. Acta.* 368 (2021) 137620. 10.1016/j.electacta.2020.137620

24. W. Zhang, Z. He, L. Yi, S. Mao, H. Li, J.M. Lin, A dual-functional microfluidic chip for on-line detection of interleukin-8 based on rolling circle amplification, *Biosens. Bioelectron.* 102 (2018) 652–660. 10.1016/j.bios.2017.12.017

25. B.B. Nunna, D. Mandal, J.U. Lee, H. Singh, S. Zhuang, D. Misra, M.N.U. Bhuyian, E.S. Lee, Detection of cancer antigens (CA-125) using gold nano particles on interdigitated electrode-based microfluidic biosensor, *Nano Converg.* 6 (2019). 10.1186/s40580-019-0173-6

26. D. Evans, K.I. Papadimitriou, N. Vasilakis, P. Pantelidis, P. Kelleher, H. Morgan, T. Prodromakis, A novel microfluidic point-of-care biosensor system on printed circuit board for cytokine detection, *Sensors (Switzerland).* 18 (2018) 1–14. 10.3390/s18114011

27. C.R.F. Caneira, R.R.G. Soares, I.F. Pinto, H.S. Mueller-Landau, A.M. Azevedo, V. Chu, J.P. Conde, Development of a rapid bead-based microfluidic platform for DNA hybridization using single- and multi-mode interactions for probe immobilization, *Sensors Actuators, B Chem.* 286 (2019) 328–336. 10.1016/j.snb.2019.01.133

28. A.S. Ghrera, C.M. Pandey, B.D. Malhotra, Multiwalled carbon nanotube modified microfluidic-based biosensor chip for nucleic acid detection, *Sensors Actuators, B Chem.* 266 (2018) 329–336. 10.1016/j.snb.2018.03.118

29. J.P. Pursey, Y. Chen, E. Stulz, M.K. Park, P. Kongsuphol, Microfluidic electrochemical multiplex detection of bladder cancer DNA markers, *Sensors Actuators, B Chem.* 251 (2017) 34–39. 10.1016/j.snb.2017.05.006

30. R. Funari, K.Y. Chu, A.Q. Shen, Detection of antibodies against SARS-CoV-2 spike protein by gold nanospikes in an opto-microfluidic chip, *Biosens. Bioelectron.* 169 (2020) 112578. 10.1016/j.bios.2020.112578

31. J. Liu, I. Jasim, Z. Shen, L. Zhao, M. Dweik, S. Zhang, M. Almasri, A microfluidic based biosensor for rapid detection of Salmonella in food products, *PLoS One.* 14 (2019) 1–18. 10.1371/journal.pone.0216873

32. Y. Jiang, S. Zou, X. Cao, A simple dendrimer-aptamer based microfluidic platform for E. coli O157:H7 detection and signal intensification by rolling circle amplification, Sensors Actuators, *B Chem.* 251 (2017) 976–984. 10.1016/j.snb.2017.05.146

33. P. Rewatkar, M. Bandapati, S. Goel, Optimized bucky paper-based bioelectrodes for oxygen-glucose fed enzymatic biofuel cells, *IEEE Sens. J.* 18 (2018) 5395–5401. 10.1109/JSEN.2018.2837092

34. D. Nath, P. Sai Kiran, P. Rewatkar, B. Krishnamurthy, P. Sankar Ganesh, S. Goel, Escherichia coli Fed Paper-Based Microfluidic Microbial Fuel Cell with MWCNT Composed Bucky Paper Bioelectrodes, *IEEE Trans. Nanobioscience.* 18 (2019) 510–515. 10.1109/TNB.2019.2919930

35. P. Rewatkar, S. Goel, Next-Generation 3D Printed Microfluidic Membraneless Enzymatic Biofuel Cell: Cost-Effective and Rapid Approach, *IEEE Trans. Electron Devices.* 66 (2019) 3628–3635. 10.1109/TED.2019.2922424

36. U.S. Jayapiriya, S. Goel, Flexible and optimized carbon paste electrodes for direct electron transfer-based glucose biofuel cell fed by various physiological fluids, *Appl. Nanosci.* 10 (2020) 4315–4324. 10.1007/s13204-020-01543-3

37. E.M. McConnell, J. Nguyen, Y. Li, Aptamer-Based Biosensors for Environmental Monitoring, *Front. Chem.* 8 (2020) 1–24. 10.3389/fchem.2020.00434

38. W. Song, S. Wei, H.-X. Yu, M. Vuki, D. Xu, Biosensor Arrays for Environmental Monitoring, *Environ. Monit.* (2011). 10.5772/26494

39. A. Avramescu, S. Andreescu, T. Noguer, C. Bala, D. Andreescu, J.L. Marty, Biosensors designed for environmental and food quality control based on screen-printed graphite electrodes with different configurations, *Anal. Bioanal. Chem.* 374 (2002) 25–32. 10.1007/s00216-002-1312-0

40. K.C. Honeychurch, Screen-printed Electrochemical Sensors and Biosensors for Monitoring Metal Pollutants, *Insciences J.* 2 (2012) 1–51. 10.5640/insc.020101

41. S. Laschi, I. Palchetti, G. Marrazza, M. Mascini, Disposable electrochemical sensors and biosensors for environmental and food analysis, Indian J. Chem. - Sect. A Inorganic, *Phys. Theor. Anal. Chem.* 42 (2003) 2968–2973.

42. L.M. Brennan, M.W. Widder, M.K. McAleer, M.W. Mayo, A.P. Greis, W.H. van der Schalie, Preparation and testing of impedance-based fluidic biochips with RTgill-W1 cells for rapid evaluation of drinking water samples for toxicity, *J. Vis. Exp.* 2016 (2016) 1–8. 10.3791/53555

43. Y.H. Lin, S.H. Chen, Y.C. Chuang, Y.C. Lu, T.Y. Shen, C.A. Chang, C.S. Lin, Disposable amperometric immunosensing strips fabricated by Au nanoparticles-modified screen-printed carbon electrodes for the detection of foodborne pathogen Escherichia coli O157:H7, *Biosens. Bioelectron.* 23 (2008) 1832–1837. 10.1016/j.bios.2008.02.030

44. R.K. Mishra, L.J. Hubble, A. Martín, R. Kumar, A. Barfidokht, J. Kim, M.M. Musameh, I.L. Kyratzis, J. Wang, Wearable Flexible and Stretchable Glove Biosensor for On-Site Detection of Organophosphorus Chemical Threats, *ACS Sensors.* 2 (2017) 553–561. 10.1021/acssensors.7b00051

45. N. Yildirim-Tirgil, J. Lee, H. Cho, H. Lee, S. Somu, A. Busnaina, A.Z. Gu, A SWCNT based aptasensor system for antibiotic oxytetracycline detection in water samples, *Anal. Methods.* 11 (2019) 2692–2699. 10.1039/c9ay00455f

46. Y. Huang, X. Dong, Y. Liu, L.J. Li, P. Chen, Graphene-based biosensors for detection of bacteria and their metabolic activities, *J. Mater. Chem.* 21 (2011) 12358–12362. 10.1039/c1jm11436k

47. M. Park, L.N. Cella, W. Chen, N. V. Myung, A. Mulchandani, Carbon nanotubes-based chemiresistive immunosensor for small molecules: Detection of nitroaromatic explosives, *Biosens. Bioelectron.* 26 (2010) 1297–1301. 10.1016/j.bios.2010.07.017

48. J.L. Gong, T. Sarkar, S. Badhulika, A. Mulchandani, Label-free chemiresistive biosensor for mercury (II) based on single-walled carbon nanotubes and structure-switching DNA, *Appl. Phys. Lett.* 102 (2013) 2012–2015. 10.1063/1.4773569

49. C. García-Aljaro, L.N. Cella, D.J. Shirale, M. Park, F.J. Muñoz, M. V. Yates, A. Mulchandani, Carbon nanotubes-based chemiresistive biosensors for detection of microorganisms, *Biosens. Bioelectron.* 26 (2010) 1437–1441. 10.1016/j.bios.2010.07.077

50. F. Liu, Y.H. Kim, D.S. Cheon, T.S. Seo, Micropatterned reduced graphene oxide based field-effect transistor for real-time virus detection, *Sensors Actuators, B Chem.* 186 (2013) 252–257. 10.1016/j.snb.2013.05.097

23

Conducting Polymer-Based Biocomposites in Flexible Bioelectronics

Ragavi Rajasekaran

School of Medical Science and Technology, Indian Institute of Technology Kharagpur, West Bengal, India

Rajendra Mishra school of Engineering and Entrepreneurship, Indian Institute of Technology Kharagpur, West Bengal, India

Atul Kumar Ojha and Gaurav Kulkarni

School of Medical Science and Technology, Indian Institute of Technology Kharagpur, West Bengal, India

Jhansi L. Parimi

Rajiv Gandhi School of intellectual property, Indian Institute of Technology Kharagpur, West Bengal, India

Baisakhee Saha

School of Medical Science and Technology, Indian Institute of Technology Kharagpur, West Bengal, India

Mamoni Banerjee

Rajendra Mishra school of Engineering and Entrepreneurship, Indian Institute of Technology Kharagpur, West Bengal, India

Santanu Dhara

School of Medical Science and Technology, Indian Institute of Technology Kharagpur, West Bengal, India

CONTENTS

23.1 Introduction 374
23.2 Materials 375
    23.2.1 PTh 375
    23.2.2 PANi 376
    23.2.3 PPy 376
    23.2.4 PA 377
    23.2.5 PEDOT 377
    23.2.6 PVDF 377
23.3 Flexible Bioelectronics Synthesis, Fabrication, and Structural Design 377
    23.3.1 PANi 378
    23.3.2 PPy 380
    23.3.3 PA 382
    23.3.4 PEDOT 382
    23.3.5 PVDF 383

23.1 Introduction

Flexible bioelectronics (FB) using electroactive polymer-based biocomposites have been attracting researchers' attention recently and garnering great interest as they offer tunable mechanical flexibility, electrically conducting substrate, biocompatibility, and tailorable surface functionality, which support the different human tissue or organ along with the interface to machine [1]. In a biological system, cell function is modulated by various cues, and among them, bioelectricity affects abundant cellular functions such as proliferation, differentiation, signal transduction, DNA repair, etc. The ion channels and gap junctions are some of the instructive signals that employ voltage and current in the complex bioelectronics mechanism where the receptor or transporters ions participate to interface with organs and regulate the biological development [2]. Intimate integration with the human body requires mechanical flexibility for shape-matching with the biological landscape, compatibility with interface stiffness, tissues, and body fluids apart from maintaining high electrical conductivity and stability. The thinner and more flexible the device, the less the insertion trauma, damage, and chronic inflammation at the insertion site. Modern-day wearable electronics have made outstanding strides towards medical diagnostics with advanced design, extremely thin, stretchability, flexibility, and very high precision in real-time monitoring.

In recent years, a conducting polymer (CP) blends with a traditional polymer matrix have been extensively explored and have shown good cell-matrix interaction due to their chemical stability along with the mechanically soft property of the substrate. This has reduced the inflammatory response along with enhanced physiological signal interface in the biological environment, and thereby high reproducibility is observed and is proved to be a promising factor for bioactive devices [2]. Electroactive or CP-based scaffolds are developed for a multitude of biomedical applications such as tissue engineering, biosensors, energy storage, actuators, electrotherapeutic devices, drug delivery system, and neural interfaces (Figure 23.1) [3]. The CP displays hybrid ionic-electronic conductivity, biocompatibility and responds to electrochemical oxidation-reduction processes by a reversible change in conductivity, color, dimension, etc. Superior electrocatalytic activity and strong adsorptive ability are also the reasons in their favor over metal electrodes. Their facile synthetic processes and ease of functionalization and hybridization with other materials add up to their popularity in the development of FB. CPs and their derivatives are appropriate for neural interfaces and dry electrodes for biomonitoring since most of the biological signals, including neural transduction, occur via ionic transport processes. Bioelectronics devices should be thin, imperceptible, comfortable, and low rigidity and elastic range, commensurating with the tissue containing crack-onset strain equal to or greater than that of the skin vis-a-vis substrate where these are integrated. Interestingly, even the food processing industry can benefit from their use in the storage and fermentation processes of starch-based food [4]. This chapter focuses on CP-based biocomposite material and fabrication techniques highlighting the design of the substrate towards bioelectronic applications along with future challenges.

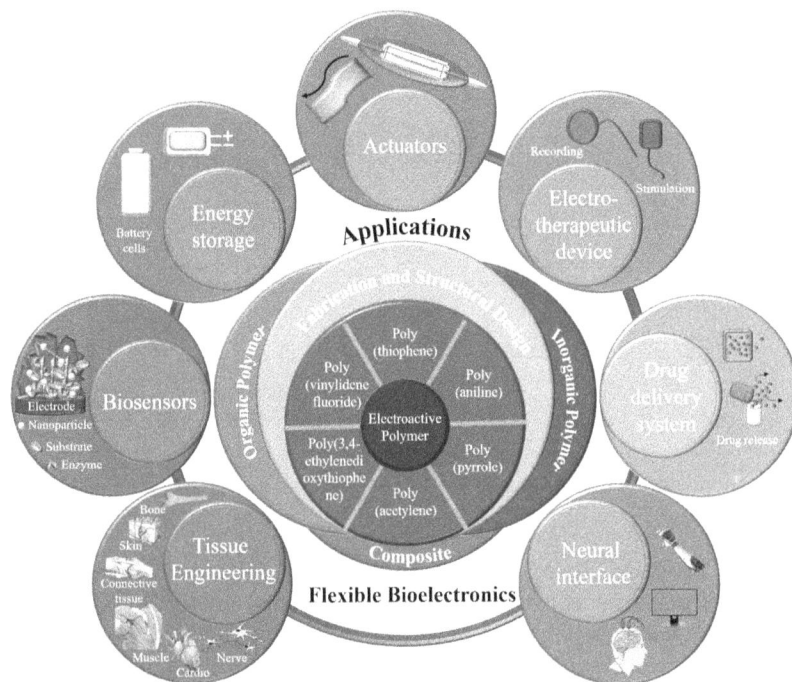

FIGURE 23.1
Illustrative image of the overall view.

23.2 Materials

CPs have tunable physicochemical and electrical properties and can be surface engineered by antibodies and other biological moieties according to the need of their application. Further, they can be altered through various cues such as electrical, pH, thermal, electromechanical, etc. CPs are used as flexible strain sensors due to their extreme sensitivity in capacitance or resistance change [5]. One of the important factors for deformable applications is the tensile modulus, where the CP can be tuned by composite biomaterials to minimize the interfacial stresses such as between layers of the material or between the device-tissue interactions. Among the CPs, this chapter focused on poly (thiophene) (PTh), poly(aniline) (PANi), poly(pyrrole) (PPy), polyacetylene (PA), poly (3,4-ethylene dioxythiophene) (PEDOT), and poly (vinylidene fluoride) (PVDF) that are a few of the well-explored techniques. Figure 23.2 explains fundamental factors to fabricate flexible bioelectronics and their structural design.

23.2.1 PTh

Due to its aromatic nature, thiophene, an organosulfur heterocyclic compound, offers the scope of many substitution reactions. PTh finds enormous usage in organic electronic devices due to its mechanical flexibility, low-cost synthesis, high electrical conductivity (10^3 S/cm), environmental and thermal stability under both doped and dedoped states, good optical property, and processability. The rigidity of PTh materials is ascribed to its

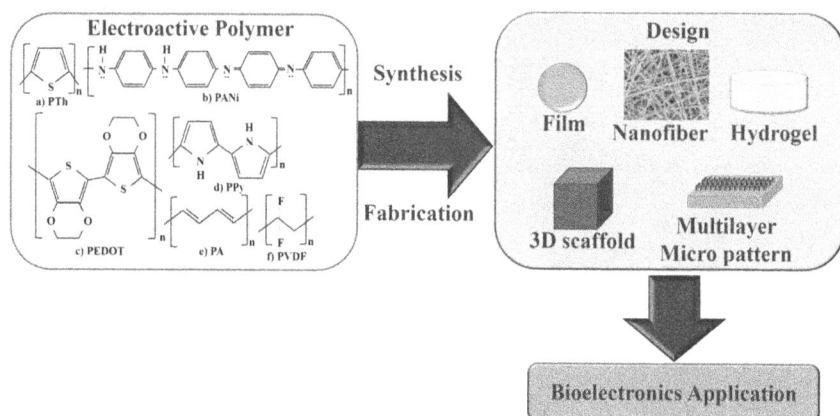

FIGURE 23.2
Schematic representation of fundamental factors to fabricate flexible bioelectronics and their structural design.

π-conjugated backbone structure. The disruption of this structure improves its flexibility but significantly lowers its conductivity. PTh is a conjugated polyelectrolyte with a pendant sulfonate group, capable of detecting a biological molecule/event due to its high-performance accumulation-mode organic electrochemical transistor mode in aqueous media [6]. Its electronic properties can be modulated by doping and/or chemical modifications.

23.2.2 PANi

PANi is considered as one of the well explored and first tested microelectronic devices owing to its easy synthesis, low cost, and environmentally friendly nature. PANi has been widely explored in the last decade for various applications due to its good optoelectrical properties. PANi is now gaining more importance in the field of bioelectronics. The combination of mechanical flexibility along with conductivity is an important prerequisite factor for organic electronic interfaces [7]. PANi exhibits both properties of electrically conductive and insulating material, which is dependent upon its oxidation state. It can be observed or detected in the form of leucoemeraldine (LE, yellow), pernigraniline (PG) purple, and emeraldine (EM) dark green.

23.2.3 PPy

One of the most promising CP variants for bioelectronic application is PPy. With the advances in the development of electron-conducting materials, PPy with high conductivity, excellent biocompatibility, and good mechanical stability were synthesized [8]. Therefore, PPy and its biocomposites were explored as sensors, actuators, and electrodes. To develop human skin–like materials for modern flexible electronics, PPy-based materials must be modified due to their high brittleness, non-transparent nature, and lower solubility in aqueous solutions, restricting the use of PPy for stretchable electronics and becoming one of the areas to explore more [8]. The selection of synthesis strategies and composite matrix varies based on their application such as wearable electronics, supercapacitors, electrodes for energy conservation, etc.

23.2.4 PA

PA, previously known as polyene, was synthesized by polymerization of acetylene and was reported by Natta et al. through a noble lecture in 1963 [9]. Shirakawa et al., in their noble lecture, mentioned that the discovery of the PA film was a fortuitous error and possess intrinsic electrical properties, which didn't vary between its powder and film form [10]. Later, due to carbocation of PA, the charge carrier was termed a conducting polymer. Synthesis of PA is mainly being carried out by three processes: a) catalytic polymerization, b) non-catalytic polymerization, and c) precursor assisted synthesis. Ziegler–Natta catalysts offer a good choice for catalytic polymerization owing to good solubility in organic solvents. For a high molecular weight PA, a luttinger catalyst is used, which utilizes acetonitrile and other hydrophilic solvents. Further, non-catalytic polymerization of the PA includes electrochemical polymerization, where aniline monomers are deposited on the metallic electrode to get a uniform PA film. Ring-opening polymerization is another method of synthesis, which doesn't require any catalyst and electro-machine setup.

23.2.5 PEDOT

PEDOT is a popular member of this group and the very first material used as an electrode on the human brain [11]. The PEDOT properties depend on the chemical structure, fabrication condition, incorporation of surfactants or doping, polymer composition, post-treatment, and polymerization. PEDOT is both n- and p-dopable and also displays electronic, electrical, and magnetic properties akin to metals and semiconductors. To develop PEDOT with mechanical stability, conductivity, and degradation under a change in temperature, pressure, or time strategies of both fundamental and practical are ensured according to the application. PEDOT itself and its derivatives are highly transparent in the visible range therefore suitable as flexible transparent electrodes.

23.2.6 PVDF

PVDF is a widely explored piezoelectric, thermo-mechanically stable, organic polymer for bioelectronic applications because of its flexible electroactive and processing properties. It exists in three dominant polymorphic forms, α, β, and γ. Among the three phases, the β-phase is for the most part electroactive because of the all-trans (TTTT) configuration and high dipole moment induced from CH_2-CF_2 [12]. The copolymerization of vinyl difluoride with trifluoroethylene (PVDF-TrFE) also enhances the piezoelectric response inducing chain alignment and high crystallinity [13].

23.3 Flexible Bioelectronics Synthesis, Fabrication, and Structural Design

PTh: Samanta et al. doped PTh with poly(ethylene glycol) (PEG)2000 and sodium p-toluene with synthesized PTh-g-poly (dimethylamino ethylmethacrylate) using atom transfer radical polymerization (ATRP) technique. The graft copolymer using methylcellulose gel was investigated the result showed photoluminescence property with change in temperature and pH. The graft copolymer showed similarity to AND logic gate functions, whereas the change in polarity in hydrogel at microenvironment was altered by the temperature and pH, which acted as an input, therefore resulting in fluorescent output [14]. The conductive film, fabricated with thin PTh-nanofibrillated cellulose synthesized by one-step oxidative polymerization of 3-methyl thiophene onto nanocellulose film using $FeCl_3$ as oxidant. The fabricated film displayed good flexibility, high electrical conductivity, and mechanical strength [15].

In an experimental-cum-theoretical study by Brazilian and Italian researchers, the electronic and optical properties of PTh were enhanced by patterning resulting in an organized internal structure of the material. A droplet of PTh solution deposited on a surface was allowed to evaporate, during which a pattern of parallel strips was made on it by an elastomeric stamp placed over it. This process made the atom chains linear to each other, as they bring atoms and hold very close to each other in the same chain. After migration, the electrons return to their starting point, where they emit and absorb light. This nanostructured PTh is suitable for active photonic devices [16]. Owyeung et al. fabricated a 3D transistor with multifilament threads, which was interconnected to logic gates and an integrated circuit that paved a way for smart sutures and wearable technology for transdermal application. The multiplexed diagnostic device was created by colloidal nanoparticles of silica supported with ion gel gated, linen thread-based transistors using P3HT which have been integrated with thread-based electrochemical sensors, which are thin and flexible [17].

An atom transfer radical polymerization initiator-functionalized PTh was grafted with a low glass transition temperature (T_g) (9.5°C) and hydrogen-bonded poly(acrylate urethane) side chains of varying lengths. It was observed that with increasing chain lengths, the graft polymer became softer and stretchable, resulting in higher strain and lower Young's modulus, respectively, these properties are more desirable for flexible and wearable electronics. Poly[5,5'-bis(2-butyloctyl)-(2,2'-bithiophene)-4,4'-dicarboxylate-alt-5,5'-2,2'-bithiophene] substituted PTh derivative displays better charge mobility of >0.1 $cm^2/V.s$ and stretchability of 400 stretch–release cycles than native PTh [18]. Doping of PTh with PEG2000 and sodium p-toluene sulfonate as polymeric and anionic surfactant dopants imparted superior mechanical flexibility (elongation-at-break of 110%), good tensile strength (160 MPa), and tensile toughness of 133 MJ/m^3, comparable to that of spider silk (100–160 MJ/m^3) [19]. Zokaei et al. fabricated PTh-based conducting fiber, where PTh with tetraethylene glycol side chains (p(g42T-T) blended with PU which is a combination of a semiconductor and insulator resulted with microfibers using the wet spinning technique, as shown in Figure 23.3a [20]. Using dimethylformamide (DMF) as a common solvent (p(g42T-T) and PU was dissolved, blended, and extruded in a coagulation bath where the fibers are further collected by a take-up roller. With different concentrations, microfibers with different diameters are fabricated as shown in Figure 23.3(b–d). The fibers are collected in a collector as shown in Figure 23.3e and showed the best reversible deformation and mechanical stability, as presented in Figure 23.3f. Additionally, by doping with iron(III) p-toluenesulfonate hexahydrate fibers exhibited conductivity up to 7.4 S/cm, flexibility up to 480%, and retained their conductivity until elongation at break.

23.3.1 PANi

PANi for flexible bioelectronics relevance to applications that are specifically related to the epidermal layer of tissue could be fabricated via 3D printing, electrospinning, laser ablation, and lithography. 3D printing is an additive manufacturing technique that is related to layer-by-layer fabrication. Among several subtypes available fused deposition printing, inkjet printing, direct printing, and stereolithography are widely used. Metallic

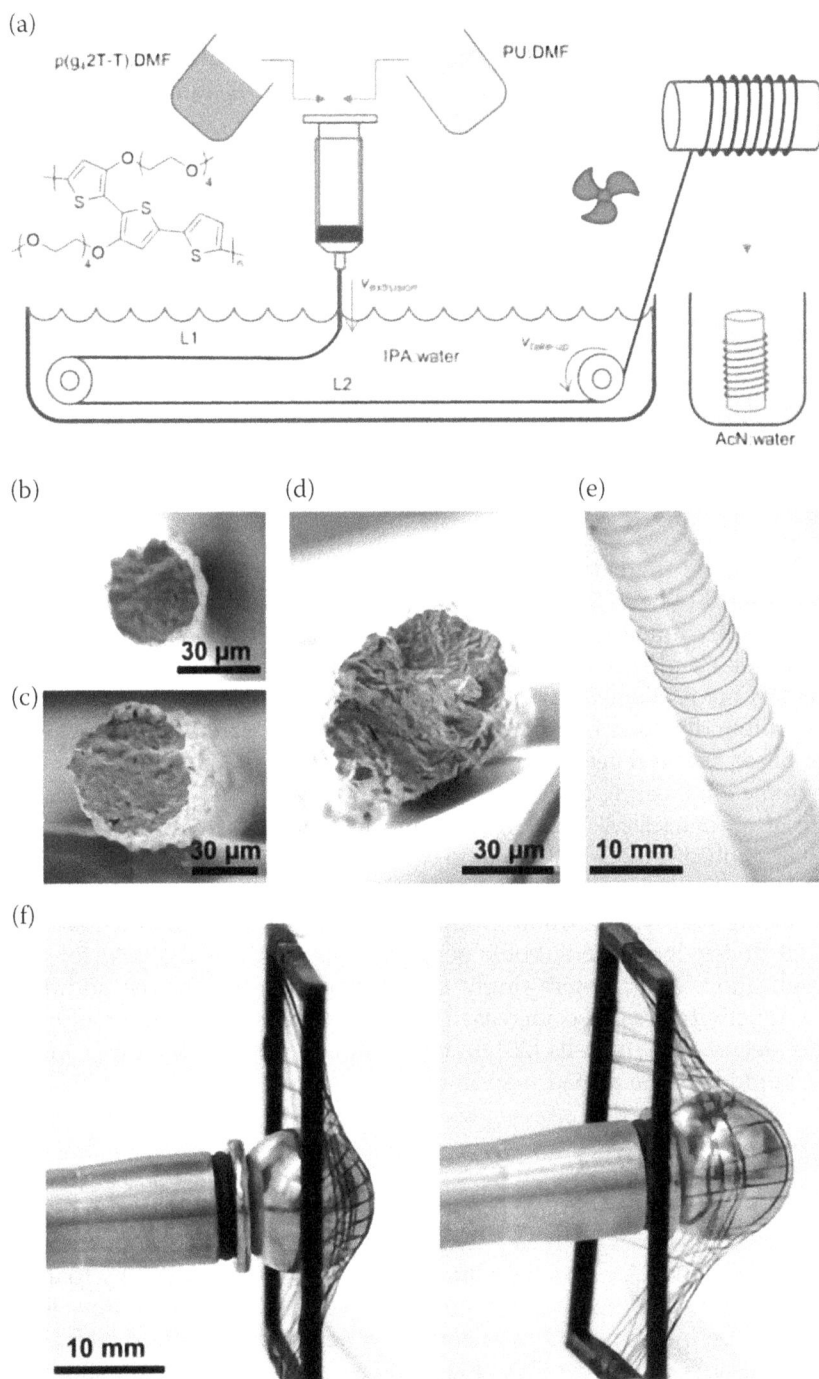

FIGURE 23.3
(a) Schematic illustration of wet-spinning, (b) thin-sized fiber, (c) thick-sized fiber, (d) medium-sized fiber, (e) rolled fibers, and (f) showing the reversible deformation on weaved fibers [20]. Copyright (2021). The article was printed under a CC-BY license (https://creativecommons.org/licenses/by/4.0/).

electrodes like platinum, carbon electrode, and gold are conductive and well explored as implantable devices and proved with long-term stimulation performance. Here comes a need for 3D printable hydrogel with properties of mimicking extracellular matrix, with water retention. Furthermore, PANi-based electric conductive hydrogels can be utilized as electrodes for amplification of signals at the bioelectrode interface and have been reported to have enhanced cellular adhesion, proliferative, and differentiation [21]. Pan et al. fabricated PANi hydrogels via direct inkjet printing with different layers of phytic acid and for glucose sensing, which resulted in good electronic conductivity. Owing to PANi low processibility for bioink, it is often mixed or blended with different biocompatible polymers like silk fibroin (SF), polycaprolactone (PCL), and gelatin methacrylate (GelMA). GelMA/PANi hybrid matrix hydrogel was fabricated with micro-architecture showed enhanced electrical properties than GelMA, a form of denatured collagen, and biocompatible with 10T1/2s cells [22].

For damaged cardio myocardium, bioelectric patches are required to restore the electric signals and it should be operational for a longer duration. Hoang et al. fabricated the laser-ablated chitosan sutureless patches with PANi on its surface with micro-architecture-controlled porosity, good mechanical strength, and large surface area. Here, porosity varied to nearly 40% and with good conductivity, these adhesive patches can adhere to tissues after exposure to LED light [23]. Electrospinning, which is a cost-effect technique to fabricate nanofibers, has limitations in its solvent selection for PANi. With the development of recent technologies and machines, researchers can get the aligned PANi nanofibers and thereby used in many biomedical applications. Electrospun PANi and its different composites are profoundly used in biomedical applications, which not only include electrical stimulation-based tissue regeneration like neural, cardiac functionality but also have explored the tissue engineering fields.

Jiahui He et al. fabricated the skin-repairing PCL-chitosan grafted PANi via electrospinning with antibacterial as well as good cell compatibility and proliferation. Moreover, this nanofiber graft was found to be more effective than Tegaderm and pure PCL in terms of wound healing [24]. The Bertuoli group fabricated the uniaxial and coaxially aligned PANi tagged dodecylbenzene sulfonic acid with polylactic acid (PLA) for cardiac biomedical application. Later, interestingly they reported that with the addition of PLA, electrical conductivity was also increased and PANi release into the culture media attributed to a decrease in the cells [25]. In the coming years, PANi-based composites and nanofibers would provide a road map in health care applications.

23.3.2 PPy

The most common technique in general to manufacture stretchable systems is using intrinsically flexible substrates such as poly(dimethylsiloxane) (PDMS), polyurethane (PU), natural rubber (NR), etc. A nylon membrane (NM) was coated with PPy to achieve a supercapacitor with outstanding electrochemical performance [26]. The composite membrane was synthesized by interfacial polymerization, as depicted in Figure 23.4a. Utilizing this strategy, a stretchable conductive PPy/PU strain sensor was prepared using in-situ polymerization [27]. The solidified PU substrates first reacted with pyrrole monomer containing sodium salt and later ferric nitrate and 2-sulfosalicylic acid hydrate solution and used as an oxidizing and stabilizing agent, respectively to carry out oxidation. The resultant PPy/PU composite showed maximum elongation of 420% with a resistivity of 8.364 $\Omega \cdot$cm. In another report, flexible composite films were synthesized by combining PPy with a series of polyol including pentaerythritol ethoxylate (PEE), PEG, polypropylene glycol (PPG), and

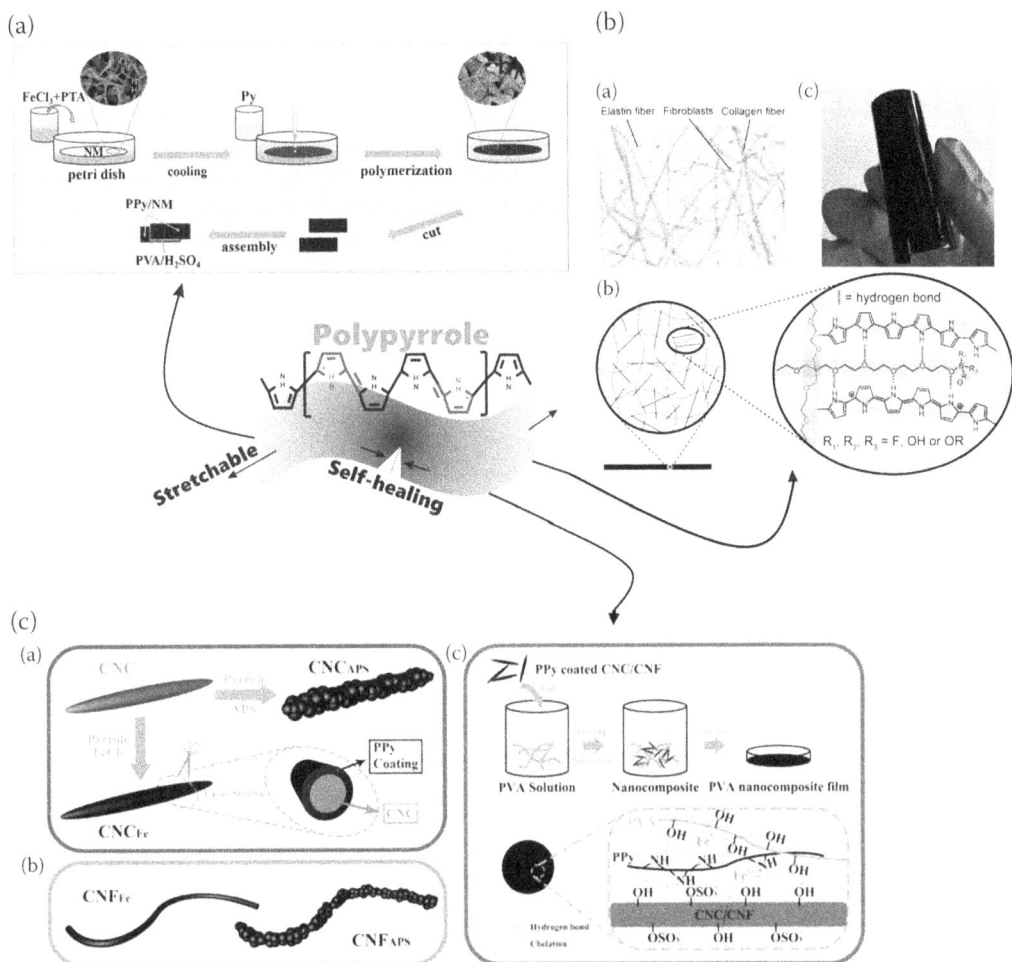

FIGURE 23.4
Illustration depicting various fabrication strategies for flexible PPy composites. (a) Schematic illustration of the fabrication of PPy/NM FSC. Reprinted with permission [26]. Copyright (2019) Elsevier B.V. (b) Structure design of polyol-PPy composites. (a) Dynamic network in the animal dermis is formed by the interconnection between collagen fibers and elastin fibers. (b) Dynamic network structure formed between polyols and polypyrrole through hydrogen bonding and electrostatic interactions. (c) Photograph of a PEE-PPy film. Reprinted with permission [28]. Copyright (2017) American Chemical Society). (c) Schematic illustration for the synthesis process of PVA nanocomposite films. (a) Synthesis of CNC PPy nanocomposites and (b) CNF PPy nano-composites. (c) Preparation and structure of a PVA nanocomposite film. Reprinted with permission [29]. Copyright (2019) American Chemical Society.

pentaerythritol propoxylate (PEP) (Figure 23.4b) [28]. All the composites were fabricated by electro-polymerization and the resulting polyol-PPy films were interconnected through hydrogen bonding forming a dynamic network structure. PEE-PPy films provided the overall best performance for flexible electronic applications.

Hydrogels were often the best choice in bioelectronics due to their inherent bio-compatibility and tunable tissue-like mechanical characteristics. In this aspect, SF films were utilized to make bilayer electrochemical actuation devices. Acid-modified SF films were coated with PPy by *in situ* polymerization in which $FeCl_3$ was oxidant and para-toluenesulfonic acid (pTSA) served as a dopant. PPy modification of SF drastically improved elastic modulus and ultimate tensile strength. Similar to SF, sodium alginate (SA) is one of the well-known biomaterials for tissue engineering applications. However, combining SA with dopamine functionalized PPy (DAPPy) nanofibers increased its stretchability by more than 800% [30]. To prepare hybrid hydrogels, different amounts of DAPPy nanofibers were added to SA and cross-linked with borax. The prepared formulation displayed fast healing capability as well as arbitrary moldable ability. Considering energy storage applications, a miniaturized device was fabricated. Peelable nickel nanocone arrays (NNAs) and polypyrrole nanotubes (PPyNTs) were used as conductive frameworks and active materials, respectively, to prepare patterned interdigital electrodes [31]. PPyNTs were deposited on the NNA using electrodeposition. The fabricated device showed superior long-term cycling performance.

On a similar note, hollow PPy/cellulose (PC) hybrid hydrogels were reported as energy storage systems. PPy was deposited electrochemically using a three-electrode system. The designed hollow PC hybrid hydrogels were found to achieve significant enhancement in terms of mechanical strength and flexibility. In an attempt to develop a material possessing human skin-like mechanical compliance, PPy-rGO-PPy nanosheets modified gelatin hydrogel was proposed [32]. The nanohybrids were synthesized by interface self-assembly, which avoided the use of oxidants and dopants. The as-prepared sandwich-like nanosheets had a wrinkled appearance and showed high stretchability and thermo-responsive behavior. PPy coated cellulose nanocrystals (CNC) and cellulose nanofibers (CNF) were used to reinforce PVA to prepare a biocompatible electronic skin sensor system, as shown in Figure 23.4c. CNC and CNF were made by ultrasonication and then PPy polymerization was initiated after mixing monomer followed by $FeCl_3$ and APS [29].

Initially, CNC and CNF suspensions were prepared by ultrasonication. Then, a pyrrole monomer was added to each dispersion to make a homogeneous mixture. Following this, the polymerization was initiated by adding $FeCl_3$ and APS. Meanwhile, a PVA solution was prepared in Milli-Q water. Finally, the nanocomposites were dropwise mixed with PVA solution. The resulting composite was proposed to show enhanced mechanical properties due to hydrogen bonds present in the PPy network, nanocomposite, and PVA. Moreover, Fe^{+3} ions present in the oxidant can chelate with the composite network further increasing its strength.

23.3.3 PA

PA is insoluble, making it very difficult to process it for a range of biomedical applications and surface modifications. Since any kind of chemical modifications in the polymer leads to a change in their electronic or mechanical properties, this, hereby hinders any possible chances for PA to bind any biological molecule.

23.3.4 PEDOT

Doping PEDOT with polystyrene sulfonate (PSS) results in PEDOT:PSS polymer with extremely high electrochemical stability, solution processability, high transparency in the visible range, and a very narrow bandgap, useful for the detection of biomolecules like uric acid, ascorbic acid (AA), glucose, dopamine (DA), metal ions, and also in tissue engineering applications like fabrication of stimuli-responsive scaffolds. Ko et al. fabricated flexible sensor PEDOT:PSS with graphene oxide (GO) to determine DA. Polymerization and simple electrophoretic deposition of GO and EDOT:PSS dispersed

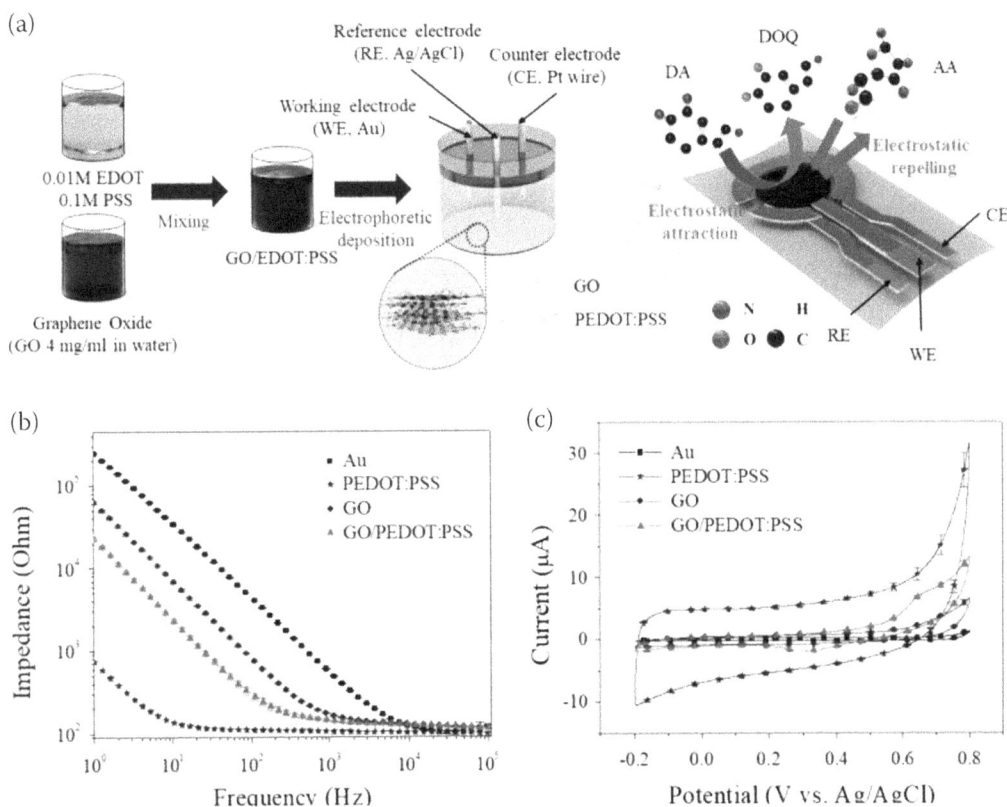

FIGURE 23.5
Illustration of (a) electro-polymerization of biocomposite flexible sensor, (b) comparative analysis of EIS, and (c) CV in .1 M phosphate buffer solution of Au, PEDOT:PSS, GO and GO/PEDOT:PSS [33]. Copyright (2021) Scientific Report. The article was printed under a CC-BY license. (https://creativecommons.org/licenses/by/4.0/).

and suspended in water (Figure 23.5a) provide a strong interaction resulting in an interfacial property with high sensitivity and careful determination of low amounts of DA. The biocomposite for detection of DA resulted in comparatively low interfacial impedance (281.46 ± 30.95 Ω at 100 Hz) in electrochemical impedance spectroscopy (EIS) analysis (Figure 23.5b), great charge storage capacity (53.94 ± 1.08 μC/cm^2) in cyclic voltammogram (CV) (Figure 23.5c), and presented high sensitivity (69.3 μA/μMcm^2) and selectivity of detection limit (0.008 μM) using differential pulse voltammetry (DPV) characterization technique [33]. Skorupa et al. fabricated PEDOT-based film with tailorable properties through doping with PSS, ClO$_4$ (perchlorate), and PF$_6$ (hexafluorophosphate) ions. The resulting film was promising and confirmed to show different physicochemical properties according to the dopant and doping condition according to the requirement of the application and tissue interface [34].

23.3.5 PVDF

Flexible pressure sensors made of PVDF are mainly made as a film with nanopatterning, whereas piezoelectric layers were made of PVDF/BaTiO3 nanocomposite materials [35]. For obtaining high output voltages, β-phase PVDF molecules have been aligned in the perpendicular direction to the electrode surface by the technique called, poling. In addition to this surface chemical modification; "thiol modification" on the Au electrode surface for the formation of a poled β-PVDF film is an additional advantage to improve the carrier injection efficiency at the metal/organic interface of the electrode devices [36]. However, thiol modified Au electrodes presented polarization of the PVDF film-based pressure sensors performs better.

23.4 Functions and Devices in Recent Bioelectronic Application

As an advancement towards flexible and wearable bioelectronics, they also demonstrated that molecular doping of PTh with oligoethylene glycol side chains increases its degree of π-stacking, strongly modulates its electrical conductivity to >52 S/cm, the toughness from 0.5 to 5.1 MJ/m^3, and elastic modulus from 8 to >200 MPa [37]. A new-generation wearable, flexible, therapeutic photoelectronic dual-responsive wound dressing has been designed from selenoviologen-appendant polythiophene containing polyacrylamide hydrogels. This sandwich device ensures sustained *in situ* reactive oxygen species (ROS) generation in a physiological environment via six seconds short-time light irradiation with or without wireless-controlled electrification. The derivative harnessing the high conductivity and strong light absorption properties of PTh along with efficient ROS generation properties of selenoviologens was immersed in polyacrylamide hydrogels. When put directly over the bacterially infected wound, it starts generating ROS outflow under visible light and/or electrical stimulation thereby limiting the healing time of infected full-thickness wounds up to 7 days. Interestingly, this is a BlueTooth-enabled, cell phone–controlled, free-radical generation system. The green color, upon turning the cell phone on, indicated a ROS generation, which turned to yellow upon switching off. This electronic switching on and off was repeatable and had optical memory too [38].

Most of the research is limited to *in vitro* applications of PANi-based electrodes. It is widely being used for *in-vivo* applications ranging from tumor imaging and treatment, photothermal treatment, sensors, tissue regeneration, and drug delivery. It is used in tumor therapy as the image-guided phototherapeutic agent. Further, limited negligible toxicity was observed *in vivo* implantation. In another interesting work, researchers tagged iron-copper co-doped PANi nanoparticle as a metal dopant platform with PANi nanoparticles and utilized the ability of Cu to undergo redox reaction with glutathione of tumor microenvironment. This was further verified with tumor photoacoustic imaging and *in vivo* photothermal therapy [39]. The bacterial microenvironment hampers the PTT and it leads to a decreased theranostic effect of nanoparticles. Yan et al. reported the PANi and glycol chitosan functionalized core-shell nanostructures with persistent luminescent imaging and capability of pH switchable platform for *in vivo* mice photothermal therapy [40]. Another widely explored *in vivo* application is based on the utility of PANi to sense different biomolecules. Glucose biosensors based on PANi with limited interference was fabricated with double-sided flexible electrode for continuous monitoring in a rat model after 24 hours' post-implantation [41]. Nanoporous PANi membrane along with polymerized tannic acid-coated carbon fiber electrode is being used for DA sensing in rats at medial forebrain bundle in the brain. Here, the antifouling capability was observed over the membrane as bovine serum albumin (BSA) protein adsorption was found to be very low and it was then able to sense DA oxidized product on its surface with high sensitivity [42].

There are limitations associated with CP like PANi in the context of *in vivo* applications. Issues like lower stability with conjugated particles, low mechanical strength, and low sensitivity are often encountered. These problems are generally addressed by either chemical modifications on the surface of PANi or mixing/blending with biocompatible non-conductive polymers with enhanced mechanical strength.

Performance tuned stretchable biocomposites of PPy were used as a potential candidate for wearable electronics mimicking the skin-like properties. Apart from that, there are several reports where significant electronic modifications were observed after PPy incorporation into the substrate. Out of many, sensors and actuators made of PPy are trending among the research community with a flexible feature. The capability of PEE-PPy matrix to convert chemical gradient to mechanical work was demonstrated and it finds applications in sensors, switches, and ultra-low-power sources. A mechanical sensor based on PPy-SA-gelatin biocomposite was also developed. Apart from self-healing and biocompatibility, PPy incorporated sensors presented good flexibility and adjustable resistance under the bending motion of fingers. Flexible supercapacitor electrodes are one of the essential components of energy storage systems. In this regard, flexible PPy/copper sulfide (CuS) or bacterial cellulose (BC) nanofibrous composite membranes as supercapacitor electrodes were proposed [43]. The supercapacitors achieved a relatively high specific capacitance and retained their initial value even after 300 cycles. PPy and agarose composite (APY gel) electrodes were prepared for electronic skin mimicking [44]. The electrodes exhibited Young's modulus close to human skin and can be directly painted on human skin for possible bendable or stretchable electronics. Moreover, it showed properties such as thermoplasticity and self-healing. Another application, which demands precise and controllable flexibility is actuated catheter. In this perspective, PPy coated minimally invasive catheter was developed to enhance intravascular navigation during angiographic procedures [44]. A PA is insoluble, making it very much difficult to process it for biomedical applications and surface modifications. Since any kind of chemical modifications in the polymer leads to change in their electronic or mechanical properties, it hereby hinders any possible chances for PAs to bind any biological molecule.

Nanostructured PEDOT provides an adaptable neural interface coating with minimal hardness mismatch and glial reaction, improved neural electrode performance by increasing its charge storage ability, and reduced its electrical impedance without a substantial increase in the geometric surface area [6]. Parylene-based, flexible, neural PEDOT coated microelectrodes have been successfully used for electrocorticography in rat brain [45]. Khodagoly and his coworkers developed 'Neurogrid', a flexible, ultra-comfortable high density, low impedance PEDOT coated multielectrode array that was able to record spikes from individual superficial cortical neurons for one week, without any intervention [11]. As shown in Figure 23.6, the well-explored CP has established various applications and with more novel challenges can exile with enhanced properties.

Piezoelectric sensors based on a PVDF nanofibrous membrane and microporous zirconium-based metal-organic frameworks (MOFs) have been used for arterial pulse monitoring with superior flexibility over the existing wrist pulse monitoring sensors (600 mV, 5N) (Figure 23.7i) [47]. Polydopamine (PDA)-barium titanate-polyvinylidene fluoride (BTO/PVDF) piezoelectric nanocomposites in a fiber made through comprehensive phase-field simulation given maximum piezoelectric charge, voltage coefficient, and mechanical stiffness. The prepared, nonwoven piezoelectric (PMNP) textile showed outstanding sensitivity and long-term stability for wearable biomonitoring, including limb motion detection, facial expression identification, respiratory monitoring, and human-machine interfacing (Figure 23.7ii) [48]. PVDF-TrFE matrix (tuned up to 76.8 mV

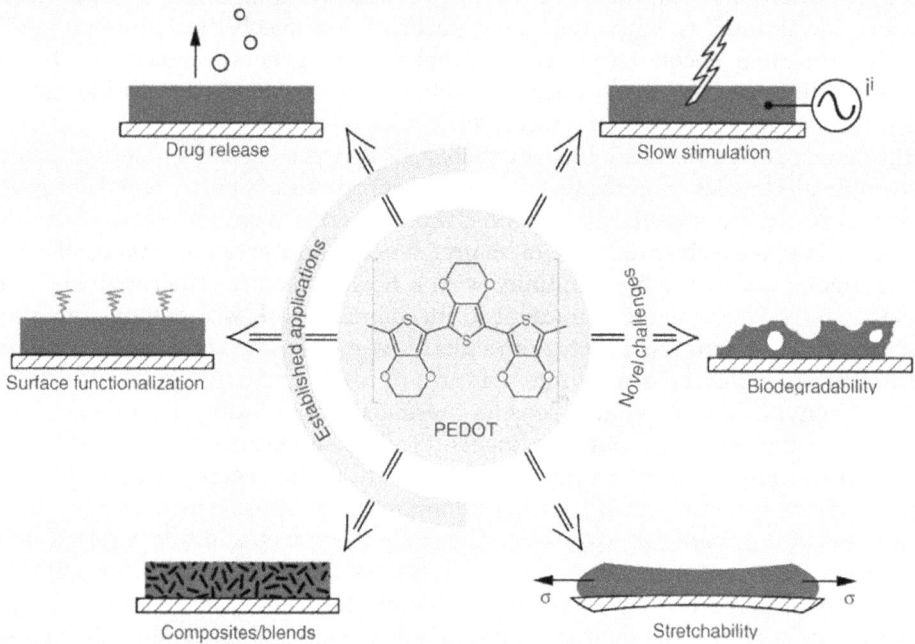

FIGURE 23.6
Representation of established application with various use of well-explored PEDOT in flexible electronics and novel challenges which could enhance the property to utilize the polymer to its fullest [46]. Copyright (2019) Advanced Science. The article was printed under a CC-BY license (http://creativecommons.org/licenses/by/4.0/).

by optimizing the composition ratio and corona poling treatment) coated with poly-dopamine $BaTiO_3$ nanoparticles showed endogenous electrical potential mimicking of the bone tissue up to 12 weeks. The resulting osteogenic differentiation gave rise to rapid bone regeneration and complete mature bone-structure formation [49].

PVDF-graphene oxide (GO) scaffold made by preferential laser sintering technique showed superior cell behavior with commendable compressive (97.9%) and tensile strength (24.5%). under the influence of electric field [50]. Ag-decorated barium titanate (BT) increases the piezoelectric effect of PVDF showed, increased proliferation and differentiation of osteosarcoma cells [51]. PVDF nanocomposites owing to their commendable electrical conductivity due to electroactive β-phase proved to be good substrates for direct stem cell differentiation [52]. $BaTiO_3$ incorporated PVDF/MWNT matrixes induce electro-physiologically distinguishable glial-like differentiation and neurogenesis of neural stem cells (Figure 23.7iii) [52] (Table 23.1).

23.5 Conclusion and Future Aspects

Further, understanding the CP-based flexible bioelectronics interaction with electro responsive tissue *in vivo* need to be explored to understand and analyze the retention of

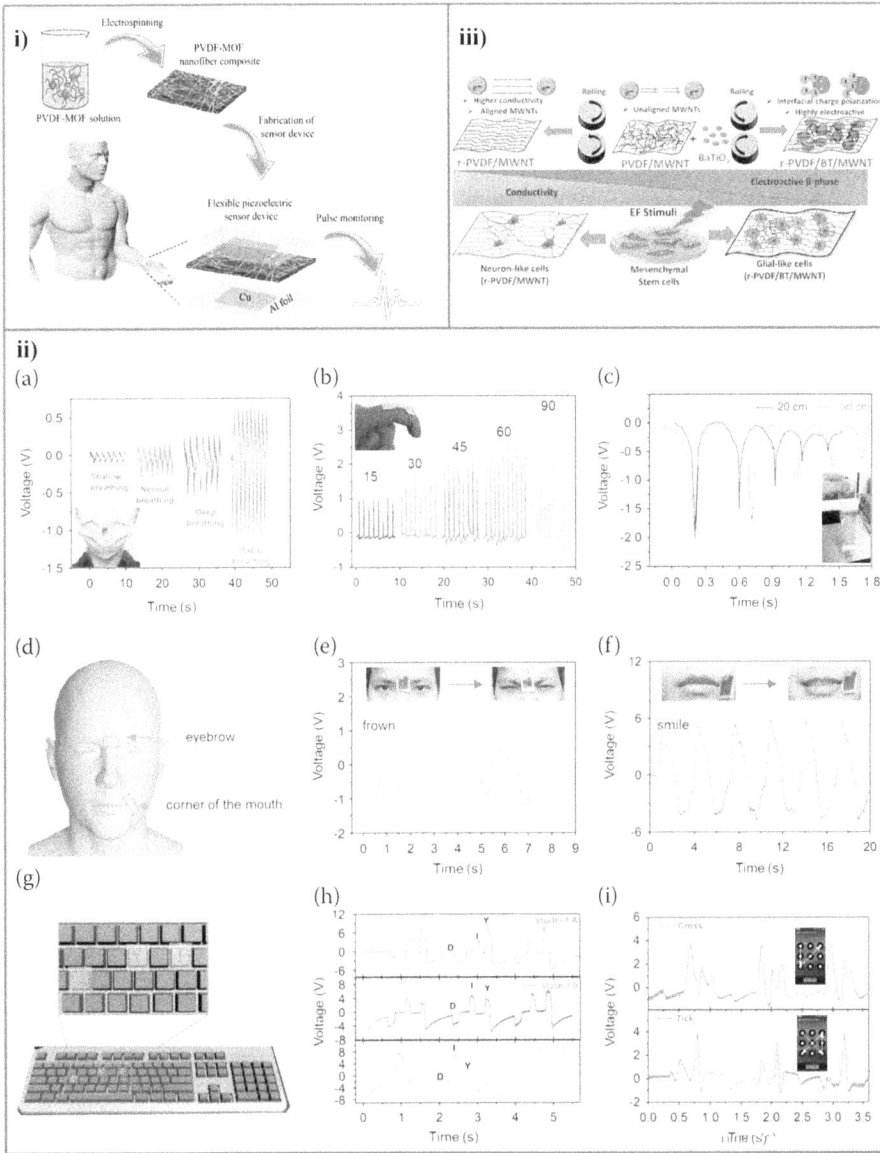

FIGURE 23.7

(i) Schematic Illustration of (a) flexible sensor assembling, (b) piezoelectric measurement setup, and (c) recording of radial artery pulse signals of a candidate, (Reprinted with permission [47],Copyright © 2020, American Chemical Society); **(ii)** sensing performance of the as-prepared PMNP textiles. (a) Real-time output voltage profile in response to various respiratory patterns, (b) dynamic output voltage waveforms of finger bending at various angles, (c) dynamic output profile for free-falling table tennis ball with different falling heights, (d) schematic illustration of PMNP textiles for active facial expression identification, (e) real-time output profile in response to frown, (f) real-time output profile in response to smiling. (g) photograph of PMNP textiles attached on the keyboard, (h) dynamic voltage profiles of three adult volunteers when typing the word "DIY," (i) dynamic voltage profiles when crossing and ticking on the touch screen of a smartphone (Reprinted with permission [48], Elsevier and Copyright clearance Center, January 26, 2022); **(iii)** schematic representation depicting the strategy adopted to guide the EF-mediated stem cell differentiation. The tailored conductivity, surface topography, and electroactivity together, could switch the EF-mediated lineage commitment toward neuron-like and glial-like cells (Reprinted with permission [66], Copyright © 2020, American Chemical Society).

TABLE 23.1

Summary of Discussed CP-Based Biocomposite with Its Strategy, Property, and Applications

Biocomposite	Synthesis strategy/ fabrication technique	Conductivity or output voltage	Flexibility	Applications	Ref.
PTh: PEG2000:	Electrochemical synthesis and film casted	9.5 S/cm	Elongation-at-break of 110%	Flexible, solid-state supercapacitor	[19]
PEDOT	Electrochemical polymerization	Lowering of impedance from 700 kΩ to 10 kΩ	Highly flexible	Implantable neural probe	[45]
PTh-nanofibrillated cellulose films	One-step oxidative polymerization	133μS/cm	Elongation at break of 12%	Potential for flexible electronics	[15]
Thread based transistors	Ionogel synthesis	Effective linear mobility of 3.2 ± 1.7 cm^2/V.s	Maintains high flexibility of thread	Sodium and ammonium ion-selective sensors as key biomarkers of the liver, kidney function and cardiovascular health	[17]
PTh	Drop casting at 40°C	to >52 S/cm	Elastic modulus: 8 to >200 MPa	Applicable in flexible and wearable bioelectronics	[37]
SeV2+PTh)	Hydrogel based anti-sandwich structure	1.77 mS/cm	Good flexibility	Photoelectronic wound dressing with antibacterial properties	[38]
GelMA–polyaniline (GelMA–Pani)	interfacial polymerization and micro-stereolithography apparatus	Resistance (165.56 ± 5.97 Ω)	Patch- maximum strain – 97.68 ± 15.25%	Development conductive hybrid composite	[22]
PANi/chitosan	Laser ablation	0.23 ± 0.05 S/cm		Repair of myocardium	[23]
GO/PEDOT:PSS	Electro-polymerization	Sensitivity 69.3 μA/μMcm^2		Flexible sensor for determination of low levels DA	[33]
PPy/PU	In-situ polymerization	The resistivity of 8.364 Ω.cm was achieved	Maximum elongation of 420%	Strain sensor for human breath detection	[27]
PPy-polyol	Elelctro-polymerization	115 S/cm for PEE-PPy film	Elongation-at-break 75%	Potential electronic material for making flexible electronics	[28]

Material	Method	Properties	Mechanical	Application	Ref.
SA-B-DAPPy	Nanofibers by precipitation	As high as 1.33 ± 0.012 S/m by modulating the weight ratio	Elongation at break beyond ~800%	Flexible electronic and biosensor systems	[30]
PPyNTs on NNAs	Electrodeposition	An areal capacitance up to 60.2 mF/cm^2	–	Flexible electronics	[31]
PPy/Agarose	In-situ polymerization	Saturated at ~1.95 × 10^{-1} S/cm at PPy concentration of 450 mM	Young's modulus close to that of human skin	Self-healable smart electrodes	[44]
PDA@BTO/PVDF	facial solution-casting method	9.3 V, high load resistance of 70 MΩ	12 N (33 KPa)	Pressure sensor human motion monitoring	[35]
PVDF-MOF (Zirconia based)	Electrospinning	568 ± 76 mV, 0.118 V/N	5 N	Arterial pulse monitoring	[36]
PVDF/BaTiO3/MWNT	Melt mixing followed by compression molding	~10 11 to ~10 4 S/cm	–	A regenerative platform for neuron-like and Glial cells	[52]
PVDF/Ag-pBT	Selective laser sintering technique	3.82 × 10 ^{8} S/m	168.5 ±1.4 MPa	Bone repair with anti-bacterial performance	[51]

substrates property like electrical, physicochemical property, etc. For impactful clinical technologies using CP-based biocomposites, it is still essential to realize the full potential of its ability and modified accordingly, without compromising the electrical property. PTh- and PANi-based biocomposite's main challenge is the mechanical stability, degradation, and cytotoxicity, where a novel approach to overcome these limitations may be with great consideration by focusing on bio-based polymers. PPy-incorporated biocomposites are one of the best choices for futuristic applications like flexible electronics. Although PPy offers higher conductivities and is easy to process, its brittleness, as well as solubility in common aqueous solvents, needs to be addressed. PPy-based biocomposites are still being explored for advanced areas such as flexible manoeuvring devices in surgery, neural interfacing electrodes, and electronic tattoos. PVDF with its flexibility and biocompatibility can be further explored for various animal trials to remotely monitor or induce stimulation with battery-less devices and should find use in a bioelectronics application. Similarly, PEDOT with its unique properties has already enabled the fabrication of futuristic bioelectronics devices with various neural interfaces. The real-time monitoring using CP-based flexible bioelectronics has proved its potential in a wide spectrum, further, clinical data is required to represent the new and promising devices for unresolved technological challenges. And some of the advantages, characteristics, and properties of CP-based composites can be more beneficial, which may even replace the metals in various bioelectronics devices.

References

1. E. Cuttaz, J. Goding, C. Vallejo-Giraldo, U. Areguela-Robles, N. Lovell, D. Ghezzi, R.A. Green, Conductive Elastomer Composites for Fully Polymeric, Flexible Bioelectronics, *Biomater. Sci.* 7 (2019) 1372–1385. 10.1039/C8BM01235K
2. O. Bettucci, G.M. Matrone, F. Santoro, Conductive Polymer-Based Bioelectronic Platforms toward Sustainable and Biointegrated Devices: A Journey from Skin to Brain across Human Body Interfaces, *Adv. Mater. Technol.* (2021) 2100293. 10.1002/ADMT.202100293
3. C. Ning, Z. Zhou, G. Tan, Y. Zhu, C. Mao, Electroactive Polymers for Tissue Regeneration: Developments and Perspectives., *Prog. Polym. Sci.* 81 (2018) 144–162. 10.1016/J.PROGPOLYMSCI.2018.01.001
4. J. Ouyang, Application of Intrinsically Conducting Polymers in Flexible Electronics, *SmartMat.* 2 (2021) 263–285. 10.1002/SMM2.1059
5. S. Wang, Y. Fang, H. He, L. Zhang, C. Li, J. Ouyang, Wearable Stretchable Dry and Self-Adhesive Strain Sensors with Conformal Contact to Skin for High-Quality Motion Monitoring, *Adv. Funct. Mater.* 31 (2021) 2007495. 10.1002/ADFM.202007495
6. S. Inal, J. Rivnay, A.O. Suiu, G.G. Malliaras, I. McCulloch, Conjugated Polymers in Bioelectronics, *Acc. Chem. Res.* 51 (2018) 1368–1376. 10.1021/ACS.ACCOUNTS.7B00624
7. K. Fidanovski, D. Mawad, Conjugated Polymers in Bioelectronics: Addressing the Interface Challenge, *Adv. Healthc. Mater.* 8 (2019) 1900053.
8. S. Li, Y. Cong, J. Fu, Tissue Adhesive Hydrogel Bioelectronics, *J. Mater. Chem. B.* 9 (2021) 4423–4443. 10.1039/D1TB00523E
9. G. Natta, From Stereospecific Polymerization to Asymmetric Autocatalytic Synthesis of Macromolecules, *Rubber Chem. Technol.* 38 (1965) 37–60.
10. H. Shirakawa, The Discovery of Polyacetylene Film – The Dawning of an Era of Conducting Polymers, *Curr. Appl. Phys.* 1 (2001) 281–286.

11. D. Khodagholy, J.N. Gelinas, T. Thesen, W. Doyle, O. Devinsky, G.G. Malliaras, G. Buzsáki, NeuroGrid: Recording Action Potentials from the Surface of the Brain, *Nat. Neurosci.* 18 (2015) 310. 10.1038/NN.3905

12. L. Ruan, X. Yao, Y. Chang, L. Zhou, G. Qin, X. Zhang, Properties and Applications of the β Phase Poly(vinylidene fluoride), *Polym.* 2018, Vol. 10, Page 228. 10 (2018) 228. 10.3390/POLYM10030228

13. J.E. Lee, Y. Guo, R.E. Lee, S.N. Leung, Fabrication of Electroactive Poly(vinylidene fluoride) through Non-isothermal Crystallization and Supercritical CO_2 Processing, *RSC Adv.* 7 (2017) 48712–48722. 10.1039/C7RA09162A

14. M. Jaymand, M. Hatamzadeh, Y. Omidi, Modification of Polythiophene by the Incorporation of Processable Polymeric Chains: Recent Progress in Synthesis and Applications, *Prog. Polym. Sci. Complete.* 47 (2015) 26–69. 10.1016/J.PROGPOLYMSCI.2014.11.004

15. O.A.T. Dias, S. Konar, A.L. Leão, M. Sain, Flexible Electrically Conductive Films Based on Nanofibrillated Cellulose and Polythiophene Prepared via Oxidative Polymerization, *Carbohydr. Polym.* 220 (2019) 79–85. 10.1016/J.CARBPOL.2019.05.057

16. A. Portone, L. Ganzer, F. Branchi, R. Ramos, M.J. Caldas, D. Pisignano, E. Molinari, G. Cerullo, L. Persano, D. Prezzi, T. Virgili, Tailoring Optical Properties and Stimulated Emission in Nanostructured Polythiophene, *Sci. Reports* 2019 91.9 (2019) 1–10. 10.1038/s41598-019-43719-0

17. R.E. Owyeung, T. Terse-Thakoor, H. Rezaei Nejad, M.J. Panzer, S.R. Sonkusale, Highly Flexible Transistor Threads for All-Thread Based Integrated Circuits and Multiplexed Diagnostics, *ACS Appl. Mater. Interfaces.* 11 (2019) 31096–31104. 10.1021/ACSAMI.9B09522

18. Y.S. Wu, Y.C. Lin, S.Y. Hung, C.K. Chen, Y.C. Chiang, C.C. Chueh, W.C. Chen, Investigation of the Mobility-Stretchability Relationship of Ester-Substituted Polythiophene Derivatives, *Macromolecules.* 53 (2020) 4968–4981. 10.1021/ACS.MACROMOL.0C00193/SUPPL_FILE/MA0C00193_SI_001.PDF

19. Q. Chen, X. Wang, F. Chen, N. Zhang, M. Ma, Extremely Strong and Tough Polythiophene Composite for Flexible Electronics, *Chem. Eng. J.* 368 (2019) 933–940. 10.1016/J.CEJ.2019.02.203

20. S. Zokaei, M. Craighero, C. Cea, L.M. Kneissl, R. Kroon, D. Khodagholy, A. Lund, C. Müller, S. Zokaei, M. Craighero, L.M. Kneissl, R. Kroon, A. Lund, C. Müller, C. Cea, D. Khodagholy, Electrically Conducting Elastomeric Fibers with High Stretchability and Stability, *Small.* 18 (2021) 2102813. 10.1002/SMLL.202102813

21. J.H. Min, M. Patel, W.-G. Koh, Incorporation of conductive materials into hydrogels for tissue engineering applications, *Polymers (Basel).* 10 (2018) 1078.

22. Y. Wu, Y.X. Chen, J. Yan, D. Quinn, P. Dong, S.W. Sawyer, P. Soman, Fabrication of Conductive Gelatin Methacrylate–Polyaniline Hydrogels, *Acta Biomater.* 33 (2016) 122–130.

23. A.-P. Hoang, H. Ruprai, K. Fidanovski, M. Eslami, A. Lauto, J. Daniels, D. Mawad, Porous and Sutureless Bioelectronic Patch with Retained Electronic Properties under Cyclic Stretching, *Appl. Mater. Today.* 15 (2019) 315–322.

24. J. He, Y. Liang, M. Shi, B. Guo, Anti-Oxidant Electroactive and Antibacterial Nanofibrous Wound Dressings Based on Poly (ε-caprolactone)/Quaternized Chitosan-Graft-Polyaniline for Full-Thickness Skin Wound Healing, *Chem. Eng. J.* 385 (2020) 123464.

25. P.T. Bertuoli, J. Ordoño, E. Armelin, S. Pérez-Amodio, A.F. Baldissera, C.A. Ferreira, J. Puiggalí, E. Engel, L.J. del Valle, C. Alemán, Electrospun Conducting and Biocompatible Uniaxial and Core–Shell Fibers Having Poly(lactic acid), Poly(ethylene glycol), and Polyaniline for Cardiac Tissue Engineering, *ACS Omega.* 4 (2019) 3660–3672. 10.1021/acsomega.8b03411

26. X. Zhang, M. Gao, L. Tong, K. Cai, Polypyrrole/Nylon Membrane Composite Film for Ultra-Flexible All-Solid Supercapacitor, *J. Mater.* 6 (2020) 339–347. 10.1016/J.JMAT.2019.11.004

27. M. Li, H. Li, W. Zhong, Q. Zhao, D. Wang, Stretchable Conductive Polypyrrole/Polyurethane (PPy/PU) Strain Sensor with Netlike Microcracks for Human Breath Detection, *ACS Appl. Mater. Interfaces.* 6 (2014) 1313–1319. 10.1021/AM4053305

28. F. Gao, N. Zhang, X. Fang, M. Ma, Bioinspired Design of Strong, Tough, and Highly Conductive Polyol-Polypyrrole Composites for Flexible Electronics, *ACS Appl. Mater. Interfaces.* 9 (2017) 5692–5698. 10.1021/ACSAMI.7B00717/SUPPL_FILE/AM7B00717_SI_004.AVI

29. L. Han, S. Cui, H.Y. Yu, M. Song, H. Zhang, N. Grishkewich, C. Huang, D. Kim, K.M.C. Tam, Self-Healable Conductive Nanocellulose Nanocomposites for Biocompatible Electronic Skin Sensor Systems, *ACS Appl. Mater. Interfaces.* 11 (2019) 44642–44651. 10.1 021/acsami.9b17030

30. Y. Li, X. Liu, Q. Gong, Z. Xia, Y. Yang, C. Chen, C. Qian, Facile Preparation of Stretchable and Self-Healable Conductive Hydrogels Based on Sodium Alginate/Polypyrrole Nanofibers for Use in Flexible Supercapacitor and Strain Sensors, *Int. J. Biol. Macromol.* 172 (2021) 41–54. 10.1016/J.IJBIOMAC.2021.01.017

31. S. Ma, W. Li, J. Cao, X. Wang, Y. Xie, L. Deng, H. Liu, Z. Huang, L. Sun, S. Cheng, Flexible Planar Microsupercapacitors Based on Polypyrrole Nanotubes, *ACS Appl. Energy Mater.* 4 (2021) 8857–8865. 10.1021/ACSAEM.1C00962/SUPPL_FILE/AE1C00962_SI_001.PDF

32. X. Yang, L. Cao, J. Wang, L. Chen, Sandwich-like Polypyrrole/Reduced Graphene Oxide Nanosheets Integrated Gelatin Hydrogel as Mechanically and Thermally Sensitive Skinlike Bioelectronics, *ACS Sustain. Chem. Eng.* 8 (2020) 10726–10739. 10.1021/ACSSUSCHEMENG.0C01998/SUPPL_FILE/SC0C01998_SI_004.ZIP

33. S.H. Ko, S.W. Kim, Y.J. Lee, Flexible Sensor with Electrophoretic Polymerized Graphene Oxide/PEDOT:PSS Composite for Voltammetric Determination of Dopamine Concentration, *Sci. Reports* 2021. 111. 11 (2021) 1–10. 10.1038/s41598-021-00712-w

34. M. Skorupa, D. Więcławska, D. Czerwińska-Główka, M. Skonieczna, K. Krukiewicz, Dopant-Dependent Electrical and Biological Functionality of Pedot in Bioelectronics, *Polymers (Basel).* 13 (2021) 1–15. 10.3390/polym13121948

35. Y. Yang, H. Pan, G. Xie, Y. Jiang, C. Chen, Y. Su, Y. Wang, H. Tai, Flexible Piezoelectric Pressure Sensor Based on Polydopamine-Modified BaTiO3/PVDF Composite Film for Human Motion Monitoring, *Sensors Actuators A Phys.* 301 (2020) 111789. 10.1016/J.SNA.2019.111789

36. H. Klauk, U. Zschieschang, J. Pflaum, M. Halik, Ultralow-Power Organic Complementary Circuits, *Nat.* 2006. 4457129. 445 (2007) 745–748. 10.1038/nature05533

37. S. Zokaei, D. Kim, E. Järsvall, A.M. Fenton, A.R. Weisen, S. Hultmark, P.H. Nguyen, A.M. Matheson, A. Lund, R. Kroon, abf L. Michael Chabinyc, E.D. Gomez, cg Igor Zozoulenko bf, C. Mü ller, Tuning of the Elastic Modulus of a Soft Polythiophene through Molecular Doping, *Mater. Horizons.* 9 (2022) 433–443. 10.1039/D1MH01079D

38. K. Zhou, D. Chigan, L. Xu, C. Liu, R. Ding, G. Li, Z. Zhang, D. Pei, A. Li, B. Guo, X. Yan, G. He, Anti-Sandwich Structured Photo-Electronic Wound Dressing for Highly Efficient Bacterial Infection Therapy, *Small.* 17 (2021). 10.1002/SMLL.202101858

39. S.L. Wang, L.L. Zhang, J.J. Zhao, M. He, Y. Huang, S.L. Zhao, A Tumor Microenvironment-Induced Absorption Red-Shifted Polymer Nanoparticle for Simultaneously Activated Photoacoustic Imaging and Photothermal Therapy, *Sci. Adv.* 7 (2021). 10.1126/sciadv.abe3588

40. L.X. Yan, L.J. Chen, X. Zhao, X.P. Yan, pH Switchable Nanoplatform for In Vivo Persistent Luminescence Imaging and Precise Photothermal Therapy of Bacterial Infection, *Adv. Funct. Mater.* 30 (2020). 10.1002/adfm.201909042

41. Y. Cai, B. Liang, S.D. Chen, Q. Zhu, T.T. Tu, K. Wu, Q.P. Cao, L. Fang, X. Liang, X.S. Ye, One-Step Modification Of Nano-polyaniline/Glucose Oxidase on Double-Side Printed Flexible Electrode for Continuous Glucose Monitoring: Characterization, Cytotoxicity Evaluation and In Vivo Experiment, *Biosens. Bioelectron.* 165 (2020). 10.1016/j.bios.2020.112408

42. T.T. Feng, W.L. Ji, A. Tang, H. Wei, S. Zhang, J.P. Mao, Y. Zhang, L.Q. Mao, M.N. Zhang, Low-Fouling Nanoporous Conductive Polymer-Coated Microelectrode for In Vivo Monitoring of Dopamine in the Rat Brain, *Anal. Chem.* 91 (2019) 10786–10791. 10.1021/acs.analchem.9b02386

43. S. Peng, L. Fan, C. Wei, X. Liu, H. Zhang, W. Xu, J. Xu, Flexible Polypyrrole/copper Sulfide/bacterial Cellulose Nanofibrous Composite Membranes as Supercapacitor Electrodes, *Carbohydr. Polym.* 157 (2017) 344–352. 10.1016/J.CARBPOL.2016.10.004

44. J. Hur, K. Im, S.W. Kim, J. Kim, D.Y. Chung, T.H. Kim, K.H. Jo, J.H. Hahn, Z. Bao, S. Hwang, N. Park, Polypyrrole/Agarose-Based Electronically Conductive and Reversibly Restorable Hydrogel, *ACS Nano.* 8 (2014) 10066–10076. 10.1021/NN502704G/SUPPL_FILE/NN502704G_SI_001.PDF

45. V. Castagnola, E. Descamps, A. Lecestre, L. Dahan, J. Remaud, L.G. Nowak, C. Bergaud, Parylene-Based Flexible Neural Probes with PEDOT Coated Surface for Brain Stimulation and Recording, *Biosens. Bioelectron.* 67 (2015) 450–457. 10.1016/J.BIOS.2014.09.004

46. X. Fan, W. Nie, H. Tsai, N. Wang, H. Huang, Y. Cheng, R. Wen, L. Ma, F. Yan, Y. Xia, PEDOT:PSS for Flexible and Stretchable Electronics: Modifications, Strategies, and Applications, *Adv. Sci.* 6 (2019) 1900813. 10.1002/ADVS.201900813

47. B.H. Moghadam, M. Hasanzadeh, A. Simchi, Self-Powered Wearable Piezoelectric Sensors Based on Polymer Nanofiber–Metal–Organic Framework Nanoparticle Composites for Arterial Pulse Monitoring, *ACS Appl. Nano Mater.* 3 (2020) 8742–8752. 10.1021/ACSANM.0C01551

48. Y. Su, W. Li, L. Yuan, C. Chen, H. Pan, G. Xie, G. Conta, S. Ferrier, X. Zhao, G. Chen, H. Tai, Y. Jiang, J. Chen, Piezoelectric Fiber Composites with Polydopamine Interfacial Layer for Self-Powered Wearable Biomonitoring, *Nano Energy.* 89 (2021) 106321. 10.1016/J.NANOEN. 2021.106321

49. X. Zhang, C. Zhang, Y. Lin, P. Hu, Y. Shen, K. Wang, S. Meng, Y. Chai, X. Dai, X. Liu, Y. Liu, X. Mo, C. Cao, S. Li, X. Deng, L. Chen, Nanocomposite Membranes Enhance Bone Regeneration Through Restoring Physiological Electric Microenvironment, *ACS Nano.* 10 (2016) 7279–7286. 10.1021/ACSNANO.6B02247/SUPPL_FILE/NN6B02247_SI_001.PDF

50. C. Shuai, Z. Zeng, Y. Yang, F. Qi, S. Peng, W. Yang, C. He, G. Wang, G. Qian, Graphene Oxide Assists Polyvinylidene Fluoride Scaffold to Reconstruct Electrical Microenvironment of Bone Tissue, *Mater. Des.* 190 (2020) 108564. 10.1016/J.MATDES.2020.108564

51. C. Shuai, G. Liu, Y. Yang, F. Qi, S. Peng, W. Yang, C. He, G. Wang, G. Qian, A Strawberry-like Ag-Decorated Barium Titanate Enhances Piezoelectric and Antibacterial Activities of Polymer Scaffold, *Nano Energy.* 74 (2020) 104825. 10.1016/J.NANOEN.2020.104825

52. A.K. Panda, R. Ravikumar, A. Gebrekrstos, S. Bose, Y.S. Markandeya, B. Mehta, B. Basu, Tunable Substrate Functionalities Direct Stem Cell Fate toward Electrophysiologically Distinguishable Neuron-like and Glial-like Cells, *ACS Appl. Mater. Interfaces.* 13 (2021) 164–185. 10.1021/ACSAMI.0C17257/SUPPL_FILE/AM0C17257_SI_007.PDF

Index

For Product Safety Concerns and Information please contact our EU
representative GPSR@taylorandfrancis.com
Taylor & Francis Verlag GmbH, Kaufingerstraße 24, 80331 München, Germany

www.ingramcontent.com/pod-product-compliance
Lightning Source LLC
Chambersburg PA
CBHW080655220326
41598CB00033B/5213

9 781032 203423